CLINICAL APPLICATION OF 3D SONOGRAPHY

CLINICAL APPLICATION OF 3D SONOGRAPHY

Edited by
Asim Kurjak, MD and Sanja Kupesic, MD

Department of Obstetrics and Gynecology,
Medical School, University of Zagreb, Croatia

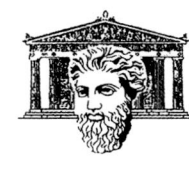

The Parthenon Publishing Group
International Publishers in Medicine, Science & Technology

NEW YORK   LONDON

Library of Congress Cataloging-in-Publication Data

Clinical application of 3D sonography / [edited] by A. Kurjak and S. Kupesic
   p. :cm.
   Includes bibliographical references and index.
   ISBN 1-84214-006-X (alk. paper)
   1. Ultrasonics in obstetrics. 2. Generative organs, Female--Ultrasonic imaging. 3. Three-dimensional imaging in medicine. 4. Diagnosis, Ultrasonic.
I. Kurjak, Asim. II. Kupesic, Sanja.
   [DNLM : 1. Genital Diseases, Female--ultrasonography. 2. Pregnancy Complications--ultrasonography. 3. Ultrasonography, Doppler--methods.
WP 141 C6407 2000]
RG527.5.U48 C55 2000
618'.047543--dc21   00-039998

British Library Cataloguing in Publication Data

Kurjak, Asim
Clinical application of 3D sonography
1. Ultrasonic imaging   2. Three-dimensional imaging in medicine   3. Ultrasonics in obstetrics
4. Generative organs, Female-Ultrasonic imaging
I. Title   II. Kupesic, S. (Sanja)
618'.1'07543

ISBN 1-84214-006-X

Published in the USA by
The Parthenon Publishing Group Inc.
One Blue Hill Plaza
PO Box 1654, Pearl River
NY 10965, USA

Published in the UK and Europe by
The Parthenon Publishing Group Limited
Casterton Hall, Carnforth
Lancs., LA6 2LA, UK

Copyright © 2000 Parthenon Publishing Group

No part of this book may be reproduced in any form without permission from the publishers, except for the quotation of brief passages for the purposes of review.

Typesetting by M₂Community, Seoul, Korea.
Printed by Naeway Communication, Seoul, Korea.

Contents

List of principal contributors	vii
Foreword	ix
1. Methodology of three-dimensional ultrasound *F. Wiesauer*	1
2. Three-dimensional and power Doppler in the study of angiogenesis *A. Kurjak, S. Kupesic and T. Zodan*	7
3. Ovarian lesions assessed by three-dimensional and power Doppler ultrasound *A. Kurjak and S. Kupesic*	23
4. The use of echo contrast in the investigation of adnexal tumors *S. Kupesic and A. Kurjak*	35
5. Three-dimensional ultrasound and the Fallopian tube *A. Kurjak, S. Kupesic and T. Zodan*	43
6. The assessment of uterine lesions *S. Kupesic, A. Kurjak and D. Bjelos*	55
7. The assessment of female infertility *S. Kupesic and A. Kurjak*	67
8. Three-dimensional ultrasound and power Doppler for the diagnosis of septate uterus *S. Kupesic and A. Kurjak*	77
9. Three-dimensional hysterosonosalpingography *S. Kupesic, A. Kurjak and D. Bjelos*	85
10. Three-dimensional imaging of intrauterine devices *R. Bauman, S. Kupesic and A. Kurjak*	97
11. Three-dimensional ultrasound in urogynecology *I. Bekavac, S. Kupesic and A. Kurjak*	103
12. Three-dimensional sonoembryology of the first trimester *A. Kurjak, T. Zodan and S. Kupesic*	109
13. The assessment of normal fetal anatomy *B. Benoit, M. Kos and A. Kurjak*	121
14. The normal and abnormal fetal face *B. Benoit, M. Kos and A. Kurjak*	127

15. The assessment of abnormal fetal anatomy — 133
    A. Kurjak, M. Kos, B. Benoit and S. Kupesic

16. Three-dimensional ultrasound markers of chromosomal anomalies — 143
    A. Kurjak and R. Matijevic

17. Three-dimensional ultrasound for nuchal translucency measurement at 10–14 weeks of gestation — 151
    B. L. Chung, Y. P. Kim and M. H. Nam

18. Three-dimensional color and power imaging: experience in prenatal diagnosis — 155
    R. Matijevic and A. Kurjak

19. Three-dimensional fetal echocardiography — 161
    G. Bega and K. Kuhlman

20. Three-dimensional power Doppler in the study of placental and umbilical cord abnormalities — 167
    A. D. Hull and D. H. Pretorius

21. Fetal brain assessment by three-dimensional ultrasound — 171
    R. K. Pooh

22. Three-dimensional neonatal neurosonography — 181
    G. Thieme, M. L. Manco-Johnson and D. Cioffi-Ragan

23. Non-gynecological three-dimensional ultrasound — 191
    A. Kratochwil

24. Three-dimensional sonography of the breast — 215
    C. F. Weismann

25. The role of three-dimensional and power Doppler ultrasound in evaluation of breast lesions — 229
    I. Bekavac, E. Cosmi and S. Kupesic

26. Three-dimensional ultrasonography in hepatogastroenterology — 235
    G. Esmat

27. Advantages, limitations and future developments of three-dimensional ultrasound in gynecology and obstetrics — 243
A. Kurjak and S. Kupesic

28. Telemedicine performed by three-dimensional ultrasound — 253
    K. Kettl

Index — 257

List of principal contributors

G. Bega
Department of Obstetrics and Gynecology
Division of Maternal–Fetal Medicine
834 Chestnut Street, Suite 400
USA

B. L. Chung
St. Luke's Obstetrics and Gynecological Clinic
34–8 Cheonho-1-Dong
Kangdong-Ku
Seoul 134–021
Korea

G. Esmat
Department of Tropical Medicine
Cairo University
98 El Tahrir street
Cairo 112411
Egypt

A. D. Hull
UCSD Medical Center 8433
200 West Arbor Drive
San Diego
CA 92103–8433
USA

K. Kettl
Kretztechnik AG
Tiefenbach 15
A–4871 Zipf
Austria

A. Kratochwil
University of Vienna
Dept. Radiation Therapy
Währingergürtel 18–21
A–1090 Vienna
Austria

S. Kupesic
Ultrasonic Unit
Department of Obstetrics and Gynecology
University of Zagreb
Sveti Duh Hospital
Sveti Duh 64
10000 Zagreb
Croatia

A. Kurjak
Ultrasonic Unit
Department of Obstetrics and Gynecology
University of Zagreb
Sveti Duh Hospital
Sveti Duh 64
10000 Zagreb
Croatia

M. L. Manco-Johnson
Department of Radiology
Health Science Center
University of Colorado
Denver
Colorado
USA

R. K. Pooh
Department of Obstetrics and Gynecology
Clinical Research Institute
National Zentsuji Hospital
2–1–1, Senyu-cho
Zentsuji City
Kangawa # 765–8507
Japan

F. Wiesauer
Kretztechnik AG
Tiefenbach 15
A–4871 Zipf
Austria

C. F. Weismann
Department of Diagnostic Radiology
St. Johanns Hospital
Landeskliniken Salzburg
Muellner Hauptstrasse 48
5020 Salzburg
Austria

Foreword

Recent technological breakthroughs in diagnostic ultrasound have surpassed all expectations. With these advances, clinicians now have the tools needed to contend with many significant diagnostic challenges. At the same time, these new technologies are so numerous and have been introduced in such rapid succession that considerable confusion surrounds these technologies concerning how they work and how they should best be used.

Similarly, the professional milieu around us all is moving rapidly, and we have to run faster and faster just to keep the external environment in focus. We are working ever harder just to keep up. We are advancing rapidly, but, because our surroundings are changing at a similar rate, we do not seem to be moving at all.

The rapid improvement in ultrasound image quality that has occurred, particularly over the past 10 years, has enabled us all to a degree that was thought inconceivable a short while ago. The dramatic changes brought about by the advent of color Doppler, power Doppler and, more recently, 3D imaging are undeniable. The simultaneous development of ultrasound contrast has also widened the diagnostic armamentarium at our disposal. These developments now occur at such a rapid pace that unless we keep up with developing technology we will inevitably fall behind. Professional obsolescence or irrelevance is merely a stumble away. Hence, all of us need to run harder and harder just to stand still.

Three-dimensional ultrasound has become a valuable medical imaging modality within recent years. It combines the advantages of 3D-data acquisition, as known from other tomographic imaging technologies such as computed tomography, magnetic resonance imaging and positron emission tomography, with the unique features of ultrasound technology, a non-invasive, non-radiation and inexpensive method with an excellent imaging capability in soft tissues.

Three-dimensional sonography has, in a relatively short period of time, evolved from crude laboratory experiments to its present level of sophistication. Useful clinical applications have already been reported from almost all sections of clinical medicine. It is our belief that to publish this book illustrating the initial results from the clinical application of this exciting technology is justified.

The contributors in this book have all been selected for their special expertise in their own fields, their access to outstanding material and their ability to explain the significance of the subject in an effective and lucid way. We are extremely grateful for their assistance and pleased to be able to present such a truly international authorship.

A. Kurjak
S. Kupesic
Zagreb, April 2000

Methodology of three-dimensional ultrasound

F. Wiesauer

Introduction

Three-dimensional (3D) imaging is well known. The reconstruction of computed tomography (CT) and magnetic resonance data in three dimensions has been performed for more than a decade. The first application was the reconstruction of bony structures based on parallel CT slices with a known distance between them. This technology was used for a few applications such as the planning of radiation therapy and craniofacial reconstructive surgery[1].

During the 1980s some laboratories used 3D acquisition and reconstruction techniques for echo data which were based on reflected ultrasound waves. Systems have been described for echocardiography[2], intravascular ultrasound[3] and peripheral vascular ultrasound[4]. The methods for determining the spatial position of the echo data included mechanical arms[5] and acoustic triangulation[6]. In 1989 Kretztechnik AG launched the Combison 330, which acquired the 3D data set by using special 3D probes for transabdominal and transrectal scanning and which introduced the multiplanar reconstruction of the 3D data set in three orthogonal planes.

Basics of three-dimensional ultrasound

The aim of 3D ultrasound is the representation of the morphology of an organ of interest (Figure 1)[7]. To achieve these results, the following steps are necessary:

(1) Echo data processing along an ultrasound beam;

(2) Movement of the ultrasound beam over the area of interest. The 3D data set is created by the translation/rotation of the axis from the ultrasound beam and the flight time of the reflected sound waves, which is converted into distance information by the assumption of the speed of sound within the volume of interest;

(3) Storage of data and gap-filling procedure;

(4) Data representation/visualization.

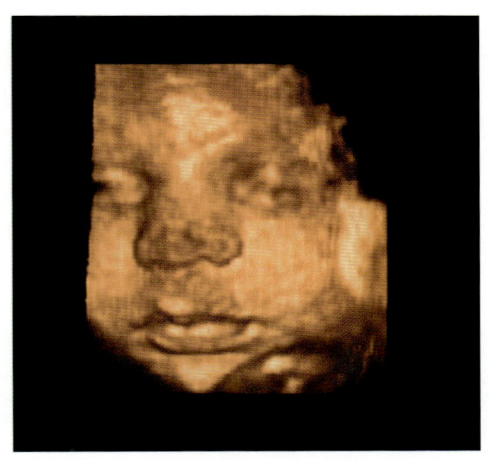

Figure 1 Fetal face reconstructed from a three-dimensional echo data set. From reference 7

Echo data processing

This procedure is well known from two-dimensional (2D) ultrasound. The reflected ultrasound waves can be processed according to their amplitude (B-mode imaging), their frequency shift compared to the frequency that has been transmitted (Doppler imaging), their energy in spectral components that were shifted by moving targets (angiography, power Doppler) or their amplitude on harmonic components of the reflected echo signal (harmonic imaging). All modalities of 2D ultrasound can also be applied to 3D ultrasound.

Scanning procedure

There are two technologies for moving the ultrasound beam over the object of interest: the scanning movement can be done manually or automatically. Some systems combine these two components.

System with automated scanning movement

Systems with fully automated scanning movement use ultrasound probes that include the scanning mechanism. Because the movement is controlled by precise mechanics and/or electronics, the accuracy of the 3D data set is excellent and corresponds to the position accuracy which is standard in 2D ultrasound. This system also ensures that the information density is determined so that no area within the region of interest is skipped (producing lack of information) and no area is scanned several times (producing motion artifacts).

The automated scanning movement can be achieved by mechanical gears and/or electronic scanning techniques such as steered phased arrays and/or curved/linear arrays with different groups of elements excited. Different types of probes are available which are optimized for different applications (Figure 2). A preferred type uses an electronic array in one direction that is mechanically swept in the orthogonal direction.

To realize both scanning components electronically, a so-called 2D-array is necessary. Such an array consists of a transducer mosaic and increases the number of information channels for the ultrasound echo processing exponentially. One method for reducing the number of channels – and thereby also reducing the costs – is the sparse array technology, which uses only some of the available channels, thus compromising the image quality.

Mixed systems

In a mixed system one component of the scanning movement is carried out in an automated scanning mode the other component is performed manually. A typical application is the scanning movement with a hand-held B-mode transducer.

The position in the manual scanning direction is unknown. Therefore, we can differentiate between two basic methods:

(1) Freehand scanning without detection of the position;

(2) Freehand scanning with detection of the position.

In freehand scanning without position detection, the reconstruction algorithm assumes a certain geometry, e.g. parallel slices with a distance of 1 mm. The user must try to match these assumptions with his manual scanning movement. Any deviation from the assumed algorithm results in inaccuracy of the 3D data set; therefore, this method allows only a qualitative representation of a scanned volume. Any measurement that includes data points that are not within the same B-mode image is inaccurate.

For position detection different methods are possible. All these methods need one or more reference points on the probe which must be measured from a reference position. The measurement must include the translation of the probe – the distance and direction of the movement from a reference position – as well as the rotation of the probe. The detection methods are based on different physical effects such as optical detection, acoustic detection (measurement of flight-time of an acoustic signal between a group of generators in the reference position and a group of microphones on the probe) and position detection, by evaluating the signals in orthogonal antennas within an electromagnetic reference field (Figure 3).

One problem is that all these methods can easily show interference from environmental conditions. The acoustic and optical method is sensitive to shadowing of the position sensors from the user, the probe or the patient. With the electromagnetic sensor any metallic part in the reference field disturbs the field and results in inaccurate measurements.

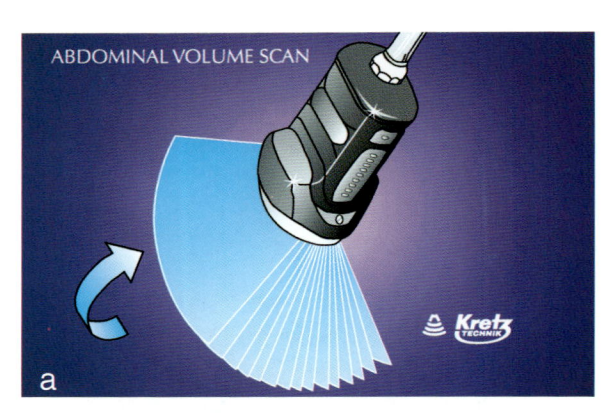

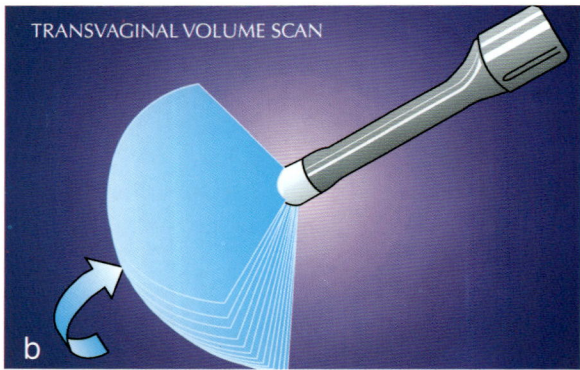

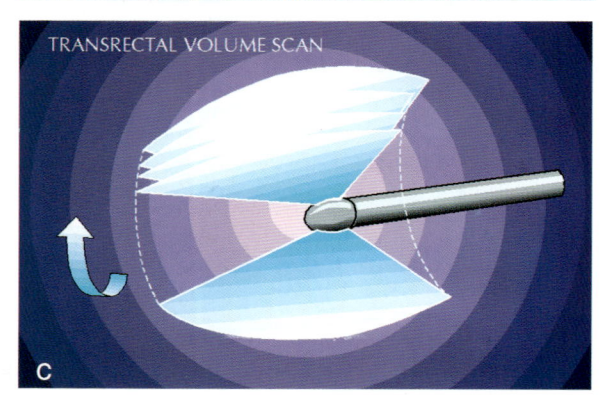

Figure 2 Scanning methods for the transabdominal (a), transvaginal (b) and transrectal (c) probes

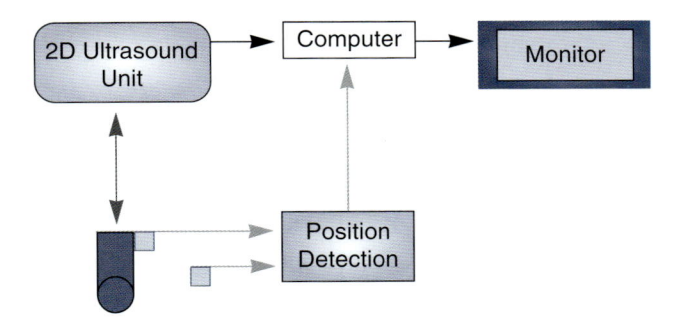

Figure 3 Diagram of a freehand scanning system with position detection

Manually moved systems

Such a system consists of a single transducer – producing one single line of ultrasound information – which is moved by hand for position detection. (This method has no real significance and is only mentioned for completeness.)

Storage of data

For the visualization process all echo data must be stored in a memory where the address of the data element must have a clear connection to its spatial coordinates. Different coordinate systems can be used: polar coordinates, spherical coordinates or, the most often used, Cartesian coordinates. In this chapter the detailed descriptions are based on Cartesian coordinates, but all the described procedures have their equivalent representation in the other coordinate systems.

One echo value represents the information from the scanned volume in its environment. Such a data element is called a voxel. This name is analogous to the word that designates a 2D picture element as a pixel (Figure 4).

If the echo data are transferred into memory according to their spatial coordinates, then it is obvious that not all voxels are crossed by the ultrasound beam; therefore, these voxels contain no information, or the value is zero. On the other hand, the value zero can mean that the voxel is crossed by an ultrasound beam but there has been no echo in this site. The reconstruction of such a data set is full of artifacts because there is no differentiation between a cystic object (low echo amplitude) and a hyperechoic (high echo amplitude) region which is located between two scanning lines. Therefore, 3D ultrasound requires a step to fill the gaps between adjacent ultrasound beams within the voxel with interpolated data. The interpolation algorithm compromises the calculation speed and quality.

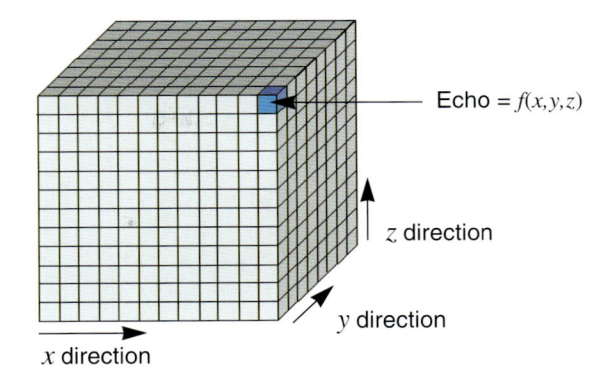

Figure 4 Three-dimensional data set in Cartesian coordinates. 'Echo' can signify amplitude (B-mode), average flow (CFM) or the energy of moving echoes (angiography)

Data presentation

Data are presented on a 2D display – such as a monitor. A holographic presentation of 3D data sets is conceivable but has not yet been used. The stereoscopic presentation of data can be led back to 2D displays, which are combined by human visual perception into a 3D impression.

The normal representation of a 3D data set is the multiplanar representation. This uses echo information from the three planes that cut the voxel and which are orthogonal to each other. Figure 5 illustrates the three orthogonal planes after data acquisition has been accomplished.

The position of these planes can be shifted and rotated with reference to the 3D data set (Figure 6). This method is analogous to the representation of organs in a book of anatomy which are mostly shown by their cross-sectional views through the axis of

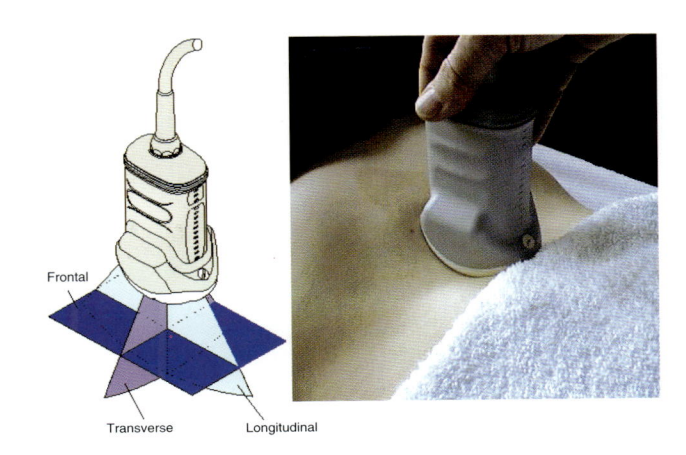

Figure 5 The three orthogonal planes in reference to the probe

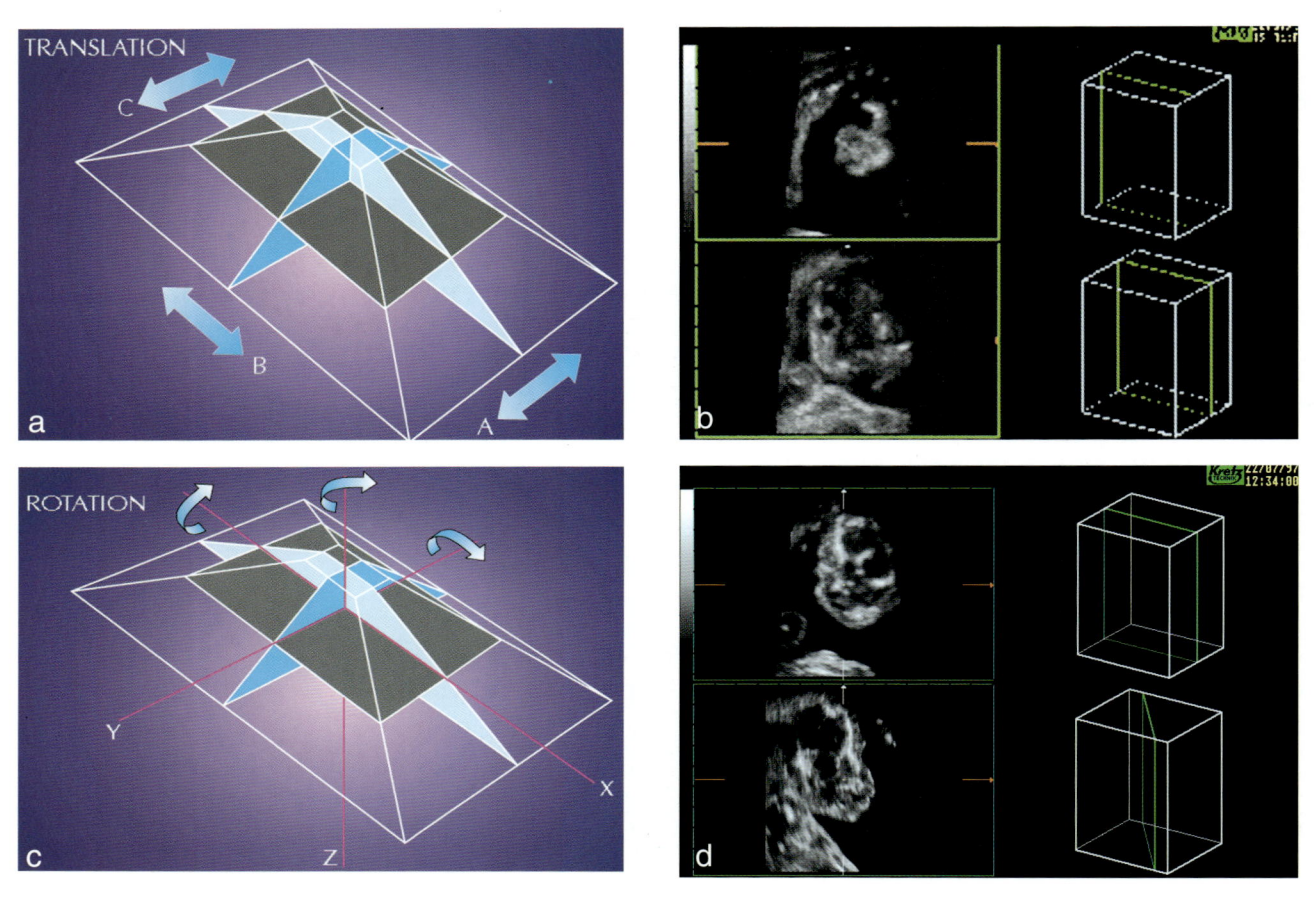

Figure 6 (a) Translation of orthogonal planes with reference to a scanned volume; (b) parallel movement to the frontal plane; (c) rotation of orthogonal planes with reference to a scanned volume; (d) rotation around the vertical axis

symmetry (e.g. a kidney in longitudinal, transverse and coronal views). The result is very detailed concerning the information within these planes but does not represent any information about the object outside these planes. It does not stimulate the visual perception of the observer to produce a 3D impression of the object.

A second family of algorithms for visualization of a 3D data set is ray tracing (also known as ray casting)[8]. The data set is seen as an optically transparent block whereby the optical parameters such as reflectivity and transparency are strictly dependent on the echo data inside this block. Ray tracing involves an imaginary ray of light being traced from the object to the viewer's eye and, depending on the algorithm that is used to determine the intensity of the light, results

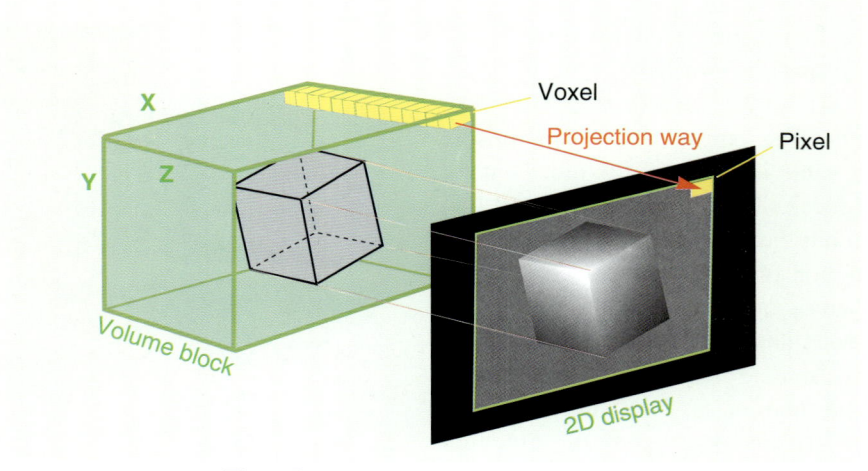

Figure 7 The principle of volume rendering

METHODOLOGY OF THREE-DIMENSIONAL ULTRASOUND

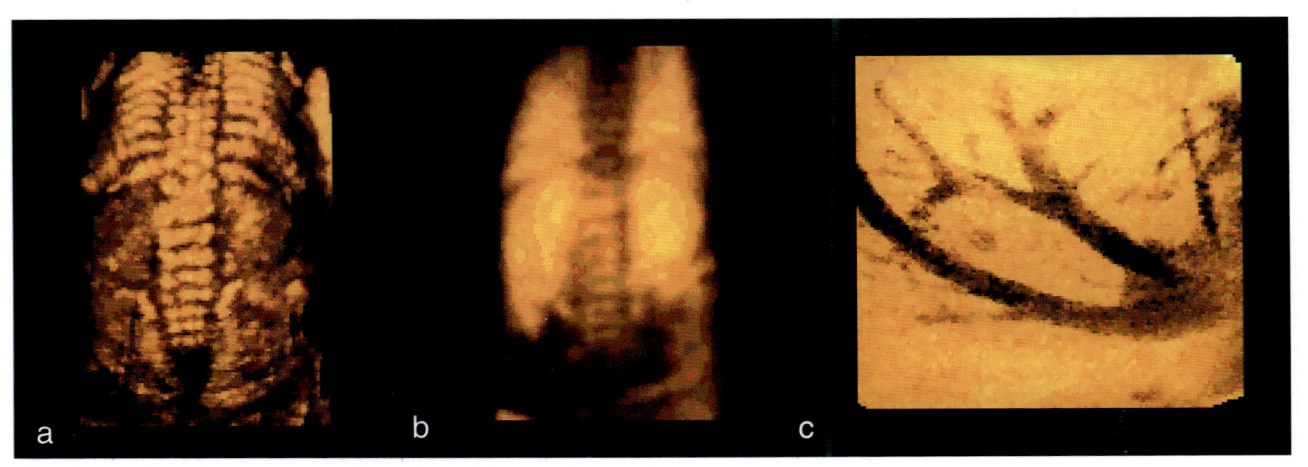

Figure 8 (a) Detection of bony structures; (b) transparent mode; (c) detection of hypoechoic structures (liver vessels)

in one stimulated light-sensitive cell on the retina of the observer. The retina is replaced by the 2D monitor and a light-sensitive cell is one pixel on this monitor. A bundle of different rays result in a complete picture (Figure 7). The different ray-tracing algorithms apply different mathematical methods for determining the resulting light stimulation from one ray of light. We can differentiate between algorithms that result in a transparent view through the object (Figure 8b), those that detect hyperechoic structures (e.g. the bones of a fetus) (Figure 8a) and those that detect hypoechoic structures (e.g. the vessels in the liver) (Figure 8c).

Impressive results can be achieved with methods that are able to detect the surface of an object. With these algorithms the object can be represented similarly to an optical visualization even if the representation is based on reflected sound waves and not reflected light. This effect can be extended by the use of imaginary light-reflection effects – the part of a surface that is perpendicular to the ray reflects with higher intensity than the part of an object that has an oblique angle to the ray of light (Figure 9).

For all the visualization processes described above, the echo signal is reflected in the image of the object.

The segmentation process uses the echo data only for determining 3D areas which are classified as part of a certain structure[9]. For example, all echoes coming from inside the prostate are classified as 'tumor'. Now the virtual object tumor can be described by a mathematical formula with the means of analytic geometry – e.g. the surface of the prostate obeys a certain function: $f(x,y,z)$. This function can be visualized by all the algorithms which are well known from computer-aided design (CAD) software. This includes light effects, textures, etc. For this visualization method the original data set no longer influences the result of the image – the data set is replaced by the virtual object 'tumor' (Figure 10).

Recent progress in visualization technology allows the evaluation of echo data inside a shell around the volume of interest. This method seems to have huge potential in collecting reliable and robust parameters regarding the perfusion and blood supply of certain areas in a tissue such as a tumor. Figure 11 illustrates the definition and representation of such an object.

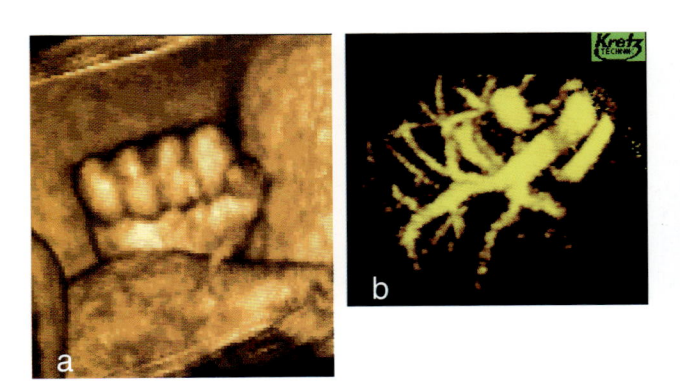

Figure 9 Surface-sensitive reconstruction: (a) fetal extremities; (b) ultrasound angiogram of liver vessels

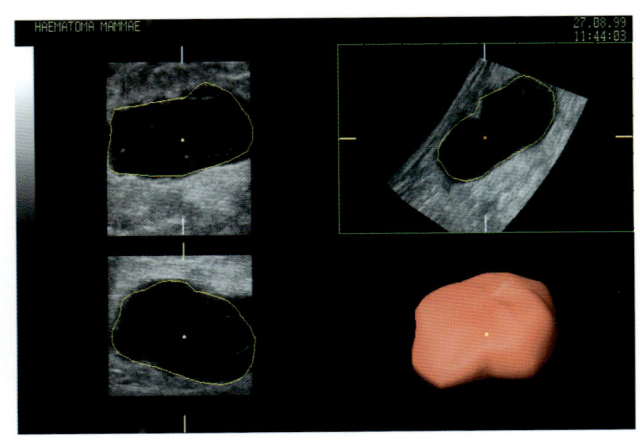

Figure 10 Segmentation of tissue: the contour of segmented region controlled in multiplanar mode; and surface repre segmented sentation of the segemented region with light effects (lower right)

5

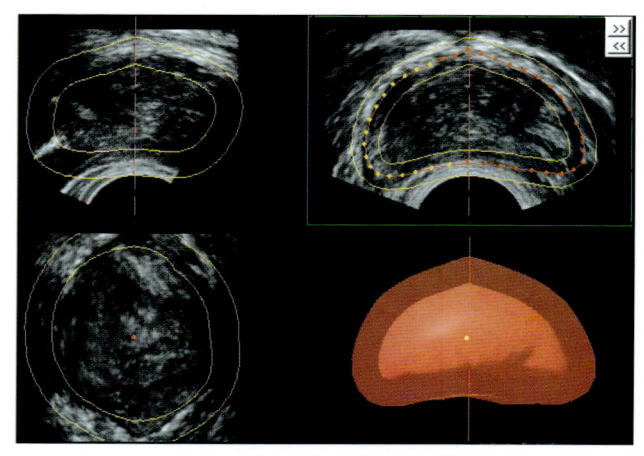

Figure 11 Definition and representation of a shell around a prostate

Conclusions

Three-dimensional ultrasound needs the processing technology of 2D ultrasound as a basis. Beyond that it needs new competencies in transducer design and in the design of position detection systems. It needs high-level software to implement all the visualization algorithms under the constraint of execution time and it needs a great deal of system and application knowledge from the designer of such 3D ultrasound systems to make this powerful tool valuable for the user.

New technologies in probe design, memory bandwidth and processing speed will allow the continuous acquisition and visualization of volumes. The selection of volumes of interest can then be done interactively, causing the examination time to speed up dramatically. This is similar to the impact of real-time ultrasound compared to the static compound mode.

References

1. Kossoff G. Three-dimensional ultrasound – technology push or market pull? *Ultrasound Obstet Gynecol* 1995;5:217–18
2. Levine RA, Weyman AE, Handschumacher MD. Three dimensional echocardiography; techniques and applications. *Am J Cardiol* 1992;69:121–34
3. Kitney R, Moura L, Straughan K. 3-D visualization of arterial structures using ultrasound and voxel modeling. *Int J Card Imaging* 1989;4:135–43
4. Schrank E, Phillips DJ, Moritz WE, *et al*. A triangulation method for the quantitative measurement of arterial blood velocity magnitude and direction in humans. *Ultrasound Med Biol* 1990;16:499–509
5. Blankenhorn DH, Chin HP, Strikwerda S, *et al*. Common carotid artery contours reconstructed in three dimensions from parallel ultrasonic images. *Radiology* 1983;148:533–7
6. King DL, Shao MY, Evaluation of *in vitro* measurement accuracy of a three dimensional ultrasound scanner. *J Ultrasound Med* 1991;10:77–82
7. Merz E, Gritzky A, Brandl H. *3-D Ultrasound in Obstetrics and Gynecology*. Philadelphia, PA: Lippincott Williams & Wilkins, 1998
8. Foley J, van Dam A, Feiner S, *et al. Computer Graphics*. Reading, MA: Addison Wesley, 1987
9. Sakas G, Walter S. Extracting surfaces from fuzzy 3D-ultrasound data. *Computer Graphics Proceedings*, 1995

Three-dimensional and power Doppler in the study of angiogenesis

A. Kurjak, S. Kupesic and T. Zodan

Introduction

The formation of new blood vessels (angiogenesis) results in neovascularization. It has been established that new blood vessels arise from postcapillary venules in response to an angiogenic stimulus. After proteolysis of the basement membrane and degradation of the interstitial matrix, endothelial cells migrate towards the angiogenic stimulus. These cells form a capillary bud, which is later canalized to form a tubule. As the endothelial cells of the tubule proliferate, they join the adjacent capillary bud and form a loop. At this point, blood begins to flow and a new vessel is formed.

Every tissue shows its own pattern of angiogenesis. In the female reproductive system, the angiogenesis of follicular development has been studied extensively. The characteristic vascular pattern starts as a simple capillary network around the primary follicles. A multilayered and complicated vascular system develops, surrounding the follicles; the largest vascular network is that around the Graafian follicle. Just before the rupture, a marked dilatation of the vessels occurs and they become 'leaky'. Angiogenesis in the follicle is limited to the theca, but following follicular rupture the thecal vessels invade the granulosa layer to give rise to the luteal vascular network[1–4].

The endothelial cells of the endometrium are estrogen receptor-negative[5]. It seems that the angiogenic response to estrogen must come from the estrogen receptor-positive epithelium or the stromal component of the endometrium.

Despite their low turnover, adult endothelial cells are not postmitotic but can form new blood vessels. The mechanisms underlying physiological angiogenesis during the ovarian cycle and pathological angiogenesis in tumors, ophthalmic and rheumatic diseases[6] are not fully understood. In pathological conditions and in wound healing, angiogenesis is a complex process accompanied by, and possibly requiring, inflammation. Nevertheless, those factors known to be necessary for adult angiogenesis also regulate embryonic angiogenesis. Indeed, vascular endothelial growth factor (VEGF), first found to affect angiogenesis in malignant gliomas[7], also regulates angiogenesis in many different tumors, and inhibition of VEGF signalling inhibits both tumor angiogenesis and the growth of experimental solid tumors[8–10]. However, the mechanisms responsible for the vascularization of tumors growing *in situ*, rather than as a transplant under the skin of mice, are still poorly understood. Although the sequence of events superficially resembles that in embryonic angiogenesis, the additional events in an established quiescent vessel are probably necessary, involving cell-cycle progression, remodelling of cell adhesions and junctions, induction of proteolytic activities and neutralization of inhibitors. In physiological processes, such as corpus luteum development or ovulation, angiogenesis subsides or terminates once the process is completed. In contrast, tumor angiogenesis is never self-limited. Once tumor-induced angiogenesis is initiated, it continues indefinitely until tumor growth is restrained and neovascularization interrupted[11–14]. Whilst in healthy adult tissues endothelial cells have a low mitotic rate and form a quiescent population, tumor-induced endothelium undergoes rapid mitoses and proliferation.

Recent work has emphasized genetic switches regulating angiogenesis[15], but the detailed genetic changes and their effects on angiogenesis must still be identified. Oncogenic, tumor-suppressive or mutant forms of mitogenic signalling pathways and cell-cycle control switches probably regulate the genes involved in angiogenesis[6], but whether they act directly or by way of the changing microenvironment in a growing tissue mass remains unclear. Malignant cells with mutations in the p53 gene, for example, can survive hypoxic conditions that kill less malignant cells[16], indicating that the supply of nutrients and oxygen to a growing tumor can affect its growth, malignancy and metastatic potential. An improved understanding of normal angiogenesis may suggest new approaches to therapy.

It has been over 100 years since it was first observed that tumors had an increased vascularity compared to normal tissues[17]. It was long believed that simple dilatation of existing host blood vessels accounted for tumor hyperemia[18]. Vasodilatation was generally thought to be a side-effect of tumor metabolites released from necrotic parts of the tumor. However, some authors suggested that tumor hyperemia could be related to the growth of new blood vessels, i.e. neovascularization, rather than to dilatation. A report published in 1945 revealed that new vessels in the neighborhood of a tumor implant arose from host vessels and not from the tumor itself[19]. This report initiated much discussion, which continued in the literature for two more decades, about whether tumors were supplied by existing vessels or by neovascularization[20].

A new concept that tumor growth is restricted in the absence of a vascular response was developed in the 1960s. Experiments with isolated perfused organs revealed that tumor growth was severely limited because of the absence of neovascularization[11-14]. A series of experiments in the following decade showed that tumors implanted into animals consistently induced the growth of new capillaries. Viable tumor cells were found to release diffusible angiogenic factors that stimulated new capillary growth and endothelial mitosis[21,22], even when tumor cell proliferation had been arrested by irradiation[23]. However, the products of necrotic tumors did not show any angiogenic properties.

On the basis of these observations, Judah Folkman proposed a hypothesis that once a tumor had occurred, every further increase in the tumor cell population had to be preceded by an increase in new capillaries, which sprouted towards the early growth of the tumor[21]. According to this concept, a small focus of tumor cells (containing less than 10^6 cells in a volume of a few cubic millimeters) could not increase without the induction of angiogenesis. Folkman's hypothesis was proved by the following experimental evidence:

(1) A tumor implanted in a subcutaneous transparent chamber grows very slowly; its volume increases linearly before vascularization takes place. After vascularization, tumor growth is rapid and tumor volume may increase exponentially[19].

(2) Tumor growth in the avascular rabbit cornea proceeds slowly and at a linear rate, but switches to exponential growth as soon as vascularization occurs[24].

(3) Tumors suspended in the aqueous fluid of the anterior chamber of the rabbit eye remain viable, avascular and limited in size (less than 1 mm^3). These tumors induce neovascularization of iris vessels, but are too remote from these vessels to be vascularized by them. Once a tumor is implanted in the vicinity of the proliferating iris vessels, it may enlarge its original volume up to 16 000 times within 2 weeks[25].

(4) Human retinoblastomas that have metastasized to the corpus vitreum are viable, avascular and growth-restricted.

The density of the capillary network seems to be one of the factors determining the malignancy of a tumor. Metastases of highly vascularized tumors appear earlier than those of poorly vascularized tumors[26-28]. The reason for this is not simply the capillary permeability that enables the shedding of tumor cells into the bloodstream, but also a fine regulatory angiogenic mechanism between the primary tumor and its distant metastases. In the majority of cases, metastases inherit the angiogenic properties of the primary tumor. However, clinical research has shown that this need not always be the case. Sometimes, when a primary tumor is removed, distant metastases disappear, while in other cases, even when the primary tumor is not particularly aggressive, distant metastases spread rapidly[3]. This has given rise to a hypothesis that only a certain subtype of tumor cells possesses angiogenic properties. Others, having the same karyotype, do not have these angiogenic factor genes switched on, and therefore do not take part in the angiogenic process. What triggers a cell to activate its angiogenic potential is still unknown.

Electron microscopy, *in vitro* cultures and experiments in animal models have enabled us to understand the visible part of the angiogenic process. The angiogenic factors, powerful molecules that control the formation of new blood vessels, are still a mystery. Compelling data indicate an interaction between positive and negative regulatory factors and the extracellular tissue matrix as a key event in the process of neovascularization.

The molecular basis of tumor angiogenesis

In recent years, cancer scientists have used molecular and biochemical knowledge, as well as insight into tumor physiology, to bridge the gap between preclinical and clinical work. Those factors most frequently found in human cancers are p16, p53 and Ras.

In 1993 it was reported that a small protein of approximately 16 kDa encoded from the MTS1 tumor suppresser locus on chromosome 9p21 had the capacity to block progression through the G$_1$ phase of the cell cycle by inhibiting cell cycle kinases (CDKs)[29] that phosphorylate the retinoblastoma protein (pRb), thereby preventing the release of pRb-associated transcription factors necessary for initiating DNA replication[30,31]. In the following few years, it was shown that this protein, p16 INK4a, has three closely related homologs: p15, p18 and p19[32-34]. Interestingly, all four family members have the capacity to block kinase activity derived from the cyclin D-dependent kinases cdk4 and cdk6, but it is only p16 function that is lost with high frequency in human cancers[35]. Reports have also shown that p16 is lost in late and invasive stages of melanoma and glioblastoma tumor development, but this does not exclude a role for p16 in regulating tumor cell spreading[36,37].

In vitro studies have shown that p53 is kept in a latent, non-DNA-binding form through its C-terminal domain and can be activated by small peptides derived from the C-terminus[38]. It is believed that activation mutations in the Ras genes (Ha-, Ki- and N-*ras*) contribute to the formation of some 30% of human malignancies, including 95% of pancreatic and 50% of colon cancers[39]. There is considerable evidence that activated Ras proteins promote tumor formation and growth by induction of cell proliferation and inhibition of apoptosis. While activated Ras is capable of transforming most immortalized cell lines, transformation of normal primary cell lines requires co-operating oncogenes and the loss of specific tumor suppresser genes[40].

Angiogenic factors

The first indication of the importance of angiogenesis for tumor growth came from observations in the early 1980s that tumors secreted soluble factors that could stimulate vascular endothelial growth[41]. The basic and acidic fibroblast growth factors were among the first to be identified and were soon followed by many others such as vascular endothelial growth factor/vascular permeability factor (VEGF/VPF) and transforming growth factors (TGF-α and -β), to mention some of the more important.

The major role in vasodilatation and angiogenesis during ovulation may be attributed to the action of the prostaglandins PGE$_2$ and PGI$_2$, assumed to be potent vasodilators[42], but also to angiogenic stimulants, especially PGE$_1$ and PGE$_2$[43]. These prostaglandins are produced by small luteal cells and markedly increase the local blood flow in corpora lutea, causing vascular 'luteal conversion'. Because prostaglandins correlate with corpus luteum production of prostaglandins[44], it is assumed that abundant corpus luteum vascularity is caused by the local action of prostaglandins. Based on the assumption that angiogenesis is a uniform process, a newly formed vascular network should yield no difference in blood flow parameters if detected in the early stage of its development in folliculogenesis, in the corpus luteum or in benign and malignant lesions. Regarding the blood flow characteristics of early angiogenesis observed with the vasodilatation and opening of arteriovenous shunts by the action of prostaglandins at local levels, it is reasonable to believe that certain benign tumors, and some normal conditions, have high angiogenic potential and/or intense local production of prostaglandins.

Tumor neovascularization

In general, tumor vasculature consists of the vessels recruited from the pre-existing network of the host vasculature and the vessels grown from the host vessels under the influence of the angiogenic factors of cancer cells[45,46]. Although the tumor vasculature originates from the host vasculature, its organization may be completely different, depending upon the tumor type, its growth rate and its location. The architecture differs not only among various tumor types, but also between the primary tumor and its transplants[47]. Macroscopically, tumor vasculature can be studied in terms of two categories: peripheral and central. In tumors with peripheral vascularization, the centers are usually poorly perfused. In those with central vascularization, one would expect the opposite. However, a tumor may consist of many territories, each exhibiting one or the other type of vascular pattern. Microscopically, tumor vasculature is highly heterogeneous and does not conform to the standard vascular organization[48]. The main characteristics of tumor vasculature include:

(1) A single branch, varying in caliber, being formed of narrow and dilated segments;

(2) Elongation and coiling;

(3) A non-hierarchical vascular network, vascular rings and sinusoids;

(4) No normal precapillary architecture with dichotomous branching, and no decrease in size and diameter of the higher-order branches;

(5) An incomplete vascular wall: various gaps in the endothelium, discontinuity of the basal membrane and no muscular layer except in pre-existing vessels encased by the tumor.

A key difference between normal and tumor vessels is that the latter are dilated, saccular and tortuous, and may contain tumor cells within the endothelial lining of the vessel wall[47]. The amount of structural abnormalities depends on how rapidly a tumor grows. Well-differentiated, slow-growing tumors are expected to have a less disturbed vessel architecture, because angiogenesis can keep pace with the slow tumor growth. Anaplastic, poorly differentiated tumors grow so rapidly that the angiogenic process creates chaotic, vessel-like spaces lacking mature elements. In addition, unlike normal tissue with a relatively fixed route between the arterial and venous circulation, a tumor may have blood flowing from one venule to another via a series of vessels or directly via an arteriovenous shunt. Furthermore, owing to the peculiar nature of the vasculature, the organization of vessels may differ from one location to another and from one phase to the next. As regards perfusion rates, four regions can be recognized in a tumor: an avascular (necrotic) region; a seminecrotic (ischemic) region; a stabilized microcirculation; and an advancing front as a region of tumor hyperemia.

Functional impairments caused by structural abnormalities

Structural abnormalities of capillaries formed in tumor angiogenesis can cause numerous functional impairments[48]:

(1) The transcapillary permeability is increased (up to eight times normal). Mural defects may even be large enough to allow extravasation of red blood cells. Generally, increased permeability causes hemoconcentration and increased viscous flow resistance. A different mechanism appears to be related to vesicovascular organelles. They cause substances to pass across the endothelial cell itself and may, in addition to mural defects, be involved, for example, in the transcapillary exchange of contrast agents. VEGF has been shown to be present in increased vascular permeability[49].

(2) In highly vascularized tumors the total vascular cross-sectional area is increased. This will lower the peripheral flow resistance. However, lumen irregularities may regionally increase flow resistance. Along with hemoconcentration and increased interstitial pressure, this may even lead to local stasis.

(3) Interstitial pressure is near atmospheric values in normal tissue, whereas in tumors it may reach 50 mmHg or even more. The main factors attributed to interstitial hypertension are increased vascular permeability and lack of lymphatic drainage. Furthermore, the interstitial space is usually three to five times larger than normal. High interstitial pressure leads to compression of vessels inside the tumor.

(4) Where arteriovenous shunts develop, a fraction of blood will bypass the capillary bed. Consequently, despite a low global flow resistance and a high global blood flow, a variable proportion of the tumor may be deprived of its blood supply. Shunt fractions are estimated to range between 8 and 43%. Tissue with only venous–venous flow will be hypoxic, owing to slow flow velocity and low oxygen saturation of the supplied blood.

The effect of such functional mechanisms is not constant throughout the tumor but highly inconstant, spatially and temporally. There may be stasis in one part and maintained flow in another part of the lesion. It is estimated that only between 20 and 80% of the tumor vessels are actually patent. Considering also local factors, such as invasion by tumor cells, or variations in intercapillary distance, it is not surprising that vessel density and blood flow can differ between tumors by a factor of 100, and even inside a tumor by a factor of 55[48]. Information on global blood flow and flow resistance may be of limited relevance regarding local oxygen and nutrient supply.

According to histomorphometric studies of tumor vasculature, the microvessel density appears to be a major factor determining the aggressiveness of the disease. With highly vascular tumors, distant metastases occur significantly earlier and more frequently than with poorly vascularized tumors, independent of the risk factors[25–28,50–57]. Not only is neovascularization necessary to enable tumor cells to be shed into the bloodstream, but distant metastases also need angiogenesis if they are to grow beyond a clinically undetectable size[54]. The most supported hypothesis is that both the primary tumor and the distant metastases are involved in complex regulation by angiogenic and antiangiogenic factors. In the most simple case, metastases inherit the angiogenic properties of the primary tumor. They may, however, also lose the capability of angiogenesis and entirely depend on systemically distributed angiogenic factors produced by the primary tumor. Conversely, they may remain dormant under the antiangiogenic control by the primary tumor.

These are models to explain the surprising clinical courses after removal of the primary tumor, such as the disappearance of overt metastatic disease, or rapidly progressive distant metastases of a primary lesion which itself did not appear to be particularly aggressive[3]. Only a subfraction of the tumor cells appears to be angiogenic. It is thus far unknown what triggers a cell to switch to the angiogenic state.

It has been known for over 25 years that the development of new blood vessels is necessary to sustain the growth, invasion and metastasis of tumors[58–60]. Angiogenesis is crucial for sustaining tumor growth, as it allows oxygenation and nutrient perfusion of the tumor as well as removal of waste products. Moreover, increased angiogenesis coincides with increased tumor cell entry into the circulation and thus facilitates metastasis[61,62]. Cancer cells activate the quiescent vasculature to produce new blood vessels via an 'angiogenetic switch' often during the premalignant stages of tumor development. Data suggesting that control of angiogenesis is separate from control of cancer cell proliferation raise the possibility that drugs inhibiting angiogenesis could offer a treatment that is complementary to traditional chemotherapy, which directly targets tumor cells[58–60,63]. This exciting possibility has prompted current research on tumor angiogenesis[64–68].

Studies and quantification of angiogenesis

Not so long ago, the only features assessed when studying an organ or a tumor were size and shape. Conventional ultrasound imaging, although an important innovation, relies on the same features. This tool can tell us the size, shape and location, but cannot describe the physiology, the inner life within a neoplasm. Neovascularization is not displayed on the screen and the only vessels shown are those of large diameter. They are depicted as hollow, hypoechogenic structures with clear hyperechogenic borders. Smaller vessels remain hidden.

The 1980s were characterized by the development of high-resolution real-time gray-scale imaging, the transvaginal approach and spectral and color Doppler sonography. In the early 1990s better sensitivity was achieved in color Doppler sonography. In contrast to frequency-based color Doppler sonography, which analyzes the frequency shift of blood velocity information, power Doppler sonography uses the amplitude component of the signals received to represent the number of moving blood cells. Power Doppler sonography has been found to be superior to frequency-based color Doppler sonography, especially in situations of low-velocity blood flow[69], with the potential to detect alterations in blood flow[70], because it is more sensitive, less angle-dependent and not susceptible to aliasing[69,71]. This allows visualization of small vessels and lower flows[72].

All these features make this new method optimal for three-dimensional (3D) reconstruction of vessels. The diagnostic accuracy of impedance values in differentiating benign from malignant lesions has ranged considerably from over 96% to less than 40%. Statistical analyses of the data from various reports are confounded by non-universal selection of Doppler parameters (resistance vs. pulsatility index), choice of the highest, lowest or mean impedance values and selection of vessels for interrogation. Differences in operator variance and system sensitivity contribute to an already confusing analysis of parameters[73]. It is clear that there is a need for further improvement in the ultrasonic assessment of pelvic tumor angiogenesis and, to this end, there has been a growing interest in 3D power Doppler ultrasound.

Ultrasound images are shown on a monitor screen and are thus inherently two-dimensional (2D). Data from the body, however, are inherently 3D. New 3D scanners have the ability to collect 3D infomation and represent it on the 2D screen.

Power Doppler ultrasound, also known as color power angiography or Color Doppler Angio®, has been in clinical practice for several years[69,70,74–76]. In this technique the hue and brightness of the color signal represent the total energy of the Doppler signal. Power Doppler ultrasound has the advantage that it is more sensitive to low flow and thus overcomes the angle-dependence and aliasing of standard color Doppler. It displays the total flow in a confined area, giving an impression similar to that of angiography. Power Doppler involves an upgrade of the existing software of original color Doppler scanners. However, the experience of power Doppler in the field of obstetrics and gynecology is still limited[77–80]. The 3D capability has been extended to various diagnostic ultrasound modalities[81–84]. In the case of tumor vascularity, the 3D display allows the physician easily and quickly to visualize multiple overlapping vessels, and their relationship to other vessels and tumors or other surrounding tissues. This implementation of the 3D display permits the physician to see three dimensions on the screen interactively, rather than mentally assembling the sectional images. The 3D power Doppler system may enable physicians to study the region of interest in more detail, and speed up the entire patient management process.

For example, conventionally we follow up the blood flow of a transplanted kidney by calculating the impedance indices of interlobular branches[85]. The calculation of power signal intensities in serial image sections may also help in the detection of chronic rejection[86,87]. Now we can generate 3D vascular images that display the morphology and branching patterns of intrarenal vessels, and the presence or absence of avascular areas (possibly indicating infarction) within a graft. Three-dimensional vascular imaging may be a means of triaging patients to optimize management.

Image acquisition and equipment for three-dimensional ultrasound

Two main types of equipment for the 3D display of vascular structures are currently available. The first kind is a computer program that does not require additional hardware (e.g. Color Power Angio in HDI-3000 or 5000 by ATL or SSD-1700, Volume mode by Aloka). This kind of program that does not need upgraded hardware does not perform a complicated calculation of spatial information for each acquired 2D image. The data acquisition is by freehand scanning and, in this type of acquisition, the XY plane is fixed (equal to the width of each single 2D view). However, the moving path and speed of the transducer in the Z dimension is not defined. Therefore, imaging of the vascular architecture is sometimes less accurate. Varying the manual movement of the probe over the same vascularized area will produce different images of the vascular architecture with this processing method. Since the processing of this type of acquisition does not deal with the calculation of spatial information, the 3D reconstruction time is short, usually less than 30 s (depending on the frames reconstructed).

The second kind of 3D machine operates with fully digitized processing of power Doppler data and complete storage of 3D data. Examples of commercially available systems are the 3D ultrasound scanner by Kretz 530D (Medison) and the off-line workstation 3D FreeScan® (Echo-Tech Inc., Germany). In this type of acquisition each originally acquired 2D view contains its own positional information. Therefore, the 3D reconstruction is more accurate but is also more time-consuming. The data are acquired with mechanical 3D probes (Kretz 530D) or a remote magnetic positioning sensor (3D FreeScan) lined up to the 2D probe. The mechanical 3D probe contains a normal 2D probe that is driven in the third dimension with a motor. During the 3D data acquisition, the mechanical 3D probe must be kept still. The relationships between acquired 2D images are constant. On the other hand, the magnetic positioning sensor of the off-line fully digitized workstation (3D®) attaches to the conventional transducer, and provides spatial information for each of the captured 2D images. The movement of the transducer is free.

Types of display for three-dimensional vascular images

With the built-in program of HDI-3000 or 5000, 3D vascular images are viewed as multi-sided objects with the vascular architecture mapped on multiple planes. The 3D multi-sided objects can be rotated horizontally.

The fully digitized data with spatial information from Kretz 530D or Echo-tech 3D FreeScan are interpolated with the 'ray-casting' technique. A minimum-intensity projection of vascular images is used for creation of a translucent vascular image, and a maximum-intensity projection (rarely used) is for surface-rendered vascular images[88,89].

With freehand 3D compounding (HDI 3000 or Aloka 1700 Volume mode) the operator must take care to move the transducer at a constant rate. The resulting image is quite good for visualization of the 3D architecture of the vasculature, but not for distance or volume measurement. Fully digitized processing with spatial information (e.g. Kretz 530D) allows a more accurate 3D display. It is also possible to evaluate the corresponding 3D gray-scale image. It takes longer than the freehand system. In addition, the operator needs more technical knowledge and a sense for the complex computing.

Various investigators[81,89–91] have found that multi-slice viewing, maximum-intensity projection and surface-rendering of vasculature all have some role in displaying the vascular data. However, it has been suggested that the last two methods are more effective in displaying large-vessel flow, with multi-slicing being reserved for assessment of the microcirculation.

Problems in data interpretation of three-dimensional power Doppler imaging

Although power Doppler has several advantages over conventional color Doppler ultrasound, it is still a kind of color Doppler imaging and therefore subject to some of the limitations of the conventional technique. For example, various parameters of color Doppler ultrasound, such as pulse repetition frequency (PRF), wall filter, priority, power gain, color persistence and frame rate must be optimized for 3D display, as well as for qualitative and quantitative analysis of these power Doppler data. A change in color setting may lead to a totally different 3D vascular image and dissimilar quantitative results. In addition, since now both color and power Doppler can be combined with more complex computing, the frame rate will be significantly reduced (usually down to 2–3 Hz) when the power/color Doppler mode is active. Therefore, if a mechanical 3D probe (e.g. in Kretz 530D) is used, some tiny vessels may escape from image capture. The effects of ultrasound attenuation can sometimes cause different 'power intensity' and hence vessel detection between nearer and deeper parts of the tissue being explored.

Ultrasound technology in tumor diagnostics

In our work towards finding ways of early cancer detection we use various ultrasound modalities. Studying the morphology by ultrasound echography represented the first approach and, in fact, there is evidence of morphology and attenuation of tumors in the very early stages of ultrasound diagnosis[92]. However, the specificity of such an approach used alone continues to be insufficient[93]. It is therefore common to assess both the morphology and the flow characteristics of various structures for their characterization. A number of scoring methods have been in existence for some time, but none has been widely accepted.

Morphological analysis of the blood vessel system represents another approach to tumor diagnosis which, so far, has not been extensively evaluated. However, there is a distinct subjective impression that the distribution and branching pattern of blood vessels that supply fast-growing tumors differ from those of the normal blood supply to normal organs. The blood vessel distribution therefore seems to carry additional information that is missed in the present diagnostic approaches. However, describing branching structures such as the blood vessel tree is a mathematically complicated task that calls for the most recent mathematical apparatus. This aspect will be dealt with in more detail.

The branching pattern is a result of some principle (mathematical law) that acts repeatedly upon the blood vessels so that they branch out in similar ways at different scale factors. The process is, presumably, similar to processes that govern the branching in actual trees. If the underlying rule changes, the branching pattern must change too. It is this change in the branching pattern that we wish to quantify and make use of in early cancer detection. The novelty in our proposal is the application of such new mathematical analysis and concepts to data acquired with the newly developed 3D ultrasound imaging system. We are in a unique situation to apply a new technological development to contribute to solving a crucial medical problem using a truly novel mathematical approach.

Ovarian malignancy as well as other gynecological malignancies have low prevalence and are elusive and deadly diseases, requiring studies of a large number of patients (conforming to the prevalence and development time) for a long period[94,95]. Many other tumors fall into this category, which warrants a completely new approach in ultrasound diagnosis and other imaging methods. Before describing our work-in-progress we must give a short description of the fundamentals.

A short outline of the mathematical basis

Mathematical knowledge usually becomes general knowledge centuries after its first discovery[96–98]. It is not surprising, therefore, that the knowledge of non-linear processes that has been gained in the past 36 years has not yet reached all the technology and science faculties, let alone the majority of practical applications. On the other hand, it has received much attention in the research of population dynamics, ecology, meteorology and fluid dynamics. Large companies, particularly oil companies and the aerospace industry, invest large sums of money in projects that apply this mathematical methodology.

Processes in time or space can be described either with linear or with non-linear equations and formulae. Linear mathematical models can very often be solved so that the complete behavior of a linear system is known. Non-linear systems, e.g. virtually all biological systems, present tremendous mathematical problems and are often only partially solved by treating a small part of the non-linear process as linear; this, therefore, yields only a partial insight into the process. The main difference between the two types of system is that, in linear systems, a small change in some parameter results in a small change in the end results, while in non-linear systems a small change in some parameter can yield large, hardly predictable, changes in the outcome. Many processes in nature are recursive; i.e. the generations of results are obtained by applying the same mathematical law (formulae) over and over again (as in the calculation of the number of multiplying cells). The starting point of the next generation is the result of the same type of calculation for the preceding generation. The outcomes (final states) after variation of some parameter may, at the first glance, look totally chaotic. However, when one maps many of the possible outcomes of such a process (e.g. blood vessel branching, animal population, climatic changes, etc.) the map may turn out to have a pattern, which is self-similar at different magnifications. Such objects that are self-similar at different scales are called fractals. A map of possible states of a system is called an attractor[96,97].

The present state of the art in blood vessel geometry and functionality diagnostics

While fractal research is new, there exist some initial results in the use of simpler vessel geometry. For example, microvessel density in ovarian and endometrial cancers has been correlated with the likelihood of recurrence[99,100]. The density (determined histologically) of microvessels irrespective of their distribution was also found to have significant implications for recurrence. In color Doppler studies the density can be determined by counting the number of color spots in a tumor area.

Our group has studied the Doppler characterization of tumors extensively. The results have been widely reported and compared to similar results by other groups. While further development and refinement of the simple color Doppler technique used alone may be feasible, our conclusion is that we must combine a geometrical feature with the existing criteria. The specificity of the Doppler approach in the early studies seemed to be high, but has turned out not to satisfy the requirements of an appropriate screening method.

Evaluation of tumoral blood vessel geometry

Our initial hypothesis was that the general view of the pattern of branching of blood vessels within 1 cm³ generally resembles that of the branching in 50 cm³ of the same tissue. Structures that look alike at different magnifications are fractal[97,98,101] and are found in natural geometric forms (trees, bird's feathers, etc.) as well as in the maps of the (apparently chaotic) outcomes of processes that have nothing to do with geometry (animal populations). The growth of blood vessels is likely to have these properties. The main property of a fractal is its fractal dimension. We postulate that blood vessel trees are an example of fractal geometry[98,101]. The normal blood vessel trees (arteries and veins) form branched structures with ever-smaller branches and diameters. They provide blood supply to the whole body while taking up less than 6% of the available space. The underlying proposition of our hypothesis is that there is a change in fractal dimension when the branching becomes unregulated by normal processes, i.e. when the ordered growth is replaced by disordered growth.

A study is already under way with our Histopathology Department that is aimed at proving the differences in the scalability aspects of blood vessel branching in malignant tumors when compared to normal vascularization. There is little doubt that any results may be of basic scientific interest, although the blood vessels found in one single specimen are too few to provide us with an attractor.

Three-dimensional modelling on a large scale is a mathematically and technologically demanding task. One important aspect of this approach is the interplay of results obtained by reconstruction of blood vessel geometry using ultrathin histological sections and the resolution of diagnostic imaging methods, particularly 3D ultrasound imaging. Although ultrasound resolution has greatly improved over the years, it is physically impossible to obtain resolutions of the order of 10 μm with any non-invasive form of ultrasonic imaging or Doppler. 3D reconstruction with ultrasound imaging and Doppler is now feasible and takes us a step nearer to this mathematical evaluation, but the resolution problems are similar in two and three dimensions. 'Cross breeding' with other fields may improve the situation[102–104].

The consequence of the resolution limitation is that we cannot follow many scale factors of magnification in the human body, because we rapidly run into the resolution limit of our imaging system. There may be ways to assess the chaos and fractal properties of blood vessel growth. It is a sensible proposition that the growth is a non-linear process and that chaotic behavior ought to be expected. Even simple non-linear functions may give rise to alternating episodes of orderly and totally chaotic behavior. If tumor blood vessel structure and population behave like this, ordinary statistics may fail. The likely problem is that an essential part of the growth occurs at the tiniest blood vessel diameters, where a further reduction in size is not possible. Blood vessels that are much smaller than erythrocytes make little sense, so there is an end to the self-similarity at these sizes. We therefore propose a combined approach that will include 3D ultrasound at larger blood vessel diameters and histology at diameters that are too small for ultrasonic imaging.

Three-dimensional power Doppler quantification of blood flow and vascularization

A new method in the field of vascular quantification, called 3D histogram, was recently introduced by Pairleitner and colleagues[105–108]. The 3D color histogram measures the color percentage and flow amplitudes in the volume of interest. Therefore, the histogram enables the quantification of vascularization and blood flow within a tissue block, in contrast to 2D color histogram measurements, where only single planes can be investigated. Here, the 3D tissue block is swept through with a volume probe to obtain the 3D information and, after that, to delineate the border of the volume of interest that contains the color information – an automatic delineation called 'shell'.

High-velocity flow vessels (such as the vasa iliaca) should be placed outside the volume of interest, if the measurement is to determine neoangiogenetic flow. Artifacts due to tissue, patient or probe movements should also be excluded. These artifacts are rather common, because of the high sensitivity of the amplitude-based color Doppler. The defined cube is then analyzed with computer algorithms to form indices of blood flow and vascularization. The vascularization index (VI) describes the color percentage within the volume of interest and therefore tells us how many vessels can be detected within the tissue block. The flow index (FI) is a mean amplitude value. The FI tells how many blood cells are transported in the moment of the 3D sweep. In this way blood flow can be estimated. The vascularization–flow index (VFI) and the flow–vessel quotient (FVQ) are a combination of the VI and FI. The VFI and FVQ combine the information of vessel presence and amount of flow by multiplying (VFI) or dividing (FVQ) the FI and VI.

Recently, Pairleitner and co-workers[106] analyzed 20 patients with adnexal masses and created the first description for the quantification of blood flow by 3D power Doppler sonography[109]. In each measurement a cube enclosing the vessels of the cyst wall, but excluding the iliac vessels or motion artifacts, was defined. This cube was stored on a hard disk as a Cartesian file for computer analysis using specially designed software.

Analogous to 2D pixels, the stored volume ultrasound information obtained using 3D power Doppler sonography was defined by voxels (smallest units of volume). Background voxels contain all the 3D gray-scale information in grades from black to white. All 3D color information is summarized by color voxels. To accentuate the difference between the amplitudes of the reflected ultrasound waves (intensity of flow), the color voxels are weighted, i.e. multiplied by a factor from 1 (= lowest amplitude) to 32 (= highest amplitude).

The 3D-View function calculates the background, gray scale and color and size parameters of the defined cube, which we used for creating three indices. These indices measure vascularization (1) or blood flow (2) or both (3):

(1) Vascularization index (VI) = color voxels/(total voxels – background voxels)

(2) Flow index 1 (FI 1) = weighted color voxels/(color voxels – border voxels)
Flow index 2 (FI 2) = weighted color voxels/color voxels

(3) Vascularization–flow index 1 (VFI 1) = weighted color voxels/(total voxels – background voxels)
Vascularization–flow index 2 (VFI 2) = (weighted voxels × cube volume)/(cyst volume × total voxels)

The VI measures the number of color voxels in the cube, representing the vessels in the tissue. The FI, a mean color value of all blood flow or induced flow intensities, represents the intensity of flow at the time of the 3D sweep. The FI is not an indicator of perfusion, so it cannot give information on the volume of blood pumped through the vessels during a certain period of time. The VFI is a combination of vascularization and flow information relating the weighted color values (weighted by their amplitudes) to the cube. Therefore, the VFI represents both blood flow and vascularization.

In FI 1 we excluded the border voxels, which contain both color and gray-scale information; they represent the virtual borders of the vessels, exceeding the real vessel borders. In VFI 2 the weighted color was related not to the cube volume but to the cyst volume, measured manually on the ultrasound unit.

The authors stressed that their data indicate that 3D power Doppler sonography combined with the cube method gives reproducible information for the vascularization and blood flow. This method relies on Cartesian analysis and thus eliminates the subjectivity that arises from depiction of randomly selected 2D slices.

Examples of three-dimensional power imaging of benign and malignant gynecological neoplasms

Different types of angiogenesis in different physiological and pathological conditions have been described. Physiological angiogenesis is seen in folliculogenesis, embryogenesis and implantation, chronic inflammation and some benign neoplasms[110]. In our relatively short experience with 3D power Doppler, we have been able to depict the mesovarium vessels entering the hilum area and extending to the stroma gradually with increasing numbers and branches of fine vessels during the preovulatory phase. After ovulation, we can sometimes disclose the luteal cyst formation. The luteal vessels are usually fewer (usually only one) and seldom have complicated branching or encircle the cyst (Figure 1), in contrast to the findings in a malignant neoplasm. In chocolate cysts the vessels are usually straight and regularly branching, and usually come from a hilar vessel then run along the surface of the tumor. Similar vascular anatomy is detected in dermoid cysts.

We observed the neovascularization in a number of cases of malignant neoplasm (Figure 2). In these cases the tumor vessels are usually randomly dispersed within the stroma and periphery, and some of them form several tangles or coils around the surface. The course of the main tumor vessel is usually irregular, with more complicated branching (Figure 3). The diameter of these vessels is felt to be more 'uneven' and 'thorn-like'. The findings can be compared to those of previous studies with conventional color Doppler ultrasound[110]. However, the appeal of the 3D display is that it is more comprehensive and allows physicians to understand the 3D architecture of the microcirculation interactively. In addition, the resolution of current power Doppler is sufficient to detect vessels of around 1 mm in diameter[52]. Therefore, we believe that 3D power Doppler is a promising tool in the evaluation of the angiogenesis of pelvic tumors, especially when a malignant neoplasm is suspected (Figures 4 and 5).

In an attempt to systematize the extent of perfusion[52] four regions of different perfusion states can be recognized: a necrotic region (central portion), a seminecrotic (ischemic) region, a stabilized microcirculation and the hyperemia region within the outermost area. Different pathological types, tumors with different growth rates, primary tumors or metastases can all exhibit different perfusion patterns. The compact type of gestational trophoblastic tumors (classification proposed by Hsieh and associates[111,112]), often choriocarcinoma, has this typical pattern of

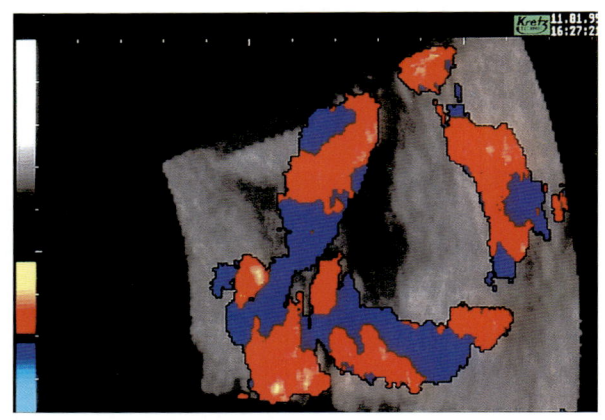

Figure 1 Three-dimensional scan displaying functional cyst and surrounding vessels. Color Doppler demonstrates regularly separated peripheral vessels typical of benign structures

Figure 2 Three-dimensional power Doppler scan of malignant tumor neovascularization. Note the three generations of vessels, areas of stenosis, microaneurysms and tumoral lakes

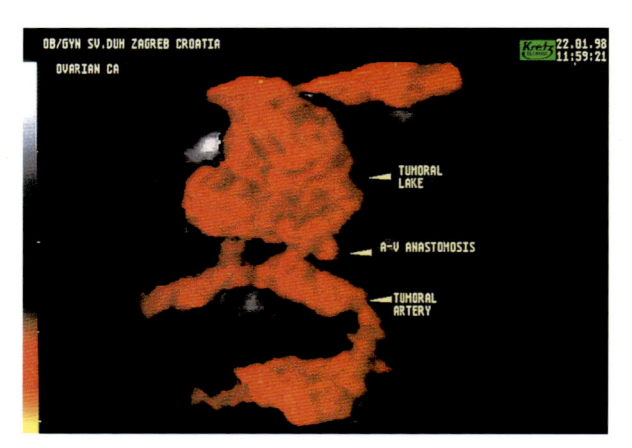

Figure 3 Malignant tumor neovascularization is characterized by arteriovenous (A-V) shunts, stenosis and blind-ending lakes. All these features can be assessed using three-dimensional power Doppler imaging

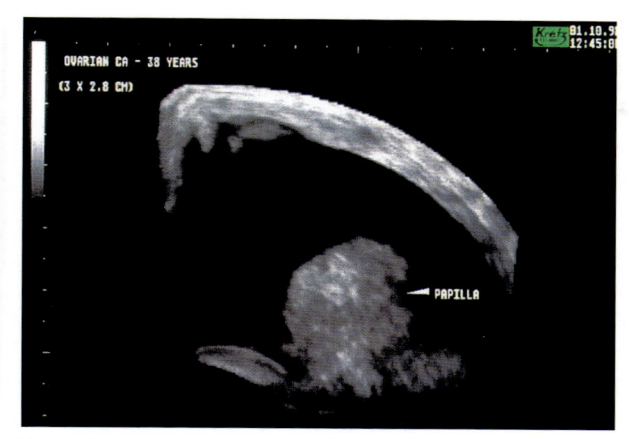

Figure 4 Complex ovarian tumor as seen by three-dimensional ultrasound. Surface view demonstrates papillary projections protruding into the cystic cavity. The morpology was suggestive of ovarian malignancy, which was confirmed by histopathology

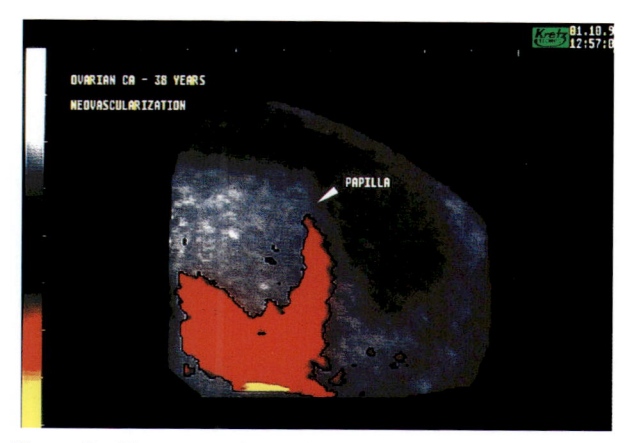

Figure 5 The same patient as in Figure 4. The volume has been rotated in all three dimensions, allowing visualization of the tumoral vessels with an irregular course and branching

tumor vascularity. 3D power Doppler imaging could provide us with a tool for *in vivo* assessment of tumor vascularity in a quantitative way.

Advances in tumor therapy

Our discussion is based on over 10 years of experience with transvaginal color and pulsed Doppler ultrasound and its correlation with macro- and microscopic pathology. However, our present studies and those of other authors on tumor-induced angiogenesis and the possible assessment of 3D chaos and fractals should be explored further, since they may offer better mathematical models of the complexity of malignant neovascularization than the simple analyses of the flow indices that have been applied to date.

The role of color Doppler sonography in the assessment of the architecture of tumor vascularity therefore seems clinically pertinent, justifying expanded research on this topic. This is based on the discovery and molecular characterization of a diverse family of regulators of angiogenesis, both stimulators and inhibitors[37]. In the case of solid tumors a shift in the balance of stimulators and inhibitors can trip the angiogenetic switch, allowing tumors to recruit new blood vessels from the surrounding host vasculature, which provides them with survival advantage. This process appears absolutely necessary for tumors to grow beyond microscopic size. It is the ultimate goal of most tumor angiogenesis research to find ways of turning off the angiogenetic switch in tumors as a form of cancer treatment. Recent results from Folkman's laboratory[77] present findings that strongly support a new treatment possibility.

Boehm and co-workers[113] have shown that three different mouse tumors treated with repeat cycles of a newly discovered angiogenesis inhibitor called endostatin regressed, did not become drug resistant and, after a characteristic number of treatment cycles, became dormant. Such a treatment strategy could help circumvent many of the problems associated with current chemotherapeutic regimens, such as acquired drug resistance, attributable to tumor cell genetic instability, or intrinsic resistance due to poor penetration of certain drugs into the tumor parenchyma[114]. The results of cyclic endostatin therapy strongly suggest that drugs targeting angiogenesis and the tumor vasculature will become a major new weapon for effectively treating, and indeed preventing, human cancer. As with any new treatment procedure there are a number of important questions for the future. A pure angiogenesis inhibitor would be expected to block new blood vessel growth, leaving quiescent blood vessels intact. Such an inhibitor should stop neovascularization in a tumor and effect a static, dormant state. The tumor should neither grow nor regress but should continue to be fed by its established vessels, remaining in a metastable state of proliferation balanced by apoptosis[115].

There is another important question. Are there tissue-specific differences in the vasculature and consequently in tumor vessel anatomy that affect a tumor's susceptibility to inhibition/disruption? Could 3D power Doppler help in answering some of these questions? It is undoubtedly a challenge for ultrasonographers, because control and perhaps cure of human cancers are surely on the horizon.

References

1. Kanzaki H, Okamura H, Okuda Y. Scanning electron microscopic study of rabbit ovarian follicle microvasculature using resin injection–corrosion casts. *J Anat* 1982;134:697–704
2. Murakami T, Ikebuchi Y, Ohtusuka A. The blood vascular wreath of rat ovarian follicle, with special reference to its changes in ovulation and luteinization: a scanning electron microscopic study of corrosion casts. *Arch Histol Cytol* 1988;51:299–313
3. Basset DL. The changes in the vascular pattern of the ovary of the albino rat during the estrous cycle. *Am J Anat* 1943;73:252–92
4. Brambell FWR. Ovarian changes. In Parkes AS, ed. *Marshall's Physiology of Reproduction*. London: Longmans and Green, 1956;1:397–542
5. Perrot-Applanat M, Groyer-Picard MT, Garcia E. Immunocytochemical demonstration of estrogen and progesterone receptors in muscle cells of uterine arteries in rabbits and humans. *Endocrinology* 1988;123:1511–19
6. Folkman J. Angiogenesis in cancer, vascular, rheumatoid and other disease. *Nature Med* 1995;1:27–31
7. Plate KH, Breier G, Weich HA, Rissau W. Vascular endothelial growth factor is a potential tumor angiogenesis factor in human gliomas *in vivo*. *Nature (London)* 1992;359:845–8
8. Kim KJ. Inhibiton of vascular endothelial growth factor-induced angiogenesis suppresses tumor growth *in vivo*. *Nature (London)* 1993;362:841–4
9. Millauer B, Shawver LK, Plate KH, Rissau W, Ullrich A. Glioblastoma growth inhibited *in vivo* by a dominant negative Flk-1 mutant. *Nature (London)* 1994;367:576–9
10. Millauer B, Longhi MP, Plate KH, et al. Dominant-negative inhibition of Flk-1 suppresses the growth of many tumor types *in vivo*. *Cancer J Res* 1996;56:1615–20
11. Folkman J, Long D, Becker F. Growth and metastasis of tumor in organ culture. *Tumor Res* 1963;16:453–67
12. Folkman J, Cole P, Zimmerman S. Tumor behavior in isolated perfused organs: *in vitro* growth and metastasis of biopsy material in rabbit thyroid and canine intestinal segment. *Ann Surg* 1966;164:491–502
13. Folkman J, Gimbrone M. Perfusion of the thyroid. *Acta Endocrinol* 1971;4:237–48
14. Folkman J. The intestine as an organ culture. In Burdette J, Thomas CC, eds. *Carcinoma of the Colon Antecedent Epithelium*. Springfield, IL: 1970:113–27
15. Hanahan D, Folkman J. Patterns and emerging mechanisms of the angiogenic switch during tumorigenesis. *Cell* 1996;86:353–64
16. Graeber TG, Osmanian C, Jacks T, et al. Hypoxia-mediated selection of cells with diminished apoptotic potential in solid tumors. *Nature (London)* 1996;379:88–91
17. Warren BA. The vascular morphology of tumors. In Peterson HI, ed. *Tumor Blood Circulation: Angiogenesis, Vascular Morphology and Blood Flow of Experimental Human Tumors*. Boca Raton, FL: CRC Press, 1979:1–47
18. Coman DR, Sheldon WF. The significance of hyperemia around tumor implants. *Am J Pathol* 1946;22:821–6
19. Algire GH, Chalkley HW, Lagallais FY, Park HD. Vascular reactions of mice to wounds and to normal and neoplastic transplants. *J Natl Cancer Inst* 1945;6:73–85
20. Day ED. Vascular relationships of tumor and host. *Prog Exp Tumor Res* 1946;4:57–9
21. Folkman J, Merler E, Abernathy C, Williams G. Isolation of a tumor factor responsible for angiogenesis. *J Exp Med* 1971;133:275–88
22. Klagsbrun M, D'Amore PA. Regulators of angiogenesis. *Annu Rev Physiol* 1991;53:217
23. Auerbach R. Angiogenesis-inducing factors: a review. In Pick E, ed. *Lymphokines*. London: Academic Press, 1981;4:69–88
24. Gimbrone MA Jr, Cotran RS, Folkman J. Endothelial regeneration and turn over. Studies with human endothelial cell cultures. *Serol Haematol* 1973;6:453–5
25. Gimbrone MA Jr, Leapman S, Cotran RS, Folkman J. Tumor dormancy *in vivo* by prevention of neovascularization. *J Exp Med* 1972;136:261–76
26. Gasparini G, Weidner N, Maluta S, et al. Intratumoral microvessel density and p53 correlation with metastasis in head-and-neck squamous-cell carcinoma. *Int J Cancer* 1993;55:739–44
27. Gasparini G, Weidner N, Bevilacqua P, et al. Tumor microvessel density, p53 expression, tumor size, and peritumoral lymphatic vessel invasion are relevant prognostic markers in node-negative breast carcinoma. *J Clin Oncol* 1994;12:454–66
28. Jaeger TM, Weidner N, Chew K, et al. Tumor angiogenesis correlates with lymph node metastases in invasive bladder cancer. *J Urol* 1995;154:69–71
29. Serrano M, Hannon GJ, Beach D. A new regulator motif in cell-cycle control causing specific inhibition of cyclin D/cdk4. *Nature (London)* 1993;366:704–7
30. Weinberg R. The retinoblastoma protein and cell control. *Cell* 1995;81:323–30
31. Sherr C, Roberts J. Inhibition of mammalian G1 cyclin-dependent kinases. *Genes Dev* 1995;9:1149–63
32. Hannon G, Beach D. p15[INK4b] is a potential effector of TGF-beta-induced cell cycle arrest. *Nature (London)* 1994;371:257–61
33. Hirai H, Roussel M, Kato J, Ashmun R, Sherr C. Novel INK4 proteins p19 and p18, are specific inhibitors of cyclin dependent kinases cdk4 and cdk6. *Mol Cell Biol* 1995;15:2672–81
34. Chan F, Zhang L, Chen L, Shapiro D, Winoto A. Identification of human mouse p19, a novel cdk4/cdk6 inhibitor with homology to p16[INK4a]. *Mol Cell Biol* 1995;15:2682–8
35. Hall M, Peters G. Genetic alterations of cyclins, cyclin-dependent kinases, and Cdk inhibitors in human cancers. *Adv Cancer Res* 1996;68:67–108

36. Ichimura K, Schmidt EE, Goike HM, Collins VP. Human glioblastomas with no alterations of the CDKN2A$^{(p16\ INK4/MTS1)}$ and CDK4 genes have frequent mutations of the retinoblastoma gene. *Oncogene* 1996;13:1065–72
37. Reed JA, Loganzo F, Shea CR. Loss of expression of the p 16/cyclin-dependent kinase inhibitor 2 of tumor suppressor gene in melanocytic lesions correlates with invasive stages of tumor progression. *Cancer Res* 1995;55:2713–18
38. Hupp T, Sparks A, Lane D. Small peptides activate the latent sequence-specific DNA-binding function of p53. *Cell* 1995;83:237–45
39. Bos JL. Ras oncogenes in human cancer: a review. *Cancer Res* 1989;49:4682–9
40. Lloyd AC. Ras versus cyclin-dependent kinase inhibitors. *Curr Opin Genet Dev* 1998;8:43–8
41. Folkman J, Klagsburn M. Angiogenic factors. *Science* 1987;235:442–7
42. Raud J. Vasodilatation and inhibition of mediator release represent two distinct mechanisms for prostaglandin modulation of acute mast cell dependent inflammation. *Br J Pharmacol* 1990;99:449–54
43. Jaffe BM. Prostaglandins and cancer. An update. *Prostaglandins* 1974;6:453–61
44. Alila HW, Corradino RA, Hansel W. A comparison of the effects of cyclooxygenase prostanoids on progesterone production of small and large bovine luteal cells. *Prostaglandins* 1988;36:259–70
45. Guilino PM. Extracellular compartments of solid tumors. In Becker J, ed. *Cancer*. New York: Plenum Press, 1975:327
46. Jain RK. Determination of tumor blood flow: a review. *Cancer Res* 1988;48:2641–6
47. Jain RK, Ward-Harley K. Tumor blood flow characterization, modifications and role in hyperthermia. *Trans Sonics Ultrasonics* 1984;31:504–9
48. Less JR, Skalak TC, Sevick EM, Jain RK. Microvascular architecture in a mammary carcinoma: branching patterns and vessel dimensions. *Cancer Res* 1991;51:262–73
49. Dvorak HF, Brown LF, Detmar M, Dvorak AM. Vascular permeability factor/vascular endothelial growth factor, microvascular hyperpermeability, and angiogenesis. *Am J Pathol* 1995;146:1029–39
50. Leedy DA, Trune DR, Kronz JD, Weidner N, Cohen JI. Tumor angiogenesis, the p53 antigen, and cervical metastasis in squamous carcinoma of the tongue. *Otolaryngol Head Neck Surg* 1994;111:417–22
51. Roychowdhury DF, Tseng A Jr, Fu KK, Weinburg V, Weidner N. New prognostic factors in nasopharyngeal carcinoma. Tumor angiogenesis and C-erbB2 expression. *Cancer* 1996;77:1419–26
52. Weidner N, Folkman J, Pozza F, *et al*. Tumor angiogenesis: a new significant and independent prognostic indicator in early stage breast carcinoma. *J Natl Cancer Inst* 1992;84:1875–87
53. Weidner N, Carroll PR, Flax J, Blumenfeld W, Folkman J. Tumor angiogenesis correlates with metastasis in invasive prostate carcinoma. *Am J Pathol* 1993;143:401–9
54. Weidner N. Tumor angiogenesis: review of current applications in tumor prognostication. *Semin Diagn Pathol* 1993;10:302–13
55. Weidner N, Gasparini G. Determination of epidermal growth factor receptor provides additional prognostic information to measuring tumor angiogenesis in breast carcinoma patients. *Breast Cancer Res Treat* 1994;29:97–107
56. Weidner N. Prognostic factors in breast carcinoma. *Curr Opin Obstet Gynecol* 1995;7:4–9
57. Weidner N, Folkman J. Tumoral vascularity as a prognostic factor in cancer. *Important Adv Oncol* 1996:167–90
58. Folkman J. What is the evidence that tumors are angiogenesis dependent? *J Natl Cancer Inst* 1989;82:4–6
59. Rak JW, St Croix DB, Kerbel RS. Consequences of angiogenesis for tumor progression, metastatis and cancer therapy. *Anti-Cancer Drugs* 1995;6:3–18
60. Skobe M, Rockwell P, Vosseler S, Fusenig NE. Halting angiogenesis suppresses carcinoma cell invasion. *Nature Med* 1997;3:1222–7
61. Weidner N. Intratumor microvessel density as a prognostic factor in cancer. *Am J Pathol* 1995;147:9–15
62. Liotta L, Kleinerman J, Saidel F. Quantitative relationships of intravascular tumor cells, tumor vessels, and pulmonary metastases following tumor implantation. *Cancer Res* 1974;34:997–1004
63. Hanahan D, Folkman J. Parameters and emerging mechanisms of the angiogenic switch during tumorigenesis. *Cell* 1996;86:353–4
64. Kurjak A, Kupesic S, Ilijas M, Sparac V, Kosuta D. Preoperative diagnosis of primary Fallopian tube carcinoma. *Gynecol Oncol* 1998;68:29–34
65. Kurjak A, Jukic S, Kupesic S, Babic D. A combined Doppler and morphopathological study of ovarian tumors. *Eur J Obstet Gynecol Reprod Biol* 1997;71:147–50
66. Emoto M, Iwasaki H, Mimura K, Kawarabayashi T, Kikuchi M. Differences in the angiogenesis of benign and malignant ovarian tumors, demonstrated by analyses of color Doppler ultrasound, immunohistochemistry, and microvessel density. *Cancer* 1997;80:899–907
67. Suren A, Osmers R, Kuhn W. 3D Color Power Angio™ imaging: a new method to assess intracervical vascularization in benign and pathological conditions. *Ultrasound Obstet Gynecol* 1998;2:133–8
68. Kupesic S, Kurjak A, Zodan T. Staging of the endometrial adenocarcinoma by three-dimensional power Doppler ultrasound. *Gynaecol Perinatol* 1999;8:1–7
69. Rubin JM, Bude RO, Carson PL, Bree RL, Adler RS. Power Doppler US: a potentially useful alternative to mean frequency-based color doppler US. *Radiology* 1994;190:853–6
70. Rubin JM, Adler RS, Fowlkes JB, *et al*. Fractional moving blood volume: estimation with power Doppler US. *Radiology* 1995;197:183–90
71. Meyerowith CB, Fleischer AC, Pickens DR, *et al*.

Quantification of tumor vascularity and flow with amplitude color Doppler sonography in an experimental model. *J Ultrasound Med* 1996;15:827–33
72. Chaoui R, Kalache K. Three-dimensional color power imaging: principles and first experience in prenatal diagnosis. In Merz E, ed. *3D Ultrasound in Obstetrics and Gynecology*. Philadelphia, PA: Lippincott Williams & Wilkins, 1998:135–41
73. Fleischer AC. Color Doppler sonography of benign and malignant adnexal masses: a spectrum of findings. In Kurjak A, Fleischer AC, eds. *Doppler Ultrasound in Gynecology*. Carnforth UK: Parthenon Publishing, 1989:27–36
74. Bude RO, Rubin JM, Adler RS. Power versus conventional color Doppler sonography in the depiction of normal intrarenal vasculature. *Radiology* 1994;192:777–80
75. Winsberg F. Power Doppler sonography. *J Ultrasound Med* 1996;15:164
76. Babcock DS, Patricuin H, LaFortune M, Dauzat M. Power Doppler sonography: basic principles and clinical applications in children. *Pediatr Radiol* 1996;26:109–15
77. Fortunato SJ. The use of power Doppler and color power angiography in fetal imaging. *Am J Obstet Gynecol* 1996;174:1828–33
78. Fox DB, Bruner JP, Fleischer AC. Amplitude-based color Doppler sonography of fetus with sacrococcygeal teratoma. *J Ultrasound Med* 1996;15:785–7
79. Pooh RK, Aono T. Transvaginal power Doppler angiography of the fetal brain. *Ultrasound Obstet Gynecol* 1996;8:417–21
80. Papadimitriou A, Kalogirou D, Antonio G, Petridis N, Kalogirou O. Power Doppler ultrasound: a potential useful alternative in diagnosing pelvic pathological conditions. *Clin Exp Obstet Gynecol* 1996;23:229–32
81. Downey DB, Fenster A. Vascular imaging with a three-dimensional power Doppler system. *Am J Roentgenol* 1995;165:665–8
82. Wagner S, Gebel M, Bleck JS, Magnus MP. Clinical application of three-dimensional sonography in hepatobiliary disease. *Bildgebung* 1994;61:104–9
83. Baba K, Satoh K, Sakamoto S, Okai T, Ishii S. Development of an ultrasonic system for three-dimensional reconstructions of the fetus. *J Perinat Med* 1989;17:19–24
84. Fine D, Perring S, Herbetko J, Hacking CN, Fleming JS, Dewburz KC. Three-dimensional (3D) ultrasound imaging of the gall-bladder and dilated biliary tree: reconstruction from real time B scans. *Br J Radiol* 1991;64:1956–7
85. Kelcz F, Pozniak MA, Pirsch JD, Oberly TD. Pyramidal appearance and RI: intensitive and non-specific sonographic indicators of renal transplant rejections. *Am J Roentgenol* 1990;155:531–5
86. Akiyama T, Ikegami M, Hara Y, *et al*. Hemodynamic study of renal transplant chronic rejection using power Doppler sonography. *Transplant Proc* 1996;28:1458–60
87. Martinoli C, Crespi G, Bertolotto M, *et al*. Interlobular vasculature in renal transplants: a power Doppler US study with MR correlation. *Radiology* 1996;200:111–17
88. Robb RA. *Three-dimensional Biomedical Imaging: Principles and Practice*. New York: VCH Publishers, 1995
89. Rankin RN, Fenster A, Downey DB, Munk PL, Levin MF, Vellet AD. Three-dimensional sonographic reconstruction: techniques and diagnostic applications. *Am J Roentgenol* 1993;161:695–702
90. Tong S, Downey DB, Cardinal HN, Fenster A. A three-dimensional ultrasound prostate imaging system. *Ultrasound Med Biol* 1996;22:735–46
91. Guo Z, Fenster A. Three-dimensional power Doppler imaging: a phantom study to quantify vessel stenosis. *Ultrasound Med Biol* 1996;22:1059–69
92. Kratochwil A. *Ultraschalldiagnostik in Geburtshilfe und Gynaekologie*. Stuttgart: Georg Thieme Verlag, 1986:84
93. Buy JN, Ghossain MA, Hugol D, *et al*. Characterization of adnexal masses: combination of color Doppler and conventional sonography compared with spectral Doppler analysis alone and conventional sonography alone. *Am J Roentgenol* 1998;166:385–94
94. Woolf SH, Battista RN, Anderson GM, Logan AG, Wang E. Force on the Periodic Health Examinations: assessing the clinical effectiveness of preventive maneuvers: analytic principles and systematic methods in reviewing evidence and developing clinical practice recommendations. *J Clin Epidemiol* 1990;43:891–905
95. Parkes C, Wald NJ. Screening for ovarian cancer. In Kurjak A, ed. *An Atlas of Transvaginal Color Doppler*. Carnforth, UK: Parthenon Publishing, 1994:317–28
96. May R. Biological populations with non-overlapping generations: stable points, stable cycles and chaos. *Science* 1974;186:645–7
97. Mandelbrot B. *Fractals: Form, Chance and Dimension*. New York: WH Freeman, 1977
98. Breyer B, Kurjak A. Tumor vascularization Doppler measurements and chaos: what to do? *Ultrasound Obstet Gynecol* 1995;5:209
99. Hollingworth H, Kohn E, Steinberg S, Rothenberg ML, Merino MJ. Tumor angiogenesis in advanced stage ovarian carcinoma. *Am J Pathol* 1995;147:33–41
100. Kirschmer CV, Alamis-Amezcus JM, Martin VG, *et al*. Angiogenesis factor in endometrial carcinoma: a new prognostic indicator? *Am J Obstet Gynecol* 1996;174:1879–84
101. Schoenfeld A, Levavi H, Tepper R, Breslavski D, Amir R, Ovadia J. Assessment of tumor induced angiogenesis by three dimensional display: confusing Doppler signals in ovarian cancer screening? *Ultrasound Obstet Gynecol* 1994;4:516–18
102. Kurjak A, Shalan H, Kupesic S, *et al*. Transvaginal color Doppler sonography in the assessment of pelvic tumor vascularity. *Ultrasound Obstet Gynecol* 1993;3:137–54
103. Breyer B, Ferek-Petric B, Cikes I. Properties of ultrasonically marked leads. *PACE* 1989;12:1369–80
104. Nissen SE, Gurley JC. Application of intravascular ultrasound for detection and quantitation of coronary

atherosclerosis. *Int J Cardiac Imaging* 1991;6:165–7
105. Pairleitner H. Three-dimensional color histogram using three-dimensional power Doppler. In Kurjak A, ed. *Three-dimensional Power Doppler in Obstetrics and Gynecology*. Carnforth, UK: Parthenon Publishing, 1999:35–9
106. Pairleitner H, Steiner H, Hasenoehrl G, Staudach A. Three-dimensional power Doppler sonography: imaging and quantifying blood flow and vascularization. *J Ultrasound Obstet Gynecol* 1999;14:139–43
107. Fleischer AC, Pairleitner H. 3D tranvaginal Doppler assesses ovarian flow. *Diagn Imaging* 1999;9:47
108. Fleischer AC, Pairleitner H. 3D transvaginal color Doppler sonography: current and potential applications. *Med Imaging Int* 1999;9:10–13
109. Cameron JR, Warren, SE, Laurence AM, Dale RC, Yongmin K. Three-dimensional ultrasonic angiography using power-mode Doppler. *Ultrasound Med Biol* 1996;3:277–86
110. Kurjak A, Schulman H, Predanic M. Pelvic tumor neovascularity. In Kurjak A, ed. *An Atlas of Transvaginal Color Doppler: Current State of the Art*, 2nd edn. Carnforth, UK: Parthenon Publishing, 1993:231–46
111. Hsieh FJ, Wu CC, Lee CN, *et al*. Vascular pattern of gestational trophoblastic tumors by color Doppler ultrasound. *Cancer* 1994;74:2361–5
112. Hsieh FJ, Liu CH, Chang FM, *et al*. Ultrasonography in the diagnosis and management of invasive gestational trophoblastic disease. *J Formosa Med Assoc* 1988;87:139–45
113. Boehm T, Folkman J, Browder T, O'Reilly MS. Antiangiogenic therapy of experimental cancer does not induce acquired drug resistance. *Nature* (*London*) 1997;390:404–7
114. Kerbel RS. Inhibition of tumor angiogenesis as a strategy to circumvent acquired resistance to anticancer therapeutic agents. *BioEssays* 1991;13:31–6
115. Holmgren L, O'Reilly MS, Folkman J. Dormancy of micrometastases: balanced proliferation and apoptosis in the presence of angiogenesis suppression. *Nature Med* 1995;1:149–53

Ovarian lesions assessed by three-dimensional and power Doppler ultrasound

A. Kurjak and S. Kupesic

Transvaginal ultrasonographic characterization of ovarian lesions by gray-scale imaging proved to be feasible[1,2]. By using different scoring systems based on visualization of the inner wall irregularities, the wall thickness, the presence of thick septations or solid components, evaluation of the echogenicity of the lesion and analysis of the distal shadowing, identification of the ovarian malignancy became more accurate[3,4] (Figure 1). The introduction of color-coded flow studies represents another diagnostic modality that, if added to morphological gray-scale evaluation of ovarian lesions, may improve our capability of diagnosing ovarian malignancy[5] (Figure 2). Color Doppler examination of flow velocity and the resistance to blood flow allows identification of fast-growing tumoral capillaries. Since these newly formed vessels are devoid of the muscular layer, the downstream resistance measured by color flow determinations such as

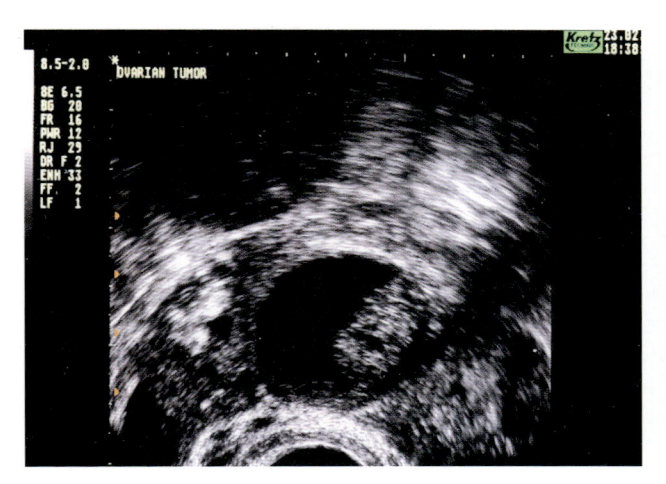

Figure 1 Transvaginal scan of a cystic–solid ovarian tumor measuring 3 cm. Note the papillary protrusion on the right side of the tumor

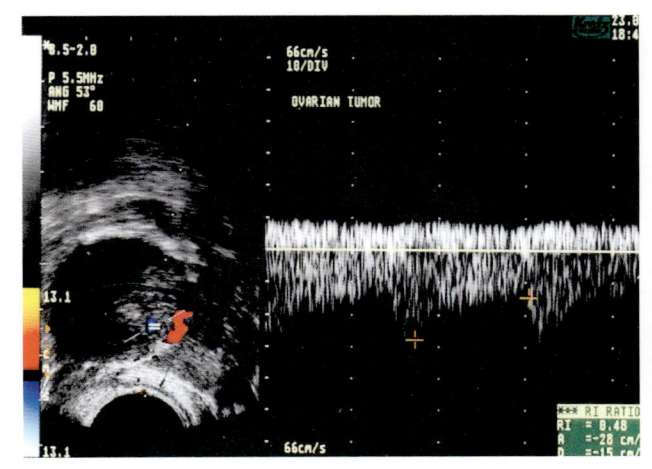

Figure 2 Pulsed Doppler sonogram (right) from the vessels displaced at the base of the papillary protrusion in Figure 1, demonstrating moderate vascular resistance (RI = 0.48)

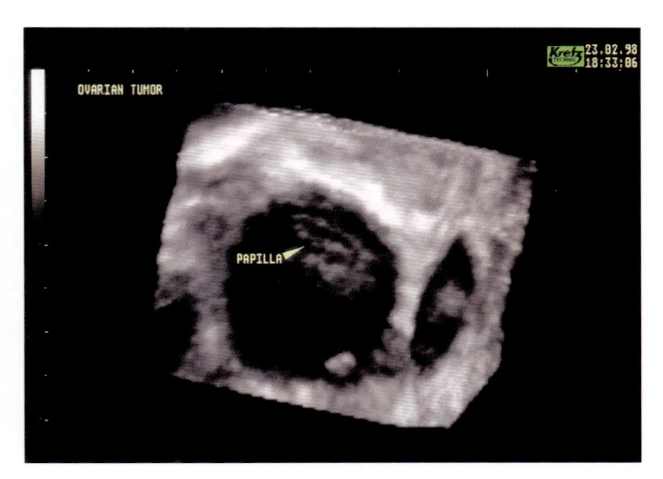

Figure 3 Three-dimensional scan of the same patient as in Figures 1 and 2. The papillary projection protruding into the cystic cavity is clearly demonstrated

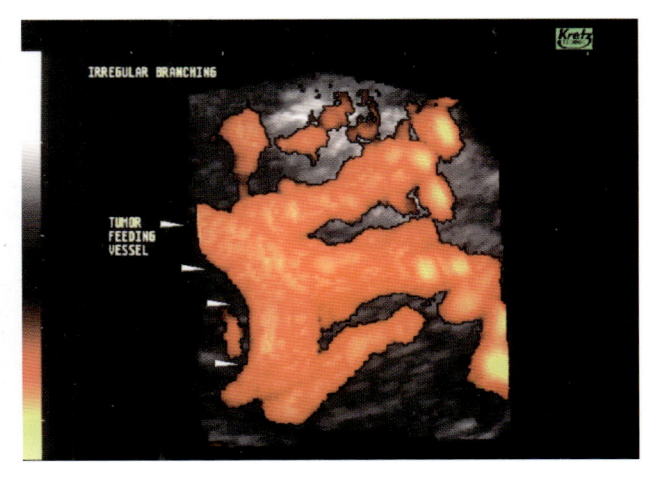

Figure 4 Numerous randomly dispersed vessels are shown within the papilla in Figures 1–3, by three-dimensional power Doppler imaging. This feature is suggestive of ovarian malignancy, which was confirmed by histopathology

resistance (RI) and pulsatility index (PI) is low and can be potentially used to predict ovarian malignancy.

Three-dimensional (3D) ultrasound is a new, emerging technology that provides additional information for the evaluation of ovarian tumors. Multiplanar and volume-rendering display methods combined with the ability to rotate volume data into standard orientations are essential components of the current and future success of 3D ultrasound[7] (Figure 3).

Increasing knowledge about 3D ultrasound, as well as improved handling, allow application of this method to the field of gynecological oncology. The recent development of real-time 3D ultrasound imaging will further advance the clinical applications, particularly in the assessment of pelvic tumors. The introduction of the 3D power Doppler systems may improve the information available on ovarian tumor vascularity and speed up the entire patient management process[8,9] (Figure 4).

In this chapter we discuss the advantages of 3D and power Doppler ultrasound in the assessment of ovarian lesions.

Own results on characterization of ovarian lesions

Our group recently performed a study on 120 ovarian masses prospectively evaluated by both transvaginal color Doppler ultrasound and 3D ultrasound with power Doppler facilities[10].

Seventy-six of the women studied were premenopausal (mean age 34, with a range between 18 and 48 years). Seven women were perimenopausal (mean age 49, with a range between 47 and 54 years). The remaining 37 women were postmenopausal (mean age 61, with a range between 50 and 77 years).

An experienced sonographer used B-mode transvaginal sonography to evaluate the morphology of both adnexal regions. The two-dimensional (2D) sonographic parameters used for distinguishing between benign and malignant ovarian lesions were wall structure, shadowing, septa, solid parts, echogenicity and the presence of peritoneal fluid.

B mode was used to evaluate the morphology of both adnexal regions, while color flow imaging was superimposed to detect vascularized areas. Pulsed repetition frequencies used in Doppler studies ranged from 2 to 42 kHz. The spatial peak temporal average range intensity was approximately 80 mW/cm. Wall filters (50 Hz) were used to eliminate low-frequency signals occurring from noise. Finally, pulsed Doppler was used to analyze blood velocity in the area of interest and the Pourcelot resistance index (RI) was used as the calculation measurement of the flow velocity waveform (systole minus diastole divided by systole). In order to reduce false positives caused by increased vascularity of the corpus luteum and/or follicular structure, all examinations in the premenopausal patients were performed during the early proliferative phase of the menstrual cycle.

Sonographic criteria used for diagnosing ovarian malignancy were based on the scoring system listed in Table 1. A score of 5 or greater was associated with a high risk for adnexal malignancy.

Three-dimensional studies of the adnexa were performed using a B-mode scanner that monitors the spatial orientation of the images and stores these as a volume set in the memory of the computer (Voluson 530,

Table 1 Two-dimensional sonographic and color Doppler criteria for diagnosis of ovarian malignancy. From reference 10, with permission

	Criteria	*Score*
Wall structure	smooth/irregularities ≤ 3 mm	0
	papillarities > 3 mm	2
Shadowing	present	0
	absent	1
Septa	none/thin ≤ 3 mm	0
	thick > 3 mm	1
Solid parts	absent	0
	present	2
Echogenicity	sonolucent/low-level echo	0
	mixed or high	2
Peritoneal fluid	absent	0
	present	1
Tumoral blood flow	RI > 0.42	0
	RI ≤ 0.42	2
Total score		

Total score is the sum of individual scores. The cut-off score, ≥ 5, is associated with a high risk for ovarian malignancy

Kretztechnik, Austria). Once the region of interest had been identified, the volume box was superimposed, the ultrasound probe was kept steady and the patient was asked to lie still on the examination bed. The volume mode was switched on, and the 3D ultrasound volume was generated by the automatic rotation of the mechanical transducer through 360°. The acquisition time ranged between 2 and 11 s, depending on the size of the volume box. Three perpendicular planes were displayed simultaneously, thus enabling better understanding of the morphology of the ovarian lesion. Evaluation of the stored volumes took between 15 and 25 min, depending on the number of slices, rotation angle and rendering modes used. Since the number and orientation of reformatted planes are not limited, meticulous evaluation of numerous sections through the tumor becomes possible. From the stored image, in each case we obtained a plastic image of the ovarian mass as well as surface rendering. The surface rendering mode allowed exploration of the outer wall surface of the tumor, while in patients with a certain amount of free fluid we were able to evaluate the relationship with surrounding structures. The niche aspect enabled detection and analysis of the selected sections of ovarian lesions such as papillary projections, septa and solid parts. Application of the 'transparent maximum–minimum' mode enabled visualization of the intratumoral calcification or identification of the bone structures in dermoid tumors. At the end of each examination, the combined angiographic and rendering mode was used, allowing simultaneous analysis of the morphology, texture and vascularization.

Comprehensive 3D display allowed interactive analysis of the architecture of the tumor microcirculation: irregular and randomly dispersed vessels with complex branching were suggestive of ovarian malignancy. We postulated that tumoral blood vessel trees do not follow the geometry of the normal pre-existing vasculature with ever-smaller branches and diameters. Tumoral blood vessels branch with chaotic outcome, which has nothing to do with regular geometry. Three-dimensional power Doppler projections highlight the tumor-feeding vessels and multiple tortuous intralesional vessels of varying caliber with abnormal branching patterns. Morphological criteria analyzed by 3D ultrasound for diagnosing ovarian malignancy are listed in Table 2. Six morphological criteria (wall structure, shadowing, septa, solid parts, echogenicity and peritoneal fluid) were involved in both 2D and 3D ultrasound scoring systems. A total score of 7 or greater was associated with a high risk for ovarian malignancy.

All cases were operated on by the same surgical team (laparotomy or laparoscopy) and histopathological diagnosis was considered final. Malignant tumors were classified according to the International Federation of Gynecology and Obstetrics (FIGO) system. The study protocol was approved by the hospital's ethics committee, and all patients consented to participate in the study.

Table 2 Three-dimensional sonographic and power Doppler criteria for diagnosis of ovarian malignancy. From reference 10, with permission

	Criteria	*Score*
Wall structure	smooth/irregularities ≤ 3 mm	0
	papillarities	2
Shadowing	present	0
	absent	1
Septa	none/thin ≤ 3 mm	0
	thick > 3 mm	1
Solid parts	absent	0
	present	2
Echogenicity	sonolucent/low-level echo	0
	mixed or high	2
Peritoneal fluid	absent	0
	present	1
Surface	regular	0
	irregular	2
Relationship with surrounding structures	normal	0
	disturbed	2
Vessels' architecture	linear vessel arrangement	0
	chaotic vessel arrangement	2
Branching pattern	simple	0
	complex	2
Total score		

Total score is the sum of individual scores. The cut-off score, ≥ 7, is associated with a high risk for ovarian malignancy

CLINICAL APPLICATION OF 3D SONOGRAPHY

A total of 109 patients had benign ovarian conditions (Table 3; Figures 5 and 6). The most common ovarian lesions in premenopausal patients were ovarian endometrioma (35/76) (Figures 7, 8 and 9) and dermoid cysts (26/76) (Figures 10, 11, 12 and 13), while the most common ovarian tumor during the postmenopausal period was serous cystadenoma (28/37). The most common ovarian malignancy was serous cystadenocarcinoma (Figure 14) detected in six postmenopausal patients (6/37), one perimenopausal

Table 3 Histopathological diagnoses of ovarian lesions (n = 120). From reference 10, with permission

	Number
Benign ovarian lesions (n = 109)	
Simple ovarian cyst	2
Dermoid cyst	26
Serous cystadenoma	30
Mucinous cystadenoma	9
Endometrioma	36
Fibroma	5
Cystadenofibroma	1
Malignant ovarian tumors (n = 11)	
Serous cystadenocarcinoma	8
Mucinous cystadenocarcinoma	3

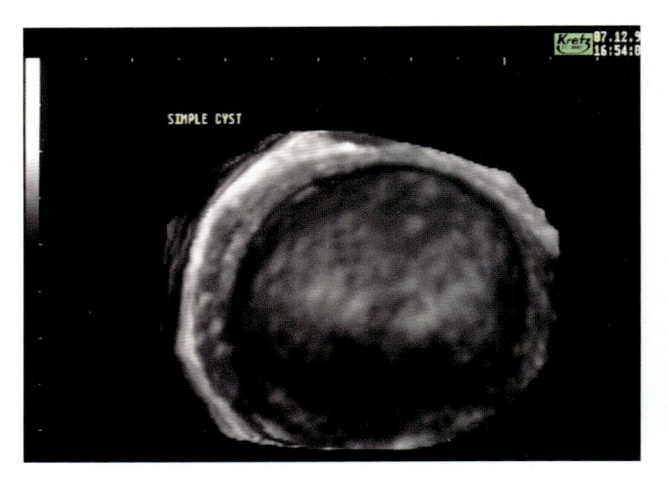

Figure 5 Three-dimensional scan of an ovarian cyst. Note the regular walls of the cyst, typical of a benign lesion

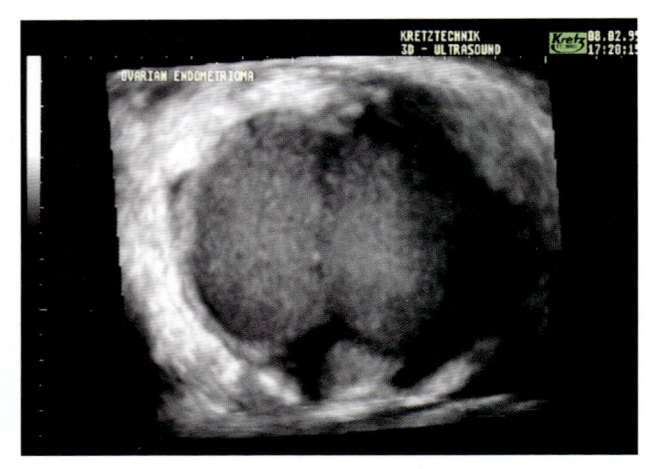

Figure 7 Three-dimensional scan of an ovarian endometrioma. Homogeneous high-level internal echoes are clearly visualized by this technique

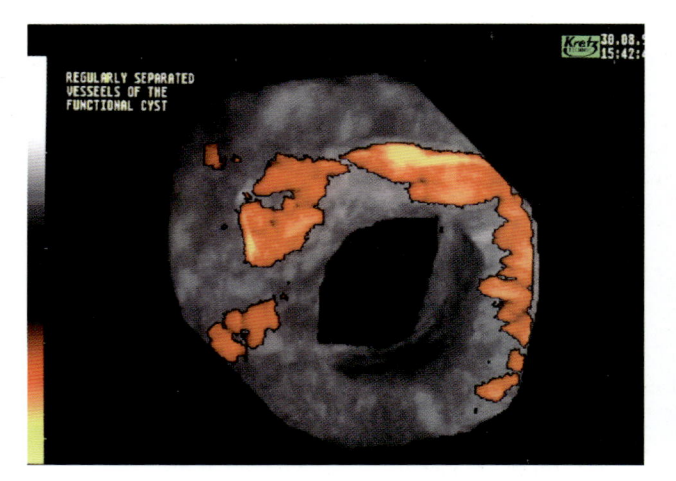

Figure 6 Three-dimensional power Doppler image of an ovarian cyst and pericystic blood flow

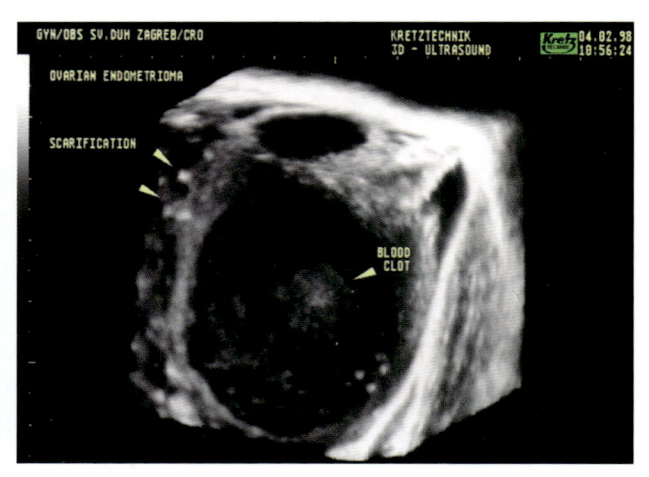

Figure 8 Three-dimensional scan of an ovarian endometrioma. Note some blood clots within the 'chocolate' paste-like fluid and regular echogenicities at the periphery, indicative of scarification

ASSESSMENT OF OVARIAN LESIONS

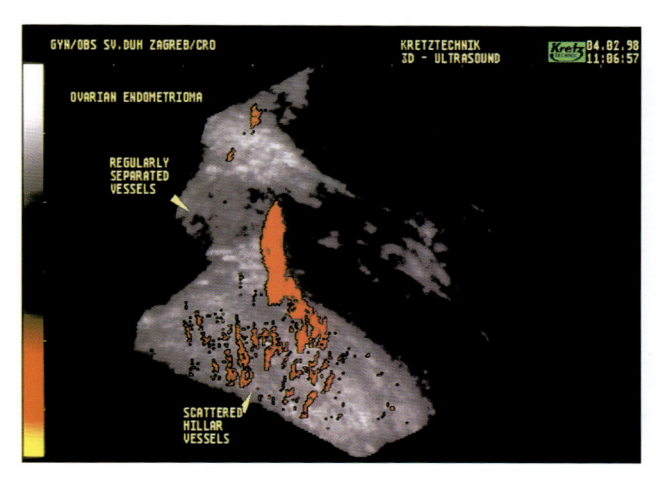

Figure 9 The same patient as in Figure 8. Note the scattered vascularity at the level of the ovarian hilus and the regularly separated peripheral vessels. Both vascular features are typical of an ovarian endometrioma and are easily depicted by power Doppler three-dimensional imaging

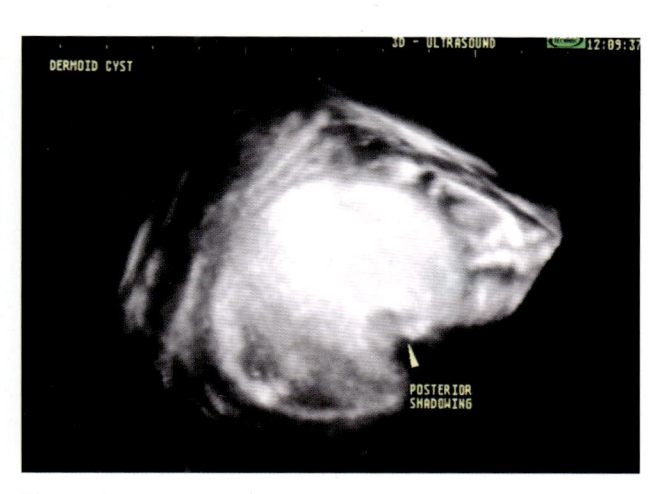

Figure 12 Three-dimensional image of a dermoid cyst. Note the posterior shadowing due to the presence of bone structures

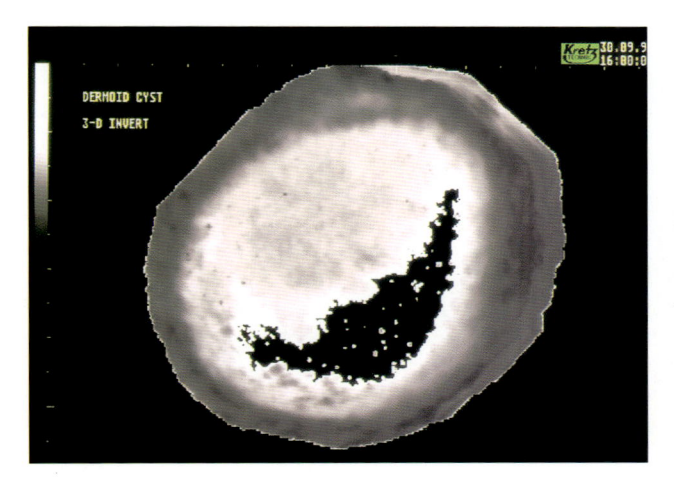

Figure 10 Three-dimensional scan of a bizarre ovarian tumor containing echogenic fluid and intracystic echoes

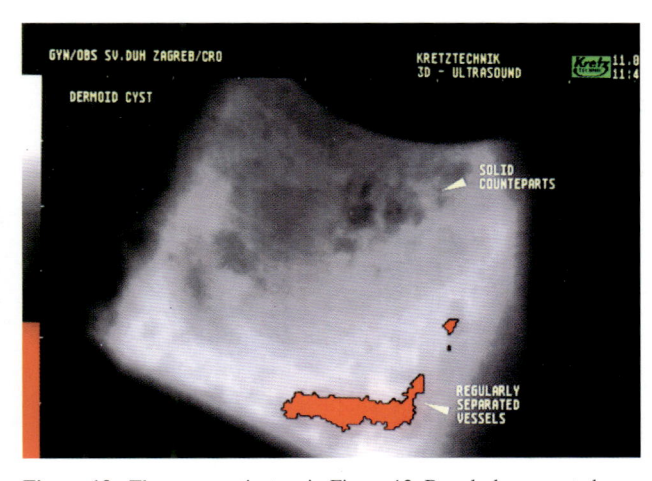

Figure 13 The same patient as in Figure 12. Regularly separated vessels are detected at the periphery of the dermoid cyst by three-dimensional power Doppler imaging

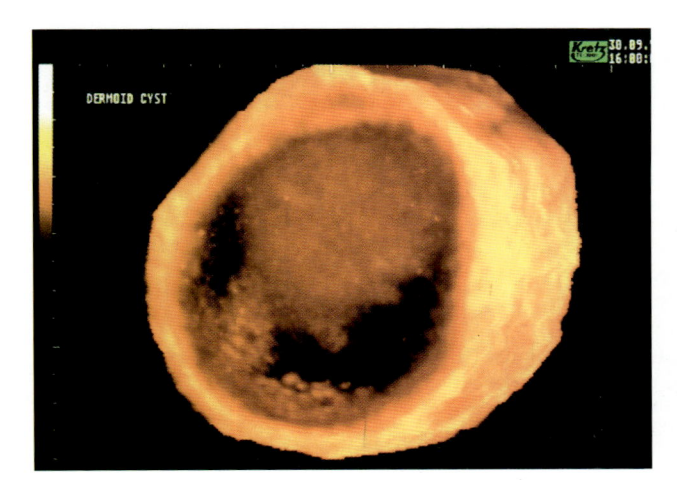

Figure 11 The same tumor as in Figure 10. The hyperechoic solid part and speckled appearance of the sebaceous contents are seen with the use of the minimum–maximum mode. A dermoid cyst was confirmed by histopathology

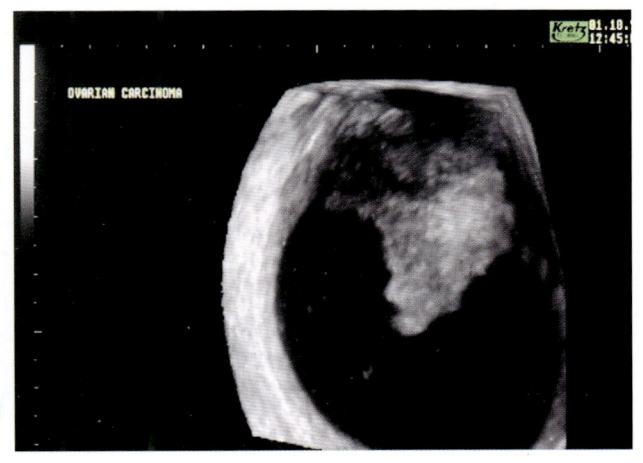

Figure 14 Three-dimensional view of a cystic–solid ovarian tumor. Papillary projections protruding into the cystic cavity indicate ovarian malignancy. Serous cystadenocarcinoma was confirmed by histopathology

27

patient (1/7) and one premenopausal patient (1/76). Mucinous cystadenocarcinoma was diagnosed in three postmenopausal patients (3/37).

Transvaginal color Doppler accurately predicted ten cases of ovarian malignancy (10/11), while all cases of ovarian malignancy were correctly diagnosed with 3D power Doppler (11/11). A case of serous cystadenocarcinoma in a 38-year-old patient measured only 3 cm and was missed by 2D transvaginal color Doppler (Figures 1 and 2), but was successfully identified by 3D power Doppler ultrasound (Figure 4). Transvaginal sonography did not demonstrate small papillary projections (< 5 mm in maximum diameter) extending the cystic wall. Although pulsed Doppler waveform analysis demonstrated peripheral vascularity, RI values were above the cut-off value proposed for the diagnosis of ovarian malignancy and measured 0.48. Three-dimensional ultrasound clearly depicted papillary protrusions and power Doppler enabled detection of tiny irregular vessels within the papillary protrusion.

By performing 2D transvaginal color Doppler, three benign ovarian lesions were wrongly interpreted as malignant: one was a dermoid cyst, one an ovarian fibroma and one an ovarian cystadenofibroma. The last lesion was the only false-positive finding by 3D power Doppler ultrasound (Figure 15).

The dermoid cyst contained a heterogeneous solid core at the periphery and irregular inner contents. Additionally, peripheral vessels with low vascular resistance (RI = 0.42) and a certain amount of peritoneal fluid raised the suspicion of ovarian malignancy. Three-dimensional transparent maximum–minimum mode revealed high echogenicity within the tumor typical for the presence of bone and teeth (Figure 12), while power Doppler showed a linear appearance and regular branching of the peripheral vessels indicative of a benign lesion (Figure 13).

The ovarian fibroma was a predominantly solid tumor with mixed echogenicity. The presence of peritoneal fluid and low vascular resistance in both central (RI = 0.39) and peripheral vessels (RI = 0.42) was associated with a high risk of ovarian malignancy.

Three-dimensional ultrasound allowed detection of the regular tumoral surface and normal relationship with surrounding pelvic structures. Demonstration of the linear vessels throughout the mass using multiplanar images, together with recognition of the regular type of branching, guided the ultrasonographer performing 3D ultrasound to an accurate diagnosis of a benign adnexal mass.

The cystadenofibroma presented as a complex solid–cystic mass of mixed echogenicity with thick septa. Low vascular resistance obtained from solid (RI = 0.36) and septal areas (RI = 0.39) incorrectly indicated ovarian malignancy. Three-dimensional transparent maximum–minimum mode for reconstruction clearly depicted thick septa and mixed echogenicity of the solid part. Although the regular surface of the tumor and undisturbed anatomic relationships were suggestive of benign ovarian pathology, power Doppler provided clues to the malignant vessels' architecture: chaotic vessels with irregular branching and disproportional calibration of the vessels. This was the only false-positive finding of 3D power Doppler in our study (Figure 15).

The sensitivity, specificity and positive and negative predictive values of transvaginal color and pulsed Doppler, as well as 3D static and power Doppler, are listed in Table 4.

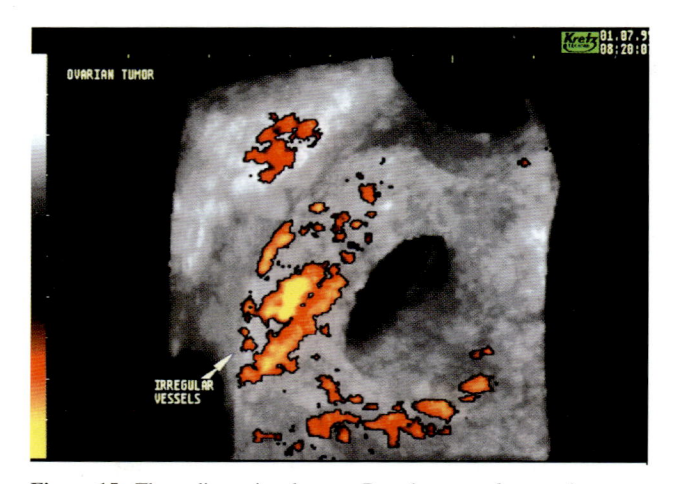

Figure 15 Three-dimensional power Doppler scan of a complex ovarian lesion. Thick septa, mixed echogenicity of the solid part and chaotic vessels with dichotomous branching indicated ovarian malignancy. Histopathology revealed ovarian cystadenofibroma, and this was the only false-positive finding of three-dimensional power Doppler in our study

Table 4 Sensitivity, specificity, positive predictive value (PPV) and negative predictive value (NPV) of two-dimensional (2D) transvaginal color Doppler and three-dimensional (3D) static and power Doppler ultrasound in detection of ovarian malignancy. From reference 10, with permission

	Sensitivity (%)	Specificity (%)	PPV (%)	NPV (%)
2D transvaginal color Doppler	90.90	97.25	76.92	99.06
3D power Doppler	100	99.08	91.67	100

Advantages of three-dimensional power Doppler ultrasound

Sonomorphological evaluation of ovarian tumors using parameters such as the presence of papillary protrusions, solid parts, thick septa and high echogenic reflection patterns is useful in assessing the risk of ovarian malignancy[3]. Our results indicate that 3D ultrasound scanning, by meticulous investigation of the ovarian lesion, reduces false-positive findings (Figures 16, 17 and 18). This technique is especially useful in the evaluation of complex ovarian lesions (such as ovarian dermoids, endometriomas, fibromas and corpus luteum cysts), which may give a wrong impression of malignancy when using conventional transvaginal sonography and color Doppler ultrasound (Figures 19 and 20). We detected a significant reduction in the rate of false-positive findings between 2D

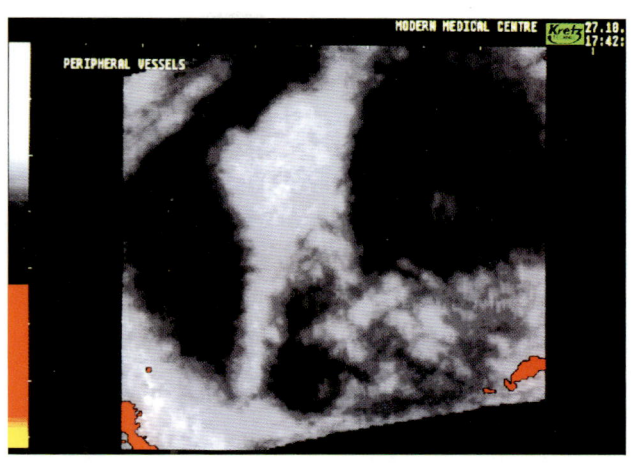

Figure 18 The same patient as in Figures 16 and 17. Regularly separated peripheral vessels and absence of intratumoral flow indicated a benign lesion. Serous cystadenoma was confirmed by histopathology

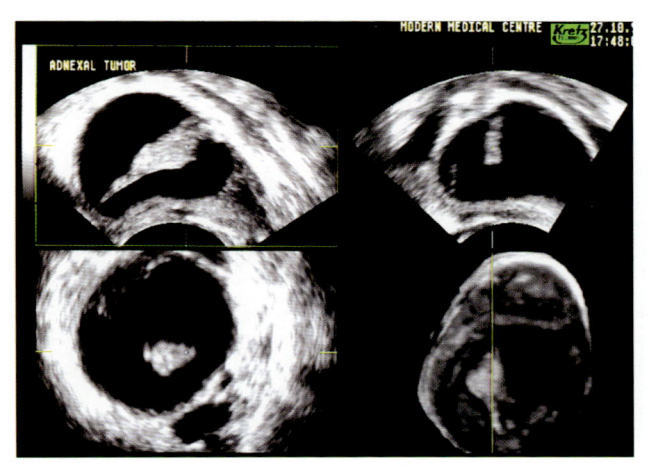

Figure 16 Simultaneous rendering of all three orthogonal sectional planes, demonstrating a complex adnexal tumor. Note the three-dimensional surface view of the same tumor (lower right)

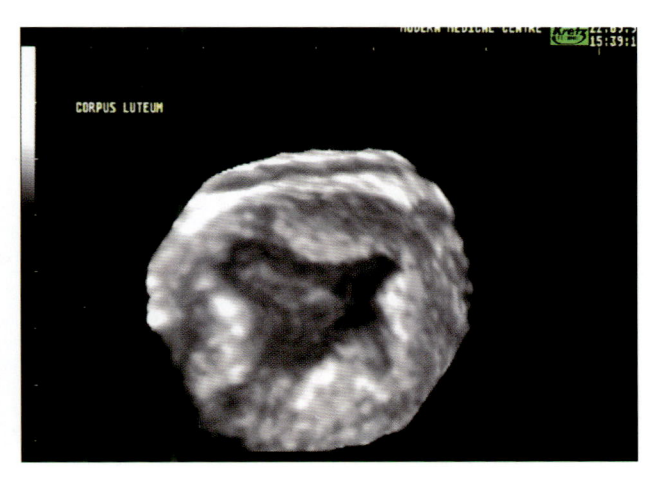

Figure 19 Three-dimensional scan of a corpus luteum. Note the blood-filled cavity of the ruptured follicle and the echogenic clots

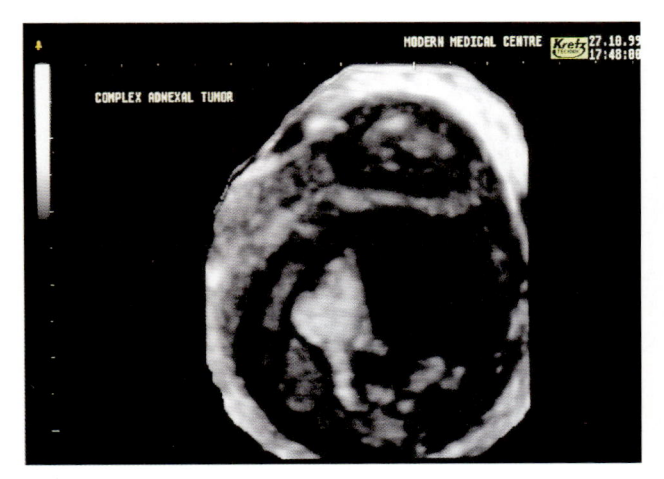

Figure 17 Three-dimensional surface view of an irregular wall proliferation in a cystic ovarian tumor

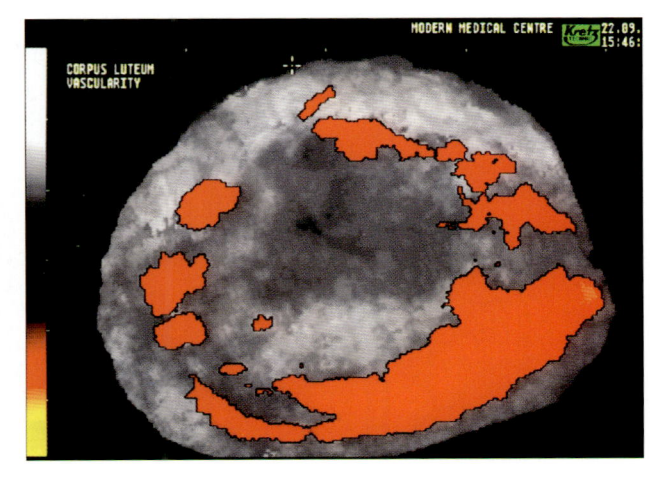

Figure 20 The same patient as in Figure 19. The power Doppler image depicts capillaries penetrating the cystic cavity. Note the regular arrangement of the vessels located pericystically. Blood clots are displayed as heterogeneous avascularized areas within the corpus luteum

transvaginal color Doppler and 3D power Doppler in our study: 76.92% vs. 91.67%[10]. However, we are aware of the small numbers included in our study, which limit the applicability of the sensitivity, specificity and positive and negative predictive values.

Obvious advantages of 3D ultrasound are improved recognition of the anatomy of ovarian lesions, accurate characterization of surface features, determination of the extent of tumor infiltration through the capsule and clear depiction of the size and volume of the mass (Figures 21 and 22). Shortened scanning time and detailed analysis of the stored data by an experienced ultrasonographer allow detection of small lesions that may even be missed during the initial scan by 2D and 3D imaging[7]. Although the first six characteristics were identical in both 2D and 3D scoring systems, 3D ultrasound appears to be better in evaluation of the architecture of tumors. In our study, 3D transvaginal ultrasound demonstrated papillary projections extending from the cystic wall in an ovarian lesion measuring 3 cm which were not demonstrated by conventional transvaginal sonography[10] (Figures 23 and 24). Multiple sections of the tumor, rotation, translation and reconstruction of 3D plastic images allowed more precise evaluation of the tumor without increasing the scanning time or patients' discomfort.

Color Doppler sonography is capable of supplying useful additional information in tumors with solid parts and in those with simple morphology assessed by ultrasound[11]. However, this supplementary information is of limited value, since there are no generally accepted cut-off values for the RI or PI or flow velocity[12]. Differences in operator variance and system sensitivity contribute to an already confusing analysis of variables. Overlap in blood flow parameters between benign and malignant ovarian tumors is another element of the current debate regarding attempts to achieve accurate differentiation of ovarian tumors on

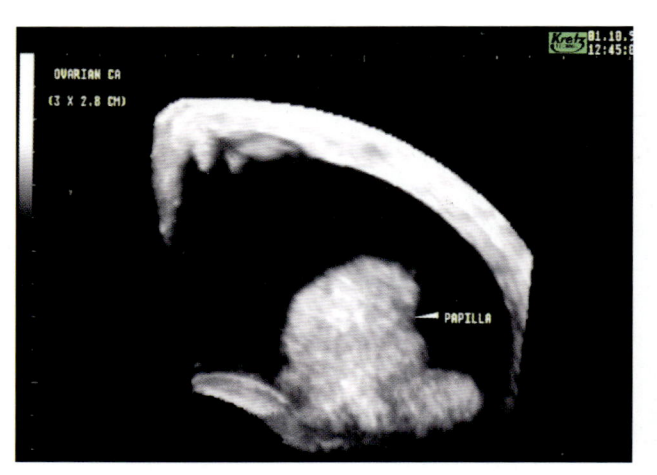

Figure 21 Three-dimensional scan of a complex ovarian tumor. A papillary projection protruding into the cystic cavity is clearly demonstrated

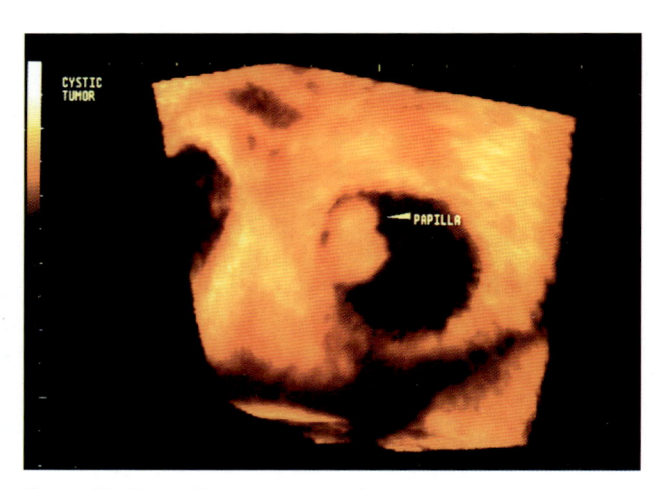

Figure 23 Three-dimensional scan of an early stage of ovarian carcinoma. Note the papillary projection on the left side of the lesion

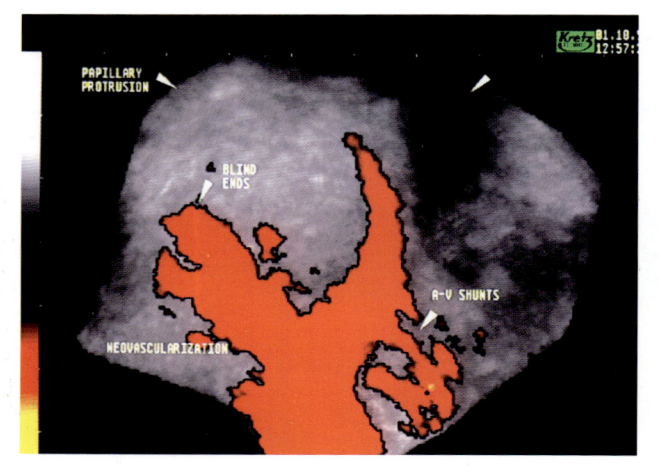

Figure 22 Numerous randomly dispersed vessels within the papilla indicate the malignant nature of an ovarian tumor. Ovarian adenocarcinoma was confirmed by histopathology

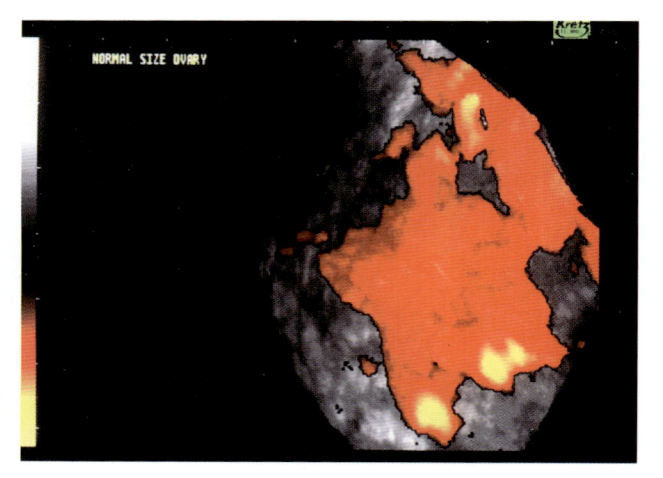

Figure 24 The same patient as in Figure 23. Three-dimensional power Doppler imaging visualizes the tumoral vessels with irregular course and complicated branching. Ovarian cystadenocarcinoma was confirmed by histopathology

the basis of their vascular characteristics. Further development of technology and the introduction of 3D power Doppler may improve our ability to differentiate between benign and malignant neoplasms, predict tumor prognosis and determine treatment options[13].

Difficulties and outlook for further developments

Currently, the application of this modality in the evaluation of neoplasms is mainly qualitative or semi-quantitative (for example, for the determination of whether the vascularity is present or not)[14] (Figures 25–29). Power Doppler imaging at this stage can accurately detect characteristic structural abnormalities of malignant tumor vessels such as microaneurysms, arteriovenous shunts, tumoral lakes, disproportional calibration, elongation, coiling and dichotomous branching[15] (Figure 30). Arteriovenous shunts, which are pathognomonic for ovarian malignancy, can be initially diagnosed by pulsed Doppler

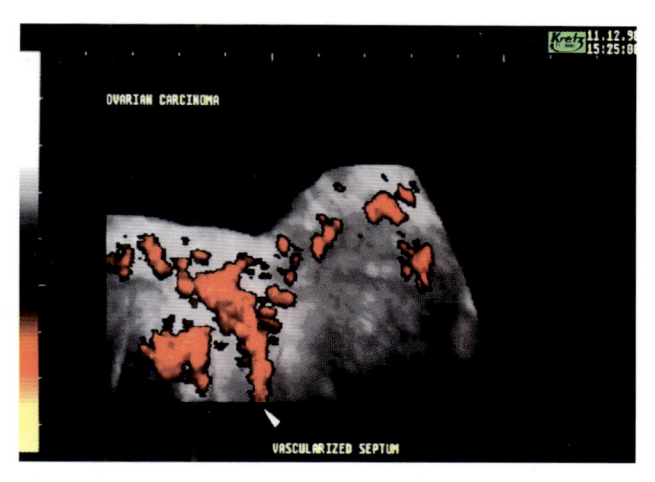

Figure 27 Another case of ovarian carcinoma. Note the irregular, thorn-like vessels in septal areas of the malignant ovarian tumor

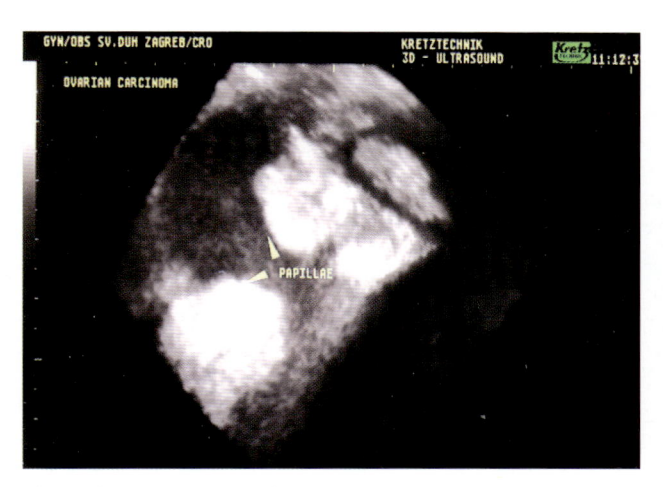

Figure 25 Complex ovarian tumor as seen by three-dimensional ultrasound. Surface view revealed irregular wall proliferations suggestive of ovarian malignancy

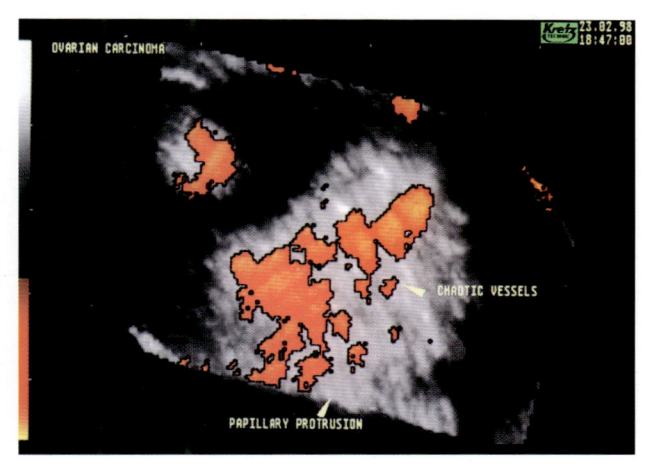

Figure 28 Three-dimensional power Doppler scan of malignant tumor vessels located in a papillary projection. Note their irregular course and branching

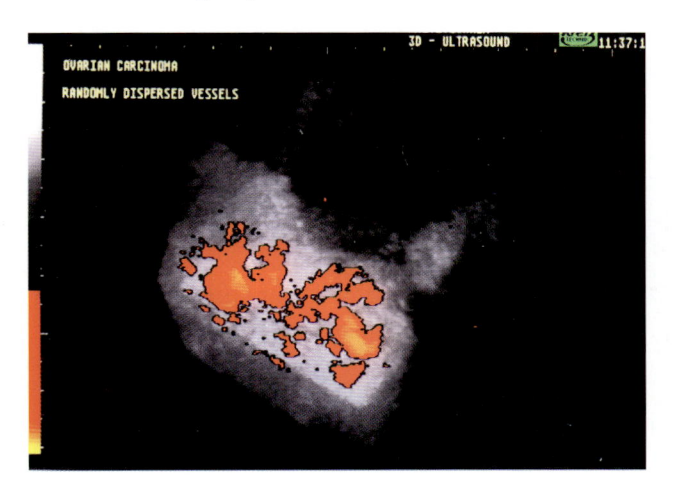

Figure 26 The same patient as in Figure 25. Randomly dispersed vessels with dichotomous branching are clearly illustrated by three-dimensional power Doppler ultrasound

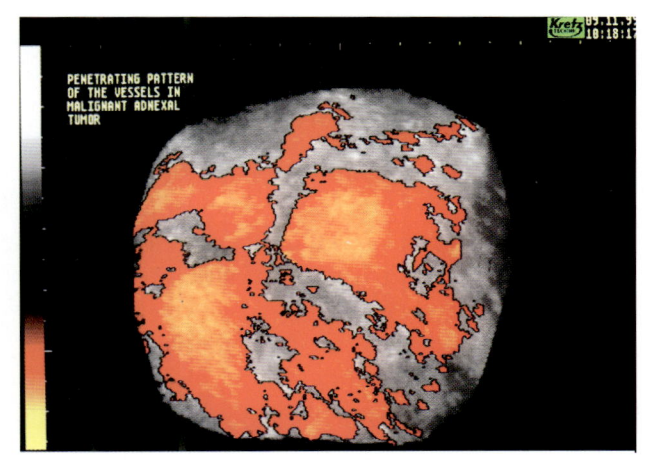

Figure 29 Three-dimensional power Doppler scan of a solid ovarian tumor. The penetrating pattern of the vessels, areas of arteriovenous shunts, microaneurysms and tumoral lakes are clearly illustrated and suggest ovarian malignancy

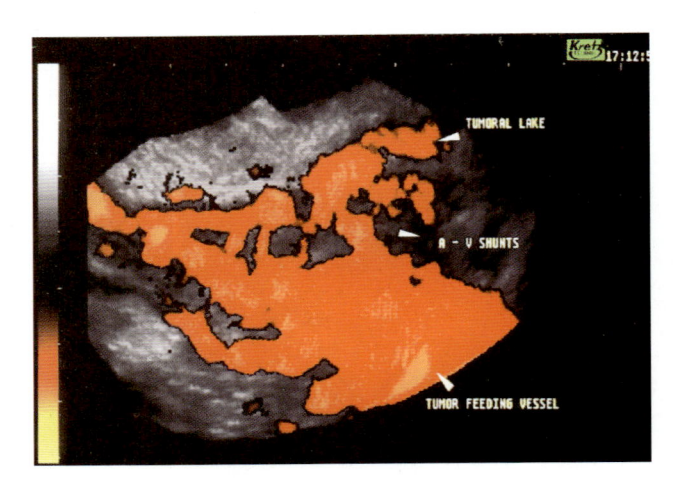

Figure 30 An illustrative example of a complex branching pattern in a malignant ovarian tumor as shown by three-dimensional power Doppler. Note the irregular course of the main tumoral artery, shunts and blind-ending 'ponds'

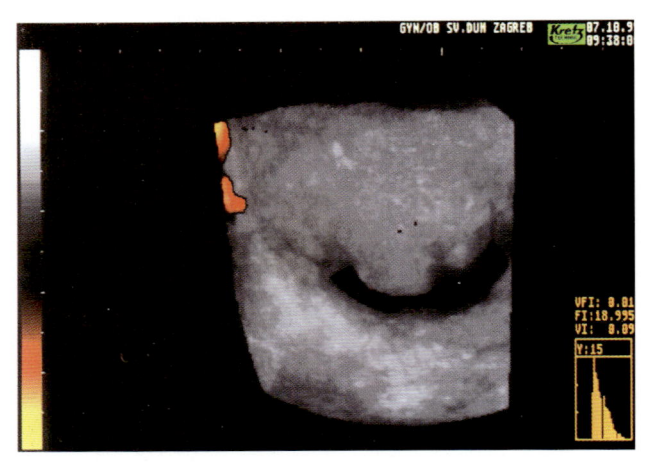

Figure 31 Three-dimensional power Doppler scan of a complex ovarian tumor. The cube method for measurement of blood flow and vascularization reveals low values of the vascularization flow index (VFI = 0.018) and vascularization index (VI = 0.09). In contrast, the flow index was high, and reached the value of 18.995. Histopathology confirmed a benign lesion

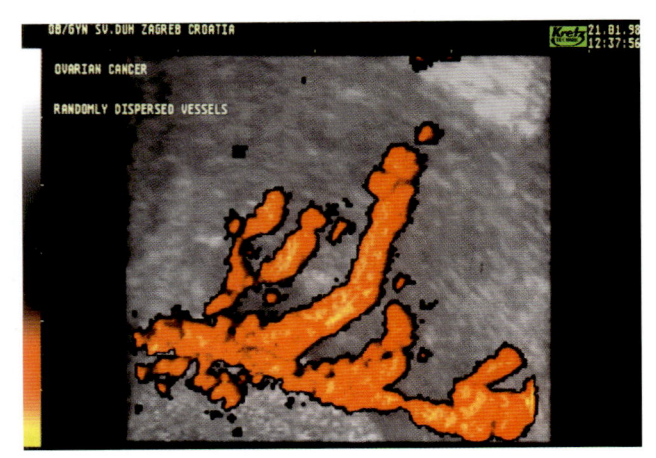

Figure 32 Three-dimensional power Doppler imaging enables effective targeting and rendering of ovarian tumor vasculature. Note the irregular course of the vessels, their dichotomous branching and disproportional calibration, indicative of ovarian malignancy

analysis by visualization of both arterial and venous blood flow patterns. Three-dimensional power Doppler ultrasound can confirm this finding, by demonstrating communications between two vessels within the adnexal tumor. Our study showed that a qualitative analysis of the tumor vascular architecture added to morphological parameters is clinically pertinent, reaching a sensitivity and specificity of 100 and 99.08%, respectively[10].

Further development of the technology and the introduction of 3D quantification of blood flow may improve our ability to differentiate between benign and malignant tumors and predict tumor prognosis. Pairleitner and co-workers[16] recently reported on the use of the cube method for measurement of blood flow and vascularization in the 3D perspective. The vascularization index (VI) represents the vessels in the tissue and is important for diagnosing both high and low vascularization. The flow index (FI), a mean color value, is important for characterizing high flow intensities (presumably tumors). The vascularization flow index (VFI) is a combination of VI and FI, and identifies the extremes between low vascularization and low blood flow on the one hand, and high vascularization and high blood flow on the other hand. While both VI and FI showed excellent reproducibility, VFI did not achieve an accurate agreement between two observations, which will lead to unreliable measurement. It is expected that VI and FI will become good predictors for tumoral neovascularization, and that they will replace qualitative or semi-quantitative 3D power Doppler evaluation[17] (Figure 31).

Conclusions

The use of B-mode transabdominal and transvaginal ultrasound has not been significantly accurate in differentiating benign from malignant ovarian tumors. The advent of transvaginal color and pulsed Doppler ultrasound has improved the situation, although its predictive role is dependent upon selection of the Doppler parameters (cut-off values of RI and PI), the experience of the sonographer and the sensitivity of the equipment. Three-dimensional transvaginal sonography allows simultaneous rendering of all three vertically superimposed sectional planes in the female pelvis (Figure 16). Sections through the ovarian tumor can be reconstructed three-dimensionally in the surface and transparent modes (Figure 17).

The use of 3D power Doppler ultrasound permits effective targeting and rendering of ovarian tumor

ASSESSMENT OF OVARIAN LESIONS

vasculature, thus providing new diagnostic possibilities for differentiating benign from malignant ovarian pathology (Figure 32). The higher detection rate of small vessels after injection of contrast agents may allow application of mathematical models assessing 3D vascular chaos and fractals (Figures 33–37). This is further discussed in Chapter 2.

Future 3D power Doppler units with high-resolution 3D gray-scale information and simultaneous Doppler shift spectrum analysis will probably increase the usefulness of this method. Undoubtedly, further technological development and introduction of real-time 3D ultrasound imaging will contribute to more objective evaluation of tumor morphology and vascularity, which might lead to a significant reduction of morbidity and mortality from ovarian cancer.

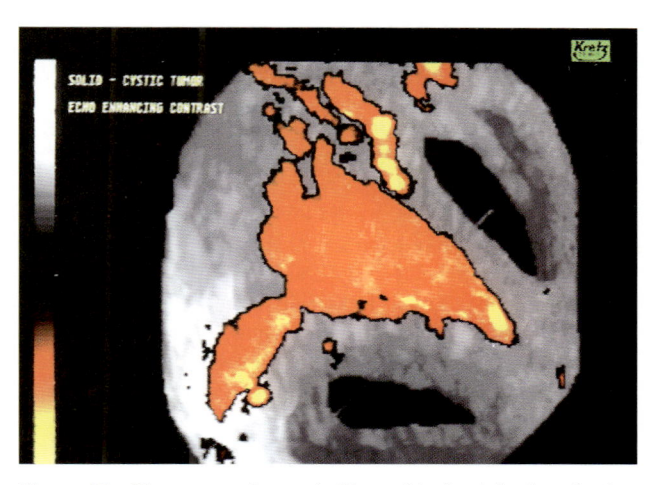

Figure 35 The same patient as in Figure 34 after injection of echo-enhancing contrast. This method facilitates visualization of the main tumoral vessel and depicts its irregular course and complicated branching typical of ovarian malignancy. Ovarian carcinoma was confirmed by histopathology

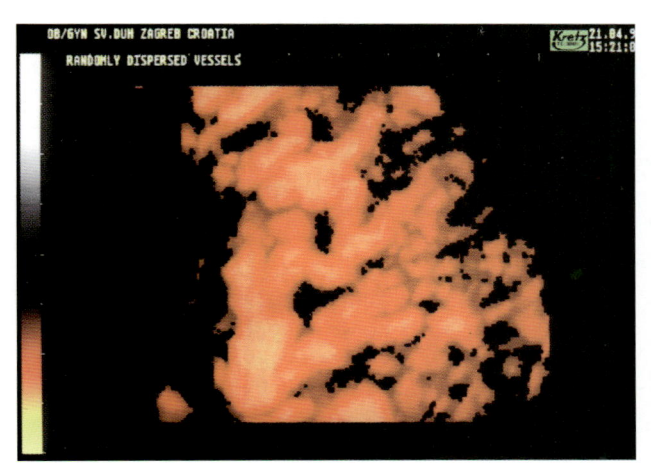

Figure 33 Echo-enhanced three-dimensional power Doppler imaging of malignant ovarian tumor microcirculation. Note three and more generations of tumor feeding vessels, areas of stenoses, shunting and tumoral lakes

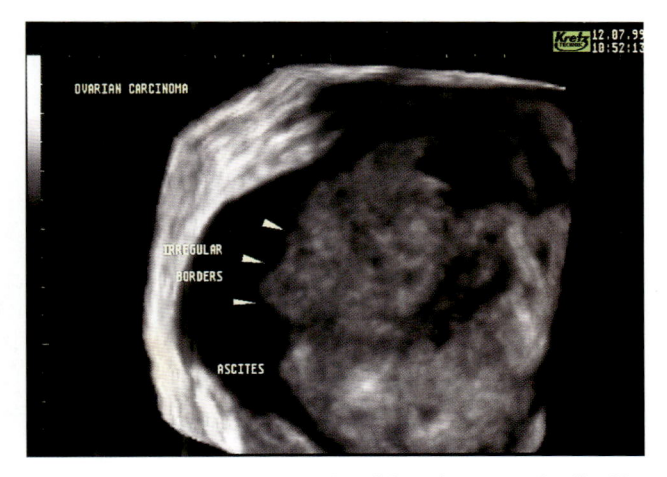

Figure 36 Complex, predominantly solid ovarian tumor visualized by three-dimensional ultrasound

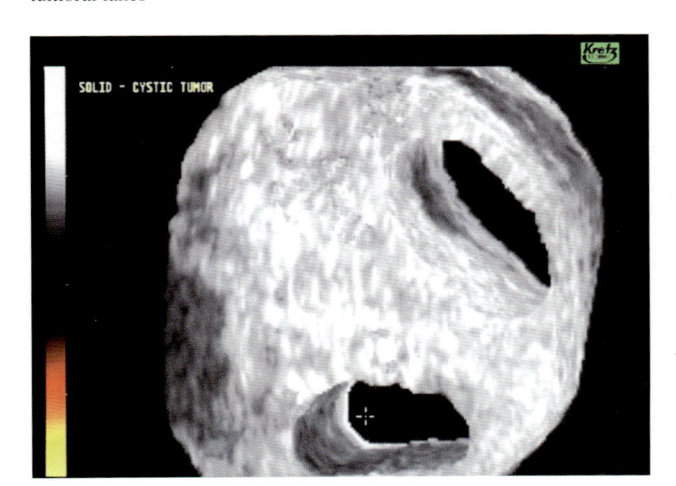

Figure 34 Non-enhanced three-dimensional power Doppler image of a complex adnexal tumor. Absence of tumoral vasculature suggests a benign ovarian lesion

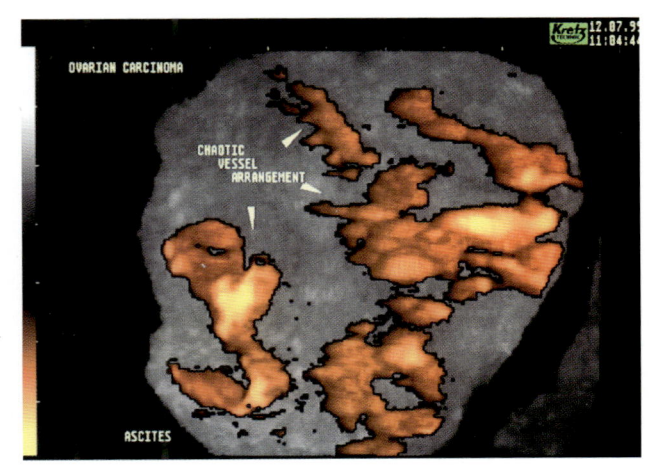

Figure 37 Enhanced three-dimensional power Doppler scan depicts the penetrating intratumoral vessels with irregular course and numerous shunts. Histopathology revealed ovarian malignancy

References

1. Granberg S, Norstrom A, Wikland M. Tumors in the lower pelvis as imaged by vaginal sonography. *Gynecol Oncol* 1990;37:224–9
2. Benacerraf BR, Finkler NJ, Wojchiechowski C, Knapp RC. Sonographic accuracy in the diagnosis of ovarian masses. *J Reprod Med* 1990;35:491–5
3. Sassone AM, Timor-Tritsch IE, Artner A, Westhoff C, Warren B. Transvaginal sonographic characterization of ovarian disease: evaluation of a new scoring system to predict ovarian malignancy. *Obstet Gynecol* 1991;78:70–6
4. Lerner JP, Timor-Tritsch IE, Federman A, Abramovich G. Transvaginal sonographic characterization of ovarian masses using an improved, weighted scoring system. *Am J Obstet Gynecol* 1994;170:81–5
5. Kurjak A, Predanic M. New scoring system for prediction of ovarian malignancy based on transvaginal color Doppler sonography. *J Ultrasound Med* 1992;11:631–5
6. Kurjak A, Kupesic S. Transvaginal color Doppler and pelvic tumor angiogenesis: lessons learned and future challenges. *Ultrasound Obstet Gynecol* 1995;6:145–59
7. Bonilla Musoles F, Raga F, Osborne NG. Three-dimensional ultrasound evaluation of ovarian masses. *Gynecol Oncol* 1995;59:129–35
8. Downey BD, Fenster A. Vascular imaging with a three dimensional power Doppler system. *Am J Roentgenol* 1995;165:665–8
9. Chan L, Lin WM, Verpairojkit B, Hartman D, Reece EA. Evaluation of adnexal masses using three-dimensional ultrasonographic technology: preliminary report. *J Ultrasound Med* 1997;16:349–54
10. Kurjak A, Kupesic S, Anic T, Kosuta D. Three-dimensional ultrasound and power Doppler improve the diagnosis of ovarian lesions. *Gynecol Oncol* 2000;76:28–32
11. Fleischer AC, Cullinan JA, Peery CV, Jones JW III. Early detection of ovarian carcinoma with transvaginal color Doppler ultrasound. *Am J Obstet Gynecol* 1996;174:101–6
12. Kurjak A, Shalan H, Kupesic S, *et al.* Transvaginal color Doppler sonography in the assessment of pelvic tumor vascularity. *Ultrasound Obstet Gynecol* 1993;3:137–54
13. Kurjak A, Kupesic S. Three-dimensional ultrasound and power Doppler in assessment of uterine and ovarian angiogenesis: a prospective study. *Croat Med J* 1999;40:413–20
14. Suren A, Osmers R, Kuhn W. 3D color power Angio imaging: a new method to assess intracervical vascularization in benign and pathological conditions. *Ultrasound Obstet Gynecol* 1998;11:133–7
15. Kurjak A, Kupesic S, Breyer B, Sparac V, Jukic S. The assessment of ovarian tumor angiogenesis: what does three-dimensional power Doppler add? *Ultrasound Obstet Gynecol* 1998;12:1–11
16. Pairleitner H, Steiner H, Hasenoehrl G, *et al.* Three-dimensional power Doppler sonography: imaging and quantifying blood flow and vascularization. *Ultrasound Obstet Gynecol* 1999;14:139–43
17. Pairleitner H. Three-dimensional color histogram using three-dimensional power Doppler. In Kurjak A, ed. *Three-dimensional Power Doppler in Obstetrics and Gynecology*. Carnforth, UK: Parthenon Publishing, 1999:35–9

The use of echo contrast in the investigation of adnexal tumors

S. Kupesic and A. Kurjak

Color Doppler imaging has been useful in the evaluation of adnexal lesions, and the color Doppler appearances of both malignant and benign lesions have been previously described[1-3]. Power Doppler imaging is more sensitive in detecting flow than color Doppler imaging, and this results in a greater resemblance between power Doppler sonograms and angiograms[4]. Nevertheless, power Doppler imaging lacks sufficient sensitivity to detect a very small amount of blood flow.

The development of three-dimensional (3D) ultrasound color imaging displays has allowed a more complete visualization of ovarian blood vessels, both normal and abnormal. Not only has it been possible to study the pathways of normal vessels and to see their branching within a total volume of information as opposed to individual planes, but it is also possible to demonstrate normal variations as well as such vascular abnormalities as varices and arteriovenous malformations. The ability to display objects in multiple planes as well as in a reconstructed 3D display often provides a better understanding of the patterns of both normal and abnormal vessels.

Intravenous contrast agents for ultrasound studies have recently become commercially available. They are of particular importance in cases of 'slow flow, low flow and no flow'. One of the most exciting areas is the potential for using 3D color/power Doppler with contrast agents which enhance the ability to see many more vessels and, in particular, smaller vessels in many regions throughout the body[5] (Table 1). Contrast experiments in animals, and to a limited extent in humans, have shown the capability of imaging much smaller vessels than is possible even with the most sensitive color Doppler instrumentation. In this chapter we discuss the possible improvements of echo-enhancing 3D power Doppler imaging in identifying and differentiating adnexal tumors.

Ultrasound contrast agents

Several contrast agents for the enhancement of Doppler ultrasound signals have been developed in the past decade. These contrast agents consist of tiny microbubbles of gas that are confined to the intravascular space. They increase the reflectivity of blood and, thus, enhance spectral and color Doppler signals[5].

SHU 508A (Levovist; Schering, Berlin, Germany) is a galactose-based echo-enhancing contrast agent. When mixed with water, it produces microbubbles of air covered by a thin layer of palmitic acid. It has been shown to provide clinically useful enhancement of Doppler signals in the heart from intracranial and peripheral arteries and veins, as well as from tumor vessels. SHU 508A, like other contrast agents, is injected as a bolus over a few seconds. This results in a typical wash-in–wash-out enhancement curve: a rapid increase is followed by a short peak of strong enhancement, with subsequent decay over a few minutes. This enhancement pattern means that the duration of diagnostically useful enhancement is relatively short (of the order of 2–5 min), and repeat bolus injections may be required when a clinical question cannot be answered within this time. Furthermore, undesired saturation artifacts (e.g. blooming) that compromise image quality are not infrequently encountered during peak enhancement.

Table 1 Applications of echo-enhanced three-dimensional power Doppler sonography

Demonstration of vascular architecture
  normal vessels
  abnormal vascular morphology
  regional flow differences within an organ
Evaluation of tumors
  identification of the tumor vessels
  evaluation of the surrounding normal vessels
Identification of bleeding sites

It might be possible to overcome these disadvantages with continuous infusion of the agents by using pump injection[6]. As long as the maximum permitted dose and the lifetime of the prepared agent are not exceeded, the infusion could be continued for as long as necessary to answer the clinical question. This may not only prolong the enhancement duration but, provided an adequate infusion rate is selected, avoid saturation artifacts and provide a constant plateau of enhancement throughout the duration of the infusion. Contrast-enhanced power Doppler sonography enables better visualization of the tumor vasculature in complicated renal lesions[7], focal liver lesions[8,9] and solid breast lesions[10]. More recently, our group reported on the use of contrast-enhanced 3D power Doppler sonography for the differentiation of adnexal lesions (submitted for publication).

Echo-enhanced three-dimensional power Doppler sonography of complex adnexal lesions – own results

Numerous attempts have been made to distinguish ovarian malignancy from questionable ovarian lesions on the basis of gray-scale ultrasound and/or color Doppler features[1,2,11,12]. It has been reported that the presence of intratumoral papillae, solid parts and thick septa suggests ovarian malignancy (Figure 1). The detectability of these findings varies, and their diagnostic value is not established. Therefore, the diagnostic ability of gray-scale ultrasound is still limited[11,13]. To date, spectral Doppler sonography and color Doppler ultrasound have been successfully used in the evaluation of adnexal tumor vascularity[1,2] (Figures 2 and 3). Although previous studies reported that both spectral Doppler and color Doppler ultrasound could provide clinically useful information related to adnexal tumor vascularity, these imaging modalities have inherent limitations, such as lack of sensitivity to slow flow, angle dependency and aliasing[3]. Furthermore, a non-universal selection of Doppler parameters (resistance vs. pulsatility index), the choice of highest, lowest or mean impedance values and the selection of vessels for interrogation, together with operator variance and system sensitivity contribute to an already confusing analysis of parameters.

Unlike color Doppler ultrasound, which is based on mean frequency shift, power Doppler ultrasound is based on the total integrated power of the Doppler spectrum. Concurrently with the development of

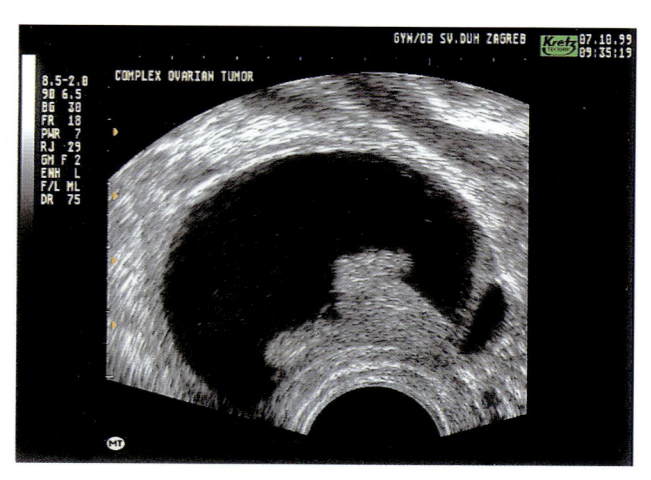

Figure 1 Transvaginal sonogram of a complex ovarian mass. Note the solid component occupying one-third of the lesion

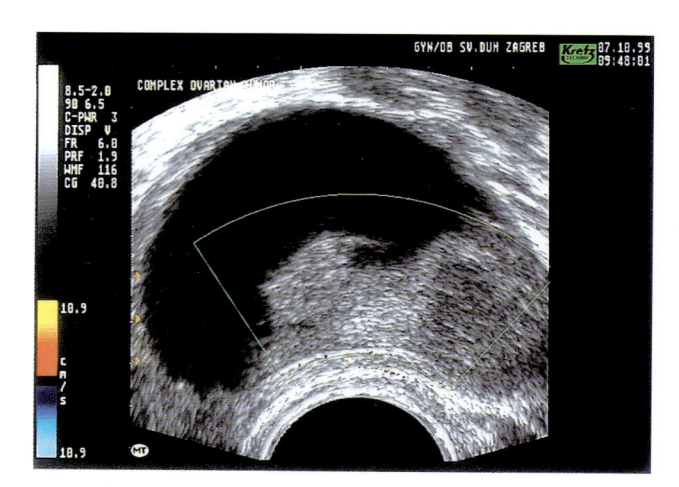

Figure 2 Transvaginal color Doppler scan of the same lesion as in Figure 1. The solid component of the lesion is free of color and indicates the absence of vascularity

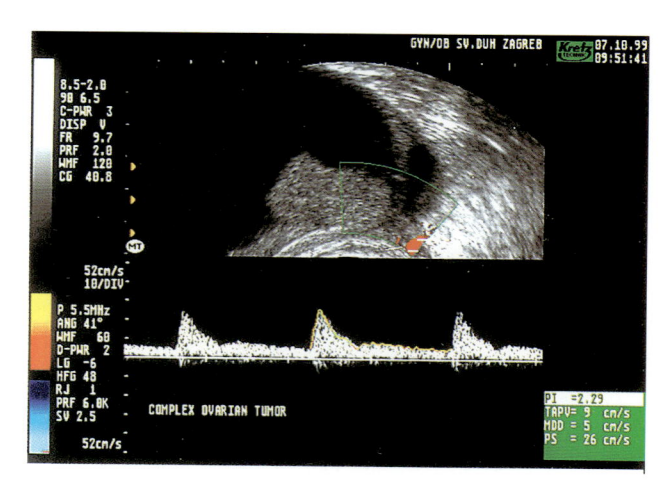

Figure 3 Transvaginal color Doppler scan of the same patient as in Figures 1 and 2. Pulsed Doppler waveform analysis demonstrates high vascular resistance (RI = 0.79, PI = 2.29), indicative of a benign lesion

various sonographic contrast agents, the potential role of power Doppler sonography has increased[6-8]. More recently, technological development enabled the physician to generate 3D vascular images that display tumor morphology and the branching pattern of intralesional vessels on the screen interactively[14-16].

The aim of our study was to evaluate the vascular pattern in questionable adnexal lesions using 3D power Doppler ultrasound with and without echo-enhancing contrast, to determine whether the imaging patterns of identified vessels could be correlated with histopathological results, and to evaluate whether the information obtained with echo-enhanced 3D power Doppler ultrasound could improve the diagnostic accuracy in adnexal lesions compared to that with unenhanced 3D power Doppler ultrasound.

The study population included a consecutive series of patients who had had problematic adnexal lesions during the preceding 12 months, which were difficult to identify as benign or malignant sonographically. Exclusion criteria were as follows: typical benign cysts with absence of internal echoes, a sharply defined smooth wall, no wall enhancement and increased sonic-through transmission. A total of 45 patients with suspicious adnexal masses were analyzed with 3D power Doppler sonography before and after injection of the sonographic contrast agent (Levovist, SHU 508A, Schering AG, Berlin, Germany). Twenty-seven of the studied women were premenopausal (mean age 34, with a range between 19 and 49 years). Three women were perimenopausal (mean age 49 with a range between 47 and 54 years). The remaining 15 women were postmenopausal (mean age 62 with a range between 51 and 77 years). All the examinations in premenopausal patients were performed during the early proliferative phase of the menstrual cycle. In all cases histopathological diagnosis was obtained after surgery, within 1 to 2 weeks after 3D power Doppler sonography.

The sonographic contrast agent used in this study (Levovist) is a suspension of monosaccharide microparticles (galactose) in sterile water. A stabilized microbubble suspension of the agent was administrated intravenously at a concentration of 300 mg/ml. An 8.5-ml dose of contrast agent was injected slowly at a rate of 0.2 ml/s by hand to reduce blooming artifacts and to prolong the duration of enhancement; this was followed by an additional 10 ml of physiological saline solution to flush the cannula, using the same injection rate.

Three-dimensional power Doppler studies were performed by a single examiner with a Voluson 530 D machine (Kretz Medison, Zipf, Austria). Volume data acquisition was performed using a 5-MHz transvaginal volume probe. The size of the volume influences the duration of the scanning procedure (acquisition time approximately 30–60 s). Fixed preinstalled instrument settings for pulse repetition frequency (1.0), signal power (2), wall motion filter (61), persistence (rise 0.1, fall 0.3), center frequency (middle), gray/color balance (G > 192), quality (4) and density (8) of the volume scan were used throughout the examinations. Only power Doppler gain was adjusted to optimize signal quality. Volumetric data were stored on a hard disk to enable full evaluation without loss of information at a later point. During each examination we defined a cube enclosing the vessels of the adnexal lesion, but excluding the iliac vessels or motion artifacts, which are very common, owing to the sensitive power Doppler.

After performing an initial scan by 3D power Doppler (Figures 4 and 5), we introduced enhancing

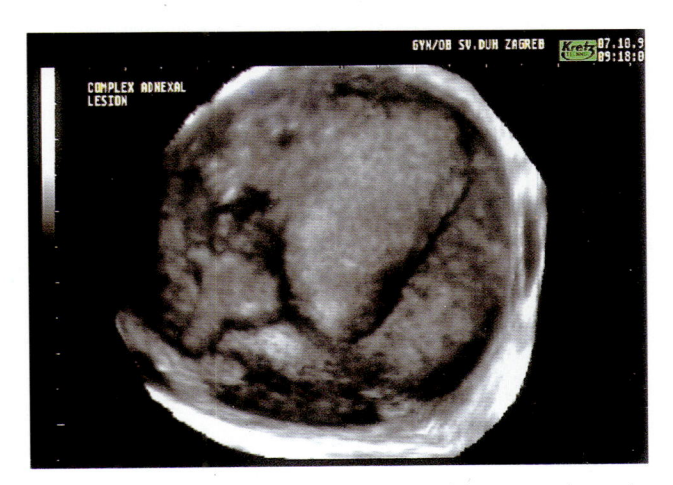

Figure 4 Three-dimensional ultrasound scan of the same patient as in Figures 1–3. Solid components protruding into the cystic cavity are easily visualized by this technique, as are their volume and relationship

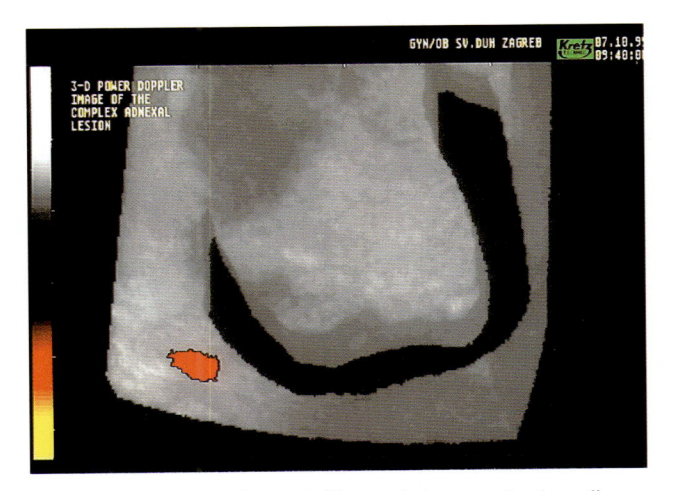

Figure 5 The same patient as in Figures 1–4, as seen by three-dimensional power Doppler. Note the regularly separated vessels at the periphery of the lesion. The solid component is free of color, indicating the absence of vascularity

CLINICAL APPLICATION OF 3D SONOGRAPHY

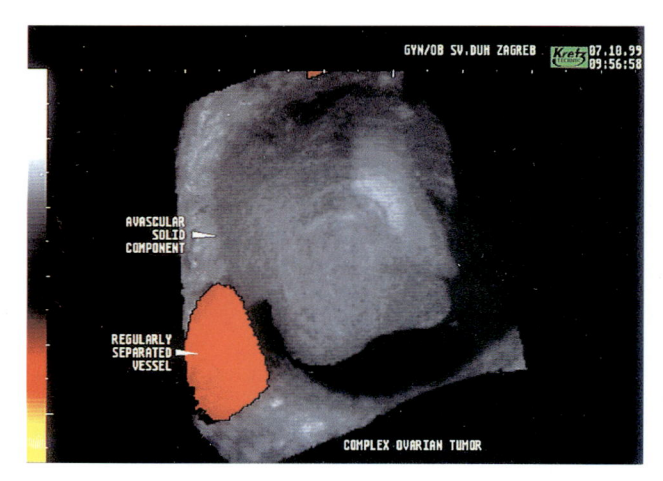

Figure 6 The same patient as in Figures 1–5, at enhanced 3D power Doppler scan. Note the improved visualization of the regularly separated peripheral vessels and absence of the vascular signals in the solid counterpart, features indicative of a benign lesion

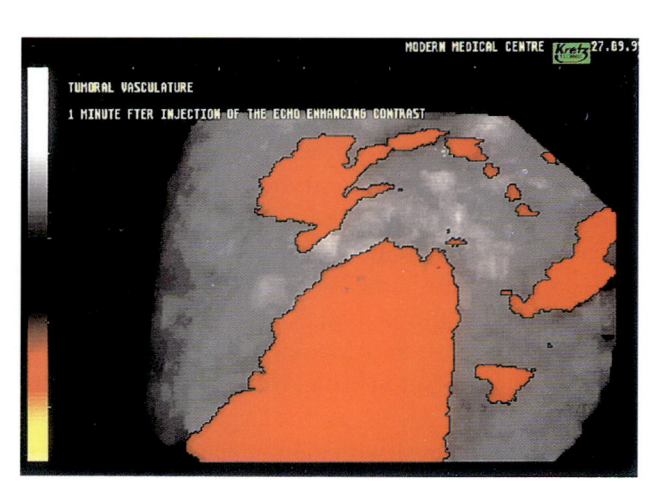

Figure 8 Enhanced three-dimensional power Doppler scan, demonstrating a mixed peripheral and penetrating vascular pattern

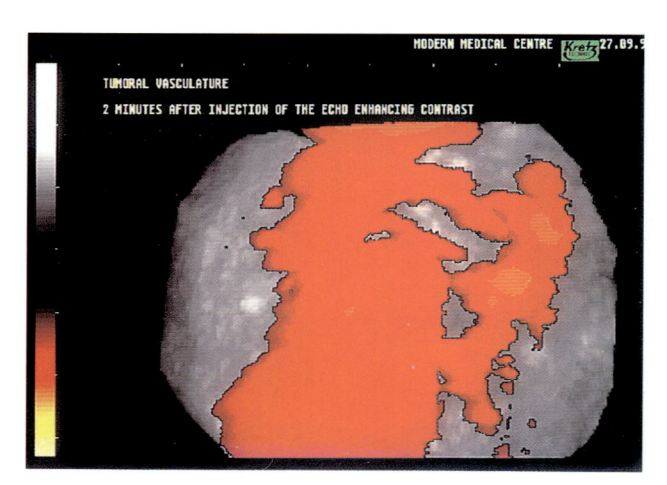

Figure 7 Enhanced three-dimensional power Doppler scan, demonstrating penetrating vessels arising outside the lesion and coursing towards the center

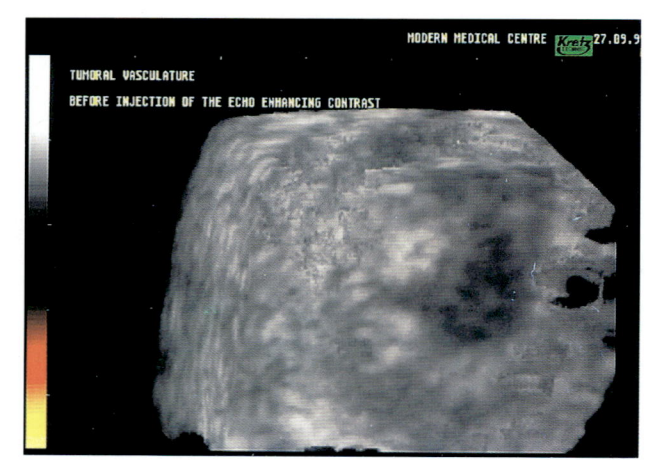

Figure 9 The same patient as in Figures 7 and 8, imaged by non-enhanced three-dimensional power Doppler sonography. Absence of the intratumoral vessels at the initial scan incorrectly indicated a benign lesion. However, contrast medium administration demonstrated stellate feeding vessels suggestive of malignancy, which was confirmed by histopathology

contrast agent (Figure 6). Thereafter, we had to reduce the power Doppler gain because power Doppler noise, such as the color blooming artifact, was produced by the effect of the contrast agent. We continuously manipulated power Doppler gain at the highest level possible that did not produce considerable artifacts, throughout the entire scanning procedure. The resultant power Doppler gains ranged from 70 to 85%. Volumetric data of power Doppler images were stored on the hard disk at 60, 120, 180, 240, 300, 360, 420 and 480 s after the initiation of the contrast agent injection.

At 3D power Doppler ultrasound examination, the vascular distribution in adnexal lesions was classified as follows: pattern 0, no signal pattern (which indicated no detectable vessels); pattern 1, peripheral pattern, which indicated that blood vessels arose outside the lesion and surrounded the lesion (Figures 5 and 6); pattern 2, penetrating pattern indicating that blood vessels arose outside the lesion and coursed towards the center (Figure 7); and pattern 3, mixed penetrating and peripheral pattern (Figure 8). Three-dimensional power Doppler findings after contrast injection were correlated with those from before the procedure (Figure 9).

Vascular features were separately analyzed for each time interval following the instillation of the contrast medium and the most representative 3D image of each patient was chosen for further interpretation. The presence of a penetrating pattern and mixed penetrating and peripheral patterns indicated adnexal malignancy.

In 39 patients the best image quality was obtained 180 s after initiation of the contrast injection, in four patients after 120 s and in two patients after 240 s.

All the cases were operated on by the same surgical team and the histopathological diagnosis was considered final. Malignant tumors were classified according to the International Federation of Gynecology and Obstetrics (FIGO) system.

Of the 12 ovarian cancers, four (33.33%) showed penetrating vessels, three (25.0%) had a mixed penetrating and peripheral pattern, three (25.0%) showed peripheral vessels and in two cases (16.67%) no flow was detected by unenhanced 3D power Doppler imaging. Malignant lesions in which penetrating vessels were found at 3D power Doppler ultrasound examination were 2.2–9.5 cm in diameter (mean 5.2 cm), lesions with a mixed penetrating and peripheral pattern were 2.5–9.2 cm in diameter (mean 5.6 cm), lesions with peripheral vessels were 3–8 cm in diameter (mean 5.4 cm) and those with no detectable vessels were 9 and 12 cm in diameter. In the group of benign lesions, no detectable flow was found in 12 (36.36%) patients, peripheral vessels were seen in 20 (60.61%) and penetrating vessels were seen in one (3.03%) case. The benign lesion with penetrating vessels was subsequently found to be cystadenofibroma.

By using the presence of penetrating vessels as the diagnostic criterion for malignancy, non-enhanced 3D power Doppler ultrasound demonstrated a diagnostic sensitivity of 58.33% and specificity of 96.97%. The positive and negative predictive values were 87.5% and 86.49%, respectively.

Contrast-enhanced 3D power Doppler sonography showed a penetrating pattern in ten (83.33%) and mixed penetrating and peripheral pattern in two (16.67%) patients with ovarian malignancy. Two malignant tumors with a lack of any signal on non-contrast 3D power Doppler sonography showed markedly increased power Doppler signals after the injection of a contrast agent. Peripheral and penetrating vessels with an irregular course were clearly visualized in these patients. In the group of benign lesions, contrast-enhanced 3D power Doppler sonography demonstrated peripheral distribution of the vessels in 29 (87.88%) cases, while two (6.07%) lesions (ovarian dermoid and chronic pelvic inflammatory disease (PID)) remained avascularized. In patients with fibroma and cystadenofibroma, contrast-enhanced 3D power Doppler sonography led to a misdiagnosis as malignant lesions owing to the frank enhancement of the vessels of the solid components which were interpreted as penetrating vessels.

With regard to the differential diagnosis between malignant and benign ovarian lesions, contrast-enhanced 3D power Doppler sonography reached the diagnostic sensitivity and specificity of 100% and 93.94%, respectively. The positive and negative predictive values of this method were 85.71% and 100%, respectively. Therefore, the diagnostic efficiency was improved with the use of the sonographic contrast agent from 86.67% to 95.56%.

Limitations and benefits of echo-enhanced three-dimensional power Doppler sonography

Although our study population included only 45 cases, the use of a contrast agent in 3D power Doppler ultrasound appeared to improve the sensitivity for differentiating benign from malignant ovarian lesions by allowing better detection of malignant tumor perfusion than is obtained by imaging without contrast. However, our results have a fundamental bias because the differential diagnosis between benign and malignant ovarian lesions was based only on the presence or absence of enhancement within the lesion. Although an optimized protocol for 3D contrast-enhanced power Doppler ultrasound has not yet been established, the selection of an optimal infusion rate and concentration of sonographic contrast agent must be very important in obtaining reliable results. Slower injection rates (approximately 0.2 ml/s) and use of a sonographic contrast agent with the concentration of 300 mg/dl can reduce the emergence of 'blooming artifacts' in early stages of the investigation[6]. It is expected that these artifacts and high sensitivity to motion may be reduced by optimization of the instrument settings[17]. In the clinical setting the enhancement provided by the contrast agents and resultant color blooming could be compensated for by reducing the scanner's color flow sensitivity soon after injection and gradually increasing the sensitivity as the effect of contrast diminishes over time.

We found that contrast-enhanced 3D power Doppler sonography provided better visualization of tumor vascularity in suspicious adnexal lesions than that obtained with non-contrast 3D power Doppler sonography, which led to a more exact differential diagnosis. In our study (submitted for publication) contrast-enhanced 3D power Doppler ultrasound showed 100% negative predictive value for malignant adnexal lesions and 85.71% positive predictive value, which were similar to non-contrast-enhanced power Doppler ultrasound. Furthermore, our results showed that the pattern of irregularly branching penetrating vessels in suspicious adnexal lesions demonstrated at 3D power Doppler ultrasound with or without contrast enhancement was an important feature that should be considered with other sonographic criteria to predict the likelihood of malignancy.

Detection of deep-lying and necrotic adnexal lesions with low-velocity blood flow profited the most through contrast-enhanced 3D power Doppler sonography. In two cases of ovarian malignancy measuring 9 and 12 cm, the initial scan by 3D power Doppler did not reveal intratumoral vessels (Figure 9). Contrast medium administration increased the strength of the returning signal, generating a clear image of central stellate feeding vessels from which a diagnosis could be made (Figures 7 and 8). Therefore, the combination of echo-enhancing contrast with the 3D power Doppler technique brought us a step closer to obtaining angiographic images.

Detectable vessels are commonly seen in benign lesions as well, and sometimes are also prominent. However, the morphology and distribution pattern of vessels in benign lesions are usually distinguishable from those in malignant tumors.

Our experience showed that contrast-enhanced 3D power Doppler ultrasound was especially useful in patients with ovarian dermoids ($n = 9$), chronic PID ($n = 9$) and organizing hematoma in a patient with hemorrhagic cyst (Figures 10 and 11). In these cases contrast-enhanced 3D power Doppler did not reveal signs of vascularity within the solid parts but visualized only peripheral vessels, which was mandatory to avoid false-positive results for malignancy. In seven patients with cystadenoma and five with endometriomas only discrete peripheral vascularization was detected, while two lesions (chronic PID and hemorrhagic cyst) remained avascularized. However, in two patients with benign lesions (one fibroma and one cystadenofibroma) contrast-enhanced 3D power Doppler sonography demonstrated penetrating vessels within the solid component, which led to misdiagnosis of ovarian malignancy. Because the treatment of benign lesions with suspicious morphology consists of surgical resection, these false-positive results did not affect the patients' management protocols.

Conclusions

It is expected that the accuracy of contrast-enhanced 3D power Doppler findings for the differentiation of adnexal tumors will be increased if it is analyzed together with morphological parameters obtained by 3D ultrasound. Using 3D power Doppler sonography it is possible to visualize vessel continuity more completely (in three orthogonal projections) and to demonstrate vessel branching (3D vascular reconstruction) more clearly. Furthermore, sonographic

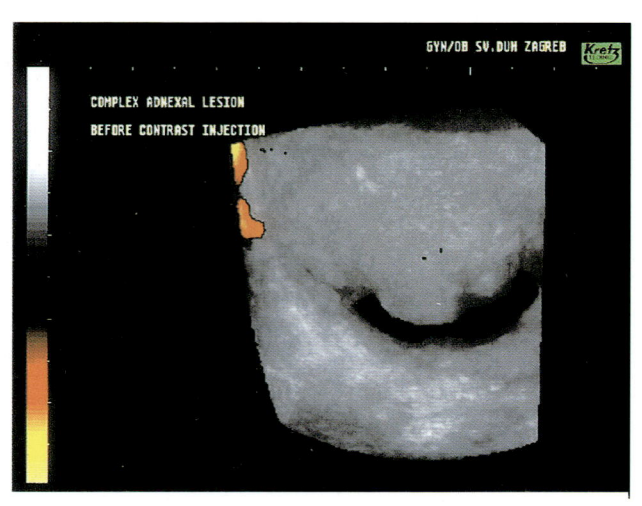

Figure 10 Three-dimensional power Doppler scan of a complex adnexal lesion. Note the avascular solid component protruding into the cystic cavity. A peripheral blood vessel is clearly depicted

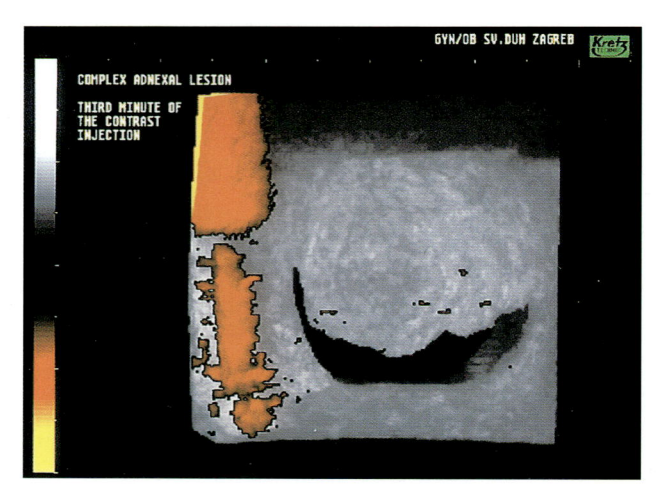

Figure 11 The same patient as in Figure 10 after injection of the echo-enhancing contrast. The solid component is free of color, indicating absence of vascularity. The peripheral vessel becomes more prominent and indicates the benign nature of the lesion which was confirmed by histopathology

findings suggesting malignancy such as irregular and thick cystic walls, a solid component, papillary protrusions, thick septa and heterogeneous echogenicity can be precisely analyzed using 3D ultrasound[18]. Therefore, we expect the combined use of 3D ultrasound and enhanced 3D power Doppler modality to be very useful in the differential diagnosis of questionable adnexal masses, particularly in discriminating malignant from benign lesions.

To determine the practical value of this modality, comparative studies of the diagnostic performance of 3D power Doppler ultrasound before and after injection of contrast agents, including evaluation of cost-effectiveness, examination time and invasiveness, need to be performed.

References

1. Kurjak A, Shalan H, Matijevic R, Predanic M, Kupesic S. Stage I ovarian cancer by transvaginal color Doppler sonography: a report of 18 cases. *Ultrasound Obstet Gynceol* 1993;3:195–8
2. Fleischer AC, Cullinan JA, Peery CV, Jones JW III. Early detection of ovarian carcinoma with transvaginal color Doppler ultrasound. *Am J Obstet Gynecol* 1996;174:101–6
3. Bourne TH. Should clinical decision be made about ovarian masses using transvaginal color Doppler? *Ultrasound Obstet Gynecol* 1994;4:257–60
4. Choi BI, Kim TK, Han JK, et al. Power versus conventional color Doppler sonography: comparison in the depiction of vasculature in liver tumors. *Radiology* 1996;200:55–8
5. Goldberg BB. 3D power/color Doppler & Contrast. 2nd World Congress on 3D Ultrasound in Obstetrics & Gynecology. *Syllabus* Las Vegas, October 1999
6. Albrecht T, Urbank A, Mahler M, et al. Prolongation and optimization of Doppler enhancement with a microbubble US contrast agent by using continuous infusion: preliminary experience. *Radiology* 1998;207:339–47
7. Kim AY, Kim SH, Kim YJ, Lee IH. Contrast-enhanced power Doppler sonography for the differentiation of cystic renal lesions: preliminary study. *J Ultrasound Med* 1999;18:581–8
8. Hosten N, Puls R, Lemke A-J, et al. Contrast-enhanced power Doppler sonography: improved detection of characteristic flow patterns in focal liver lesions. *J Clin Ultrasound* 1999;27:107–15
9. Kim YA, Choi BI, Kim TK, et al. Hepatocellular carcinoma: power Doppler US with contrast agent: preliminary results. *Radiology* 1998;209:135–40
10. Raza S, Baum JK. Solid breast lesions: evaluation with power Doppler ultrasound. *Radiology* 1997;203:164–8
11. Benacerraf BR, Finkler NJ, Wojchiechowski C, Knapp RC. Sonographic accuracy in the diagnosis of ovarian masses. *J Reprod Med* 1990;35:491–5
12. Sassone AM, Timor-Tritsch IE, Artner A, Westhoff C, Warren B. Transvaginal sonographic characterization of ovarian disease: evaluation of a new scoring system to predict ovarian malignancy. *Obstet Gynecol* 1991;78:70–6
13. Granberg S, Norstrom A, Wikland M. Tumors in the lower pelvis as imaged by vaginal sonography. *Gynecol Oncol* 1990;37:224–9
14. Kurjak A, Kupesic S, Breyer B, Sparac V, Jukic S. The assessment of ovarian tumor angiogenesis: what does three-dimensional power Doppler add? *Ultrasound Obstet Gynecol* 1998;12:1–11
15. Suren A, Osmers R, Kuhn W. 3D color power Angio™ imaging: a new method to assess intracervical vascularization in benign and pathological conditions. *Ultrasound Obstet Gynecol* 1998;11:133–7
16. Pairleitner H, Steiner H, Hasenoehrl G, Staudach A. Three-dimensional power Doppler sonography: imaging and quantifying blood flow and vascularization. *Ultrasound Obstet Gynecol* 1999;14:139–43
17. Goldberg BB, Merton AD, Forsberg F, Liu J, Rawool N. Color amplitude imaging: preliminary results using vascular sonographic contrast agents. *J Ultrasound Med* 1990;15:127–34
18. Kurjak A, Kupesic S. Three dimensional ultrasound and power Doppler in assessment of uterine and ovarian angiogenesis: a prospective study. *Croat Med J* 1999;40:413–21

Three-dimensional ultrasound and the Fallopian tube

A. Kurjak, S. Kupesic and T. Zodan

The Fallopian tubes are derived from the Müllerian ducts and arise from the cornual end of the uterus. They are a paired organ and their task is to serve as a conveyer for the oocytes and the sperm for their meeting for conception. The Fallopian tubes are about 9–11 cm long and are covered by peritoneum, which duplicates to form one of its loose attachments (mesosalpinx) to the broad ligament.

The arterial blood supply to the oviducts is derived from the terminal branches of the uterine and the ovarian arteries. The branches of the uterine arteries supply the medial two-thirds of each tube. The ovarian arteries supply the lateral one-third of the tube. Venous drainage parallels the arterial supply.

The ultrasonic scanning and evaluation of the Fallopian tube present a challenge to even the best sonographers. The normal Fallopian tube can be imaged only if fluid surrounds it and creates a sonic interface to outline its boundaries[1]. The most proximal part can also be imaged in the normal state, since it is held steady by the uterus, which in this case serves as a landmark for finding the proximal part of the tube.

In certain instances some fluid is present in the pelvis. This usually sonolucent fluid acts as a contrast medium to highlight the normal Fallopian tube. At times, a certain amount of pelvic fluid is present, and this may be enough to highlight portions of the Fallopian tube. At mid-cycle, after the release of follicular fluid, at the time of ovulation or immediately after it, parts of the tube may be detectable. Blood may be present in the pelvis for various reasons, such as rupture of the corpus luteum or rupture of an ectopic pregnancy. These larger amounts of fluid in the pelvis may increase the chance to detect one or both normal Fallopian tubes. Ascites present in the pelvis, arising from ovarian hyperstimulation or other conditions, may serve as an excellent contrast medium around the Fallopian tube and the fimbriae highlighting them. Fluid originating from infectious processes may also enable us to outline the Fallopian tubes.

If there is fluid in the pelvis, placing the patient into an anti-Trendelenburg position may increase the pooling of even small amounts of fluid and therefore create the acoustic interface necessary for imaging the tube[2,3].

Pelvic inflammatory disease

Pelvic inflammatory disease (PID) is defined as 'the acute clinical syndrome associated with ascending spread of microorganisms (unrelated to pregnancy or surgery) from the vagina or cervix to the endometrium, Fallopian tubes, and/or contiguous structures'[4]. Very rarely, PID can develop as a result of surgical intervention. PID causes more morbidity than necessary for three major reasons: women are not hospitalized when they should be; many women receive inadequate or inappropriate antibiotic therapy; and the male sex partner is not treated or is treated inadequately.

The PID infection is mostly ascending and polymicrobial. Rarely, the infection is hematogenous or spreads directly from another abdominal organ (diverticulitis or appendicitis). Among the sexually transmitted pathogens, *Neisseria gonorrhoeae* and *Chlamydia trachomatis* are most commonly identified.

Over half the women suffering from PID develop tubal damage without any symptoms of the disease, *Chlamydia* being the most frequent cause of this infection. Because of this observation, PID was classified into four major groups[5]:

(1) Silent (asymptomatic) PID (tubal scarring occurs without patient knowledge);
(2) Atypical PID (patients have only minimal symptoms);
(3) Acute PID (this form is most commonly seen in patients presenting to emergency rooms);
(4) PID residual syndrome (patients suffer from chronic pelvic pain, infertility and scar tissue formation).

Chronologically, PID can be divided into acute PID, with formation of pyosalpinx and tubo-ovarian abscess; and PID residual syndrome, with hydrosalpinx and scar tissue formation.

Ultrasound findings

Fallopian tube pathology is discerned by evaluating the wall of the tube, the luminal content and the tubal motility as well as its relation to the surrounding pelvic structures.

Early in the course of acute inflammation, pelvic sonography may be entirely normal; as the process of inflammation proceeds, the tubes become thick-walled and irregular. The associated pelvic exudate allows better delineation of the organ. The inflamed tubes are represented by one of the following pictures[6]:

(1) A dilated tubular structure;

(2) An echogenic tubal wall which reflects the inflammatory process of the mucosal lining;

(3) The presence of internal echoes within the dilated tubes, indicating pyosalpinx. Sonographically guided aspiration of the pus might be helpful for diagnostic purposes and for determining the optimal antibiotic therapy;

(4) A complex adnexal mass with thickening of the ovarian capsule and loculated fluid collections in the adnexal cul-de-sac, representing the tubo-ovarian abscess.

The sonographic appearance of hydrosalpinx differs, depending on the stage of the disease. During the acute phase, the tubal wall is thick and tender to the probe touch, while in the chronic phase, hydrosalpinx shows a typically thin wall, which is not tender. Chronic hydrosalpinx is usually discovered incidentally, on a routine transvaginal scan or during an infertility procedure. The patients are often unaware of their pelvic pathology, but can recall an episode of pelvic pain or even overt pelvic inflammation.

Transvaginal sonography seems to provide an accurate identification of Fallopian tube pathology by evaluating the structure of the tubal wall and luminal contents. However, it is difficult to differentiate tubal from ovarian pathology when complex masses are found. During the acute stage of PID, the tortuous and dilated fluid-filled tube embraces the adjacent ovary. This ovary, therefore, cannot be well delineated, although visualization of the ovarian follicles enables localization of the ovarian component of the mass. During the chronic stage of PID the thin-walled hydrosalpinx is the main sonographic hallmark. Hydrosalpinx produces the typical image of a homogeneous, elongated fluid-filled mass adjacent and medial to the ovary. Incomplete and thin tubal septa are clearly distinguished from the distended tubal wall. However, when hydrosalpinx is presented as a complex mass with thick walls, septa, suspicious papillary projections and mixed echogenic structures, an incorrect diagnosis of an ovarian malignancy might be made.

Color Doppler findings

An improvement to transvaginal B-mode sonography was color Doppler imaging. Color Doppler can depict blood flow within the various tissues and tell us more about the vessel quality in a particular organ or structure. Color Doppler can also depict other kinds of moving liquid such as in the case of hydrosalpinx, which moves when compressed by a vaginal probe or slides over bowels during peristalsis. Color Doppler is very useful in making a differential diagnosis between hydrosalpinx and pelvic congestion syndrome. When the color is turned on, pelvic congestion syndrome strikes the clinician with the amount of color on the screen, while hydrosalpinx remains black and white, the amount of color depending on only peristalsis or deliberate probe movements.

Kupesic and colleagues[7] evaluated 102 women with laparoscopically proven PID. Seventy-two had acute symptoms, 11 presented with chronic pelvic pain and 19 were infertility cases suspected of tubal etiology. The mean resistance index (RI) in patients with acute symptoms was 0.53 ± 0.09. This significantly differed from the values obtained in patients with chronic stage (0.71 ± 0.07) and infertility cases (0.73 ± 0.09). Therefore, the bizarre morphology during both the chronic and acute stages of PID, if evaluated by color and pulsed Doppler, should not cause an overlap with adnexal malignancy, since vascular resistance demonstrates significantly higher values.

Many studies have been undertaken to assess blood flow-related functional changes in the ovaries since our team first introduced the technique[8]. Significant changes have been demonstrated during the menstrual cycle in the active ovary, and most of them were attributed to angiogenesis in the follicle and, subsequently, the corpus luteum[9,10]. Transvaginal color Doppler proved to be useful in infertility evaluation and management, as well as in the assessment of adnexal masses and early detection of ovarian cancer[11–14].

Kupesic and associates[7] assumed that an inflammatory process within the pelvis might affect ovarian blood flow. The ovary is in close proximity to the tube, which is the primary focus of infection, and it shares a significant part of its blood supply with the ipsilateral tube. Therefore, it can be expected that the ovarian blood flow is altered according to the changes in the inflammatory process. Their study demonstrated the correlation of intraovarian blood flow changes with pathophysiological changes. Findings obtained in the acute stage demonstrated rapidly changing patterns in this stage of the disease. The ongoing vasodilatation mediated by the local products of inflammation caused a decrease in the RI, while the subsequent edema of the ovarian parenchyma caused an increase in the RI. As the ovarian capsule may vary in its rigidity, the intraovarian pressure differs from case to case. This affects the intensity of the intraovarian blood flow, and is reflected by variable values of RI. Furthermore, fluid collection within the tubes may influence the blood flow characteristics by compressing the vessel walls. As the process advances, the proliferation of the fibroblasts and scarring tissue formation leads towards reduction of the local blood flow, which is demonstrated by the progressive increase in RI. Very similar results were obtained by other authors, but in small series of patients[5,15]. We concluded that transvaginal color Doppler (TVCD) might be used as an additional tool in evaluating patients with suspected PID. Furthermore, we noted that flow indices returned to normal values after treatment in 36 (48.65%) patients.

This method was useful in differentiating pyosalpinx from hematosalpinx in cases of ectopic pregnancy. Ectopic pregnancies are characterized by high velocity and a low-impedance (RI < 0.42) adnexal blood flow signal[10,16].

Transvaginal color and pulsed Doppler can also be helpful in differentiating between a pseudogestational sac and free endometrial fluid. In cases of endometritis, an increased endometrial vascularity can be demonstrated, while in cases with pseudogestational sac, there are no changes in endometrial blood flow.

As the inflammation may mimic a wide variety of findings, and sometimes even suggest malignancy, serial assessment by TVCD is therefore recommended, with respect to the patient's age and the phase of the menstrual cycle. Serial examination may demonstrate morphological changes as well as variations in blood flow intensity according to the stage of the disease. Doppler studies are particularly useful in the chronic stage of PID, when pseudopapillomatous structures protruding into the cystic compartment may morphologically suggest malignancy. An absence of blood flow, typical for this stage, helps to differentiate it from adnexal malignancy. In the acute stage, low resistance to blood flow that is suggestive of malignancy may be demonstrated. In these patients, it is useful to perform some additional tests (sedimentation rate, blood cell counts, CA-125, etc.) that may help in reaching the diagnosis. Serial examination in these cases will reveal the changes that correlate with the pathophysiology of the process. However, it should be borne in mind that there is no single parameter that is sufficiently reliable for the characterization of an adnexal mass[17].

In patients with tubo-ovarian abscess, abscess drainage under transvaginal sonographic guidance can hasten the recovery process and improve the efficacy of the antibiotic therapy[18]. Addition of color Doppler facilitates visualization of the large pelvic vessels and thereby may reduce the complication rate. However, a careful clinical examination, ultrasound evaluation and blood tests are required before performing the procedure, to avoid infection propagation.

Three-dimensional ultrasound

Three-dimensional (3D) ultrasound helps in spatial delineation of the inflammatory conglomerates. Any scanned volume can be rotated in all dimensions and thus it is possible to observe the borders of tissues and organs. By conventional B-mode ultrasound, hydrosalpinx can sometimes be mistaken for a multilocular cyst, but when 3D ultrasound is applied, the true spatial position and shape of the hydrosalpinx are clearly visible (Figure 1). By using 3D volume sections it is possible to visualize the tortuous structure and contiguous spread of hydrosalpinx. Three-dimensional ultrasound enables the three perpendicular planes to be visualized simultaneously. By moving the cursor, the sonographer 'sees through' the slices of the hydrosalpinx. Another useful mode is the so-called niche mode that enables the 'cut-into' view of a certain tissue. With the use of this mode we can show the spatial spreading of the hydrosalpinx, and at the same time visualize the lumen. Furthermore, pseudopapillomatous structures within the tubal lumen can be better assessed. The surface of such papillary protrusions can be thoroughly scanned by surface mode, and its subtype 'X-ray mode'. When applying this mode, the

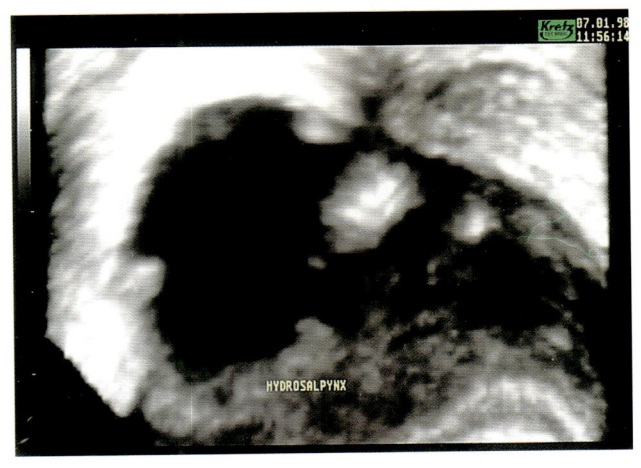

Figure 1 Three-dimensional view of a dilated tube in a patient with hydrosalpinx. Note the pseudopapillomatous projections protruding into the tubal lumen

spaces that appeared anechoic on the conventional ultrasound scan are even darker, while the echoic tissues are shown lighter, so that the whole image gains more sharpness and contrast.

Various inflammatory conglomerates sometimes pose a problem to the ultrasonographer. They may form a part of a tubo-ovarian abscess or stay encapsulated by two sheets of peritoneum in the retrouterine space. Because of echogenicity and low vascular resistance, such structures can be mistaken for malignant structures. Three-dimensional ultrasound and the various forms of its usage can define more clearly the spatial relations of such a structure and its connection to an organ system (Figure 2).

Vascularity can be assessed by superimposed 3D power Doppler. By the use of this modality it is possible to visualize a vascular pattern and to study the branching and shape of vascular structures. An interesting future possibility for the use of 3D power Doppler in the field of PID stems from work on 3D color Doppler histograms. The vascularity index (VI) measures the number of color voxels in the cube, representing the vessels in the tissue. The flow index (FI), a mean color value of all blood flow or induced flow intensities, represents the intensity of flow at the time of the 3D sweep. With these indices it is easier to quantify the flow and identify the phase of the inflammatory process. The changes caused by vasodilatation or those caused by scar tissue formation can be better understood.

Ectopic pregnancy

Ectopic pregnancy is a gestation that implants outside the uterine cavity. In the past 20 years, the rate of ectopic pregnancies has increased significantly worldwide. Between the years 1970 and 1987, there was an almost four-fold increase in the incidence of ectopic pregnancy per 1000 pregnancies.

As far as the location of ectopic pregnancies is concerned, more than 90% of ectopic pregnancies involve the Fallopian tube; the remaining ectopic gestations implant in the cornual or isthmic area of the tube, in the ovary, the cervix and different sites in the abdominal cavity.

The cause of blastocyst implantation and development outside the endometrial cavity is unknown. Abnormal tubal morphology, alterations in the hormonal environment affecting tubal motility, uterine abnormalities, foreign bodies and defects of the fertilized ovum are associated with its occurrence. Among the mechanical factors that have been implicated in the prevention of the movement of the fertilized egg

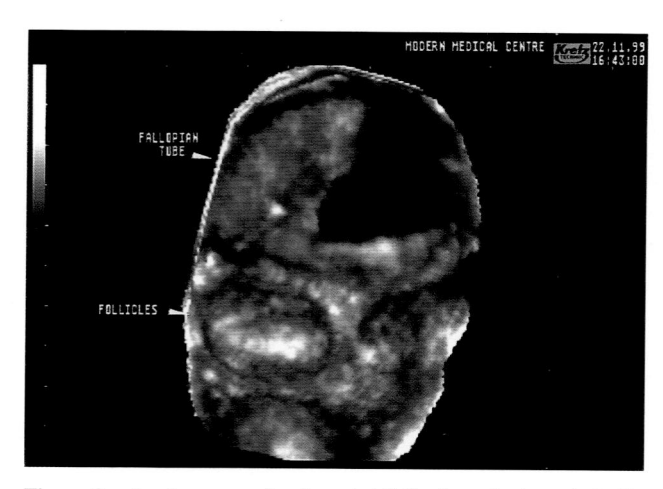

Figure 2 Another case of a distended Fallopian tube in an infertile patient. The ovary containing preovulatory follicles is clearly separated from the occluded tube. This is an illustrative example of how surface rendering defines spatial relations of a tubal lesion with a nearby ovary

are the following: low-grade infection of the pelvic contents, which is believed to be the main cause for the faulty implantation of the fertilized egg and/or the embryo; peritubal adhesions as a result of previous PID; and salpingitis, with partial or total destruction of the tubal mucosa. Early recognition of the symptoms and risk factors attributed to ectopic pregnancy and prompt application of advanced technology will result in more rapid diagnosis and allow initiation of conservative therapy to reduce the morbidity.

The most common cause of tubal pathology is PID. The risk of ectopic pregnancy increases seven-fold after acute salpingitis. Most series report a history of PID in 20–50% of patients with ectopic pregnancy. Examination of the Fallopian tube after removal or resection for ectopic pregnancy shows evidence of prior inflammation in a higher percentage (40–50%).

Symptoms of ectopic pregnancy are usually bleeding, pelvic pain and a palpable adnexal mass. Shoulder pain can also occur as a result of intraabdominal bleeding which, then, triggers the reflex pain via the phrenic nerve. Regardless of how atypical the complaints of a patient are, the good clinician gathers an initial and careful history about the menstrual periods, previous possible ectopic pregnancies, contraceptive practices, history of PID, and, above all, the patient's participation in infertility treatment or assisted reproductive technologies. If ectopic pregnancy is then suspected, a simple pregnancy test and transvaginal scan would be performed.

Ultrasound findings

The early and reliable diagnosis of extrauterine pregnancy still remains a challenge, but is essential to avoid life-threatening bleeding or consequent infertility. Although the introduction of vaginal sonography has improved diagnostic accuracy, the adnexal pathology is not seen with the conventional 2D B-mode technique in about one-quarter of ectopic pregnancies, whereas an extrauterine chorionic cavity is visible in only about half of such cases[20,21]. According to a literature review[22] an adnexal mass other than a simple cyst or intraovarian lesion in patients clinically suspected of having an ectopic pregnancy was evident in 84% of cases of ectopic pregnancy with a likelihood of 96% that this finding represented ectopic pregnancy, based on an ectopic pregnancy prevalence of 26%.

A review of the world literature indicates that transvaginal sonography has a diagnostic sensitivity between 75 and 90% for the diagnosis of ectopic pregnancy. The following images may be seen:

(1) An empty uterus (27.8%);

(2) An empty uterus and an adnexal mass (34.7%);

(3) An intrauterine sac or pseudogestational sac (25%);

(4) An empty uterus and an ectopic gestational sac (12.5%) with or without:
   (a) a yolk sac
   (b) an embryo
   (c) embryonic heart activity

(5) Images with cul-de-sac fluid (25%).

The sonographic image observed will depend both on gestational age and on whether the ectopic pregnancy is in development or in regression at the time when it is first diagnosed. The evidence is that at least 60% of ectopic pregnancies regress spontaneously. Regressive ectopic pregnancies present the images described as an empty uterus with or without a suspicious adnexal mass. In cases of early diagnosis, living embryos are observed infrequently. This observation is so well established that it can be stated with confidence that, if a living embryo is seen in a Fallopian tube, the diagnosis may have been made late.

Color Doppler findings

Ectopic pregnancy is one of the conditions changing the normal high-resistance blood flow from the uterine or ovarian artery branches. Color Doppler is essential to detect such hemodynamic changes in vessels[20]. This method is an excellent and rapid guide to search for abnormal or ectopic blood flow signals in the entire pelvic anatomy visualized by transvaginal ultrasound. When combining Doppler studies and measurement of β-human chorionic gonadotropin (β-hCG) it should be mentioned that ectopic pregnancies with higher β-hCG levels demonstrate lower resistance to blood flow and higher 'quantity' of color, and that 'live', or still actively β-hCG-producing ectopic pregnancies, show a 'hot' flow pattern in addition to a higher diastolic flow, as opposed to ectopic pregnancies in which there is long-standing embryonic demise and in which less flow and higher resistance to blood flow are seen.

Jurkovic and co-workers[23] have shown that, in both main uterine arteries, impedance to flow decreases and the calculated RI values are well within the reference ranges for normal intrauterine pregnancy. However, uterine blood flow velocity was lower in the ectopic group, indicating an overall reduction in uterine blood supply. This reduction may be a consequence of a reduced mass of viable trophoblast, or perhaps a larger contribution from the ovarian arteries to the blood supply of a tubal pregnancy.

An area of high vascularity at the periphery of the adnexal mass can be found in 94% of ectopic pregnancies. The appearance and location of blood flow in relation to the gestational sac and the flow velocity waveform characteristics are similar to those obtained from the spiral arteries in normal intrauterine pregnancies[20]. However, the decrease in the impedance to flow with gestation observed in normal intrauterine pregnancies does not occur in the ectopic group.

In maternal serum, β-hCG can be detected as early as 7–8 days after ovulation or about the day after blastocyst implantation. The term 'discriminatory β-hCG level' was coined to express the titer of this pregnancy hormone when a chorionic (gestational) sac was seen in the cavity of a normal uterus. Transabdominal and transvaginal probes have different discriminatory β-hCG levels. It should be mentioned that, using a transabdominal probe of 3.5 MHz, a normal intrauterine pregnancy is detectable at a level of 6500 mIU/ml. Transvaginal probes using 5–7.5 MHz perform much better; they detect the gestation at levels of 1000 ± 200 mIU/ml. If the ectopic pregnancy is developing and is 'alive', it is expected that a careful transvaginal scanning will detect the ectopic sac at discriminatory titers similar to those used in the case of a normal intrauterine pregnancy. Furthermore, if the scanning is guided by color flow, successful detection of ectopic pregnancy is possible at even lower discriminatory β-hCG titer.

Three-dimensional ultrasound

Rempen[24] conducted a prospective follow-up study in order to evaluate the potential utility of 3D ultrasound to differentiate intrauterine from extrauterine gestations. Fifty-four pregnancies with a gestational age of < 10 weeks and with an intrauterine gestational sac < 5 mm in diameter formed the study group. The configuration of the endometrium in the frontal plane of the uterus was correlated with eventual pregnancy outcome. After exclusion of three patients with a poor 3D image quality, the endometrial shape was found to be asymmetrical with regard to the median longitudinal axis of the uterus in 84% of intrauterine pregnancies, whereas the endometrium showed a symmetry in the frontal plane in 90% of extrauterine pregnancies ($p = 0.0000001$). Intrauterine fluid accumulation may distort the uterine cavity, thus being responsible for false-positive as well as false-negative results. The evaluation of the endometrial shape in the frontal plane appeared to be a useful additional means of distinguishing intrauterine from extrauterine pregnancies, especially when a gestational sac was not clearly demonstrated with conventional ultrasound.

Harika and co-workers[25] conducted a 3D imaging study on the early diagnosis of ectopic pregnancy. Twelve asymptomatic patients before 6 weeks of amenorrhea and with no feature of intrauterine or of ectopic pregnancy were examined with traditional two-dimensional (2D) ultrasound. Laparoscopy showed ectopic pregnancy in nine cases. Three-dimensional transvaginal ultrasonography preceding laparoscopy showed a small ectopic gestational sac in four cases. The Fallopian tube on the side of the ectopic pregnancy could be imaged in all cases. This was possible because the Fallopian tube was surrounded by a fine hypoechogenic border, an apparently specific feature that had not been reported previously. These preliminary data suggested that 3D ultrasonography is an effective procedure for early diagnosis of ectopic pregnancy in asymptomatic patients before 6 weeks of amenorrhea.

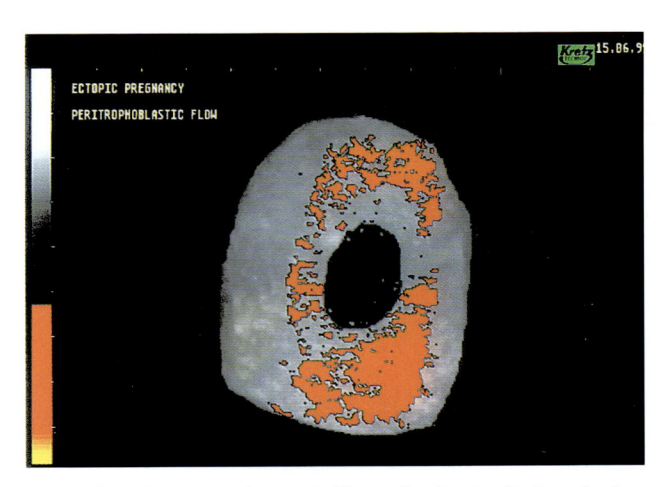

Figure 4 The same patient as in Figure 3, after instillation of echo-enhancing contrast medium. Dilated tubal arteries are clearly visualized encircling the ectopic gestational sac

The possible use of 3D power Doppler ultrasound is the monitoring of the vascularity of ectopic pregnancy (Figures 3 and 4). The hypoperfusion, quantified by indices of vascularity (VI) and flow (FI), could indicate that the ectopic pregnancy is dying off itself, and that laparoscopy should be postponed. This way, the conservative approach to ectopic pregnancy would rely on more data. Vice versa, in case of hyperperfusion, the patients should be subjected to laparoscopy or medical treatment immediately.

Benign tumors of the Fallopian tube

Although the muscles of the Fallopian tube and the uterus are of the same embryological origin (Müllerian ducts), leiomyomas of the Fallopian tube are exceptionally rare. Leiomyomas of the Fallopian tube are commonly incidental findings, as they are asymptomatic and small. However, there are reported cases of large tubal myomas associated with acute abdomen consequent to its torsion[26]. Tubal pregnancy associated with tubal leiomyomas, in which the tubal myoma was the obstructing factor, has also been reported[1,26,27].

Conventional B-mode sonography reveals little of the nature of a benign tubal tumor. A smaller papilla can resemble a chronic PID remnant, while a larger mass in the oviduct can be mistaken for an inflammatory conglomerate. Because of its limited imaging possibilities, 2D ultrasound cannot always define the borders of the lesion and delineation from the surrounding tissue.

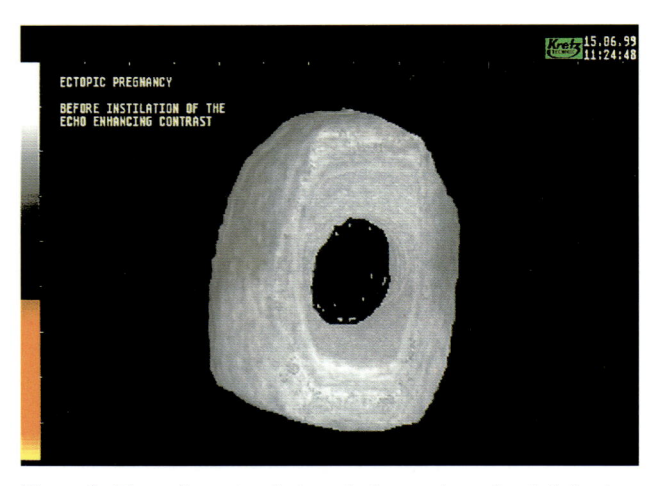

Figure 3 Three-dimensional view of a hyperechogenic tubal ring in a 6-week ectopic pregnancy. The initial three-dimensional power Doppler scan does not reveal peritrophoblastic vascularity

Color Doppler can be used for the assessment of vascularity. As with any other benign tissues, the oviduct leiomyomas would have a moderate-to-high RI. If they undergo necrosis of inflammation, they can present a true complication in the diagnostic process.

Three-dimensional ultrasound can help in the diagnosis of benign ovarian lesions by its possibility of precisely delineating and spatially defining a certain tumor. With the use of 3D power Doppler it is possible to visualize the regular branching of benign intratubal structures, and distinguish them from the uterine and ovarian vascular network.

Malignant tumors of the Fallopian tube

Although rare, tubal malignancy must be considered in the differential diagnosis of an adnexal mass. Of all gynecological cancers, malignancy of the Fallopian tube is the most rare. The triad of pain, bleeding and leukorrhea is considered pathognomonic of tubal carcinoma. Sedlis[28] defined parameters for better differentiation between ovarian and tubal malignancies. He postulated that the tumor is of Fallopian origin if:

(1) It is derived from the Fallopian tube;

(2) It has the same histological structure as oviduct mucosa;

(3) There is a clear transition zone between benign and malignant epithelium;

(4) There is no endometrial or ovarian carcinoma.

Ultrasound findings

The sonographic findings in all reported cases of Fallopian tube carcinoma were complex, predominantly cystic adnexal masses and/or sausage-shaped structures apparently separated from the uterus[29–42]. Table 1 reviews data from the literature on B-mode diagnosis of primary Fallopian tube carcinoma.

In a remarkable review of 376 cases of tubal carcinoma, McGoldrick and colleagues found only one diagnosed preoperatively[43]. More recently, Eddy and colleagues analyzed the data of 74 patients regarding tubal malignancies and only two cases of tubal carcinoma were correctly diagnosed before surgery[44].

Ayhan and colleagues reported a study of eight cases of primary Fallopian tube carcinoma[29]. Dava and colleagues describes six adenocarcinomas of the Fallopian tube that resembled the female adnexal tumor of probable Wolffian origin[30]. Microscopically, the tumors were characterized by a predominant pattern of small, closely packed cells punctured by numerous glandular spaces, which were typically small but occasionally cystically dilated. Soundara and associates published a review of Fallopian tube carcinoma over 20 years[31]. Nine cases of tubal carcinoma were found among approximately 9000 gynecological malignancies.

Unfortunately, there is no high index of suspicion for tubal malignancy, although more than 80% of patients have a pelvic mass detected before surgery. However, cervical cytology, X-ray of the pelvis, computed tomography or hysterosalpingography are usually no more specific than the pelvic examination. Conventional transvaginal sonography is one of the most important tools in preoperative diagnosis, but the efficacy of morphological scoring systems alone is hampered by the degree of overlap between benign- and malignant-appearing adnexal masses[45–47].

Color Doppler findings

Our group was the first to publish a case of primary adenocarcinoma of the Fallopian tube (stage I FIGO) preoperatively diagnosed by color and pulsed Doppler ultrasound[48]. Podobnik and co-workers published a case of a 69-year-old woman with a history of right-sided lower abdominal pain accompanied by profuse watery vaginal discharge for the prior 3 months[49]. Six years after the initial report, Kurjak and associates[50]

Table 1 Review of the literature on B-mode diagnosis of primary Fallopian tube carcinoma

Reference	No. of cases	Histopathology
Subramayon et al.[35]	3	papillary cystadenocarcinoma
Meyer et al.[36]	1	adenocarcinoma
Kol et al.[52]	1	adenocarcinoma
Ajjimakorn and Bhamarapravati[37]	4	papillary cystadenocarcinoma
Granberg and Jansson[38]	1	adenocarcinoma
Chang et al.[33]	1	mixed Müllerian tumor
Chiou et al.[32]	1	mixed Müllerian tumor
Slanetz et al.[39]	9	adenocarcinoma and mixed Müllerian tumor
Ong[40]	1	adenocarcinoma

Table 2 Review of the literature on the transvaginal color Doppler diagnosis of primary Fallopian tube carcinoma

Reference	No. of cases	Resistance index	Histopathology
Shalan et al.[48]	1	0.35	adenocarcinoma
Kurjak et al.[50]	8	0.29–0.40	adenocarcinoma and papillary cystadenocarcinoma
Podobnik et al.[49]	1	0.34	clear-cell carcinoma

reported on a series of eight cases of preoperatively diagnosed Fallopian tube malignancy (Table 2). Probably the most illustrative case of successful preoperative diagnosis of primary Fallopian tube carcinoma is a 45-year-old woman treated at our Department because of infertility problems. During the routine transvaginal ultrasound examination a pendular myoma and a complex bilateral adnexal mass were discovered. In the left adnexal region a sausage-shaped cystic structure 3.4 × 4.8 × 3.4 cm in size was present. In the upper part of the cyst a solid papillary protrusion of less than 1 cm, richly perfused, with the lowest RI of 0.37, was detected. In the right adnexal region a hydrosalpinx 3.0 × 1.6 cm was delineated from the ovary. Moderate vascular resistance (RI = 0.55) was observed in the Fallopian tube with chronic inflammatory changes. According to the visualization of the area of neovascularization and low vascular impedance, the authors suspected tubal carcinoma of the left side. Frozen section pathological examination at surgery reported papillary Fallopian tube carcinoma.

Three-dimensional ultrasound

Further progress in diagnostic procedures was made when 3D and power Doppler ultrasound were introduced. Transvaginal 3D ultrasound enables the clinician to perceive the true spatial relations and thus easily distinguish the origin of an adnexal mass, while 3D power Doppler allows detailed analysis of the neovascularization. Kurjak and associates[51] were the first to report on the preoperative diagnosis of primary Fallopian tube carcinoma by 3D power Doppler ultrasound. Three-dimensional ultrasound was used to evaluate 520 adnexal masses prior to elective surgery during a 2-year period. These lesions were originally detected with conventional transvaginal sonography and/or transvaginal color Doppler. Patients with suspicious morphology and/or Doppler findings underwent a second assessment at the referral center by an investigator performing 3D ultrasound who was unaware of the previous ultrasound examinations. Three-dimensional transvaginal ultrasound was performed using either 5- or 7.5-MHz transvaginal transducers (Voluson 530, Kretztechnik, Austria). Once the region of interest was identified, a volume box was superimposed to scan the image. The patient was asked to lie still on the examination bed, while the ultrasound probe was kept steady in the vagina. Depending on the size of the volume box the scanning procedure lasted between 5 and 13 s. The ability to store 3D data on a hard disk drive allowed the investigator to keep the examination time short (between 2 and 4 min). Detailed analysis of the adnexal tumor was performed after the patient had left, and lasted between 10 and 20 min. Rotation and translation of the stored volumes allowed different tumor sections to be evaluated in many planes. The niche mode enabled meticulous study through selected sections of the adnexal tumor and was found especially useful in evaluation of the sausage-shaped complex masses (Figure 5). The surface reconstruction allowed plastic imaging of the inner and outer walls of the tumor (Figure 6). Demonstration of the complex adnexal mass and/or sausage-shaped cystic lesions with papillary projections were the morphological criteria for detection of tubal malignancy.

After B-mode analysis, power Doppler imaging was switched on together with the volume mode. In order to reduce the acquisition time the volume of the color box and sweep angle were reduced. The color frame rate

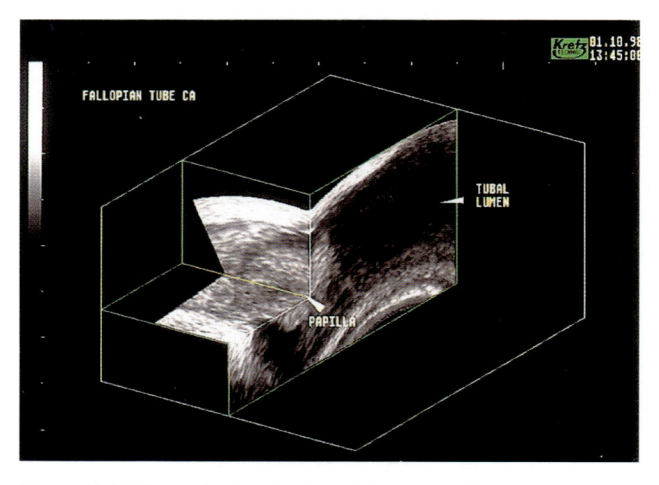

Figure 5 Niche mode visualization of the sausage-like structure in the adnexal region. Intratumoral papillae are clearly outlined in selected sections, enabling tubal pathology to be precisely evaluated

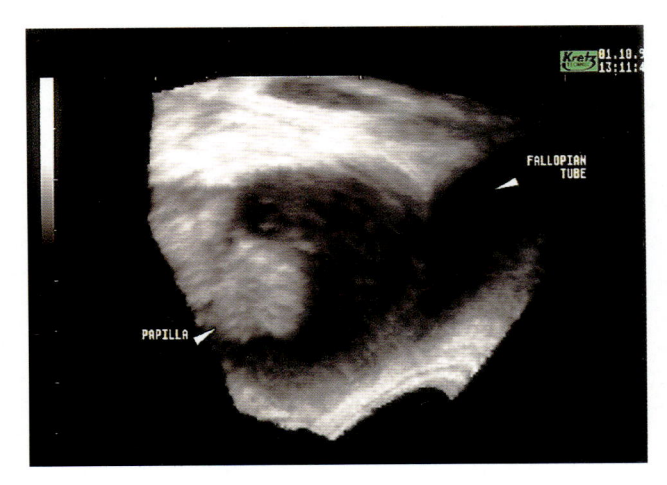

Figure 6 Transvaginal three-dimensional scan of a primary Fallopian tube carcinoma. Note the sausage-shaped structure with papillary projections protruding from the ampullar part of the tube

Figure 7 Demonstration of irregular vessels within a papillary protrusion, suggestive of tubal malignancy

was adjusted as follows: both color density and color quality were as low as necessary to obtain a good color image, while the pulse repetition frequency was as high as possible in order to display the targeted flow velocity. The spatial peak temporal average (SPTA) intensity was approximately 80 mW/cm. Wall filters (50 Hz) were used to eliminate low-frequency signals. The patient examination time by 3D power Doppler was 3 min. Using the fast line density, the average acquisition time was 48 s (range 25–88 s). At the end of each examination, combined color and gray rendering mode was used, allowing simultaneous analysis of the morphology, texture and vascularization. The subsequent analysis of the power Doppler reformatted sections lasted between 5 and 10 min. Demonstration of the chaotic, randomly dispersed vessels with irregular branching within the papillary protrusions and/or solid parts was suggestive of tubal malignancy (Figure 7). Other structural abnormalities of the malignant tumor vessels were microaneurysms, arteriovenous shunts, tumoral lakes, disproportional calibration, coiling and dichotomous branching. Using the above-mentioned criteria, five cases of Fallopian tube carcinoma were successfully identified prior to surgery. They all presented a non-pathognomonic appearance by B-mode ultrasound: the image was usually similar to that of pyosalpinx or a fluid-filled tube with a significant solid component adjacent to the tube (Figure 8). Three-dimensional transvaginal ultrasound produced a more precise distinction of the tubal mass from that of the ovary, cervix and uterus (Figure 9). Furthermore, the change in shape and size of the mass and passage of free fluid from the tubal mass through the uterine cavity could be documented dynamically. The three perpendicular planes displayed simultaneously on the screen provided the opportunity of obtaining multiple sections of the tortu-

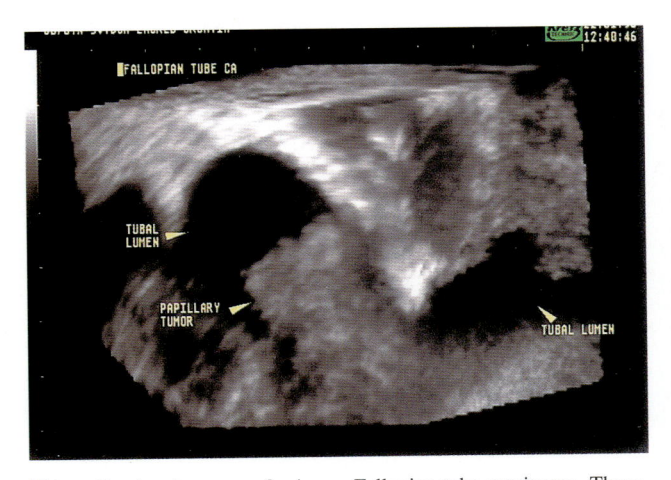

Figure 8 Another case of primary Fallopian tube carcinoma. Three-dimensional ultrasound allows papillary protrusions to be precisely depicted within the sausage-shaped structure measuring 4.0 × 3.0 × 2.6 cm. Histopathology confirmed tubal malignancy

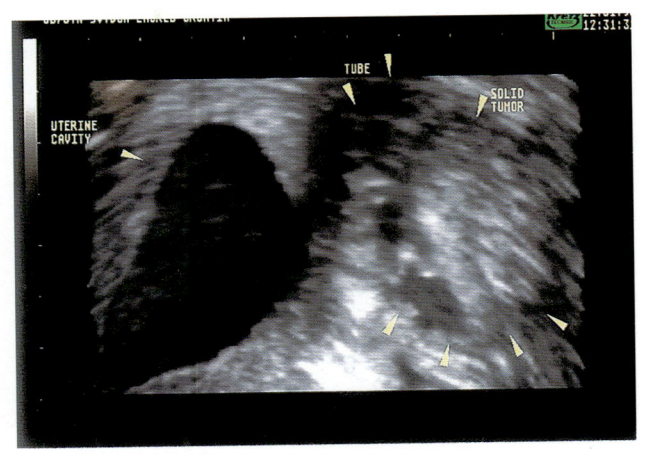

Figure 9 Transvaginal three-dimensional scan of the solid tumor within the Fallopian tube (the same patient as in Figure 8). Note the distension of the uterine cavity on the left and the irregular surface of the solid tumoral counterpart on the right

ous adnexal lesion by rotation and translation in any planes. The ability to reconstruct 3D plastic images improved the recognition of the anatomy of the adnexal lesion, characterization of the surface features and determination of the extent of tumor infiltration through the capsule (Figures 10 and 11).

The niche aspect of 3D ultrasound revealed intratumoral structures in selected sections, which was mandatory for evaluation of the tubal pathology. Multiple sections of the tumor, rotation, translation and reconstruction allowed prediction of the tumor spread to the uterus and/or the ovary or other surrounding structures. A shortened scanning time and detailed analysis of the stored data by a trained and experienced ultrasonographer were additional advantages of 3D over 2D sonography.

Indeed, tubal malignancy displays angiogenesis, which can be detected by color and pulsed Doppler[48–50]. Reports from the literature demonstrate the potential of transvaginal color Doppler to depict tumor neovascularization and low resistance indices (below 0.40) typical of tubal malignancy.

Malignant tumor vessels that are usually randomly dispersed within the central and peripheral parts demonstrate an irregular course, complicated branching and disproportional calibration – features that can be recognized using 3D power Doppler technology (Figure 12). Although it is mostly qualitative, it allows the ultrasonographer to understand the 3D architecture of the microcirculation interactively and to recognize blind ends, tumoral lakes, microaneurysms and arteriovenous shunting. It is expected that further technological development will incorporate the mathematical models assessing 3D vascular chaos and fractals in the 3D power Doppler units. Improved detection and classification of tumor architecture might contribute to better preoperative diagnosis of Fallopian tube carcinoma (Figure 13).

Figure 10 Three-dimensional image of a Fallopian tube carcinoma. Surface features such as papillary protrusions and thickened tubal wall suggest tubal malignancy

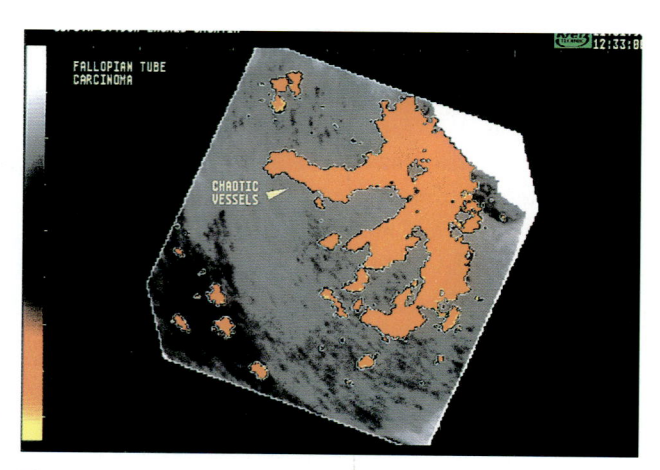

Figure 12 Vascular geometry of the vessels involved in the papillary protrusion indicates Fallopian tube malignancy. One can visualize disproportional calibration of the vessels, microaneurysms, tumoral lakes and dichotomous branching

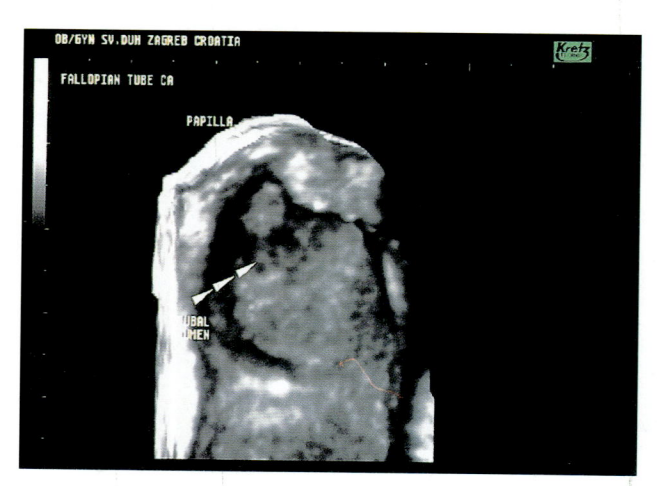

Figure 11 The same patient as in Figure 10. Three-dimensional plastic images enable visualization of the tubal wall and determination of the tumor infiltration through the capsule

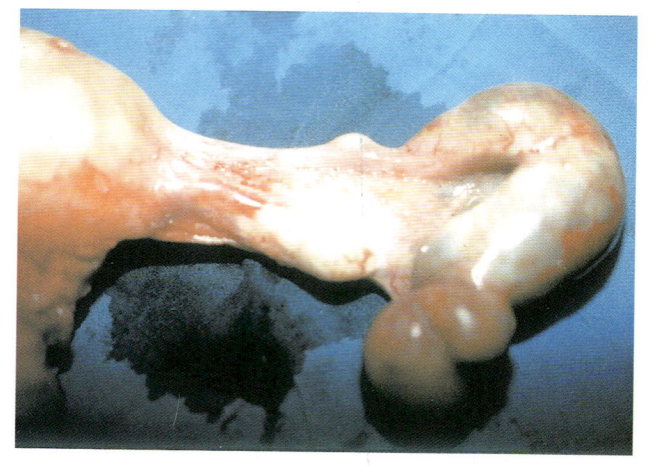

Figure 13 Primary carcinoma of the Fallopian tube. Pathological specimen showing large Fallopian tube measuring 8.4 × 4.5 × 6.0 cm and of fusiform appearance. The uterus, contralateral ovary and tube are normal

References

1. Timor-Tritsch IE, Rottem S. Transvaginal ultrasonographic study of the Fallopian tube. *Obstet Gynecol* 1987;70:424–8
2. Timor-Tritsch IE, Bar-Yam Y, Elgali S, Rottem S. The technique of transvaginal sonography with use of a 6.5 MHz probe. *Am J Obstet Gynecol* 1988;158:1019
3. Timor-Tritsch IE, Rottem S, Lewit N. The Fallopian tubes. In Timor-Tritsch IE, Rottem S, eds. *Transvaginal Sonography*, 2nd edn. New York: Elsevier, 1991:131–44
4. Westroem L, Wolner-Hanssen P. Pathogenesis of pelvic inflammatory disease. *Genitourin Med* 1993;69:9–17
5. Toth M, Chervenak FA. Color Doppler ultrasound in the diagnosis of pelvic inflammatory disease. In Kurjak A, ed. *An Atlas of Transvaginal Color Doppler*. Carnforth, UK: Parthenon Publishing, 1994:215–21
6. Patten RM, Vincent LM, Wolner-Hanssen P, Thorpe E Jr. Pelvic inflammatory disease: endovaginal sonography with laparoscopic correlation. *J Ultrasound Med* 1990;9:681–9
7. Kupesic S, Kurjak A, Pasalic L, Benic S, Ilijas M. The value of transvaginal color Doppler in the assessment of pelvic inflammatory disease. *Ultrasound Med Biol* 1995;21:733–8
8. Kurjak A, Zalud I, Jurkovic D, Alfirevic Z, Miljan, M. Transvaginal color Doppler for the assessment of the pelvic circulation. *Acta Obstet Gynecol Scand* 1989;68:131–4
9. Collins W, Jurkovic D, Kurjak A, Campbell S. Ovarian morphology, endocrine function and intrafollicular blood flow during the periovulatory period. *Hum Reprod* 1991;6:319–29
10. Kurjak A, Kupesic S, Schulman H, Zalud I. Transvaginal color Doppler in the assessment of the ovarian and uterine blood flow in infertile women. *Fertil Steril* 1991;56:870–3
11. Bourne T. Transvaginal colour Doppler in gynaecology. *Ultrasound Obstet Gynecol* 1992;80:359–73
12. Kurjak A, Zalud I, Alfirevic Z. Evaluation of adnexal masses with transvaginal color ultrasound. *J Ultrasound Med* 1991;10:295–9
13. Kurjak A, Zalud I, Schulman H. Ectopic pregnancy: transvaginal color Doppler study of trophoblastic flow in questionable adnexa. *J Ultrasound Med* 1991;10:685–9
14. Kurjak A, Predanic M, Kupesic S, Jukic S. Transvaginal color Doppler for the assessment of adnexal tumor vascularity. *Gynecol Oncol* 1993;50:3–9
15. Tinkannen H, Kujansuu E. Doppler ultrasound findings in tubo-ovarian infectious complex. *J Clin Ultrasound* 1993;21:175–8
16. Jurkovic D, Bourne TH, Jauniaux E, Campbell S, Collins WP. Transvaginal color Doppler study of blood flow in ectopic pregnancies. *Fertil Steril* 1992;57:68–73
17. Kurjak A, Predanic M. New scoring system for prediction of ovarian malignancy based on transvaginal color Doppler sonography. *J Ultrasound Med* 1992;11:631–8
18. Teisala K, Heinonen PK, Punnonen JR. Transvaginal ultrasound in the diagnosis and treatment of tubo-ovarian abscess. *Br J Obstet Gynaecol* 1990;97:178–80
19. Pairleitner, H, Steiner H, Hasenoehrl G, Staudach A. Three-dimensional power Doppler sonography: imaging and quantifying blood flow and vascularization. *Ultrasound Obstet Gynecol* 1999;14:139–43
20. Thorsen MK, Lawson TL, Aiman EJ, et al. Diagnosis of ectopic pregnancy: endovaginal vs transabdominal sonography. *Am J Roentgenol* 1990;155:307–10
21. Rempen A. Experience with 108 extrauterine pregnancies examined with vaginal sonography. *Ultrasound Obstet Gynecol* 1992;2(Suppl 1):151
22. Brown DL, Doubilet PM. Transvaginal sonography for diagnosing ectopic pregnancy: positivity criteria and performance characteristics. *J Ultrasound Med* 1994;13:259–66
23. Jurkovic D, Bourne TH, Jauniaux E, Campbell S, Collins WP. Transvaginal color Doppler study of blood flow in ectopic pregnancies. *Fertil Steril* 1992;57:68–72
24. Rempen A. The shape of the endometrium evaluated with three-dimensional ultrasound: an additional predictor of extrauterine pregnancy. *Hum Reprod* 1998;13:450–4
25. Harika G, Gabriel R, Carre-Pigeon F, Alemany L, Quereux C, Wahl P. Primary application of three-dimensional ultrasonography to early diagnosis of ectopic pregnancy. *Eur J Obstet Gynecol Reprod Biol* 1995;60:117–20
26. Woodruff JD, Pauerstein CJ. *The Fallopian Tube*. Baltimore: Williams and Wilkins, 1969
27. Mroueh J, Margono F, Feinkind L. Tubal pregnancy associated with ampullary tubal leiomyoma. *Obstet Gynecol* 1993;81:880–2
28. Sedlis A. Carcinoma of the Fallopian tube. *Surg Clin North Am* 1978;58:121
29. Ayhan A, Deren D, Yuce K, Tuncer Z, Mecan G. Primary carcinoma of the Fallopian tube: a study of 8 cases. *Eur J Gynecol Oncol* 1994;15:147–51
30. Dava D, Young RH, Scully RE. Endometrioid carcinoma of the Fallopian tube resembling an adnexal tumor of probable Wolffian origin: a report of six cases. *Int J Gynecol Pathol* 1992;11:122–30
31. Soundara RS, Ramdas CP, Reddi RP, Oumachigni A, Rajaram P, Reddy KS. A review of Fallopian tube carcinoma over 20 years (1971-90) in Pondicherry. *Indian J Cancer* 1991;28:188–95
32. Chiou YK, Su IJ, Chen CA, Hsieh CY. Malignant mixed Muellerian tumor of the Fallopian tube. *J Formos Med Assoc* 1991;90:793–5
33. Chang HC, Hsueh S, Soong YK. Malignant mixed Muellerian tumor of the Fallopian tube. Case report and review of literature. *Chang Keng I Hsueh* 1991;14:259–63
34. Tokunaga T, Miyazaki K, Okamura H. Pathology of the Fallopian tube. *Curr Opin Obstet Gynecol* 1991;3:574–9
35. Subramayon BR, Raghavendra BN, Whalen CA, Ye J. Ultrasonic features of Fallopian tube carcinoma. *J Ultrasound Med* 1984;3:391–3

36. Meyer JS, Kim CS, Price HM, Cooke JK. Ultrasound presentation of primary carcinoma of the Fallopian tube. *J Clin Ultrasound* 1987;15:132–4
37. Ajjimakorn S, Bhamarapravati Y. Transvaginal ultrasound and the diagnosis of Fallopian tubal carcinoma. *J Clin Ultrasound* 1991;19:116–19
38. Granberg S, Jansson I. Early detection of primary carcinoma of the Fallopian tube by endovaginal ultrasound. *Acta Obstet Gynecol Scand* 1997;69:667–8
39. Slanetz PJ, Whitman GJ, Halpern EF, Hall DA, Mc Carthy KA, Simeone JF. Imaging of the Fallopian tube tumors. *Am J Roentgenol* 1997;169:1321–4
40. Ong CL. Fallopian tube carcinoma with multiple tumor nodules seen on transvaginal sonography. *J Ultrasound Med* 1998;17:71–3
41. Hinton A, Bea C, Winfield AC, Entman SS. Carcinoma of the Fallopian tube. *Krol Radiol* 1988;10:113–15
42. Ekici E, Vicdan K, Danisman N, Soysal ME, Cobanoglu O, Gokmen O. Ultrasonographic appearance of Fallopian-tube carcinoma. *Int J Gynecol Obstet* 1992;49:325–9
43. McGoldrick JL, Strauss H, Rao J. Primary carcinoma of the Fallopian tube. *Am J Surg* 1943;59:559–63
44. Eddy GL, Schlaerth JB, Nalick RH, Gadis OJ, Nakamuira RM, Morrow CP. Fallopian tube carcinoma. *Obstet Gynecol* 1984;64:546–51
45. Lerner JP, Timor-Tritsch IE, Federmann A, Abramovich G. Transvaginal ultrasonographic characterization of ovarian masses with an improved weighted scoring system. *Am J Obstet Gynecol* 1994;170:81–5
46. Bourne TH, Campbell S, Steer C, Whitehead MI, Collins WP. Transvaginal color flow imaging a possible new screening technique for ovarian cancer. *Br Med J* 1994;299:1367–71
47. Kawai M, Kano T, Kikkawa F, Maeda O, Oguchi H, Tomoda Y. Transvaginal Doppler ultrasound with color flow imaging in the diagnosis of ovarian cancer. *Obstet Gynecol* 1992;79:463–6
48. Shalan H, Sosic A, Kurjak A. Fallopian tube carcinoma: recent diagnostic approach by color Doppler imaging. *Ultrasound Obstet Gynecol* 1992;2:297–9
49. Podobnik M, Singer Z, Ciglar S, Bulic M. Preoperative diagnosis of primary Fallopian tube carcinoma by transvaginal ultrasound, cytological finding and CA-125. *Ultrasound Med Biol* 1993;19:587–91
50. Kurjak A, Kupesic S, Ilijas M, Sparac V, Kosuta D. Preoperative diagnosis of primary Fallopian tube carcinoma. *Gynecol Oncol* 1998;68:29–34
51. Kurjak A, Kupesic S, Jacobs I. Preoperative diagnosis of the primary Fallopian tube carcinoma by three-dimensional static and power Doppler sonography. *Ultrasound Obstet Gynecol* 2000;15:246–51
52. Kol S, Gal D, Friedman M, Paldi E. Preoperative diagnosis of primary Fallopian tube carcinoma by transvaginal sonography and CA 125. *Gynecol Oncol* 1990;37:129–37
53. Kurjak A, Kupesic S, Breyer B, Sparac V, Jukic S. The assessment of ovarian tumor angiogenesis: what does three-dimensional power Doppler add? *Ultrasound Obstet Gynecol* 1998;12:136–46

The assessment of uterine lesions

6

S. Kupesic, A. Kurjak and D. Bjelos

The aim of this chapter is to investigate the role of three-dimensional (3D) and power Doppler ultrasound in the evaluation of uterine lesions. Morphological and vascular criteria assessed by different forms of ultrasound are listed for each type of uterine lesion.

The uterus lies in the middle of the pelvis. Its long axis is perpendicular to the ultrasound probe. Using two-dimensional (2D) ultrasound the examination of uterine lesions is limited to transverse and sagittal planes, which give an inadequate view of the uterus and uterine pathology. Three-dimensional ultrasound provides simultaneous display of coronal, sagittal and transverse planes. Volume data can be viewed using a standard anatomic orientation demonstrating the entire volume and continuity of curved structures in a single image. More accurate evaluation of sections through the studied organ becomes possible because of their unlimited number and the orientation of reformatted planes. When three perpendicular planes are simultaneously displayed on the screen, the sagittal plane is chosen for volume measurements, while the other two planes are used to ensure that the entire pathology is included in the measurement (Figure 1). The surface rendering mode allows exploration of the outer or inner contour of the lesion, while the niche aspect is used for detection and analysis of the selected sections of the uterine lesion. Three-dimensional ultrasound offers improved visualization of a lesion, more accurate volume estimation, retrospective review of stored data and assessment of tumor invasion. Using rendered images, it can more accurately locate abnormalities needing surgical intervention. Three-dimensional hysterosonography is very useful in the evaluation of the uterine cavity and is more useful than hysterosonography by 2D transvaginal ultrasound in cases of submucous myomas and polyps. The 3D power Doppler system improves the information available on tumor vascularity, enabling visualization of overlapping vessels and assessment of their relationship to other vessels or surrounding tissue. Power Doppler ultrasound compared to standard color Doppler has the advantage of greater sensitivity to low-velocity flow, overcoming angle dependence and aliasing.

In this chapter we compare findings of uterine lesions assessed with conventional B-mode and transvaginal color Doppler ultrasound on the one hand, and 3D and power Doppler ultrasound on the other.

The normal uterus

Two-dimensional ultrasound imaging of the uterus is limited by the movement of the transducer that produces sagittal and transverse planes. Three-dimensional sonography permits multiplanar display of all three perpendicular sections: coronal, sagittal and transverse. The coronal plane of the uterus is used to visualize both horns of the endometrium and the cervix at the same time. The normal uterus usually shows a convex shape of the endometrium and myometrium in the fundus (Figure 2). The endometrium appears as an echogenic interface in the central part of the uterus, but its thickness and echogenicity are dependent on the concentration of circulating estrogen and progesterone. Endometrial thickness of less than 5 mm is usually associated with the early follicular phase, whereas with approaching ovulation the expected endometrial thickness reaches about 10 mm. A triple-line endometrium is typical of the follicular phase. During the secretory phase, the endometrium becomes hyperechoic and homogeneous.

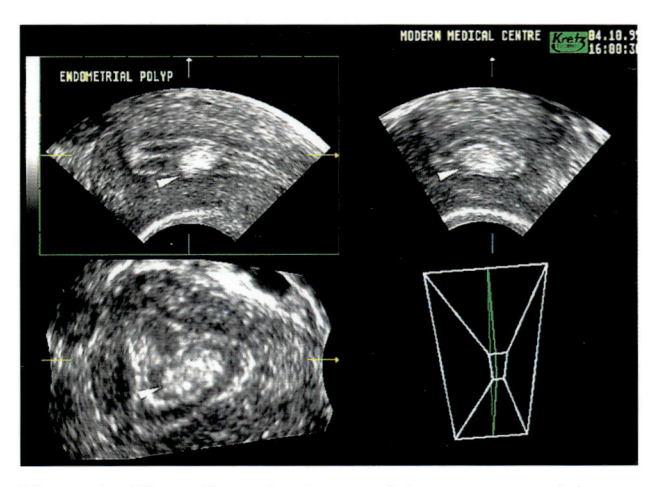

Figure 1 Three-dimensional scan of the uterus containing an endometrial polyp. Three perpendicular planes are simultaneously displayed on the screen, enabling precise exploration of the uterine cavity

CLINICAL APPLICATION OF 3D SONOGRAPHY

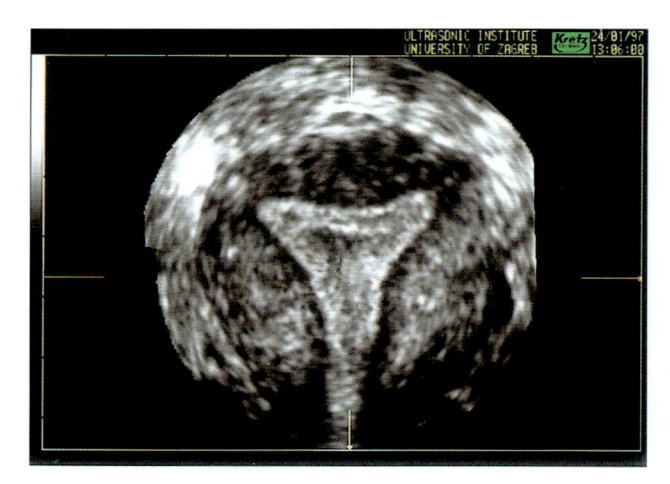

Figure 2 Planar section through a normal uterus, showing the convex shape of the uterine fundus and the straight upper border of the uterine cavity

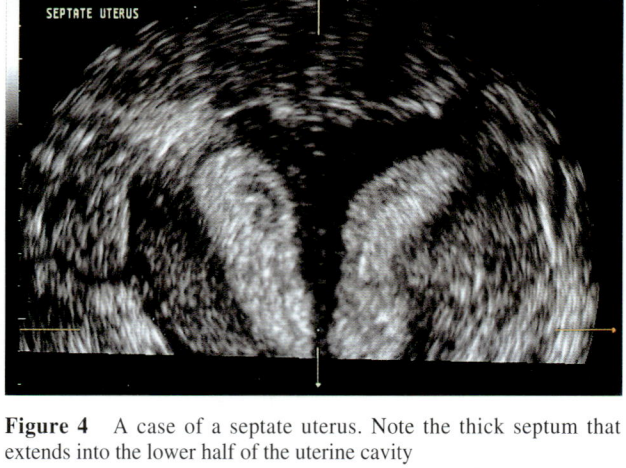

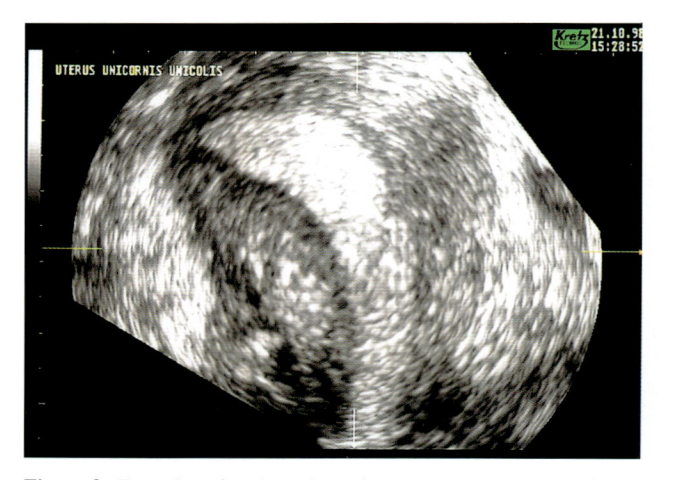

Figure 4 A case of a septate uterus. Note the thick septum that extends into the lower half of the uterine cavity

Figure 3 Frontal section through a unicornuate uterus. Note the irregular shape of the uterine cavity on the right

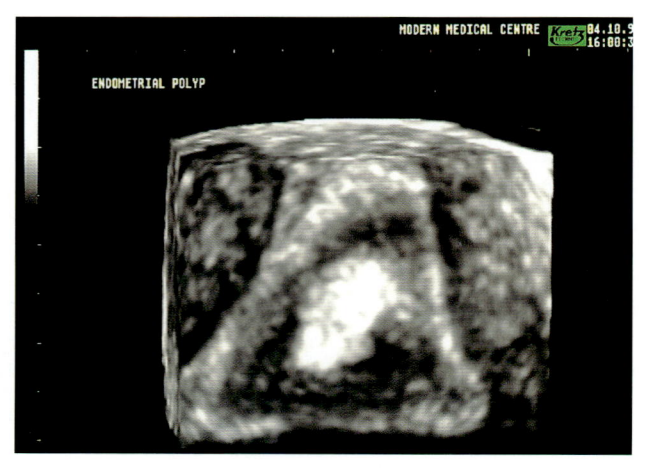

Figure 5 Surface rendering of an endometrial polyp

Since changes in the texture and volume of the endometrium can be precisely observed by 3D ultrasound, and can be retrospectively reviewed or be the subject of consultation with colleagues, this method may become the method of choice for scanning endometrial pathology in a multitude of clinical conditions (Figures 3 and 4).

Endometrial polyps

Endometrial polyps develop as solitary or multiple, soft, sessile and penduculated tumors containing hyperplastic endometrium[1,2]. Clinically, patients with endometrial polyps can be asymptomatic or show symptoms such as infertility, bleeding, infection, endometritis or pain. The ultrasonographic appearance of endometrial polyps is best imaged during the early proliferative phase of the menstrual cycle or during the secretory phase after injection of a negative contrast medium into the uterine cavity. The vascularization of polyps is supported by already existing vessels originating from terminal branches of the uterine arteries, and these can be assessed by transvaginal color Doppler ultrasound. The resistance index (RI) is moderate, usually higher than 0.45[1,3]. Infection or necrosis of polyps may lower the impedance to blood flow. The importance of endometrial polyps lies in the fact that marked reduction in blood flow impedance noted on the periphery and/or within the endometrial polyps may lead an inexperienced ultrasonographer to a false-positive diagnosis of endometrial malignancy.

Three-dimensional hysterosonography can better visualize the uterine cavity and endometrial thickness than can transvaginal sonography, transvaginal 2D hystersonography, transvaginal color Doppler, or hysteroscopy[4]. Using the multiplanar views, polypoid structures can be clearly visualized, allowing for the optimal plane to present their pedicle (Figure 1). The surface-rendering mode can suppress undesirable echoes allowing the polypoid structure to be seen in continuity with the endometrial lining[5] (Figure 5).

THE ASSESSMENT OF UTERINE LESIONS

Gruboeck and co-workers[6] measured endometrial thickness by conventional 2D ultrasound and endometrial volume by 3D ultrasound in symptomatic postmenopausal patients, and they compared the results. The volume measurement was performed using the longitudinal plane delineating the whole of the uterine cavity in a number of parallel longitudinal sections 1–2 mm apart. The endometrial volume was calculated automatically by the in-built computer software. The endometrial thickness was similar in patients with endometrial hyperplasia and polyps, but the endometrial volume in hyperplasia was significantly higher than the volume in patients with polyps. They concluded that the difference between endometrial hyperplasia and polyps cannot be detected by the measurement of endometrial thickness, but by 3D volume measurement (Figure 6). Polyps are localized thickenings of the endometrium not affecting the whole of the uterine cavity, and therefore their volume is much smaller, while the maximum thickness is similar to that of hyperplasia (Figure 7).

Intrauterine synechiae (adhesions)

Hysterosonography performed with 3D ultrasound has several advantages over that with conventional 2D ultrasound. It gives more accurate information about the location of abnormalities which is very important for preoperative assessment and the distinguishing of pathologies. Furthermore, the uterus is distended for a shorter time than that necessary for 2D examinations, resulting in better acceptance by patients. According to Momtaz and El Ebrashi[7], in cases of intrauterine adhesions the use of echogenic contrast media (e.g. Echovist, Schering) is more accurate than saline-contrast 3D hysterosonography. Intrauterine synechiae can be accurately visualized on both multiplanar and rendered imaging traversing the uterine cavity[5]. Weinraub and colleagues[5] concluded that surface rendering in cases of equivocal signals confirmed their presence, appearance, actual size, volume and relationship to the surrounding structures.

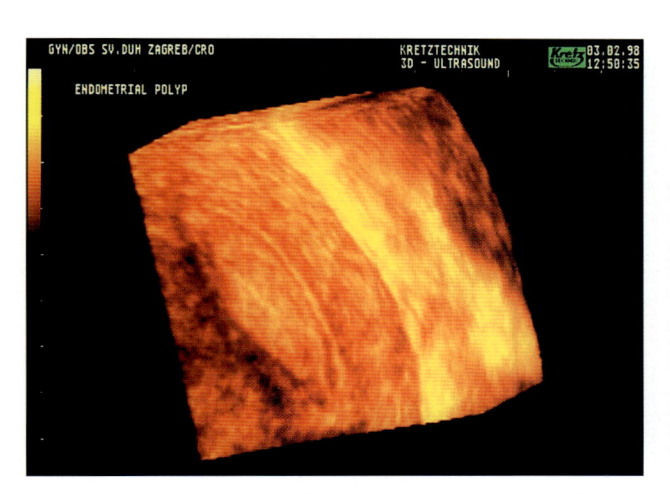

Figure 6 Another example of an endometrial polyp. Note that the uterine cavity is completely occupied by the endometrial polyp

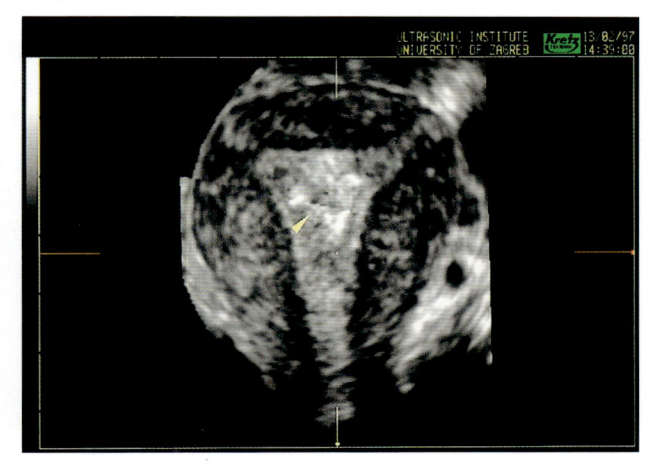

Figure 8 Frontal section through the uterus in a patient with mild intrauterine synechiae. The endometrial volume is not restricted in this particular patient

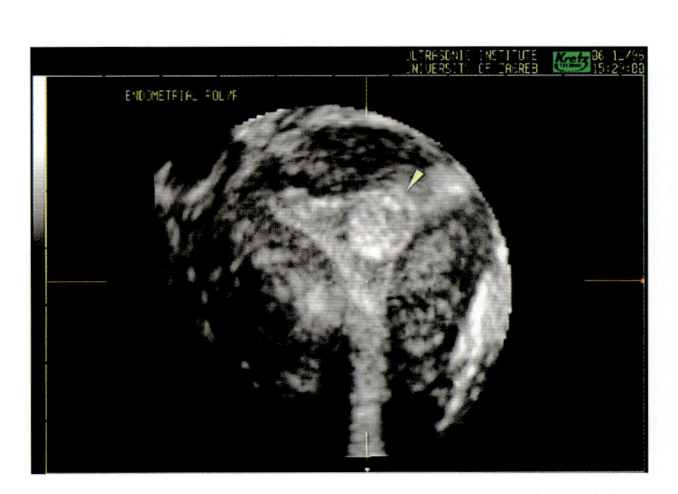

Figure 7 Frontal section through the uterus in a patient with an endometrial polyp in the left uterine cornum

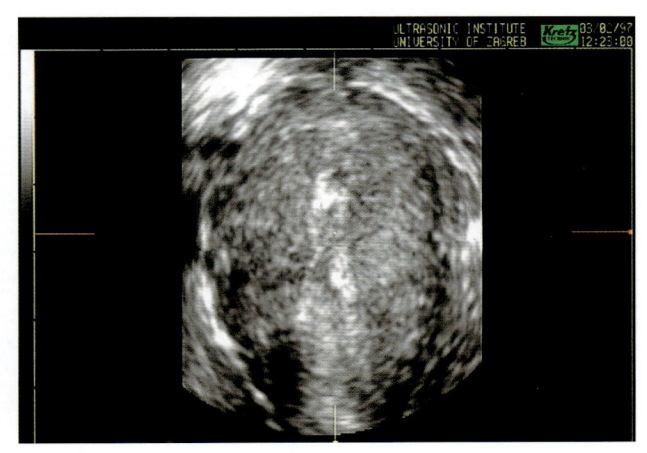

Figure 9 Irregular shape of the uterus in a patient with severe intrauterine synechiae. Note the reduced endometrial volume

Three-dimensional ultrasound is helpful in delineation of intracavitary adhesions and determination of their location which assists in surgical planning (Figure 8). In the case of bridging adhesions, the degree of cavity obliteration is accurately assessed (Figure 9). Similarly, this technique is beneficial for differentiation between small polyps and adhesions.

Adenomyosis

Adenomyosis of the uterus is a condition in which clusters of endometrial tissue ingrow into the myometrium. It may be localized close to the endometrium, or it may extend through the myometrium and serosa. Adenomyosis affects 20% of women, mainly multiparous women. The uterus can be normal-sized or enlarged with symptoms such as dysmenorrhea, pelvic pain and menometrorrhagia.

Two-dimensional ultrasound findings include the 'Swiss-cheese' appearance of the myometrium due to areas of hemorrhage and clots within the muscle (Figure 10). Disordered echogenicity of the middle layer of the myometrium is usually present in severe cases. Sometimes the uterus is generally hypoechoic, with the large cysts rarely seen. Using hysterosonography, contrast medium penetrates the myometrium. Color Doppler characteristics show increased vascularity by moderate vascular resistance within the myometrium (RI = 0.56 ± 0.12), while the RI of the uterine arteries shows decreased values compared to controls[8]. Statistically significant differences exist between adenomyosis and uterine malignancies in both RI and maximum velocity. However, no significant difference was noted between adenomyosis and myoma in the RI but a slight difference was observed in the maximum velocity[9].

In some cases, transonic areas may not represent adenomyosis, but prominent vessels, or other conditions that give rise to hyperemia. Lee and co-workers[10] performed a study that confirmed the superiority of 3D power Doppler sonography over transvaginal color Doppler ultrasound in the detection of flow in the areas of adenomyosis. Women with a provisional diagnosis of adenomyosis, listed for hysterectomy, were studied. Gray-scale ultrasound was first used to screen for the presence of adenomyosis using predetermined ultrasound criteria, and this was followed by 3D power Doppler sonography of the adenomyotic areas. The ultrasound findings such as distribution of vessels and pattern of flow in adenomyotic foci were compared with histological results. Using 3D power Doppler sonography, the authors were able to demonstrate the perfusion in adenomyotic foci as well as regular vessel distribution and branching pattern.

Endometrial hyperplasia

The endometrial thickness in postmenopausal women is no more than a thin line of 1–3 mm in thickness. Abnormal endometrial thickness may be detected in some benign uterine conditions, as well as in endometrial malignancy. Endometrial thickness greater than 14 mm in premenopausal and greater than 5 mm in postmenopausal women should be further investigated[1].

Bonilla-Musoles and co-workers suggest that, in patients on hormone replacement therapy or tamoxifen, 3D hysterosonography allowed for differentiation of normal proliferative endometrium from hyperplastic endometrium[8].

Using B-mode transvaginal sonography alone it is not possible to distinguish endometrial hyperplasia from carcinoma. More accurate diagnosis of endometrial pathology can be obtained by color and pulsed Doppler sonography[2,3]. Color Doppler findings characteristic of endometrial hyperplasia include peripheral distribution of regularly separated vessels with an RI significantly higher (mean RI = 0.65 ± 0.05) than in carcinoma (mean RI = 0.42 ± 0.02)[11]. However, reliable differentiation between endometrial hyperplasia and carcinoma is not possible, owing to an overlap in the endometrial thickness measurements, as well as to controversial results of blood flow measurements assessed by transvaginal color Doppler ultrasound. Since there is a positive correlation between arterial blood flow impedance and number of years from menopause[12], one can estimate the risk of uterine

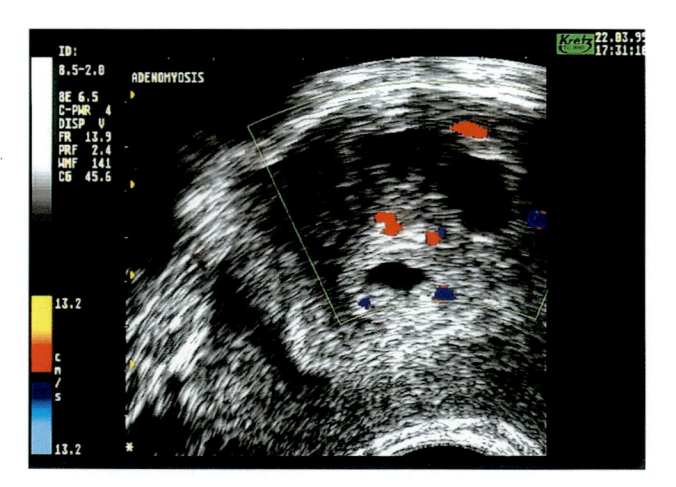

Figure 10 Transvaginal color Doppler scan of an adenomyotic uterus. Note the 'Swiss cheese' appearance of the myometrium due to areas of hemorrhage and clots within the muscle. Color Doppler reveals increased vascularity within the adenomyotic foci

malignancy in postmenopausal patients with decreased vascular resistance.

With the aid of 3D ultrasound, endometrial volume measurements have become possible (Figure 11). Gruboeck and co-workers[6] successfully measured endometrial volume in 94.2% of patients, while in others the presence of anterior uterine wall myomas caused acoustic shadowing on 3D records. The volume of the endometrium was measured by delineating the uterine cavity on parallel longitudinal sections 1–2 mm apart. The sections were added together using in-built computer software to calculate the volume. The endometrial volume was significantly lower in patients with benign pathology such as hyperplasia (mean 8.0 ml, SD 7.81 ml) than in patients with endometrial carcinoma (mean 39.0 ml, SD 34.16 ml). The normal endometrial volume of postmenopausal patients in this study was 0.9 ml (SD 1.72 ml).

Our group reported on the use of 3D power Doppler sonography in patients with endometrial hyperplasia[13]. We were able to demonstrate regularly separated vessels at the periphery of the hyperplastic endometrium.

Endometrial carcinoma

Endometrial carcinoma is the most common gynecological malignancy in many countries, with a reported incidence of about 10% in postmenopausal patients presenting uterine bleeding. Early transabdominal sonographic investigations demonstrated that increased endometrial thickness is associated with endometrial neoplasms in postmenopausal women[14,15], but the quality of transabdominal sonographic images is affected by obesity, retroversion of the uterus and an unfilled bladder, factors that do not influence transvaginal sonographic visualization of the endometrium[16–18]. Ultrasound findings assessed by conventional B-mode sonography include increased endometrial thickness of > 5 mm in postmenopausal women or > 8 mm in perimenopausal women, hyperechoic endometrium, free fluid in the cul-de-sac, intrauterine fluid or possible invasion in patients with a disrupted endometrial–subendometrial layer. In addition, color and pulsed Doppler improves diagnostic accuracy, because the endometrial carcinoma shows abnormal blood flow due to tumor angiogenesis[19]. Endometrial blood flow is absent in normal, atrophic and most cases of endometrial hyperplasia, whereas, according to our investigation[11], in 91% of the cases of endometrial carcinoma, areas of neovascularization were demonstrated as intratumoral or peritumoral. Neovascular signals from the central parts of the lesion demonstrated low vascular resistance (RI = 0.42 ± 0.02), while increased vascularity signals surrounding the lesion are suspicious of invasion. If the myometrial vessels are invaded, low vascular resistance is detected, owing to incomplete or absent membrane and leaky structure.

Conventional 2D ultrasound measurements of endometrial thickness have disadvantages in distinguishing patients with benign and malignant endometrial pathology, owing to varying thickness and interference of other pathologies such as polyps or hypoplasia (Figure 12).

In disinguishing cancer from benign pathology, endometrial volume measurements assessed by 3D ultrasound seem to be more helpful. Gruboeck and associates[6] compared endometrial thickness and volume in patients with postmenopausal bleeding and examined the value of each parameter in differentiat-

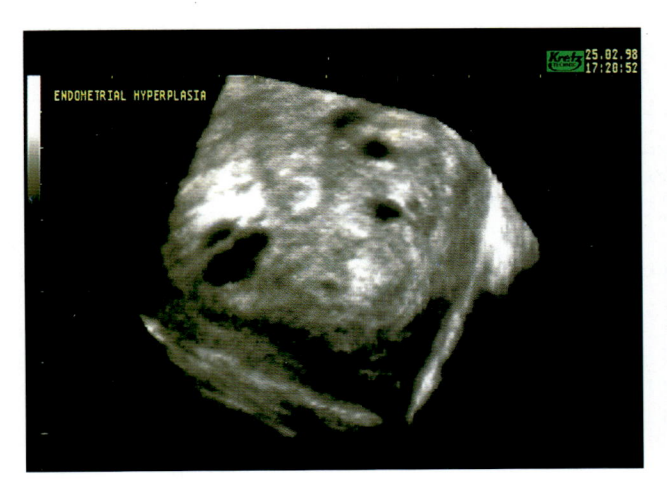

Figure 11 Three-dimensional image of a thick endometrium in a postmenopausal patient. Cystic inclusions are clearly displayed and indicate endometrial hyperplasia

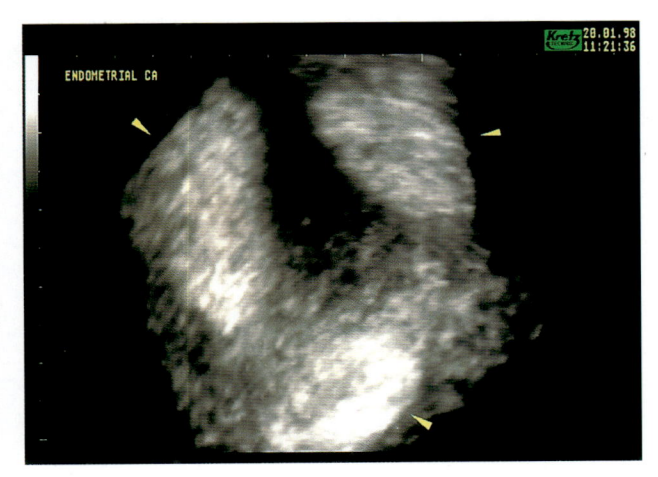

Figure 12 Increased endometrial volume in a patient with endometrial carcinoma

ing between benign and malignant endometrial pathology. Each patient underwent 3D ultrasonography for the measurement of endometrial thickness and volume. The results were compared to the histological diagnosis after endometrial biopsy or dilatation and curettage. The mean endometrial thickness in patients with endometrial cancer was 29.5 mm (SD 12.59) and the mean volume was 39.0 ml (SD 34.16). The optimal cut-off value of endometrial thickness for the diagnosis of cancer was 15 mm, with the test sensitivity of 83.3% and positive predictive value of 54.4%. With a cut-off level of 13 ml, the diagnosis of cancer was made with a sensitivity of 100%. One false-positive result in a patient with hyperplasia gave a specificity of 98.8% and positive predictive value of 91.7%. According to Gruboeck and co-workers[6] the endometrial volume was significantly higher in patients with carcinoma than in those with benign lesions. The measurement of endometrial volume was superior to that of endometrial thickness as a diagnostic test for endometrial cancer in symptomatic postmenopausal women. Increasing volume is associated with the severity or higher grade of the endometrial carcinoma, and also with progressive myometrial invasion. The depth of myometrial invasion showed a positive correlation with both endometrial thickness and volume. However, according to these authors, it is unlikely that measurement of tumor size will be more useful for the diagnosis of invasion than B-mode imaging. Only patients with a tumor volume larger than 25 ml had evidence of pelvic node involvement at operation.

Bonilla-Musoles and co-workers[4] suggest that 3D hysterosonography allowed for better visualization of myometrial invasion, and would play a significant role in the staging of malignant tumors in the future. With simultaneous display of the transverse plane with 3D ultrasound it is possible to detect the infiltration of cervical or endometrial carcinoma into the bladder or rectum.

In our study[13], apart from endometrial volume, other 3D sonographic and power Doppler criteria for the diagnosis of endometrial malignancy included regularity of the subendometrial halo, the presence of intracavitary fluid, chaotic vessel architecture and branching pattern (Table 1). In patients with endometrial carcinoma, the mean endometrial volume was 37.0 ± 31.8 ml (Table 2). The endometrial volume in hyperplasia had the mean value of 7.82 ± 7.60 ml and was significantly higher than the volume in patients with polyps (mean 2.63 ± 2.12 ml). In patients with normal or atrophic endometrium, the mean volume was 0.8 ± 1.51 ml. The subendometrial halo was regular in all patients with benign endometrial pathology,

Table 1 Three-dimensional sonographic and power Doppler criteria for the diagnosis of endometrial malignancy. From reference 13, with permission

	Criteria	*Score*
Endometrial volume	<13 ml	0
	>13 ml	2
Subendometrial halo	regular	0
	disturbed	2
Intracavitary fluid	absent	0
	present	1
Vessel architecture	linear vessel	0
	chaotic vessel arrangement	2
Branching pattern	simple	0
	complex	2
Total score		

Total score is the sum of individual scores. The cut-off score, ≥ 4 is associated with a high risk of endometrial malignancy

Table 2 Volume and vascularity of the endometrial lesions (*n* = 57) obtained by three-dimensional power Doppler sonography. From reference 13, with permission

Histopathology	*n*	*Volume* (SD) ml	*Regular endometrial halo (%)*	*Intracavitary fluid (%)*	*Neovascular signals (%)*
Normal and/or atrophic endometrium	10	0.8 (1.51)	100	20.00	0
Endometrial hyperplasia	27	7.82 (7.60)	100	37.00	0
Endometrial polyp	28	2.63 (2.12)	100	35.71	3.57
Endometrial carcinoma	12	37.0 (31.8)	66.67	41.67	100

whereas eight out of 12 patients with endometrial carcinoma had an irregular endometrial–myometrial border (Figure 13). Intracavitary fluid was present in four patients with benign endometrial lesions and in five patients with endometrial malignancy. Dichotomous branching and randomly dispersed vessels were detected in 91.67% of the patients with endometrial carcinoma, while single vessel arrangement and regular branching were pathognomonic for benign lesions. Three-dimensional power Doppler sonography accurately detected structural abnormalities of the malignant tumor vessels such as microaneurysms, arteriovenous shunts, tumoral lakes, elongation and coiling (Figure 14). When morphological and power Doppler criteria were combined, the diagnosis of endometrial carcinoma had a sensitivity of 91.67%. One false-positive result was obtained in a patient with endometrial hyperplasia and one false-negative result in a patient with endometrial carcinoma receiving tamoxifen therapy. In this case the endometrial lesion demonstrated regularly separated peripheral vessels and was falsely interpreted as hyperplasia.

Kupesic and colleagues[20] performed staging of endometrial carcinoma by 3D power Doppler. The objective of this study was to evaluate the accuracy of 3D power Doppler in determining the depth of myometrial invasion in patients with proved adenocarcinoma of the endometrium, relative to the amount of myometrial invasion measured in histopathological analysis (Table 3). Eighteen patients with histologically proved adenocarcinoma of the endometrium were analyzed. Deep myometrial invasion (> 50%) was present at postoperative histology in five of 22 (22.73%) women (Figure 15), while superficial invasion was reported in 17 of 22 (77.27%) (Figure 16). Three-dimensional power Doppler demonstrated a sensitivity of 100% (4/4) and a specificity of 94.44% (17/18) for deep invasion, with a positive predictive value (PPV) of 83.33% (5/6) and a negative predictive value (NPV) of 100% (17/17). In only one patient with adenomyosis was invasion overestimated by 3D power Doppler. Data showed acceptable accuracy in determining the depth of myometrial invasion in patients with adenocarcinoma (Figure 17). Three-dimensional power Doppler can potentially detect lesions that require aggressive intervention and thus prompt appropriate treatment.

Leiomyoma

Leiomyomas are the most common tumors of the female pelvis and occur in 20–25% of women of reproductive age. They arise mostly from the smooth

Figure 13 The relationship between endometrial carcinoma and surrounding myometrium can be precisely assessed on reformatted sections. The frontal section enables analysis of the irregular endometrial contours indicative of endometrial carcinoma invasion

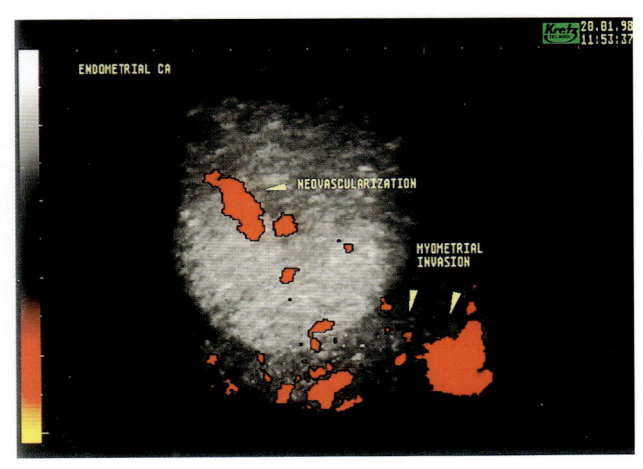

Figure 14 Three-dimensional power Doppler scan of an invasive endometrial carcinoma. Note the areas of neovascularization clearly displayed within the proximal portion of the myometrium

Table 3 Invasion of endometrial carcinoma assessed with the aid of three-dimensiinal (3D) power Doppler sonongraphy and tested by histopathology. From reference 20, with permission

Invasion	3D power Doppler	Histopathology
Superficial*	17	18
Deep†	5	4

* Invasion into less than half of the total myometrial thickness; † invasion into more than half of the myometrial thickness

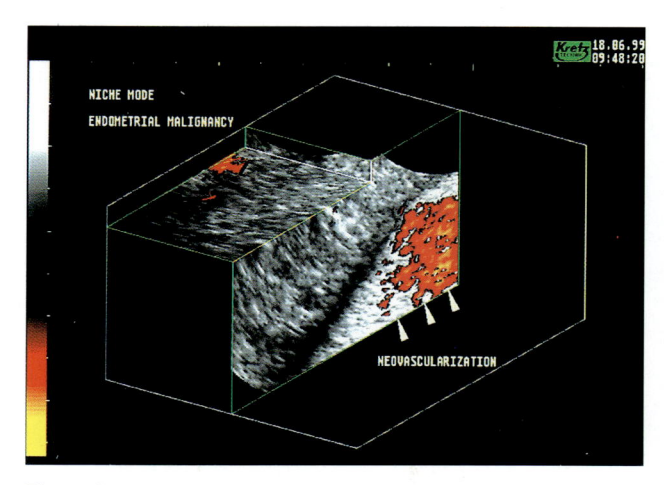

Figure 15 Reformatted sections (niche imaging) allow more precise estimation of the tumor spread by visualization of the affected myometrial vessels. Note the irregular course of the vessels within the distal half of the myometrium. Deep invasion by endometrial carcinoma was confirmed at the time of histopathology

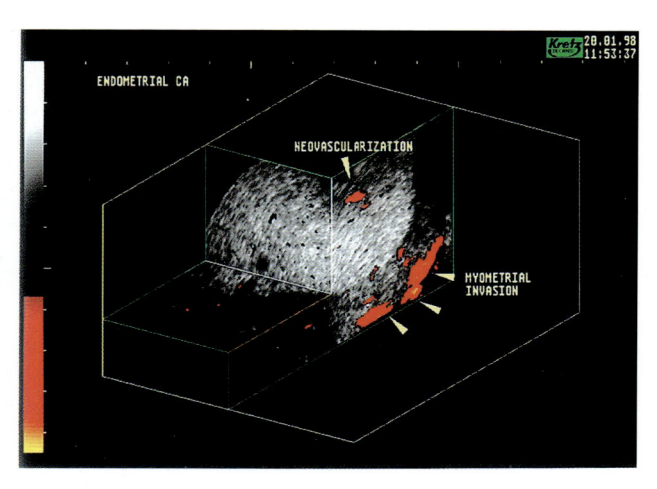

Figure 17 Another case of invasive endometrial carcinoma. Centrally located vessels are demonstrated by a frontal reformatted plane. Niche imaging allows simultaneous visualization of the irregular vessels within the myometrial portion of the uterus with the use of the longitudinal plane. Invasive endometrial carcinoma was confirmed by histopathology

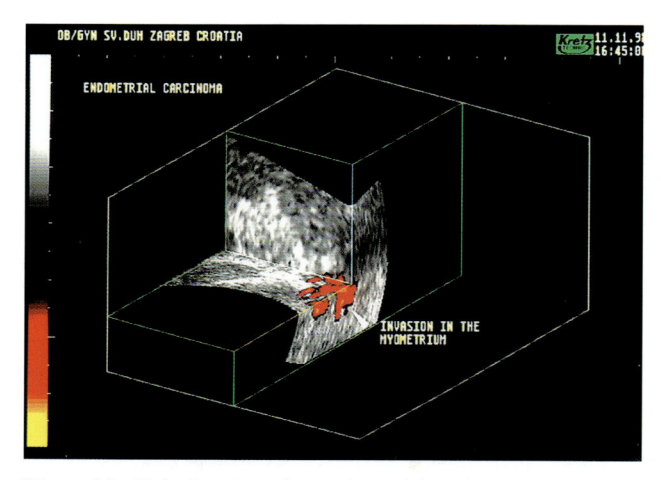

Figure 16 Niche imaging of an endometrial carcinoma with superficial myometrial invasion. Careful observation of the posterior uterine wall reveals an abnormal vascular pattern within the proximal portion of the myometrium, indicative of myometrial invasion

muscle and soft tissue of the uterine fundus and corpus, but 3% originate from the cervix[21]. Myomas are usually multiple and of various sizes. Intramural tumors are the most common, while the submucosal are the least common. If they extend outward, they become pedunculated or subserosal[22]. Symptoms of submucous leiomyomas include metrorrhagia, pelvic pain or infertility, whereas most subserosal leiomyomas are asymptomatic.

On gray-scale ultrasound imaging, the uterine leiomyomas may show uterine enlargement, distortion of the uterine contour and varying echogenicity, depending on the amount of connective or smooth muscle tissue.

Transvaginal color Doppler sonography demonstrates vascularization on the periphery of the myoma of uterine origin, with an RI of 0.54 ± 0.08, allowing better delineation of the tumor. Blood vessels in the central part of the myoma in case of necrosis, inflammation or other degenerative changes demonstrate lower RI. Uterine arteries present lower impedance to blood flow in patients with myomas (RI = 0.74 ± 0.09) than in normal women (RI = 0.84 ± 0.09)[23].

The simultaneous display of three perpendicular planes enables the accurate location of myomas, evaluation of their size and estimation of the relationship to the endometrium which is very important in therapy planning. Patients receiving medical therapy such as gonadotropin releasing hormone may be followed with serial 3D ultrasound scans to estimate myoma size and effectiveness of therapy. The size of myomas should be evaluated more accurately with 3D ultrasound using volume estimation than with 2D ultrasound, according to the reports of volume measurements in other organs, such as the liver[24] and bladder[25]. Hysterosonography by 3D ultrasound is valuable in obtaining submucosal myomas[4,5,26,27] (Figure 18). Balen and associates[26] found that 3D ultrasound and hysterosonography was useful in demonstrating the position of submucosal myomas (Figure 19). They studied both saline and a positive ultrasound contrast agent (Echovist) and found the positive contrast superior when looking at the cavity wall. Weinraub and colleagues[5] found that the negative contrast was better for evaluating the contents of the uterine cavity and delineating the outer surface of lesions, whereas positive contrast only created a cast of the cavity (Figure 20).

THE ASSESSMENT OF UTERINE LESIONS

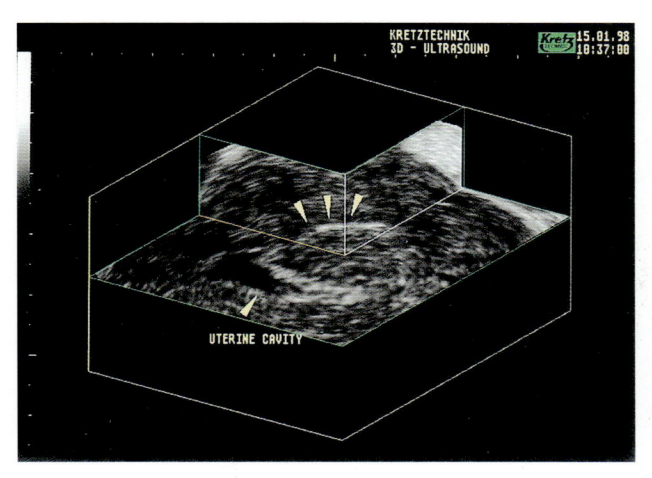

Figure 18 Niche imaging of a submucous leiomyoma occupying the majority of the uterine cavity

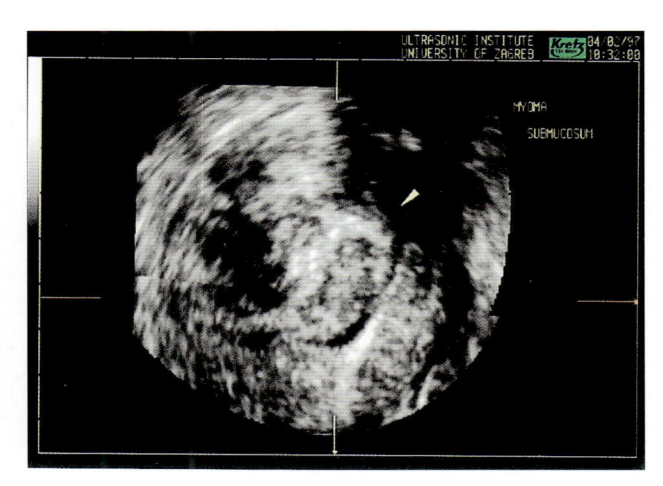

Figure 20 Another case of a submucous leiomyoma in an infertile patient. Anechoic contrast medium injected into the uterine cavity facilitates visualization of an intracavitary structure. A submucous leiomyoma was confirmed by hysteroscopy

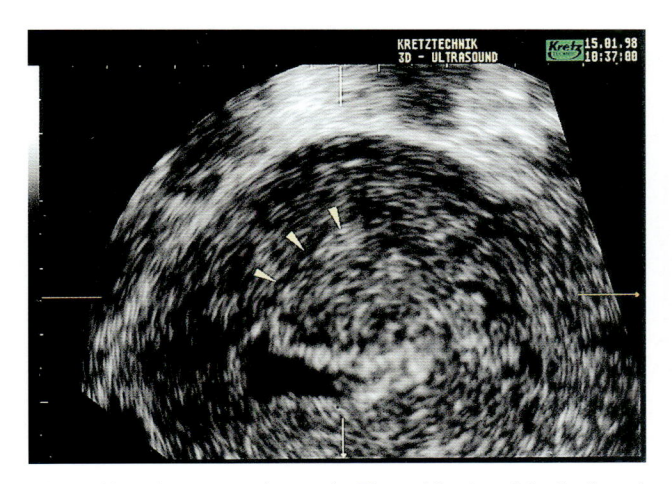

Figure 19 The same patient as in Figure 18, viewed in the frontal plane. Three-dimensional hysterosonography facilitates visualization of the submucous leiomyoma

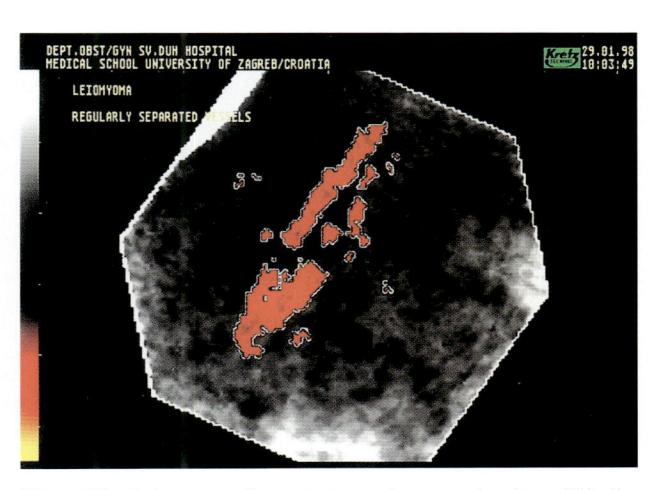

Figure 21 Leiomyoma demonstrates a clear vascular ring within the capsule

One limitation to scanning the uterus with myomas by 3D or 2D ultrasound is the significant shadowing from calcification. In our recent study[13] we evaluated myometrial lesions, morphology, volume and vascularization with 3D ultrasound and power Doppler sonography. The mean volume of the leiomyomas undergoing surgery was 78.52 ± 51.8 ml. In 84.38%, 3D power Doppler detected regular vascularity at the periphery (Figures 21 and 22), while in cases of secondary degenerative lesions the findings were suggestive of neovascularity, irregular branching and chaotic vascular arrangement, because necrosis, inflammation and degeneration altered the leiomyoma vasculature. In conclusion, because of the low PPV of 16.67%, this method should not be used for the evaluation of myometrial pathology, either benign or malignant.

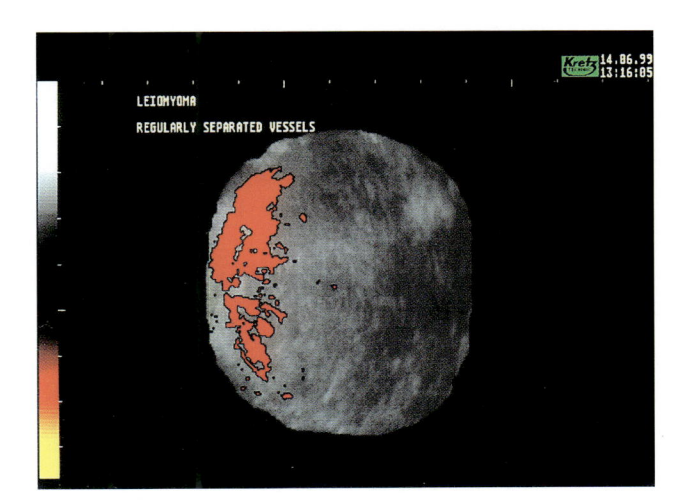

Figure 22 Another case of regularly separated vessels encircling the leiomyoma, as shown by three-dimensional power Doppler

Leiomyosarcoma

Uterine sarcoma is a rare tumor, accounting for only 1–3% of all genital tract tumors and 3–7.4% of malignant tumors of the uterine corpus[28], characterized by early dissemination and poor prognosis for survival. Through the years, several questions regarding these tumors have remained unanswered, and a method for their early and correct diagnosis is still unknown. Furthermore, uterine sarcoma is expected to become more common in the near future, as gynecologists are more frequently using conservative treatment for uterine myomas. Abnormal vaginal bleeding is the most common presenting symptom in patients with uterine sarcoma. Lower abdominal pain or pressure and a palpable abdominal mass are additional findings. An enlarged bulky uterus is palpated, and/or the tumor may be seen protruding through the cervix. Dilatation and curettage may be helpful in distinguishing benign from malignant pathology only if the tumor is submucosal. Clinically, a rapid increase in the size of a uterine tumor after the menopause arouses suspicion of sarcoma.

Ultrasonically, leiomyosarcoma is presented as a solid or solid–cystic structure, altering the echogenicity of the myometrium. On transvaginal color Doppler, the neovascularization of a leiomyosarcoma is detected at the border or in the center of the tumor with high blood flow velocity and low impedance to blood flow (RI = 0.37 ± 0.03), with irregular, thin, randomly dispersed vessels[29]. When a cut-off value for the RI of < 0.40 was used, this method reached a sensitivity of 90.91%, specificity of 99.82%, PPV of 71.43% and NPV of 99.96%[29]. Because of their rarity, uterine sarcomas are not suitable for screening. Transvaginal ultrasound can detect differences in myometrial tissue density, and therefore can be used for detection of uterine sarcoma, but because of low specificity this method is not appropriate as a screening procedure.

In our study[13], one patient with uterine leiomyosarcoma was examined with 3D and power Doppler ultrasound. Enlarged volume of the tumor (97.2 ml) and irregular, randomly dispersed vessels both in the central and in the peripheral parts of the tumor were detected using this method (Figure 23). The diameters of these vessels were 'uneven', with numerous microaneurysms and stenoses. Because of the same problems mentioned in the section about leiomyoma and the low PPV of 3D power Doppler, this technique is not acceptable for the evaluation of myometrial lesions.

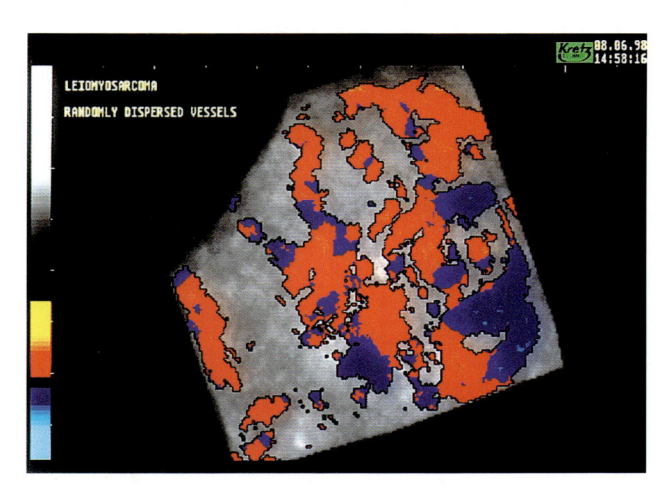

Figure 23 Three-dimensional color Doppler scan of the uterine leiomyosarcoma. Randomly dispersed vessels with complicated branching and uneven diameter are clearly demonstrated. Uterine leiomyosarcoma was confirmed by histopathology

Conclusions

Three-dimensional and power Doppler ultrasound is a new diagnostic technique and its role in the assessment of uterine lesions has yet to be investigated. Three-dimensional ultrasound offers improved visualization of uterine lesions, providing simultaneous display of coronal, sagittal and transverse planes. It displays an entire volume, demonstrating continuity of curved structures in a single image. It offers more accurate volume estimation, using a standard anatomic orientation; retrospective review of stored data, more complete viewing of pathology, using rendered images to identify the location of abnormalities, and assessment of tumor invasion. Three-dimensional hysterosonography demonstrates the exact location of intrauterine pathology. It seems that 3D power Doppler sonography has brought us a little closer to better understanding of uterine tumor angiogenesis. Interactive rotation of power Doppler rendered images provides improved visualization of the tumor vasculature. This method permits the ultrasonographer to view structures in three dimensions interactively, rather than having to assemble the sectional images mentally. Contrast agents are another possibility for enhancing the 3D power Doppler examination by increasing the detection rate of small vessels. This study is now in progress in our Department.

References

1. Kurjak A, Kupesic S, Zalud I, Predanic M. Transvaginal color Doppler. In Dodson MG, ed. *Transvaginal Ultrasound*. New York: Churchill Livingstone, 1995: 325–39
2. Fleischer AC, Kepple DM, Entman SS. Transvaginal sonography of uterine disorders. In Timor-Tritsch IE, Rottem S, eds. *Transvaginal Sonography*, 2nd edn. New York: Elsevier, 1991:109–30
3. Kurjak A, Kupesic S. Transvaginal color Doppler and pelvic tumor vascularity: lessons learned and future challenges. *Ultrasound Obstet Gynecol* 1995;6:1–15
4. Bonilla-Musoles F, Raga F, Osborne N, Blanes J, Coelho F. Three-dimensional hysterosonography for the study of endometrial tumors: comparison with conventional transvaginal sonography, hysterosalpingography, and hysteroscopy. *Gynecol Oncol* 1997;65:245–52
5. Weinraub Z, Maymon R, Shulman A, et al. Three-dimensional saline contrast hysterosonography and surface rendering of uterine cavity pathology. *Ultrasound Obstet Gynecol* 1996;8:277–82
6. Gruboeck K, Jurkovic D, Lawton F, Savvas M, Tailor A, Campbell S. The diagnostic value of endometrial thickness and volume measurements by three-dimensional ultrasound in patients with postmenopausal bleeding. *Ultrasound Obstet Gynecol* 1996;8:272–6
7. Momtaz M, El Ebrashi A. 3D sonohysterography in the evaluation of the uterine cavity. Presented at the 2nd World Congress on 3D Ultrasound in Obstetrics and Gynecology. *Syllabus* Las Vegas, October 1999
8. Fedele I, Bianchi S, Dorta M, Arcaini L, Zanotti F, Carinelli S. Transvaginal ultrasonography in the diagnosis of diffuse adenomyosis. *Fertil Steril* 1992;58:94
9. Hirai M, Shibata K, Sagai H, Sekiya S, Goldberg BB. Transvaginal pulsed and color Doppler sonography for the evaluation of adenomyosis. *J Ultrasound Med* 1995;14:529–32
10. Lee SL, Busmanis I, Tan A. 3D-angio of adenomyotic uteri. Presented at the 2nd World Congress on 3D Ultrasound in Obstetrics and Gynecology. *Syllabus* Las Vegas, October 1999
11. Kupesic-Urek S, Shalan H, Kurjak A. Early detection of endometrial cancer by transvaginal color Doppler. *Eur J Obstet Gynecol* 1993;49:46–9
12. Kurjak A, Kupesic S. Ovarian senescence and its significance on uterine and ovarian perfusion. *Fertil Steril* 1995;3:532–7
13. Kurjak A, Kupesic S. Three-dimensional ultrasound and power Doppler in assessment of uterine and ovarian angiogenesis: a prospective study. *Croat Med J* 1999;40:51–8
14. Chambers CB, Unis JS. Ultrasonographic evidence of uterine malignancy in the postmenopausal uterus. *Am J Obstet Gynecol* 1986;154:1194–9
15. Fleischer AC, Mendelson EB, Bohm-Velez M, Entman SS. Transvaginal and transabdominal sonography of the endometrium. *Semin Ultrasound Comput Tomogr Magn Reson* 1988;9:81–101
16. Mendelson EB, Bohm-Velez M, Joseph N, Neiman HL. Gynecologic imaging: comparison of transabdominal and transvaginal sonography. *Radiology* 1988;166:321–4
17. Coleman BG, Arger PH, Grumbach K. Transvaginal and transabdominal sonography: prospective comparison. *Radiology* 1988;168:639–43
18. Nasri MN, Shepherd JH, Setchell ME, Lowe DG, Chard T. Sonographic depiction of postmenopausal endometrium with transabdominal and transvaginal scanning. *Ultrasound Obstet Gynecol* 1991;1:279–93
19. Folkman J, Cole D, Becker F. Growth and metastasis of tumor in organ culture. *Tumor Res* 1963;16:453–67
20. Kupesic S, Kurjak A, Zodan T. Staging of endometrial carcinoma by 3-D power Doppler. *Gynecol Perinatol* 1999;8:1–5
21. Kurjak A, Zalud I. Uterine masses. In Kurjak A, ed. *Transvaginal Color Doppler*. Carnforth, UK: Parthenon Publishing, 1991:123
22. Fleischer AC, Entman SS, Porrath SA, James AE. Sonographic evaluation of uterine malformations and disorders. In Sanders RC, ed. *The Principles and Practice of Ultrasonography in Obstetrics and Gynecology*. Norwalk: Appleton Century Crofts, 1985:531
23. Kurjak A, Kupesic-Urek S, Miric D. The assessment of benign uterine tumor vascularization by transvaginal color Doppler. *Ultrasound Med Biol* 1992;18:645–8
24. Goswamy RK, Steptoe PC. Doppler ultrasound studies of the uterine artery in spontaneous ovarian cycles. *Hum Reprod* 1988;3:721–6
25. Kurjak A, Kupesic-Urek S, Schulman H, Zalud I. Transvaginal color Doppler in the assessment of ovarian and uterine perfusion in infertile women. *Fertil Steril* 1991;6:870–3
26. Balen FG, Allen CM, Gardener JE, Siddle NC, Lees WR. 3-Dimensional reconstruction of ultrasound images of the uterine cavity. *Br J Radiol* 1993;66:588–91
27. Lev-Toaff AS, Rawool NM, Kurtz AB, Forssberg F, Goldberg BB. Three-dimensional sonography and 3D transvaginal US: a problem solving tool in complex gynecological cases. *Radiology* 1996;201:384
28. Olah KS, Gee H, Blunt S, Dunn JA, Chan KK. Retrospective analysis of 318 cases of uterine sarcoma. *Eur J Cancer* 1991;27:1095–9
29. Kurjak A, Kupesic S, Shalan H, Jukic S, Kosuta D, Ilijas M. Uterine sarcoma: a report of 10 cases studied by transvaginal color and pulsed Doppler sonography. *Gynecol Oncol* 1995;59:342–6

The assessment of female infertility

S. Kupesic and A. Kurjak

Recent advances in three-dimensional (3D) ultrasound have made accurate non-invasive assessment of the pelvic organs feasible. The ability to visualize the oblique or coronal plane allows accurate volume measurements to be made, especially of irregularly shaped objects[1,2]. Owing to accurate recording of individual variations in structure by 3D ultrasound, these measurements are considered reliable and highly reproducible[3,4]. These improvements enable precise assessments to be made of follicular volume[2] and prediction of the follicular fluid volume at the time of follicular aspiration[5], but these methods are unlikely to become routine.

Storage capacities, reconstruction of the volume image, simultaneous viewing of all the orthogonal planes, image projections of congenital uterine anomalies[6,7] and accurate detection of uterine causes of infertility are the main advantages of this method in the field of infertility.

In this chapter we review the potential of 3D ultrasound in the evaluation of the infertile woman. Table 1 lists the clinical applications of 3D ultrasound in assisted reproductive technology.

Three-dimensional ultrasound monitoring of the ovarian response

The accuracy of diagnosis and monitoring of infertility treatments such as ovulation induction has increased greatly because of the availability of sophisticated ultrasound technology[2]. The images produced by transvaginal ultrasound are superior to those produced by transabdominal ultrasound, because vaginal transducers are in closer proximity to the tissues under scrutiny. This permits the use of higher ultrasound frequencies. Furthermore, artifactual echoes caused by multiple reflections from intervening tissues are minimized[8]. Accurate folliculometry is essential for safe and effective infertility treatment. In *in vitro* fertilization–embryo transfer (IVF-ET) cycles, follicles with a mean diameter of 12–24 mm are associated with optimal rates of oocyte recovery, fertilization and cleavage[9]. This corresponds to follicular volumes of between 3 and 7 ml. In the hands of experienced operators, ultrasound alone suffices for cycle monitoring, with no necessity for additional hormonal estimations[10–12].

The basic structural information provided by conventional scans in the longitudinal and transverse planes can now be augmented by new 3D ultrasound systems that provide an additional view of the coronal or C plane, which is parallel to the transducer face[2]. The computer-generated scan is displayed in three perpendicular planes. Translation or rotation can be carried out in one plane, while maintaining the perpendicular orientation of all three so that serial translation will result in an ultrasound tomogram from which volumetric data can be captured[13].

Kyei-Mensah and colleagues[2] evaluated the accuracy of 3D ultrasound measurement of follicular volume compared with current standard 2D techniques by comparing the volume of individual follicles estimated by both methods with the corresponding follicular aspirates, using the formula $0.52 \times (D_1 \times D_2 \times D_3)$. Limits of agreement and 95% confidence intervals were calculated and systematic bias between the methods was analyzed. The limits of agreement between

Table 1 Clinical applications of three-dimensional ultrasound in assisted reproductive technology

- Accurate measurement of ovarian follicles and estimation of follicular volume
- Objective assessment of endometrial thickness and volume
- Measurement of ovarian volume in women with polycystic ovaries and ovarian hyperstimulation syndrome
- Improved non-invasive diagnosis of congenital uterine anomalies
- Objective evaluation of endometrial shape
- Detection of the uterine causes of infertility (endometrial polyps, uterine leiomyoma, uterine anomalies, Ashermann's syndrome)
- More accurate differentiation of the hydrosalpinx from ovarian pathology
- Evaluation of tubal patency by three-dimensional hysterosalpingography

the volume of follicular aspirate and follicular volume determined by ultrasound were +0.96 to −0.43 ml for 3D measurements and +3.47 to −2.42 ml for 2D measurements.

The high accuracy of 3D measurement of follicular volume was demonstrated clearly in this study by the limits of agreement, which were within 1 ml of the true volume. These limits encompassed 95% of the volume measurements. On the other hand, the 2D method produced limits of agreement that were up to 3.5 ml above or 2.5 ml below the true volume within the most important clinical range.

Therefore, the reliability of the standard 2D ultrasound technique of follicular volume measurement is influenced by the shape and number of the follicles. There may be technical difficulty in measuring the diameters of a follicle when its shape is distorted because of compression by adjacent follicles (Figure 1). Penzias and co-workers[14] showed that mean follicular diameter accurately predicted volume in round and polygonal follicles but not in those that were ellipsoid. Round follicles were most prevalent in patients with the fewest follicles. The patients selected for this study had produced fewer follicles than normal and therefore represented the group in which the conventional technique was likely to be most accurate. Kyei-Mensah and associates[2] found that 3D assessment of follicular volume produced a more accurate reflection of the true volume. This is because 3D measurement is not affected by follicular shape, since the changing contours are outlined serially to obtain the specific volume measurement. The disparity in accuracy between 3D assessment of follicular volume and the conventional approach is therefore likely to increase significantly if there is a florid multifollicular ovarian response, because the conventional formula is less precise with ellipsoid follicles, which are likely to predominate in these cases. One limitation of 3D volume assessment is that follicles with a mean diameter of < 10 mm cannot be assessed accurately, because the limits of agreement are too wide in this range.

Feichtinger[15] found that 3D ultrasound may be useful for distinguishing ovarian cysts from ovarian follicles. Since both ovarian cysts and follicles demonstrate an elevation of serum estradiol levels, it is difficult to distinguish between them by estradiol assay alone. For the purpose of the prospective observational study, the author evaluated 50 IVF patients after ovulation induction. Three-dimensional ultrasound was used to search for the presence of cumuli in follicles greater than 15 mm (Figure 2). Only cumuli demonstrable in all three planes by multiplanar imaging predicted the recovery of mature oocytes. Follicles without visualization of the cumulus in all three planes were not likely to contain mature fertilizable oocytes.

Lass and co-workers[16] tested the hypothesis that small ovaries measured by transvaginal sonography are associated with a poor response to ovulation induction by human menopausal gonadotropin (hMG) for IVF. A total of 140 infertile patients with morphologically normal ovaries undergoing IVF were studied. The mean ovarian volume of each patient was measured by transvaginal sonography before they started hMG. Subsequent routine IVF management was conducted without knowledge of the results of transvaginal sonography. Patients (n = 17) with small ovaries of ≤ 3 cm³ represented group A. The remaining patients with normal ovarian volume represented group B. Both groups were of similar age (mean 35.8 vs. 34.4 years). Early basal follicle stimulating hormone (FSH) concentrations were increased in group A

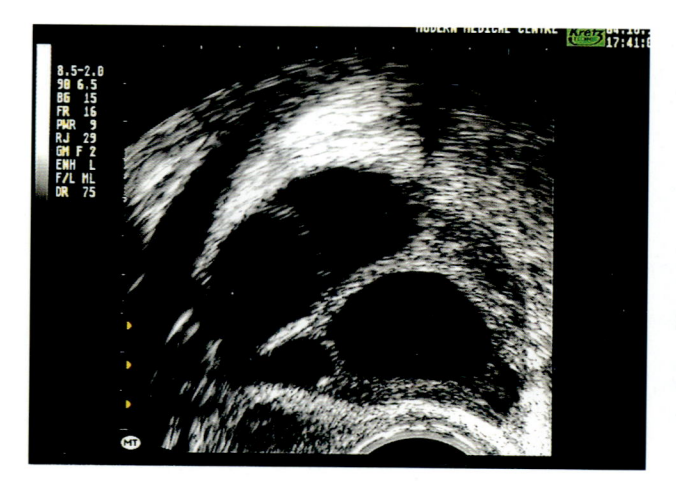

Figure 1 Transvaginal sonogram of an ovary containing three preovulatory follicles in a patient receiving clomiphene citrate for induction of ovulation

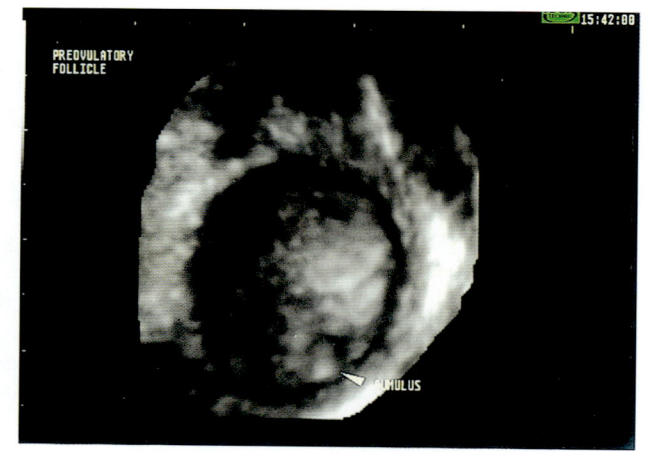

Figure 2 Surface rendering of the preovulatory ovarian follicle. Visualization of the cumulus oophorus enables the ovarian cyst to be distingushed from the ovarian follicle

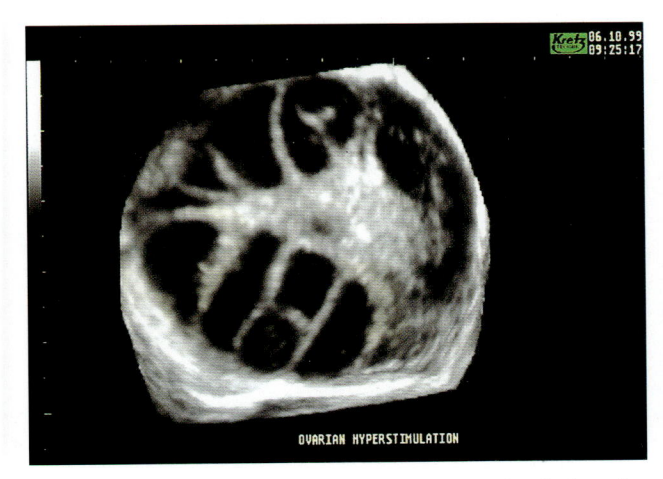

Figure 3 Three-dimensional image of the ovary on day 8 of ovarian stimulation by exogeneous gonadotropins in a patient undergoing *in vitro* fertilization

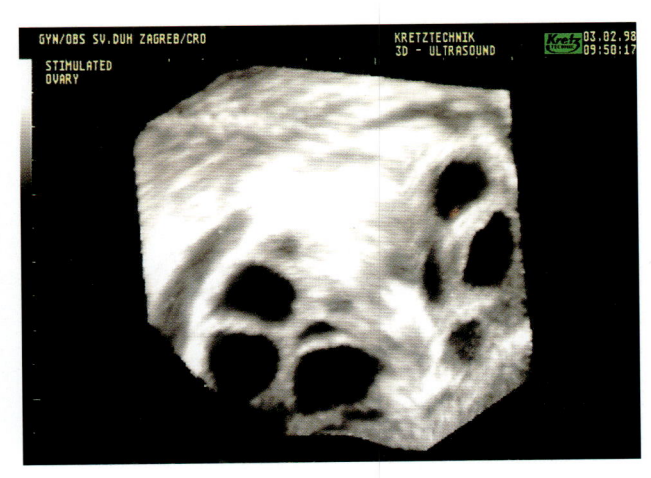

Figure 5 Three-dimensional image of the ovary in a patient receiving exogeneous gonadotropins. Note the clear distinction between the ovarian capsule and the developing follicles

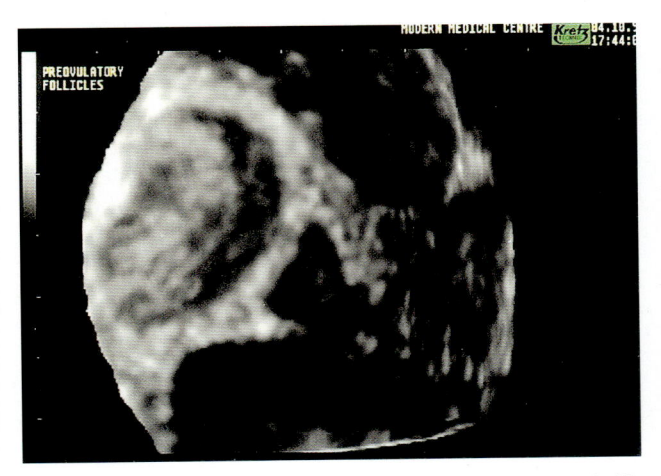

Figure 4 The same patient as in Figure 1. Surface rendering facilitates visualization of the follicles

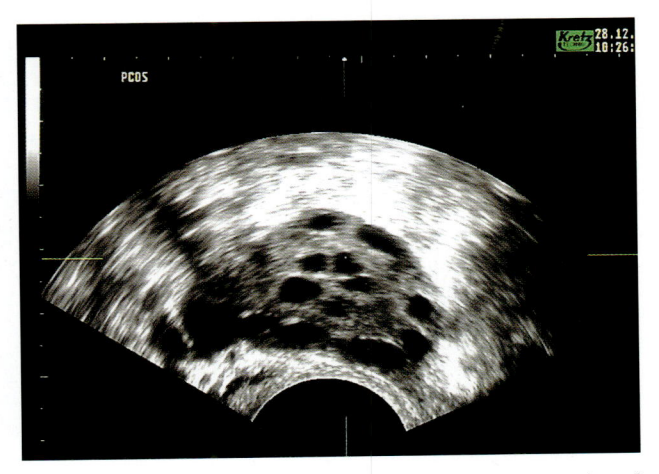

Figure 6 Transvaginal scan of a polycystic ovary. A large number of small cystic structures are crowded together and stand out from the surface of an enlarged ovarian stroma

(9.5 vs. 7.0 mIU/ml; $p = 0.025$). The cycle was abandoned before planned oocyte recovery in nine patients (52.9%) from group A and in 11 patients (8.9%) from group B, because of poor response to ovulation induction.

Oyesanya and associates[17] measured total ovarian volumes before the administration of human chorionic gonadotropin (hCG) in 42 women undergoing treatment for infertility by IVF-ET and who were considered to have an exaggerated response to stimulation (> 20 follicles). Seven women who subsequently developed moderate or severe ovarian hyperstimulation syndrome (OHSS) ($n = 7$; group 1) were compared with 35 matched controls (five matched controls per case; $n = 35$; group 2) of similar age, number of follicles and duration of infertility who underwent follicular stimulation, oocyte recovery and IVF-ET during the same period but did not develop moderate or severe OHSS. The mean age, duration of infertility and total number of follicles were similar, but the mean total ovarian volume was significantly higher in the group of women who developed moderate or severe OHSS compared with controls (271.00 ± 87.00 vs. 157.30 ± 54.20 ml) (Figures 3 and 4).

Clearly, there is a place for 3D ultrasound in the assessment of the ovaries prior to ovulation induction and medically assisted reproduction. Ovarian volume measurements can predict the ovarian response to stimulation and the risk of ovarian hyperstimulation (Figure 5).

Ovarian volume measurement in patients with polycystic ovary syndrome

Wu and co-workers[18] studied 44 women who presented with a history of irregular menstrual periods; the conditions of most of the women had been diagnosed as polycystic ovary syndrome (PCOS) (Figure 6). The

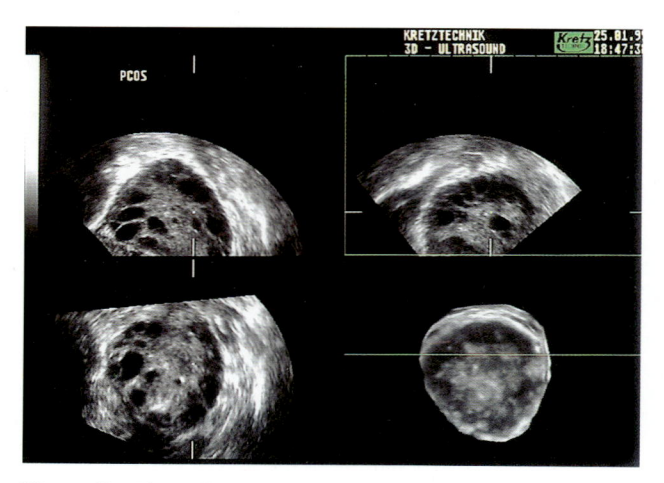

Figure 7 Three-dimensional image of a polycystic ovary. This method allows direct measurement of the total ovarian volume and estimation of the ovarian stromal volume

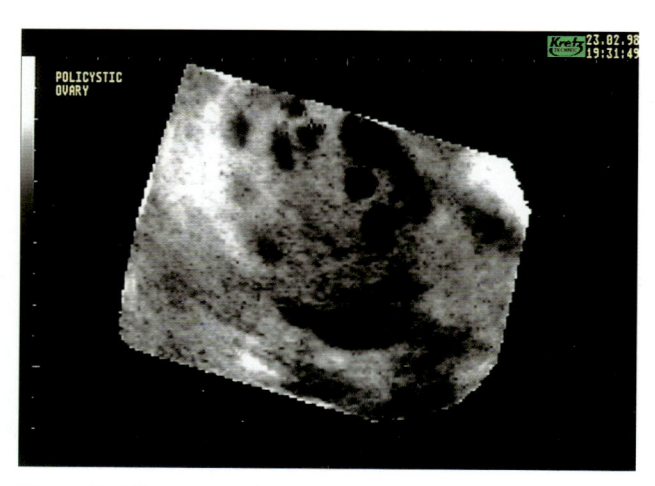

Figure 8 Minimum–maximum mode facilitates visualization of the enlarged and hyperechoic ovarian stroma and subcapsular follicles, features typical of polycystic ovaries

diagnosis of PCOS was based on the clinical symptoms (e.g. menstrual problems, obesity, acne, hirsutism), endocrinological data (all with reversed serum luteinizing hormone (LH)/FSH ratio) and ultrasonographic features (increased ovarian stroma and volume, subcapsular cysts and thickened capsule). Another 22 women with regular ovulatory cycles were recruited as normal controls. There was no statistically significant difference in age (range 17–35 years) between the groups. Three-dimensional ultrasonography was performed to store and document whole volumes of the ovaries for evaluation. Three perpendicular planes of bilateral ovaries were rotated to obtain the largest dimensions (Figure 7). The 3D volume was measured using the formula for a trapezoid. The ovaries of the patients with PCOS were larger in size, area and volume than those of the controls (Figure 8).

The mean ovarian volumes (three dimensions; mean ± SD) were 11.3 ± 3.5 cm^3 in patients with PCOS and 5.5 ± 1.4 cm^3 in the controls ($p < 0.0001$). The volumes of the right ovary were 12.2 ± 4.7 cm^3 and 5.3 ± 2.0 cm^3, and of the left ovary were 10.5 ± 3.6 cm^3 and 5.7 ± 1.6 cm^3 in the PCOS and normal groups, respectively. The right ovary demonstrated a larger volume than the left ovary in women with PCOS ($p < 0.0001$); however, the left ovary was significantly larger than the right ovary in the controls ($p < 0.0001$).

The ovaries in PCOS patients were significantly increased in size, stroma and volume ($p < 0.0001$) compared with those of the controls. Cut-off values for ovarian area, stroma and volume in PCOS were 5.2 cm^2 (sensitivity 93%, specificity 91%), 4.6 cm^2 (sensitivity 91%, specificity 86%) and 6.6 cm^3 (sensitivity 91%, specificity 91%), respectively. The stroma, total ovarian area and volume detected by careful rotation and outlining of the longitudinal ovarian cut were increased in 84% (37 of 44), 89% (39 of 44) and 80% (35 of 44) of the patients with PCOS, respectively, in comparison with controls. The total ovarian area was strongly correlated with the stromal area ($r^2 = 0.66$).

Undoubtedly, 3D ultrasonography facilitates non-invasive retrospective evaluation and volume calculation. The examination time is short, without increasing patient discomfort. Three maximal dimensions of the ovaries can be measured easily once the digital volume is documented from either transvaginal or transabdominal 3D ultrasonography, and superior volume determination can be obtained from 3D images. The volume measurement in 3D ultrasonography is accurate and highly reproducible. The volume of follicles can be determined precisely, and the volume of the ovary from 3D sonography correlates better with direct measurement of the surgical specimen than that from 2D ultrasonography[2,19] (Figure 7). Undoubtedly, the ability of reconstruction increases the diagnostic potential for PCOS.

The ovaries in PCOS are usually enlarged bilaterally, but they may be about normal size (up to 20% in our study). The stromal areas in PCOS are hypertrophic, and provide yet another subjective ultrasonographic criterion that could differentiate PCOS from the multifollicular ovary. The multifollicular ovary demonstrates a normal or slightly increased size, but an increased number of follicles is noted without an increased amount of stroma. However, the results are usually subjective and not quantitative. Using the computerized quantification measurement, an increased total ovarian area of > 5.5 cm^2 correlates strongly with increased ovarian stroma at a strict longitudinal ovarian section in the diagnosis of PCOS[20].

THE ASSESSMENT OF FEMALE INFERTILITY

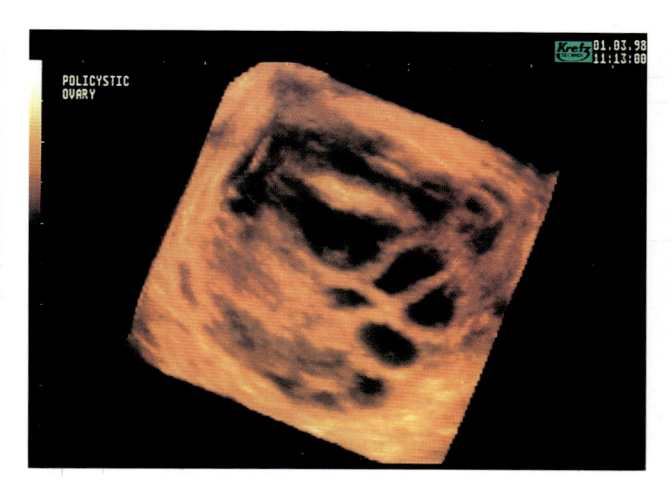

Figure 9 Polycystic ovary undergoing stimulation with gonadotropins. Note the numerous follicles at the periphery of the hyperechoic ovarian stroma

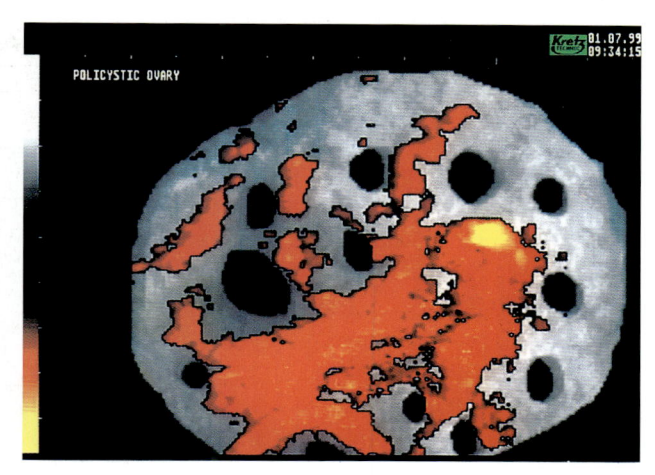

Figure 10 Three-dimensional power Doppler scan of the polycystic ovary. Increased ovarian stromal blood flow may become a new parameter to assist in the ultrasound diagnosis of polycystic ovary syndrome

Three-dimensional ultrasonography allows careful and objective evaluation of the ovaries and can repeatedly follow the outline of the ovarian area even after the examination. The value for the ovarian stroma can be obtained after subtracting the area of the ovarian follicles from the total area (Figure 9). The 3D scanning can obtain more accurate volume data by outlining the contour of the target organ, which is better than traditional 2D ultrasonographic scanning calculated by the ellipsoid formula (height × width × thickness × 0.523).

Apart from morphological and volume measurements, assessment of ovarian and uterine vessels can be added to the traditional endocrinological and ultrasonographic parameters used clinically for diagnosis of PCOS. Battaglia and colleagues[21] performed ultrasonographic evaluation of ovarian volume, echodensity and follicle number by transvaginal color Doppler measurement of the uterine and intraovarian vessel variations in 32 hirsute, oligomenorrheic patients and 18 volunteer women in the early follicular phase.

Doppler analysis of patients with PCOS (increased LH/FSH ratio, elevated androstenedione levels, high number of subcapsular follicles by ultrasonography-augmented ovarian volume and echodensity) ($n = 22$), the authors observed significantly elevated uterine artery pulsatility index values associated with a typical low resistance index of stromal ovary vascularization. The uterine artery pulsatility index was positively correlated with the LH/FSH ratio, while the resistance index of the intraovarian vessels was negatively correlated. The elevated uterine artery resistance was correlated with androstenedione levels.

Similar results in the uterine circulation were obtained by Zaidi and colleagues[22], who at the same time found significantly greater ovarian stromal blood

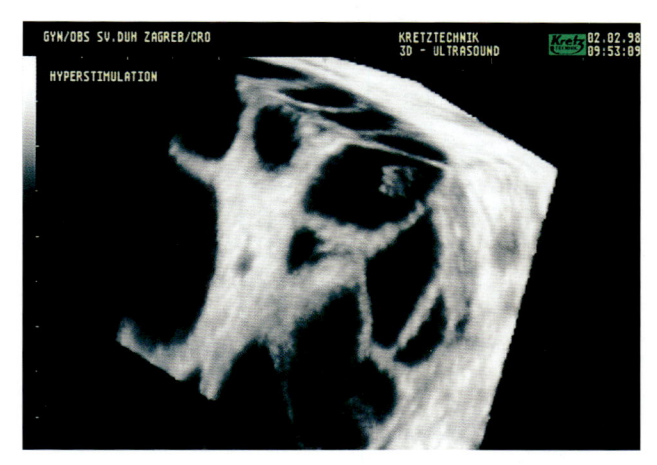

Figure 11 Three-dimensional image of the hyperstimulated polycystic ovary. Massive ovarian arrangement and numerous follicles are easily visualized by this technique. Three-dimensional ultrasound appears to give reproducible volume measurement and, therefore, can be used to predict ovarian hyperstimulation syndrome

flow velocity in women with polycystic ovaries. Increased ovarian stromal blood flow detected by 3D power Doppler ultrasound may be a new parameter to assist in the ultrasound diagnosis of PCOS (Figure 10).

Patients with PCOS undergoing ovulation induction for IVF are more likely to develop a greater number of follicles and generate more oocytes compared with women with normal ovaries, even though they require less gonadotropin stimulation[23] (Figure 11). Furthermore, since they develop more follicles of all sizes and, in particular, small- and medium-sized follicles, women with PCOS are at greater risk of OHSS[24]. This suggests that PCOS is more sensitive to gonadotropin stimulation. The exact mechanism is unknown, although it is possible that the increased ovarian stromal blood flow velocity, in combination with a relatively unchanged impedance to blood flow, may reflect increased intraovarian perfusion and thus a greater delivery of gonadotropins to the granulosa cells of the developing follicles (Figure 12). This theory may help to explain the greater likelihood of a multifollicular response (Figure 13). Using transvaginal color Doppler ultrasound, Collins and associates[25] demonstrated blood vessels in the region of the granulosa/thecal cell interface after the LH rise. Furthermore, red cells have been seen on histological examination of the granulosa cell layer of preovulatory human follicles[26]. Increased ovarian stromal blood flow velocity in patients with PCOS may help to explain the excessive response when they are administered gonadotropins. The presence of increased stromal blood flow velocity in both the groups with polycystic ovaries and PCOS compared to women with normal ovaries supports the notion that PCOS is a primary disorder of the ovary. Furthermore, the detection of increased ovarian stromal blood flow velocity by color and pulsed Doppler ultrasound may be a marker in the diagnosis of PCOS.

In conclusion, 3D ultrasonography can complement 2D ultrasonography for the diagnosis of PCOS. It allows excellent spatial evaluation of the ovaries with direct quantitative computations from the data. Evaluation of the ovarian stromal vascularity by 3D power Doppler will further increase our knowledge of this enigmatic syndrome.

Puncture procedures by three-dimensional ultrasound

Feichtinger[5] evaluated the possibility of performing puncturing procedures under 3D ultrasound control in close to real time using a new commercially available system. Transvaginal needle-guided aspiration of ten follicles using a newly developed ultrasound machine with built-in rapid and powerful calculation software for 3D interactive volume and flow translation during operation was used. Interactive 3D imaging was carried out during the aspiration of each follicle. Oocyte recovery was successful from all follicles. There was a mean ($\pm$ SD) delay of 5.00 ± 1.22 s from coasting to resuming real-time ultrasound scanning during interactive volume calculation and the search for the needle tip in the 3D mode. This did not delay the procedure remarkably but enabled the precise localization of both the needle and its tip after each penetration. The integration of flow signals produced an impressive color-coded demonstration of the needle within the tissue, but the delay was significantly longer for color-coded volume acquisition (18.40 ± 4.56 s).

The interactive mode permits the immediate observation of the effects of rotation and translation on the volume in real time, and the rapid acquisition and calculation time allow puncturing procedures to be performed in close to real time, with tolerable delays between coasting and resuming real-time scanning. It is expected that puncture under control of 3D ultrasound will be more useful in the field of perinatal medicine and gynecological oncology.

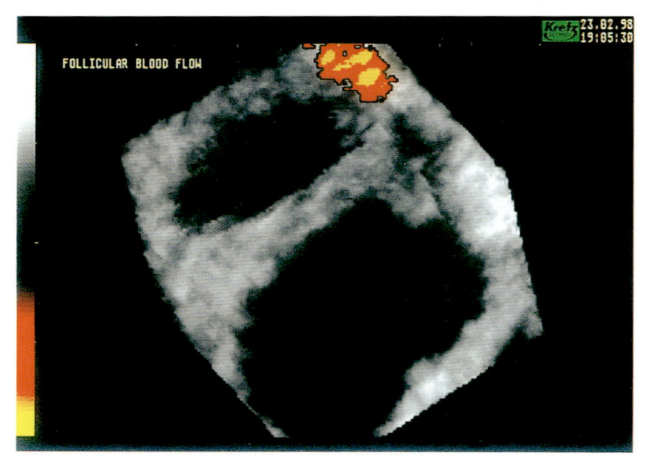

Figure 12 Three-dimensional power Doppler image of the preovulatory follicle and its vascular supply

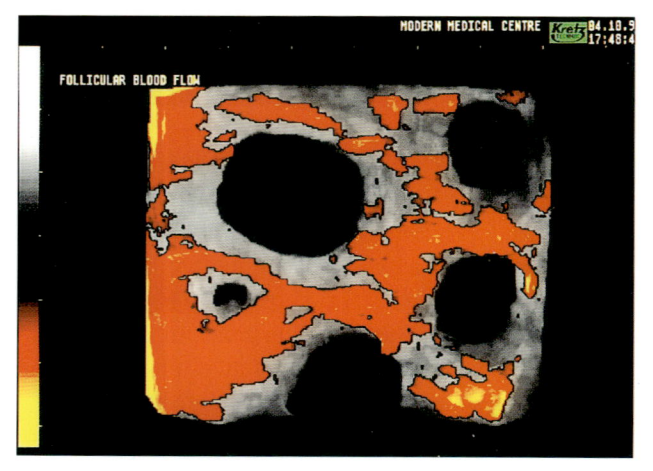

Figure 13 Three-dimensional power Doppler image of the hyperstimulated ovary. Dilated perifollicular vessels reflect increased intraovarian perfusion and the likelihood of a multifollicular response

Endometrial volume measurement

The endometrium has been a focus of interest since the beginning of ultrasound diagnosis in gynecology. Deichert and co-workers[27] described three to four typical forms of the endometrium depicted from 2D ultrasound images. Ultrasound study of the uterus and endometrial layer is now a routine procedure in gynecological investigation.

Generally the endometrium shows good contrast to the myometrium and therefore, measurements of endometrial growth can be performed easily. Endometrial thickness obtained by 2D sonography is considered the most important parameter of endometrial growth. However, this parameter does not include the total volume of the endometrium. For certain diagnoses, endometrial volume measurement can be important. Especially in postmenopausal patients, increased endometrial volume has been considered to be a marker of endometrial pathology[28].

Furthermore, retarded endometrial development can be associated with primary infertility[29,30]. Several studies have measured the impact of endometrial thickness on unexplained infertility[31]. Considerable interest has been shown in studying the endometrium in hyperstimulated menstrual cycles[32,33]. However, conflicting results have been obtained. Therefore, having an accurate means to evaluate endometrial and uterine growth is of value.

There is no general consensus on the importance of endometrial thickness for prediction of implantation and pregnancy rates in assisted conception therapy. Some studies have suggested that measurement of endometrial thickness is a useful parameter[34], whereas other studies have disputed its value[35]. The ability to quantify the volume of the endometrium using 3D ultrasound may help to resolve this issue, because cycle outcome can be correlated with a quantitative parameter rather than endometrial thickness, which is prone to greater subjective variation in measurement[3].

Study of the uterus and the endometrium seems to be an ideal application for 3D visualization[36]. Three-dimensional ultrasound has also brought the possibility of easily calculating the volume of the endometrium. By stepping through the volume in plane mode, the outer limits of the endometrium are traced, and volume calculations can be performed immediately. The accuracy of this method has already been described[1,37,38]. To obtain the best results, stepping through the volume should be performed in small units. In each new plane the area tracing has to be corrected to its new extent. Low contrast in ultrasound data can increase the error of volume estimation. In general, the endometrium shows a good contrast to the surrounding myometrial tissue and therefore, in most cases, volume estimation can be performed. Measurements can best be reproduced in longitudinal and transverse viewing planes. Other sources of measuring error may derive from the low contrast of the caudal end of the endometrium and the uterus. Endometrial fluid may also increase measuring error, because the fluid volume may be too small to be measured accurately by 3D ultrasound.

Lee and associcates[36] were the first to demonstrate volume estimation of the endometrium by 3D ultrasound. Using the same method, Kyei-Mensah and colleagues[2] assessed the reliability of 3D ultrasound in measuring endometrial volume in 20 patients undergoing ovarian stimulation. Endometrial volumes of these patients were obtained on the day of hCG administration. The intraobserver and interobserver coefficients of variation were 8 and 11%, respectively. Repeatability within and between investigators was also expressed as the IntraCC and InterCC. The coefficients describe the proportion of variation in a measurement caused by true biological subject differences. For a single measurement of endometrial volume, the IntraCC was 0.90 and the InterCC was 0.82. These results clearly demonstrate that 3D ultrasound volume measurements are highly reliable, with a small measurement error. However, one could expect higher interobserver differences in accurate locating of the internal os and endometrial margins, which may

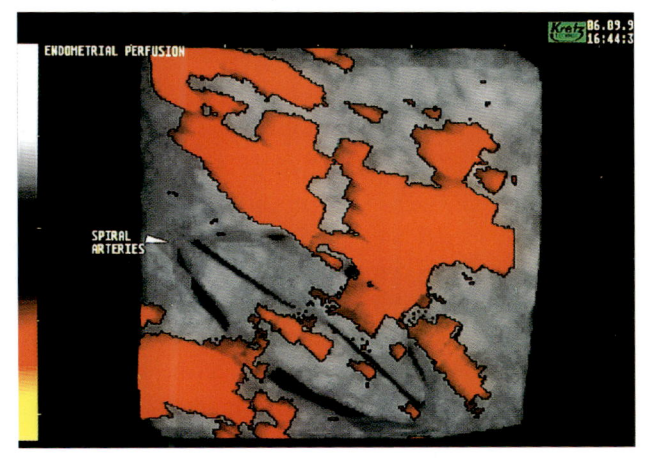

Figure 14 Three-dimensional power Doppler scan of the periovulatory endometrium. Power Doppler indicates coiling of the spiral arteries

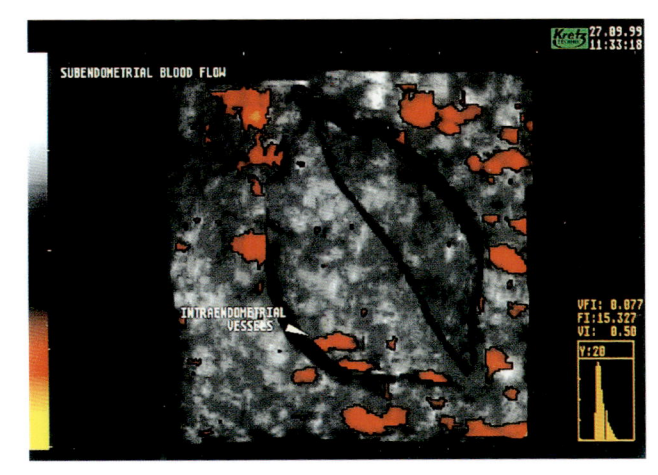

Figure 15 Color Doppler histogram enables measurement of endometrial blood flow and vascularization in the three-dimensional perspective

explain the greater interobserver variability for endometrial volume than for ovarian volume. Since the method is applied in the same manner as 2D transvaginal ultrasound it does not cause additional discomfort.

It is expected that 3D endometrial volumetry studies will increase diagnostic potential and give additional information to that from 2D ultrasound. Furthermore, quantification of endometrial volume by 3D ultrasound in combination with blood flow studies may be the best way to predict pregnancy rates (Figures 14 and 15).

Uterine causes of infertility

Assessment of uterine morphology and exclusion of endometrial pathology are essential before commencement of treatment during assisted reproduction treatment. It is clear that anatomic uterine abnormalities, including submucous leiomyomas, intrauterine adhesions and congenital uterine anomalies interfere with the implantation of the developing embryo and may cause recurrent pregnancy loss.

Since 3D ultrasound provides images of the uterine cavity in multiple tomographic sections, intracavitary structures become clearly visible. Uterine causes of infertility which were hidden until now can be non-invasively detected, measured and localized.

Leiomyomas are commonly associated with second-trimester pregnancy loss and infertility if the tubal ostia are occluded. Three-dimensional ultrasound can provide accurate diagnosis of the uterine leiomyoma at any location. Storage of volume data enables the data to be analyzed at a later date and 3D ultrasound volume measurements to be compared with intraoperative findings. If an endometrial polyp or intrauterine adhesions are detected, operative hysteroscopy should be performed before any treatment for assisted reproduction is commenced.

Our results on early pregnancy loss and complications during the second half of pregnancy in patients with septate uterus are presented in Chapter 3 together with the data on the accuracy of 3D ultrasound in detection of the uterine causes of infertility[7,39].

Although 3D ultrasonography may be the investigation of choice to assess the morphology of the uterus and its cavity, multicenter studies are required to determine the potential and cost effectiveness of the routine use of this rapidly developing technique.

Conclusions

Three-dimensional ultrasound is an exciting new technology that provides valuable information in the investigation and management of infertile patients. In the not too distant future this examination may become the method of choice for assessing morphology of the uterus and its cavity. In the context of follicular monitoring in assisted conception, planar reformatted sections allow more accurate volumetric assessment of the leading follicles, which are not always spherical.

Furthermore, the multiplanar view of the stimulated ovary may distinguish accurately between follicles and cysts. Transvaginal ultrasound-directed follicular aspiration under 3D control improves the operator's spatial evaluation of the stimulated ovary and allows precise follicular localization prior to aspiration. Furthermore, it ensures aspiration of all the follicles in each ovary. The use of 3D transvaginal ultrasonography after injection of saline solution or an echo-contrast agent may produce high diagnostic accuracy, in particular an improved assessment of the lateral portion of the uterine cavity close to the tubal ostia.

References

1. Riccabona M, Nelson TR, Pretorius DH. Three-dimensional ultrasound: accuracy of distance and volume measurements. *Ultrasound Obstet Gynecol* 1996; 4:29–34
2. Kyei-Mensah A, Zaidi J, Pittrof R, Shaker A, Campbell S, Tan S-L. Transvaginal three-dimensional ultrasound: accuracy of follicular volume measurements. *Fertil Steril* 1996;65:371–6
3. Kyei-Mensah A, Maconochie N, Zaidi J, Pittrof R, Campbell S, Tan S-L. Transvaginal three-dimensional ultrasound: reproducibility of ovarian and endometrial volume measurements. *Fertil Steril* 1996;66:718–22
4. Tan SL. Clinical applications of Doppler and three-dimensional ultrasound in assisted reproductive technology. *Ultrasound Obstet Gynecol* 1999;13:153–6
5. Feichtinger W. Follicle aspiration with interactive three-dimensional digital imaging (Voluson®): a step toward real-time puncturing under three-dimensional ultrasound control. *Fertil Steril* 1998;70:374–7
6. Jurkovic D, Geipel A, Gruboeck K, Jauniaux E, Natucci M, Campbell S. Three-dimensional ultrasound for the assessment of uterine anatomy and detection of congeni-

tal anomalies: a comparison with hysterosalpingography and two-dimensional sonography. *Ultrasound Obstet Gynecol* 1995;5:233–7

7. Kupesic S, Kurjak A. Diagnosis and treatment outcome of the septate uterus. *Croat Med J* 1998;39:185–90
8. Kossoff G, Griffiths KA, Dixon CE. Is the quality of transvaginal images superior to transabdominal ones under matched conditions? *Ultrasound Obstet Gynecol* 1991;1:29–35
9. Wittmack FM, Kreger DO, Blasco L, Tureck RW, Mastroianni L Jr, Lessey BA. Effect of follicular size on oocyte retrieval, fertilization, cleavage, and embryo quality in *in vitro* fertilization cycles: a 6-year data collection. *Fertil Steril* 1994;6:1205–10
10. Golan A, Herman A, Soffer Y, Bukovsky I, Ron-El R. Ultrasonic control without hormone determination for ovulation induction in *in-vitro* fertilization/embryo-transfer with gonadotrophin-releasing hormone analogue and human menopausal gonadotrophin. *Hum Reprod* 1994;9:1631–3
11. Shoham Z, DiCarlo C, Pater A, Conway GS, Jacobs HS. Is it possible to run a successful ovulation induction program based solely on ultrasound monitoring? The importance of endometrial measurements. *Fertil Steril* 1991;56:836–41
12. Tan SL. Simplification of IVF therapy. *Curr Opin Obstet Gynecol* 1994;6:111–14
13. Steiner H, Staudach A, Spitzer D, Schaffer H. Three-dimensional US in obstetrics and gynaecology: technique, possibilities and limitations. *Hum Reprod* 1994;9:1773–8
14. Penzias AS, Emmi AM, Dubey AK, Layman LC, DeCherney AH, Reindollar RH. Ultrasound prediction of follicle volume: is the mean diameter reflective? *Fertil Steril* 1994;62:1274–6
15. Feichtinger W. Transvaginal three-dimensional imaging for evaluation and treatment of infertility. In Merz E, ed. *3-D Ultrasound in Obstetrics and Gynecology*. Philadelphia: Lipincott Williams & Wilkins, 1998;37–43
16. Lass A, Skull J, McVeigh E, Margara R, Winston RM. Measurement of ovarian volume by transvaginal sonography before ovulation induction with human menopausal gonadotrophin for *in-vitro* fertilization can predict poor response. *Hum Reprod* 1997;12:294–7
17. Oyesanya OA, Parsons JH, Collins WP, Campbell S. Total ovarian volume before human chorionic gonadotrophin administration for ovulation induction may predict the hyperstimulation syndrome. *Hum Reprod* 1995;10:3211–12
18. Wu M-H, Tang H-H, Hsu C-C, Wang S-T, Huang K-E. The role of three-dimensional ultrasonographic images in ovarian measurement. *Fertil Steril* 1998;69:1152–5
19. Bonilla-Musoles F, Raga F, Osborne NG. Three-dimensional ultrasound evaluation of ovarian masses. *Gynecol Oncol* 1995;59:129–35
20. Robert Y, Dubrulle F, Gaillandre L, Ardaens Y, Thomas-Desrousseaux P, Lemaitre L. Ultrasound assessment of ovarian stroma hypertrophy in hyperandrogenism and ovulation disorders: visual analysis versus computerized quantification. *Fertil Steril* 1995;64:307–12
21. Battaglia C, Artini PG, D'Ambrogio G, Genazzani AD, Genazzani AR. The role of color Doppler imaging in the diagnosis of polycystic ovary syndrome. *Am J Obstet Gynecol* 1995;172:108–13
22. Zaidi J, Campbell S, Pittfor R, *et al.* Ovarian stromal blood flow in women with polycystic ovaries – a possible new marker for diagnosis? *Hum Reprod* 1995;10:1992–6
23. MacDougall MJ, Tan SL, Balen A, Jacobs HS. A controlled study comparing patients with and without polycystic ovaries undergoing *in-vitro* fertilization. *Hum Reprod* 1993;8:233–7
24. MacDougall MJ, Tan SL, Jacobs HS. *In-vitro* fertilization and the ovarian hyperstimulation syndrome. *Hum Reprod* 1992;7:597–600
25. Collins WP, Jurkovic D, Bourne T, Kurjak A, Campbell S. Ovarian morphology, endocrine function and intra-follicular blood flow during the peri-ovulatory period. *Hum Reprod* 1991;6:319–24
26. Bomsel-Helmreich O, Gougeon A, Thebault A, *et al.* Healthy and atretic follicles in the pre-ovulatory phase: differences in evolution of follicular morphology and steroid content of follicular fluid. *J Clin Endocrinol Metab* 1979;48:686–94
27. Deichert U, Hackeloer BJ, Daume E. The sonographic and endocrinologic evaluation of the endometrium in the luteal phase. *Hum Reprod* 1986;1:219–22
28. Gruboeck K, Jurkovic D, Lawton F, Savvas M, Tailor A, Campbell S. The diagnostic value of endometrial thickness and volume measurements by three-dimensional ultrasound in patients with postmenopausal bleeding. *Ultrasound Obstet Gynecol* 1996;8:272–6
29. Morgan PM, Hutz RJ, Kraus EM, Bavister BD. Ultrasonographic assessment of the endometrium in rhesus monkeys during the normal menstrual cycle. *Biol Reprod* 1987;36:463–9
30. Sachiko N, Tsutomu D, Toshimichi O, Hirofumi I, Shinichi Y, Yukihiro N. Relationship between sonographic endometrial thickness and progestin-induced withdrawal bleeding. *Obstet Gynecol* 1996;87:722–5
31. Li TC, Lenton EA, Dockery P, Cooke ID. A comparison of some clinical and endocrinological features between cycles with normal and defective luteal phases in women with unexplained infertility. *Hum Reprod* 1990;5:805–10
32. Randall JM, Fisk NM, McTavish A, Templeton AA. Transvaginal ultrasonic assessment of endometrial growth in spontaneous and hyper-stimulated menstrual cycles. *Br J Obstet Gynaecol* 1989;96:954–9
33. Shoham Z, DiCarlo C, Patel A. Is it possible to run a successful ovulation induction program based solely on ultrasound monitoring? The importance of endometrial measurements. *Fertil Steril* 1991;56:836
34. Gonen Y, Caspar RF. Prediction of implantation by the sonographic appearance of the endometrium during controlled ovarian stimulation for *in vitro* fertilization. *J In Vitro Fertil Embryo Transfer* 1990;7:146–52
35. Fleischer AC, Herbert CM, Sacks GA, Wentz AC, Entman SS, James AE Jr. Sonography of the endometrium during conception and nonconception cycles of *in vitro* fertilization and embryo transfer. *Fertil Steril* 1986;46:442–7

36. Lee A, Sator M, Kratochwil A, Deutinger J, Vytiska-Binsdorfer E, Bernaschek G. Endometrial volume change during spontaneous menstrual cycles: volumetry by transvaginal three-dimensional ultrasound. *Fertil Steril* 1997;68:831–5
37. Gregg AR, Steiner H, Staudach A, Weiner CP. Accuracy of 3D sonographic volume measurements. Presented at the *Annual Meeting of the Society of Perinatal Obstetricians*, San Francisco, 1993
38. Gilja OH, Smievoll I, Thune N, Matre K, Hausken T, Odegaard S. *In vivo* comparison of 3D ultrasonography and magnetic resonance imaging in volume estimation of human kidney. *Ultrasound Med Biol* 1995;21:25–32
39. Kupesic S, Kurjak A. Septate uterus: detection and prediction of obstetrical complications by different forms of ultrasonography. *J Ultrasound Med* 1998;17:631–6

Three-dimensional ultrasound and power Doppler for the diagnosis of septate uterus

S. Kupesic and A. Kurjak

Introduction

Congenital uterine malformations are variable in frequency and are usually estimated to represent 3–4%, although less than half have clinical symptoms[1-3]. The respective frequency of symptomatic malformations is dominated by septate uterus[3,4]. During the first trimester of pregnancy, the risk of spontaneous abortion in this group is between 28 and 45%. During the second trimester the frequency of late spontaneous abortions is approximately 5%[3]. Premature deliveries, abnormal fetal presentations, irregular uterine activity and dystocia at delivery are likely to prevail in cases of septate uterus[5]. Poor vascularization of the septum was proposed as a potential cause of miscarriages[4]. An electron microscopy study by Fedele and colleagues[6] indicated a decrease in the sensitivity of the endometrium covering the septa of malformed uteri to preovulatory changes. This could play a role in the pathogenesis of primary infertility in patients with a septate uterus.

It is clear that an unfavorable obstetric prognosis can be transformed by surgical correction of the intrauterine septum. Formerly, removal of the septum was performed by transabdominal metroplasty[7]. Hysteroscopic treatment is currently proposed as the procedure of choice for the management of these disorders. This simple and effective treatment has an obvious advantage, in that the uterus is not weakened by a myometrial scar. Cararach and co-workers[8] and Goldenberg and co-workers[9] reported 75% and 88.7% pregnancy rates, respectively, after operative hysteroscopy.

Clearly, the simplicity and effectiveness of hysteroscopy have faced the clinician with the need for an early and correct diagnosis of uterine anomalies. When used as a screening test for the detection of congenital uterine anomalies, transvaginal ultrasound has had a sensitivity of almost 100%[10,11]. However, making a clear distinction between different types of abnormalities was impossible and operator dependent[12,13].

X-ray hysterosalpingography (HSG) is an invasive test that requires the use of contrast medium and exposure to radiation. Although HSG provides a good outline of the uterine cavity, the visualization of minor anomalies and making a clear distinction between different types of lateral fusion disorders is sometimes impossible. Hysterosonography was introduced 15 years ago[14]. This method employs transvaginal ultrasound after distension of the uterine cavity by instillation of saline solution. This simple and minimally invasive approach allows anatomical images to be produced of endometrium and myometrium, accurate depiction of the septate uterus and even the measurement of the thickness and height of the septum[15].

Although some reports have indicated a high diagnostic accuracy of magnetic resonance imaging[16,17] in the diagnosis of congenital uterine anomalies, this technique is rarely routinely used for this indication. Three-dimensional (3D) ultrasound has shown high diagnostic accuracy in detection of the septate uterus[18], suggesting that invasive procedures such as CO_2 diagnostic hysteroscopy are not needed in patients scheduled for corrective surgery[19].

Ultrasound imaging in diagnosis and treatment of septate uterus – own results

Kupesic and Kurjak attempted to evaluate the combined use of transvaginal ultrasound, transvaginal color and pulsed Doppler sonography, hysterosonography and 3D ultrasound in the preoperative diagnosis of septate uterus[20]. A total of 420 infertile patients undergoing operative hysteroscopy were included in this study. Table 1 summarizes the intraoperative findings in 420 infertile patients undergoing hysteroscopy. The final diagnosis of the uterine disorder was confirmed by hysteroscopy, and 278 patients had the intrauterine septum corrected surgically. Forty-three of the patients with a septate uterus had a history of repeated spontaneous abortion, 71 had one spontaneous abortion (56 in the first trimester, while 15 reported spontaneous abortion during the second trimester), 82 had primary sterility and 20 had premature delivery, including six with breech and two with transverse presentation. A positive history of ectopic pregnancy was noted in 76 patients.

Each patient underwent transvaginal ultrasound and

Table 1 Intraoperative findings in 420 infertile patients undergoing hysteroscopy

Hysteroscopic finding	Number
Submucous leiomyoma	46
Endometrial polyp	35*
Intrauterine synechiae	19*
Septate uterus	278
Arcuate uterus	28
Bicornuate uterus	16†
Total	422

*One patient with endometrial polyp and one with intrauterine synechiae had an intrauterine septum; †diagnosis made by combined use of laparoscopy and hysteroscopy

transvaginal color Doppler examinations during the luteal phase of their cycle. A systematic examination of the uterine position, size and morphological characteristics was performed. With the use of B-mode transvaginal sonography, the morphology of the uterus was carefully explored, with emphasis on the endometrial lining in both sagittal and transverse sections. The septum was visualized as an echogenic portion separating the uterine cavity into two parts. Once B-mode examination was completed by an experienced sonographer, transvaginal color Doppler examination was performed by another skilled operator who was unaware of the previous finding.

Color and pulsed Doppler were superimposed to visualize intraseptal and myometrial vascularity. Flow velocity waveforms were obtained from all the interrogated vessels. For each recording, at least five waveform signals of good quality were obtained. During each procedure the resistance index (RI) was automatically calculated. The RI was calculated from the maximum frequency envelope as follows: peak systolic velocity minus end-diastolic velocity divided by peak systolic velocity. Instillation of isotonic saline (hysterosonography) was carried out on a gynecological examination table. In 76 patients the uterine cervix was exposed with a speculum disinfected with iodine solution. A catheter with external diameter of 1.6 mm and internal diameter of 1.1 mm was slowly introduced into the cervix. The balloon was insufflated with 1.5–2 ml of sterile saline solution to avoid outflow of the fluid. A syringe containing 20 ml isotonic saline solution was attached to the catheter and fluid was slowly injected. For distension of the uterine cavity about 5–10 ml of the contrast solution was required. The speculum was then withdrawn and the endovaginal probe was introduced. Transverse and sagittal sections were carefully explored, and the septum was visualized as an echogenic portion separating the uterine cavity into two parts.

Eighty-six women undergoing hysteroscopy were examined by 3D ultrasound. They all had a transvaginal scan and color and pulsed Doppler evaluation performed prior to the 3D examination. Twelve of these patients underwent an additional examination: instillation of the isotonic saline solution into the uterine cavity. The results of the previous diagnostic tests were not available to the ultrasonographer. Three perpendicular planes of the uterus were simultaneously displayed on the screen, allowing a detailed analysis to be made of the uterine morphology (Figure 1). Frontal reformatted sections were particularly useful for detection of the uterine abnormalities (Figure 2).

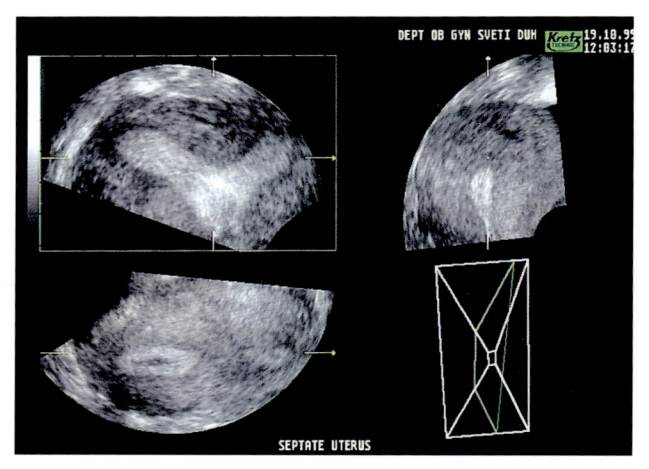

Figure 1 Three perpendicular planes of the septate uterus. Note the clear separation of the uterine cavity and absence of the fundal indentation in the myometrium

Table 2 summarizes the sensitivity, specificity, positive and negative predictive values of transvaginal sonography, transvaginal color and pulsed Doppler ultrasound, hysterosalpingography and 3D ultrasound for the diagnosis of the septate uterus.

In 264 cases septate uterus was suspected by transvaginal ultrasound, while a normal finding was reported in 14 patients. The sensitivity of transvaginal sonography in the diagnosis of septate uterus was 95.21%.

Transvaginal color and pulsed Doppler enabled the diagnosis of septate uterus to be made in 276 cases,

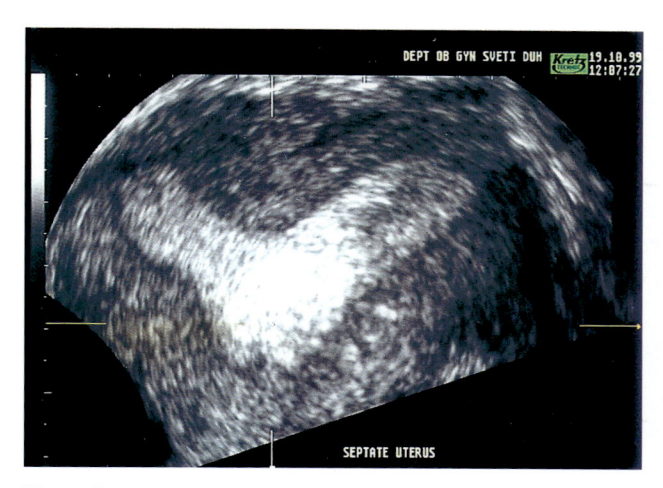

Figure 2 Frontal reformatted section of the uterus demonstrating a septate uterus. There is no fundal indentation in the myometrium, but a thick septum is seen deeply dividing the uterine cavity

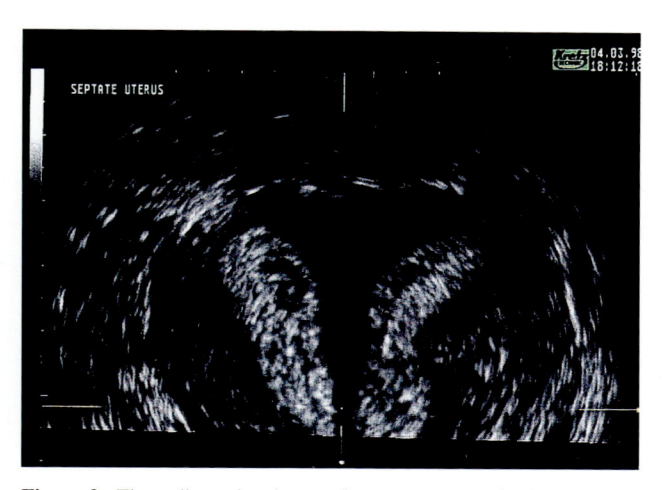

Figure 3 Three-dimensional scan of a septate uterus that is characterized by a normal outer uterine contour and thick septum extending into the uterine cavity

Table 2 Sensitivity, specificity, positive (PPV) and negative predictive value (NPV) of various imaging modalities for the diagnosis of septate uterus in 420 patients with a history of infertility and recurrent abortions. From reference 20, with permission

Imaging modality	Sensitivity (%)	Specificity (%)	PPV (%)	NPV (%)
Transvaginal sonography	95.21	92.21	95.86	91.03
Transvaginal color Doppler	99.29	97.93	98.03	98.61
Hysterosonography	98.18	100.00	100.00	95.45
Three-dimensional ultrasound	98.38	100.00	100.00	96.00

reaching a sensitivity of 99.29%. In one patient with an endometrial polyp and one with intrauterine synechiae, septate uterus was not correctly diagnosed. Thus, the reliability of color and pulsed Doppler examination was reduced if other intracavitary structures (such as endometrial polyp or submucous leiomyoma) were present.

Color and pulsed Doppler studies of the septal area revealed vascularity in 198 (71.22%) patients. The RI values obtained from the septum ranged from 0.68 to 1.0 (mean RI = 0.84 ± 0.16). Eighteen patients demonstrated absence of diastolic blood flow, while in the rest a continuous diastolic flow was present.

Hysterosonography, which was carried out in 76 patients, reached 100% specificity and positive predictive value. In one patient with extensive intrauterine synechiae, hysterosonography did not detect an intrauterine septum, although it was successful in diagnosing septate uterus in the remaining 54 patients.

Good-quality 3D images were obtained in 86 patients (Figure 2). The sensitivity and specificity of 3D ultrasonography was 98.38% and 100%, respectively. A false-negative result in one patient was caused by a fundal fibroid distorting the uterine cavity. Three-dimensional ultrasonography therefore correctly detected a septate uterus in 61 patients (Figure 3). Interestingly, in our study, septate uterus was not mistaken for bicornuate uterus. Transvaginal color Doppler sonography, hysterosonography and 3D ultrasonography were performed. However, in one patient with bicornuate uterus, transvaginal ultrasonography misinterpreted the diagnosis as septate uterus.

A total of 188 patients underwent X-ray HSG within 12 months prior to our examination. X-ray HSG made a diagnosis of septate uterus in 49 patients according to Reuter's criteria[15]. Septate uterus was suspected if the angle between the two cavities was < 75°, while a bicornuate uterus was suspected for angles of > 105°. In 15 cases (7.98%) hysterosalpingography indicated a deformed uterine cavity, but congenital anomaly of the uterus was not suspected. The sensitivity of X-ray HSG in the diagnosis of septate uterus was only 26.06%.

Our second study attempted to evaluate the obstetric complications in a population of 278 patients with septate uterus and to compare these findings with those in a control group of the general population during the 5-year period of 1992 to 1996[21]. Early abortions appeared at a rate of 114/278 (41.01%) as compared to a rate of 15% for controls. Late abortions and premature deliveries appeared at a rate of 35/278 (12.59%) as compared to a rate of 7% for pregnancies in the control group. Intrauterine growth restriction appeared in two (8.7%) pregnancies with septate uterus as compared to 6% among the general population. Intrauterine fetal death occurred in one (4.35%) patient as compared to 0.5% in our control population. Abruptio placentae was found in one (4.35%) patient with septate uterus, as well as placenta previa (4.35%). Breech presentation was found in six (26.09%) pregnancies complicated by intrauterine septum, while transverse presentation occurred in two (8.70%) patients. Since abnormal fetal presentation was significantly more frequent in patients with septate uterus, a remarkably higher rate of Cesarean section (34.78%) occurred. Cervical incompetence during pregnancy appeared in nine (25.71%) women with intrauterine septum.

Extrauterine pregnancy appeared in 76 patients at a rate of 27.34%, which was two times higher than in our control group (13.3%). Bilateral ectopic pregnancy was noted in seven patients with septate uterus.

We assessed the reproductive outcome in 116 patients (32 with primary sterility, 16 with one spontaneous abortion, 12 with premature deliveries and 26 with recurrent abortions) following operative hysteroscopy for an intrauterine septum. The prospective follow-up period was 24 months for each patient. The pregnancy rate in the studied group was 50.86%: 44 patients (74.58%) had term deliveries, 11 (18.64%) had a first-trimester abortion and four (6.78%) reported preterm delivery. Other patients ($n = 162$) are followed in the same manner, but the follow-up period is less than 24 months and therefore is not reported in this study.

New ideas on an old problem

Until now at least two procedures have been used for detection of congenital uterine anomalies. Gynecologists should be aware that long diagnostic evaluation delays the treatment and increases the cost, patient's discomfort and risk associated with each of the diagnostic procedures[15]. Therefore, quick and reliable diagnosis is important in patients with septate uterus, since surgical correction should be recommended. Fedele and colleagues[6] recently indicated that intrauterine septum may be a cause of primary infertility. They demonstrated significant ultrastructural alterations in septal endometrium compared with endometrium from the lateral uterine wall in samples obtained during the preovulatory phase. The ultrastructural alterations included a reduced number of glandular ostia distributed irregularly, ciliated cells with incomplete ciliogenesis, and a reduced ciliated/non-ciliated ratio. The ultrastructural morphological alterations were indicative of irregular differentiation and estrogenic maturation of septal endometrial mucosa. Since the hormonal levels of the patients enrolled in this study were normal for the cycle phase, the most convincing hypothesis was that the endometrial mucosa covering the septum was poorly responsive to estrogens, probably owing to scanty vascularization of septal connective tissue.

March[22] stated that the septum is built from fibroelastic tissue, while Fayez[23] believed that in the septum there are fewer muscle fibers and more connective tissue. However, our study did not confirm this statement. Color and pulsed Doppler revealed septal vascularity in 71.22% of the patients, given the fact that most of the septa comprised myometrial vessels.

Dabirashrafi and associates[24] performed a histological study of the uterine septa from 16 patients undergoing abdominal metroplasty. Four biopsy specimens were taken from the uterus in each case: from the septum near the serosal layer, at the midpoint of the septum, at the level of the tip of the septum and from the left posterior aspect of the uterus away from the septum. Statistical analysis confirmed less connective tissue in the septum compared to the amount of muscle tissue, muscle interlacing and vessels with a muscle wall, which was contradictory to the classic view about the histological features of the uterine septum.

Less connective tissue in the septum might be the reason for poor decidualization and placentation in the area of implantation[23,24]. Increased amounts of muscle tissue and muscle interlacing in the septum can cause an abortion by the higher and uncoordinated contractility of these muscles.

A recent study from our department[20] found no correlation between septal height and the occurrence of obstetric complications ($p > 0.05$). Abortions and late pregnancy complications occurred with the same rate in patients with small septa that were dividing less than one-third of the uterine cavity, and those with division of more than two-thirds of the uterine cavity (Table 3). The same was related to septal thickness: obstetric complications were found in the same proportion of the patients with tiny and those with thick septa ($p > 0.05$). Pregnancy loss correlated significantly with septal vascularity. Patients with vascularized septa had a significantly higher incidence of early pregnancy failure and late pregnancy complications than those with avascularized septa ($p < 0.05$).

By using transvaginal ultrasound it is possible to perform a precise assessment of the uterine morphology, including the endometrial lining and outer shape of the uterine muscle. The color Doppler technique allows simultaneous visualization of the morphology and vascular network, giving full information on the type of anomaly and the extent of the defect. The

Table 3 Rate of obstetric complications relating to septal morphology and vascularity. From reference 20, with permission

	Septal characteristics		Obstetric complications		Significance
	n	%	n	%	
Height					
Partial septum	126	45.32	86	68.25	$p > 0.05$
Complete septum	152	54.68	108	71.05	
Thickness					
< 1 cm (thin)	92	33.09	64	69.56	$p > 0.05$
> 1 cm (thick)	186	66.91	130	69.89	
Vascularity					
Vascularized	198	71.22	169	85.35	$p < 0.05$
Avascular	80	28.78	25	31.25	

visualization of the myometrial portion is further enhanced by detection of the myometrial vessels by the color Doppler technique. Furthermore, Doppler imaging can detect deficient intraseptal vascularity and/or inadequate endometrial development in patients with a septate uterus[25,26].

Three-dimensional ultrasound enables planar reformatted sections to be obtained through the uterus, allowing precise evaluation of the fundal indentation and the length of the septum. Based on our experience, this technique may give an incorrect impression of an arcuate uterus in patients with a fundal location of the leiomyoma. In these cases, the uterine cavity has a concave shape, while the fundal indentation is more shallow. Furthermore, shadowing caused by the uterine fibroids, irregular endometrial lining and decreased volume of the uterine cavity (in cases of intrauterine adhesions) are obvious limitations of 3D ultrasound. Recently, 3D power Doppler has been used to detect the vascularization of the uterine septa in a combined angiographic and gray rendering mode. This approach allows simultaneous analysis of the morphology, texture and vascularization (Figure 4).

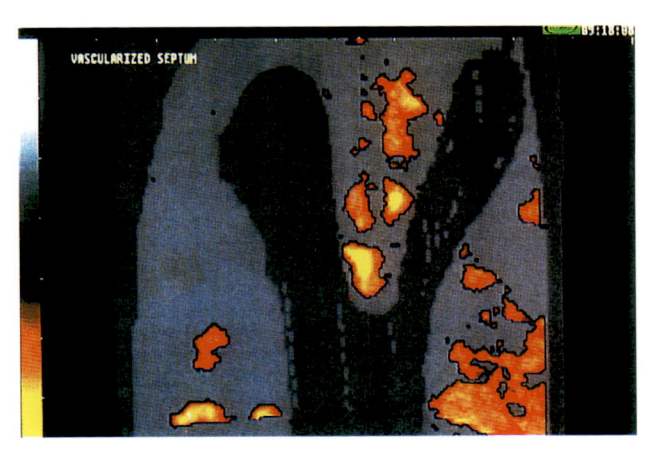

Figure 4 Three-dimensional power Doppler scan of a septate uterus. Note two separate endometria during saline-contrast hysterosonography. Power Doppler exposes vessels involving the uterine septum

Our study[21] clearly showed that obstetric complications were more frequent among patients with a septate uterus than among other women. Furthermore, it demonstrated that ectopic pregnancy occurred at double the rate (27.34%) in these patients, when compared to controls (13.3%). A possible etiology for this finding is menstrual reflux, commonly present in patients with uterine anomalies; these sequelae may interfere with passage of the fertilized egg into the uterine cavity. Furthermore, the benefit of removing the intrauterine septum in patients suffering from infertility and recurrent pregnancy wastage has been clearly demonstrated. It is expected that the cumulative pregnancy rate will be even higher, since some of the patients with primary infertility who are involved in an *in vitro* fertilization program owing to male factor await the procedure.

Three-dimensional hysterosonography

Balen and colleagues[27] described a technique of 3D reconstruction of the uterine cavity using a positive contrast medium (Echovist). The main problem that was encountered with Echovist was an acoustic shadowing artifact due to its highly reflective properties. This was especially noticeable on initial instillation of the contrast medium into the uterus. This artifact could be included in the 3D reconstruction because the region of interest was defined as being over a threshold level of echogenicity. This could ultimately lead to a false definition of the walls of the uterine cavity and, as observed in one patient, obscure a submucosal fibroid. Despite this, Echovist proved to be superior to saline as an intrauterine contrast agent for 3D reconstruction, in testing ten patients by both methods.

Weinraub and co-workers[28] applied 3D saline contrast hysterosonography in 32 volunteers, 22–65 years of age, all in good health and with no evidence of active infectious disease. Twelve patients had a history of infertility (six primary and six secondary), seven were referred because of abnormal uterine bleeding and 13 were investigated because of intrauterine abnormalities detected on routine pelvic ultrasound examination.

Two patients demonstrated uterine anomalies: one uterus was diagnosed as bicornuate, while another was didelphic. The three two-dimensional (2D) planes enabled simultaneous observation of the uterine cavity and the myometrium, which assisted in reaching the correct diagnosis. Surface rendering of those cases offered no advantages. While performing this technique, one should be aware of possible complications in patients with an overdistended cavity or occluded tubes. Owing to increased resistance, such patients may complain of dysmenorrhea-like pain, which usually resolves following decompression.

It seems that contrast 3D hysterosonography offers a more comprehensive overview of the uterine cavity and surrounding myometrium, and gives access to planes unobtainable by conventional 2D ultrasound examination. Further research is required, to document whether contrast instillation contributes to better diagnosis of uterine cavity pathology compared to an unenhanced frontal reformatted section.

Conventionally it has been agreed not to intervene until the first obstetric accidents have occurred, because a large proportion of septate uteri have no obstetric pathology[3]. However, hypofecundity in this group of patients and good results achieved by endoscopic surgical treatment oblige us to propose hysteroscopy as soon as we diagnose a septate uterus, even prior to any pregnancy[20,24,26]. It seems that septal incision eliminates an unsuitable site of implantation, through revascularization of the connective uterine fundal tissue or elimination of the unfavorable uterine contractions[6]. Since both of these events can be detected by 3D and power Doppler ultrasound, this new modality can be efficiently used for detection of congenital uterine malformations and follow-up of the patients undergoing hysteroscopy.

References

1. Ashton D, Amin HK, Richart RM, Neuwirth RS. The incidence of asymptomatic uterine anomalies in women undergoing transcervical tubal sterilization. *Obstet Gynecol* 1998;72:28–30
2. Sorensen S. Estimated prevalence of mullerian anomalies. *Acta Obstet Gynecol Scand* 1998;67:441–5
3. Gaucherand P, Awada A, Rudigoz RC, Dargent D. Obstetrical prognosis of septate uterus: a plea for treatment of the septum. *Eur J Obstet Gynecol Reprod Biol* 1994;54:109–12
4. Fedele L, Arcaini L, Parazzini F, Vercellini P, Nola GD. Metroplastic hysteroscopy and fertility. *Fertil Steril* 1993;59:768–70
5. Heinonen PK, Saarikoski S, Pystynen P. Reproductive performance of women with uterine anomalies. An evaluation of 182 cases. *Acta Obstet Gynecol Scand* 1982;61:157–62
6. Fedele L, Bianchi S, Marchini M, Franchi D, Tozzi L, Dorta M. Ultrastructural aspects of endometrium in infertile women with septate uterus. *Fertil Steril* 1996;65:750–2
7. McShane PM, Reilly RJ, Schiff L. Pregnancy outcome following Tompkins metroplasty. *Fertil Steril* 1983;40:190–4
8. Cararach M, Penella J, Ubeda J, Iabastida R. Hysteroscopic incision of the septate uterus: scissors versus resectoscope. *Hum Reprod* 1994;9:87–9
9. Goldenberg M, Sivan E, Sharabi Z. Reproductive outcome following hysteroscopic management of intrauterine septum and adhesions. *Hum Reprod* 1995;10:2663–5
10. Valdes C, Malini S, Malinak LR. Ultrasound evaluation of female genital tract anomalies: a review of 64 cases. *Am J Obstet Gynecol* 1984;149:285–90
11. Nicolini U, Bellotti B, Bonazzi D, Zamberleti G, Battista C. Can ultrasound be used to screen uterine malformation? *Fertil Steril* 1987;47:89–93
12. Reuter KL, Daly DC, Cohen SM. Septate versus bicornuate uteri: errors in imaging diagnosis. *Radiology* 1989;172:749–52
13. Randolph J, Ying Y, Maier D, Schmidt C, Riddick D. Comparison of real time ultrasonography, hysterosalpingography, and laparoscopy/hysteroscopy in the evaluation of uterine abnormalities and tubal patency. *Fertil Steril* 1986;5:828–32
14. Richman TS, Viscomi GN, Cherney AD, Polan A. Fallopian tubal patency assessment by ultrasound following fluid injection. *Radiology* 1984;152:507–10
15. Salle B, Sergeant P, Galcherand P, Guimont I, De Saint Hilaire P, Rudigoz RC. Transvaginal hysterosonographic evaluation of septate uteri: a preliminary report. *Hum Reprod* 1996;11:1004–7
16. Marshall C, Mintz DI, Thickman D, Gussman H, Kressel Y. MR evaluation of uterine anomalies. *Radiology* 1987;148:287–9
17. Carrington BM, Hricak M, Naruddin RN. Mullerian

duct anomalies: MR evaluation. *Radiology* 1990; 170:715–20
18. Jurkovic D, Giepel A, Gurboeck K, Jauniaux E, Natucci M, Campbell S. Three dimensional ultrasound for the assessment of uterine anatomy and detection of congenital anomalies: a comparison with hysterosalpingography and two-dimensional sonography. *Ultrasound Obstet Gynecol* 1995;5:233–7
19. Taylor PJ, Cumming DC. Hysteroscopy in 100 patients. *Fertil Steril* 1979;31:301–4
20. Kupesic S, Kurjak A. Septate uterus: detection and prediction of obstetrical complications by different forms of ultrasonography. *J Ultrasound Med* 1998;17:631–6
21. Kupesic S, Kurjak A. Diagnosis and treatment outcome of the septate uterus. *Croat Med J* 1998;39:185–90
22. March CM. Hysteroscopy as an aid to diagnosis in female infertility. *Clin Obstet Gynecol* 1983;26:302–12
23. Fayez JA. Comparison between abdominal and hysteroscopic metroplasty. *Obstet Gynecol* 1986;68:399–403
24. Dabrashrafi H, Bahadori M, Mohammad K, Alavi M, Moghadami-Tabrizi N, Zandinejad R. Septate uterus: new idea on the histologic features of the septum in this abnormal uterus. *Am J Obstet Gynecol* 1995;172:105–7
25. Kupesic S, Kurjak A. Uterine and ovarian perfusion during the periovulatory period assessed by transvaginal color Doppler. *Fertil Steril* 1993;3:439–43
26. Keltz MD, Olive DL, Kim AH, Arici A. Sonohysterography for screening in recurrent pregnancy loss. *Fertil Steril* 1997;67:670–4
27. Balen FG, Allen CM, Gardener JE, Siddle NC, Lees WR. 3-dimensional reconstruction of ultrasound images of the uterine cavity. *Br J Radiol* 1993;66:588–91
28. Weinraub Z, Maymon R, Shulman A, *et al*. Three-dimensional saline contrast rendering of uterine cavity pathology. *Ultrasound Obstet Gynecol* 1996:8:277–82

Three-dimensional hysterosonosalpingography

S. Kupesic, A. Kurjak and D. Bjelos

Introduction

The number of cases of tubal sterility is increasing and tubal factors, such as tubal dysfunction or obstruction, account for approximately 35% of the causes of infertility[1,2]. A history of pelvic inflammatory disease (PID), septic abortion, use of an intrauterine contraceptive device, ruptured appendix, tubal surgery, or ectopic pregnancy should alert the physician to the possibility of tubal damage. One aspect of the infertility investigation which has changed little over the past 20 years is the assessment of Fallopian tube patency. Until now, the most frequently used procedures to demonstrate tubal patency have been X-ray hysterosalpingography (HSG) and chromopertubation during laparoscopy[3].

HSG, using radio-opaque dye for X-ray studies to assess tubal and uterine anatomy, has been a standard form of investigation for several decades. The disadvantage of this type of investigation is that ionizing radiation has inherent risks to the oocyte, which may result in congenital malformations, if conception takes place in the investigatory cycle. Furthermore, known allergy to iodine-containing dyes is a contraindication to X-ray HSG. The benefit of X-ray HSG is opacification of the tubal lumen (for assessment of ampullary rugal pattern, intramural or intraluminal abnormalities of the Fallopian tube), while the risk factors include PID, dye sensitivity and infection. Anesthesia is not required.

Hysteroscopy is a technique that complements HSG. It can accurately differentiate between endometrial polyps and submucous leiomyomas, and can be used for their treatment. The same method is useful in establishing the definitive diagnosis and treatment of intrauterine adhesions and some congenital anomalies of the uterus. Risk factors include perforation, hemorrhage, infection and eventually anesthetic risk if anesthesia is required.

Hysteroscopy-directed falloposcopy can detect obstruction of the tubal ostium, and can be utilized to examine the entire length of the tubal lumen[4]. Treatment of the proximal tubal obstruction can immediately follow the diagnosis. Transcervical tubal cannulation or balloon tuboplasty performed by the hysteroscopic approach are the methods of choice[5].

Laparoscopy, to investigate tubal status, has been used as the gold standard in the past two decades, but this requires general anesthesia and carries the risk of surgical complications, such as bowel or vascular injury, hemorrhage, infection, anesthetic risk, false pneumoperitoneum and postoperative discomfort[6]. With a Jarcho-type of cannula in the uterine cavity, one can manipulate the uterus, and, by instilling indigo-carmine saline, or other tinted saline, one can test for tubal competence. Through laparoscopy it is possible to visualize the total pelvic anatomy and the upper abdominal cavity. This is also useful for evaluation of ovarian disease, genital anomalies, tubal and adnexal competence and the differentiation between pelvic distortions. Furthermore, laparoscopy is valuable for reaching an accurate classification of endometriosis of the pelvis. Laparoscopy can be used as an adjunct in assessing possible causes of pelvic pain and the extent of pelvic neoplasia, as well as for a prognostic review of a previous surgical procedure for infertility. It has also been helpful in obtaining peritoneal washings and cultures in patients with a positive history of PID.

Ultrasound imaging of the pelvic organs has improved significantly with the use of high-frequency vaginal ultrasound probes where the need for bladder filling can be avoided. The normal Fallopian tube is usually not seen by vaginal sonography unless some fluid surrounds it. The contrasting fluid may be one of the following: the normal serous fluid, follicular fluid during or after ovulation, blood, ascitic fluid, or products of an exudative or infectious process. If the Fallopian tube is not filled with fluid its lumen cannot be detected[7]. The benefits of CD HSG are: ionization or idiosyncrasy to contrast media are avoided; the test is easily repeatable; it requires the active, intraprocedural participation of the patient (increasing her knowledge of tubal status); it is a dynamic procedure, analyzing tubal motility; the procedure course is stored, reviewed, analyzed and interpreted for the infertile couple by means of a video recorder; anesthesia is not required; and it also allows collaboration with the Radiology Department.

The accuracy of sonographic HSG compared to X-ray HSG has varied from 70.37% to 90.48%[8–10] (Table

Table 1 The accuracy of sonographic compared to X-ray hysterosalpingography

Authors	Total number	Accuracy	Sensitivity (%)	Specificity (%)
Richman et al. (1984)[7]	36		100	96
Peters and Coulam (1991)[8]	27	19 (70.37%)		
Stern et al. (1992)[9]	89	72 (80.90%)		
Volpi et al. (1996)[10]	21	19 (90.48%)		

Table 2 The accuracy of sonographic hysterosalpingography compared to chromopertubation

Authors	Total number	Accuracy
Allahbadia (1993)[6]	27	25 (92.59%)
Tüfekci et al. (1992)[11]	38	37 (97.37%)
Peters and Coulam (1991)[8]	58	50 (86.20%)
Kupesic and Kurjak (1994)[12]	47	43 (91.48%)
Stern et al. (1992)[9]	121	99 (81.82%)
Deichert et al. (1992)[13]	16	16 (100.00%)
Volpi et al. (1996)[10]	29	24 (82.76%)
Holte et al. (1995)[14]	14	12 (85.71%)

1). The accuracy of sonographic HSG compared to chromopertubation has varied from 81.82% to 100.00%[6, 8–14] (Table 2).

In this chapter recent data on the use of different forms of HSG are presented, with emphasis on the three-dimensional (3D) approach. However, everybody entering this field should know the historical development of this procedure.

Historical development of the ultrasonic assessment of the Fallopian tube

In 1954, Rubin[15] published the first attempt at insufflating the Fallopian tubes. Ultrasound visualization of the internal genital tract using exogenous contrast media was described by Nanini and colleagues[16], Richman and colleagues[7] and Randolph and colleagues[17], who performed abdominal sonography after intracervical injection of fluid.

Richman and colleagues[7] were the first to report on the transabdominal sonographic evaluation of tubal patency. In their studies they used a special intrauterine catheter, the Harris uterine injector (Unimar, Canoga Park, CA). After injection of at least 20 ml of the ultrasonic contrast medium Hyskon (dextran in dextrose; Pharmacia Laboratories, Piscataway, NJ), the accumulation of the fluid in the cul-de-sac was accepted as an indicator of tubal patency.

Randolph and co-workers[17] used transabdominal ultrasound for observation of the cul-de-sac after the injection of 200 ml isotonic saline through the Rubin cannula. The presence of retrouterine fluid was accepted as a criterion for patency of one or both tubes. Tubal patency was deduced indirectly from the presence of increasing fluid in the pouch of Douglas, without differentiation of the sides.

Following instillation of dextran or saline solution into the uterine cavity it was possible to visualize lesions such as submucous myomas and polyps by sonography and subsequently to confirm their presence by hysteroscopy[17–20]. Although lesions of this type, which project into the uterine cavity, are clearly delineated by poorly echogenic or anechoic media, very small hollow cavities, such as the lumen of normal tubes, can rarely be visualized with such techniques[7,21]. Their demonstration requires visualization of the movement of a fluid, which in turn requires the use of a highly echogenic medium[22–24].

A new transvaginal ultrasonographic technique was developed in 1989 by Deichert and colleagues[25]. They visualized the patent tube directly and hence showed tubal patency by transcervical injection of an echogenic and ultrasonic contrast fluid SHU 454 (Echovist; Schering, Berlin, Germany). The method has been called transvaginal hysterosalpingocontrast sonography (HyCoSy). They used a Rubin cannula or a bladder catheter no. 8. The same researchers have continued their studies on transvaginal HyCoSy using general anesthesia[26, 27].

Tüfekci and co-workers[11] have developed an easier technique, in which the patient does not require hospitalization. By intrauterine injection of isotonic saline solution, they evaluated tubal patency directly and called this method transvaginal sonosalpingography. Transvaginal sonosalpingography performed by using isotonic saline solution without anesthesia is physiological, easy to perform, safe, cost-effective, non-invasive and more convenient than other conventional methods. Idiosyncrasy to the contrast agent cannot be expected.

Ultrasound contrast agents

All media having a different echogenicity from that of the human body can be used as contrast media. Contrast media are divided into two groups: hypoechogenic and hyperechogenic. Isotonic saline, Ringer's or dextran solutions belong to the first group. Instillation of these media facilitates the detection of echogenic border surfaces. The main disadvantage is that it is not possible to visualize the phenomena of motion and flow. Hyperechogenic contrast media enhance echo signals, allowing detection of the flow by both B-mode and Doppler ultrasound. Gramiak and Shah[28] and Meltzer and co-workers[29] found that small gas bubbles effectively reflect ultrasonic waves. Therefore, all the commercial echo contrast media contain microbubbles. The commercial products Echovist and Levovist (Schering AG, Berlin) are suspensions of microbubbles made of special galactose microparticles. The galactose microparticles are suspended either in galactose solution (Echovist) or in sterile water (Levovist)[30].

Echovist (SHU 454) is an ultrasound contrast medium consisting of a suspension of only monosaccharide microparticles (50% galactose, diameter 2 μm), in a 20% aqueous solution of galactose (w/v). The echogenic suspension is reconstituted immediately before use from granules and a vehicle solution (200 mg microparticles in 1 ml of suspension)[31]. This contrast medium has been licensed for gynecological applications on the market since 1995.

Levovist (SHU 508) microparticle granules contain in addition a very low concentration of physiological palmitic acid.

A few minutes before use, the granules have to be shaken vigorously for 5–10 s to be dissolved by an appropriate volume of aqueous galactose solution (Echovist) or sterile water (Levovist). A milky suspension of galactose microparticles in a solution is created after disaggregation of the microparticle 'snowball'. The suspension of Echovist is stable for about 5 min after preparation. Owing to its extended stability, Levovist may be administered up to 10 min after the suspension procedure.

Depending on the indication and the imaging modality (B-mode or Doppler), a clinically adequate suspension of Echovist has a concentration of 200 or 300 mg/ml. For Levovist, the maximum concentration is 400 mg/ml. The predominant limitation at concentrations lower than 200 mg/ml is the decreasing suspension stability. Concentrations exceeding 400 mg/ml are limited by a rapid increase of viscosity[31–33].

After intrauterine administration and emergence of Echovist from the fimbriae into the pelvis, the galactose microparticles dissolve. This progress is increased by warming to body temperature and dilution by the peritoneal fluid. *In vitro*, a rise in temperature of the Echovist suspension to 37 °C leads to complete dissolution within 30 min. The dissolved galactose is subsequently absorbed and metabolized.

Numerous clinical studies in the field of echocardiography, venous system analysis and HSG showed no evidence of serious side-effects. An absolute contraindication for instillation of these fluids is galactosemia (an autosomal recessive disease in which, owing to deficiency of galactose-1-phosphate uridyltransferase, galactose cannot be metabolized into glucose).

In addition, ultrasoud contrast agents are media which, when administered via the vascular system or into body cavities, change the acoustic properties of the body region under investigation. The acoustic parameters that contribute to tissue imaging by conventional sonographic units are backscatter, attenuation and the velocity of sound. Enhancement of backscatter is the most important contrast effect, since contrast agents introduce acoustic heterogeneities caused by microstructures (scatterers).

Technique of HyCoSy

Requirements

A case history must be obtained from a woman considered for examination by this technique, to rule out the possibility of the rare condition of galactosemia, which is the only absolute contraindication, apart from acute inflammatory disease of the genital organs. A gynecological and ultrasound examination prior to the procedure is necessary to define the uterine position and anomalies, if present, as well as both adnexal regions. Before any intervention, we perform a pregnancy test for legal reasons. The possibility of local or systemic infections is excluded by clinical examination (absence of elevated temperature), inspection of the genital tract and absence of signs of inflammation. The procedure should not be performed in patients with active pelvic infections, and antibiotic prophylaxis (doxycycline and metronidazole) should be used in patients with a history of PID. HyCoSy should be performed during the early follicular phase of the menstrual cycle, after the complete cessation of menses. This avoids dispersion of menstrual debris into the peritoneal cavity. Procedures carried out in this period allow absorption of the media prior to ovulation, thus avoiding the presence of a foreign substance arround the time of an imminent corpus luteum. This decreases any theoretical effect the media may have on tubal transport. HSG performed during the immediate premenstrual phase of the cycle has been advocated in the evolution of possible cervical incompetence, as that is the point in the cycle at which there is the maximum uterine constriction. Therefore, in order to maximize the information obtained, the indication for the study has an influence on timing.

Patients are informed of the benefits and the possible risks of the procedure and the procedure itself is described to them in detail. Anesthesia is generally not required for HyCoSy, and the patient can follow the results of the examination by herself on the monitor. If HyCoSy is performed without anesthesia, patients occasionally report discomfort, especially if the tubes are occluded. The degree of discomfort depends on the individual response of the patient. Premedication or sedation is routinely used: 5–10 mg of diazepam intravenously is beneficial, especially in anxious patients. Pain signifies the obstruction and potential intravasation or tubal rupture, and should not be masked by anesthesia. However, tubal spasm may occur if HyCoSy is performed without or even with anesthesia. This could mimic a tubal occlusion. Pretreatment with atropine (0.5 mg) may prevent this complication. The parenteral administration of 1 mg glucagon may relieve the spasm and allow the flow of the contrast medium[7,34,35].

Procedure

The patient voids and is positioned supine on the gynecological table. With the patients legs flexed, a speculum is inserted into the vagina and positioned such that the entire cervix is visualized and the os is easily accessible. The cervix and the vagina are then thoroughly scrubbed with Betadine solution. A tenaculum is placed on the anterior lip of the cervix, and the cannula is gently guided into the endocervical canal. Application of the contrast medium is performed via a small and very thin uterine catheter fitted with a balloon for stabilization and occlusion of the internal cervical os. The first observation to be made is of the uterine cavity, with verification of the catheter placement. After removal of the tenaculum, the transvaginal probe is gently introduced into the posterior fornix of the vagina. The contrast medium (sterile saline) is then injected slowly, under control of the ultrasound picture. Usually, no more than 5–10 ml of contrast medium is instilled into the uterine cavity. At this stage one can observe the morphology of the uterus and its endometrial lining and detect duplication anomalies of the uterus or the existence of endometrial polyps or submucous fibroids that are protruding into the uterine cavity, which is marked with anechoic contrast.

The benefits of hysterosonosalpingography include: reproducible and reliable assessment of tubal patency if used by a trained physician; avoidance of exposure to X-rays, allergic reactions and general anesthesia; the possibility of being performed as an out-patient procedure; and the fact that it is well tolerated, rapid and shows tubal patency to the patient in real time. Limitations include the possibilities that: tubal spasm may lead to misdiagnosis of tubal occlusion (spasm is also seen with other methods); tubal flow may give a false impression of tubal patency in the hydrosalpinx; intrapelvic pathology and bowel cannot be visualized; the procedure requires a degree of technical competence; and 10–20 investigations are needed to acquire facility with the new technique. The benefits and limi-

Table 3 The benefits and limitations of hysterosonosalpingography

Benefits
Provides a reproducible and reliable assessment of tubal patency if used by a trained physician
Avoids exposure to X-rays
Avoids allergic reactions
Avoids general anesthesia
Can be performed as an out-patient procedure
Is rapid
Is well tolerated, with little discomfort and few adverse events
Shows tubal patency to the patient in real time

Limitations
Tubal spasm may lead to misdiagnosis of tubal occlusion (spasm also seen with other methods)
In hydrosalpinx, tubal flow may give a false impression of tubal patency
Cannot visualize intrapelvic pathology and bowel
Requires a degree of technical competence
10–20 investigations are needed to acquire competence in the new technique

tations of hysterosonosalpingography are represented in Table 3.

Gray-scale HyCoSy (B-mode)

Deichert and colleagues[13,36] evaluated transvaginal HyCoSy for the assessment of tubal patency with gray-scale imaging (B-mode) and the additional use of pulsed wave Doppler. During the last stages of the examination the ultrasound contrast medium, Echovist, is prepared. The uterine cavity, which in most cases will still be dilated by the Ringer's solution instilled previously, is slowly filled with the echogenic ultrasound contrast medium. If the tube is patent, constant flow in a pattern resembling a point, spot or streak is seen. Further intermittent injections of volumes of 1–2 ml, given slowly and continuously, with further lateral sweeps of the ultrasound probe, allow visualization of intraluminal or intratubal flow under normal anatomical conditions via the pars intramuralis into the medial and distal segments of the tubes. For the diagnosis of tubal patency, two or three observation phases per tube are needed, with an observation period of continuous flow of about 10 s (while contrast medium is slowly injected). Although visualization of a longer segment of the tube beyond the pars intramuralis is convincing for tubal patency, one should carefully examine the adnexal regions for filling of the distal segments of the tube to exclude sactosalpinx. Examination of the pouch of Douglas for any increase in retrouterine fluid, compared with the picture at the start of the examination, completes the examination procedure.

Pulsed Doppler analysis of tubal patency

Deichert and colleagues advise confirming the findings by pulsed wave Doppler scanning, if the examination in B-mode reveals evidence suggesting tubal occlusion or if it is possible to visualize only a segment of tube of less than 2 cm in length[13,36]. After the Doppler gate has been positioned over the area to be examined, the gate width is reduced to measure only the flow noise from the pertubation and not vascular or other noise. Brief injections (about 5 s) of contrast medium are made again. The sounds heard, which are long, drawn-out and initially hissing, and the simultaneous visualization of a broad noise band on the monitor, the width of the band slowly decreasing after injection, indicate that the tube is patent. Thus, unobstructed flow is characterized by a short filling phase with a rapid, steep increase in Doppler shift and a slow, uniform fall in Doppler shift along the time axis, indicating unobstructed free distal outflow. The absence of these acoustic signals or optical tracings indicates obstruction of tubal flow or tubal occlusion. In this case there is only a short, steep Doppler shift with no subsequent noise signals. This indicates an absence of outflow of contrast medium distal to the Doppler gate. A sonographic finding of unobstructed tubes on the basis of noise band in pulsed wave Doppler sonography is more impressive than that of a shorter segment of tube in standing B-mode.

Deichert and colleagues[13] tried to determine whether the additional use of pulsed wave Doppler could improve the tubal diagnosis reached with gray-scale imaging in doubtful cases. They studied 17 patients with diagnosed sterility problems. HyCoSy by gray-scale and by pulsed wave Doppler and follow-up chromolaparoscopy ($n = 16$) or HSG ($n = 1$) were performed. The diagnostic efficacies of gray-scale and pulsed wave Doppler were compared with each other and with a conventional control procedure (chromolaparoscopy or HSG). The gray-scale findings were confirmed by pulsed wave Doppler in five cases on one side; confirmed by pulsed wave Doppler in seven cases on both sides; corrected by pulsed wave Doppler in one case on one side and confirmed on the other side by pulsed wave Doppler. In all 17 cases, the tubal findings after pulsed wave Doppler were confirmed by chromolaparoscopy or HSG. The additional use of pulsed wave Doppler in HyCoSy is recommended as a supplement to gray-scale imaging in cases of suspected tubal occlusion and in the event of intratubal flow demonstrable over only a short distance.

Deichert assessed tubal patency using HyCoSy, conventional HSG or laparoscopy with dye, in 76 women and visualized 152 Fallopian tubes. In this study, HyCoSy showed 87.5% concordance with other techniques, predicted 100% of tubal occlusions and detected 86% of patent tubes.

According to Ayida and colleagues[37], saline contrast hysterosonography, as a screening test for any cavity abnormality, had 87.5% sensitivity, 100% specificity, 100% positive predictive value and 91.6% negative predictive value.

Color Doppler hysterosalpingography

Transvaginal color Doppler HSG is a safe and efficacious method for evaluation of Fallopian tube patency without exposure to radiation or contrast dyes[38]. The cost of the procedure is significantly lower than for X-ray HSG and it gives immediate results[10]. It is advisable that all the scans be recorded on a video recorder and/or Polaroid films[25].

Further advantages of transvaginal sonosalpingography include the possibility of performing the procedure on an out-patient basis. This has significantly altered the need for in-patient facilities in some infertility departments[12]. Similar to X-ray HSG, bleeding, pregnancy and the presence of adnexal masses on pelvic or ultrasound examination are contraindications to color Doppler HSG. The equipment needed to perform color Doppler HSG includes an ultrasound unit with color Doppler capability and an intrauterine catheter[39]. The intrauterine cannula is placed into the uterus. One balloon is placed at the level of the internal cervical os, while another is fixed in the external cervical os. A tiny tubal catheter with a metal end is introduced after exploration of the uterine cavity. Sterile saline solution, 5–10 ml, is instilled into the uterine cavity. After the observation of the morphology of the uterus and endometrial lining, the color Doppler is directed at the cornual region where the tubal catheter with the metal end should be located. The exact placement of the catheter is sonographically controlled. Color signals passing through the Fallopian tube indicate its patency, and the absence of such signals is interpreted as tubal occlusion[8,40]. Accumulation of fluid in the cul-de-sac on the side of injection controlled by transvaginal color and pulsed Doppler is an accurate indicator of ipsilateral tubal patency. Selective tubal injection increases the accuracy of the procedure and appropriateness of the interpretation. The procedure is repeated for the contralateral side.

Difficulty in making the diagnosis of tubal occlusion arises in those patients with dilated hydrosalpinges, because flow through the dilated Fallopian tube may stimulate spillage on the Doppler ultrasonography screen. To avoid this error, both adnexa should be carefully observed before the procedure. In addition, the tubal architecture is not demonstrated with color Doppler flow HSG. However, a recent study has shown this information not to be useful in preoperative salpingoplasty procedures[41].

Using our modified technique, we compared the findings of color Doppler HSG from 47 patients with those of chromopertubation at the time of laparoscopy[12]. The machines used were Aloka SSD 680 and 2000. Forty-three out of 47 (91.48%) color Doppler HSG findings agreed with observations at chromopertubation. In only one patient, in whom no patency was seen in both tubes under color Doppler evaluation, was indirect diagnosis of tubal patency performed by observing free fluid in the cul-de-sac.

The increased incidence of conception during the 3 months after the procedure (in our study, two patients) may be an effect of a mechanical lavage of the uterus by dislodging the mucous plugs, breakdown of the peritoneal adhesions, or a stimulatory effect on the tubal cilia.

No serious side-effects were observed during and after the transvaginal color Doppler HSG procedure. Eighteen patients complained of pain that continued for 2–10 min after the procedure. No medication was required for these cases. The shortest time taken for the transvaginal color Doppler HSG was 5 min, and the longest time was 14 min. After removal of the instruments, the cervix is inspected for hemostasis and pressure is applied to the tenaculum site whenever necessary.

Review of the literature

To assess the accuracy of the diagnosis of tubal occlusion with the use of color Doppler flow ultrasonography and HSG, Peters and Coulam[8] studied 129 infertile women. When results of ultrasonography–HSG were compared with those of X-ray HSG and/or chromopertubation, 69 of 85 (81%) studies showed agreement, and 50 out of 58 (86%) ultrasound HSG findings agreed with observations at chromopertubation. The frequency of comparable findings between X-ray HSG and chromopertubation was 75%.

Richman and colleagues[7] evaluated tubal patency in 36 infertile women. They compared ultrasound findings with conventional hysterosalpingograms, which had been obtained simultaneously. Ultrasound demonstrated bilateral occlusion with a sensitivity of 100%, and showed tubal patency with a specificity of 96%.

Tüfekci and colleagues[11] studied 38 women with infertility complaints. The results obtained from transvaginal sonosalpingography and laparoscopy were completely consistent for 29 cases (76.32%), and partially consistent for eight cases (21.05%). Only one case showed an inconsistent result. Complete consistence indicated that the passage through both Fallopian tubes was identical by both methods. Partial consistence indicated identical results for only either the left or the right tube. Transvaginal sonosalpingography correctly indicated tubal patency or non-patency in 37 of 38 cases.

Heikkinen and co-workers[42] evaluated the advantages and accuracy of transvaginal salpingosonography in the assessment of tubal patency with regard to laparoscopic chromopertubation. Sixty-one Fallopian tubes were examined by both techniques. Concordance was 85%. By transvaginal sonosalpingography, 45 tubes were found to be patent and 16 occluded. In chromopertubation, 50 tubes were patent and 11 were occluded. Bilateral tubal patency was found by transvaginal salpingosonography in 17 cases and by laparoscopy in 22 cases. Bilateral occlusion was found in three cases using either technique. Transvaginal sonosalpingography with the combination of air and saline is a low-cost, reliable, safe and comfortable examination method and it can be used for the primary investigation of infertility on an outpatient basis.

Battaglia and co-workers[43] found that correlation between color Doppler HSG and X-ray HSG with chromolaparoscopy occurred in 86% vs. 93% of all women studied.

Stern and colleagues[9] administered saline transcervically during transvaginal color Doppler sonography in 238 women. Traditional X-ray HSG was performed in 89 women. Laparoscopy with chromopertubation was performed in 121 women. Forty-nine women had all three procedures performed. A correlation between color ultrasound HSG and X-ray findings with chromopertubation occurred in 81% vs. 60% ($p = 0.0008$) of all women studied. In the forty-nine women who had all three procedures performed, color ultrasound HSG results correlated with chromopertubation more often than did X-ray HSG (82% vs. 57%; $p = 0.0152$). In their previous report[8], discrepancies between color ultrasound HSG and chromopertubation findings involved a diagnosis of unilateral patency. They recommended repeating color ultrasound HSG before making a diagnosis of unilateral occlusion.

Allahbadia[6] reported a 92.6% agreement between color Doppler ultrasonography compared with HSG and laparoscopy. The HSG and laparoscopy findings were in 100% agreement. The same author also described the so-called Sion procedure or hydrogynecography. This procedure takes about 15 min as compared to the 5–6 min for sonosalpingography. After accomplishing sonosalpingography, sterile normal saline solution is injected until approximately 350 ml has flooded the pelvis. With the adnexa and uterus submerged in a fluid medium, the scanning of the pelvis is repeated. If there is a bilateral tubal block and reflux of the saline is seen in the stem of the Foley's catheter, the pelvis is filled by alternative means. The saline solution fills the pelvis and delineates all sorts of adhesions. All the patients undergoing this procedure are similarly given prophylactic antibiotics. Contrary to the optimistic results of different ultrasound techniques for evaluation of tubal patency[16,25], Balen and colleagues[44] found ultrasound contrast HSG using both sterile saline and Echovist contrast media insufficiently accurate and inferior to conventional X-ray HSG. False-positive rates in the range of 9% and false-negative rates in the range of 20% have been reported in the diagnosis of tubal obstruction by color Doppler HSG[9]. Therefore, all abnormal hysterosalpingogram studies deserve laparoscopic or hysteroscopic follow-up.

Normal X-ray or color Doppler HSG does not rule out the need for diagnostic laparoscopy. While X-ray HSG is the most accurate method for diagnosing intramural or intraluminal abnormalities of the Fallopian tube, color Doppler HSG is the only available non-invasive method for analyzing tubal motility.

To obtain maximum information, the procedure should be performed by a well-trained physician who is familiar with the color Doppler investigation, and who is capable of manipulating the instruments, the patient's reproductive tract and the rate of injection.

Three-dimensional hysterosonosalpingography

Currently, large technological efforts are being invested in promoting the capability of demonstrating the third dimension, although there is no doubt about the diagnostic value of two-dimensional (2D) ultrasound in obstetrics and gynecology. The 3D ultrasound image is generated by superimposing the programmed volume box over the 2D ultrasound image of the uterus[45]. The volumetric rotor is set into operation. The vaginal transducer then performs a sweep of transverse sections that are to be stored in the computer. The computer integrates the images and enables the sonographer to view three planes simultaneously. Once the perpendicular plane (plane C) to the transducer is obtained, the calculated 3D image with the complete volume scan is stored in a removable computer disk. This scanning procedure lasts between 2 and 10 s. The examination of the patient is complete, but the sonographer can analyze selected sections later. Three-dimensional images are generated only when the three planes are integrated and displayed on the screen. It is possible to rotate and translate any plane of the volume stored. To generate a final 3D image of the uterine cavity, a threshold has to be defined, up to which the echogenicity should be taken for reconstruction of the uterine cavity[45]. Depending on the structure to be studied, different 3D modes can be elaborated. The surface reconstruction mode allows study of the outer contour or profile of the uterus. The transparent maximum/minimum mode reveals objects with high echogenicity in the interior of the uterus. The basic structural information provided by conventional scans in the longitudinal and transverse planes can now be augmented by new 3D ultrasound that provides an additional view of the coronal or C plane, which is parallel to the transducer face[46]. The computer-generated scan is displayed in three perpendicular planes. The presentation of three perpendicular planes on one screen allows free scrolling of an endless amount of frames through the volume of interest. The coronal- or C-plane view allows more detailed analysis of the uterus and, for the first time, the endometrial cavity between the uterine angles can be visualized. Translation or rotation can be carried out in one plane while maintaining the perpendicular orientation of all three. The images produced by transvaginal ultrasound are superior to those produced by transabdominal ultrasound, because vaginal transducers are in closer proximity to the tissues[46]. Because of this, higher frequencies are used and artifactual echoes caused by multiple reflections from intervening tissues are minimized.

Demonstration of the coronal plane is mandatory for the diagnosis of uterine pathology, such as septate, arcuate or bicornuate uteri, and also provides the most exact measurement of the endometrial width when transsected in a midperpendicular manner. During 3D hysterosonography the typical triangulated uterine cavity appears in its full shape[47]. Surface rendering or maximal/minimal or X-ray renderings provide even more information on uterine findings, such as uterine anatomy or the uterine cavity and its content. There are two techniques to accomplish this goal: the native approach; and the use of echogenic contrast medium, which is especially useful for demonstrating the uterine cavity (Figure 1). Owing to its dual consistency of endometrium and myometrium, the uterus is an excellent ultrasonic medium. Those two tissues have different acoustic impedance which permits visualization of the size and shape of the uterus and its cavity. In addition, the use of a contrast medium is mandatory in cases where a thin endometrium or pathological content of the uterine cavity precludes its visualization.

The negative contrast medium, normal saline solution, is used for demonstration of the entire uterine cavity, its shape, pathology, and the frame of the myometrial mantle, whereas for demonstrating the permeability of the Fallopian tubes a positive contrast medium (Echovist) is used. Figure 2 demonstrates the three orthogonal planes of the uterus after instillation of the echogenic contrast agent. Power Doppler technology, sensitive to flow, was used for visualization of the echo contrast and triangular cavity of the uterus obtained by surface (color) rendering (Figure 3).

Weinraub and Herman[47] were the first to evaluate the findings of different pathology of the uterine anatomy and contents on 3D hysterosonography. Using three perpendicular planes on one screen, where

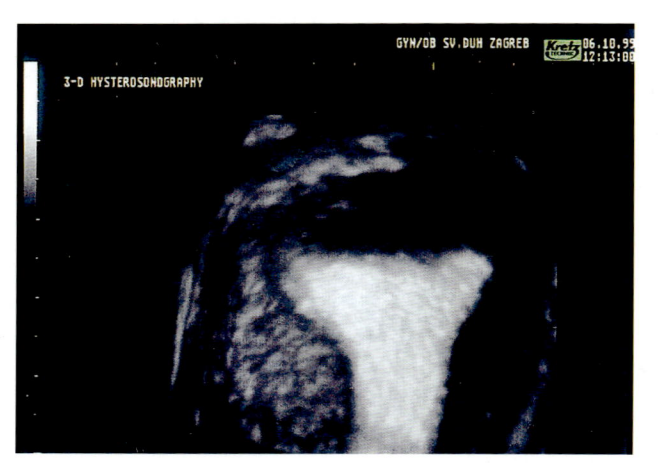

Figure 1 Frontal reformatted section of the uterus obtained after injection of the echogenic contrast agent. Note the regular contour of the uterine cavity

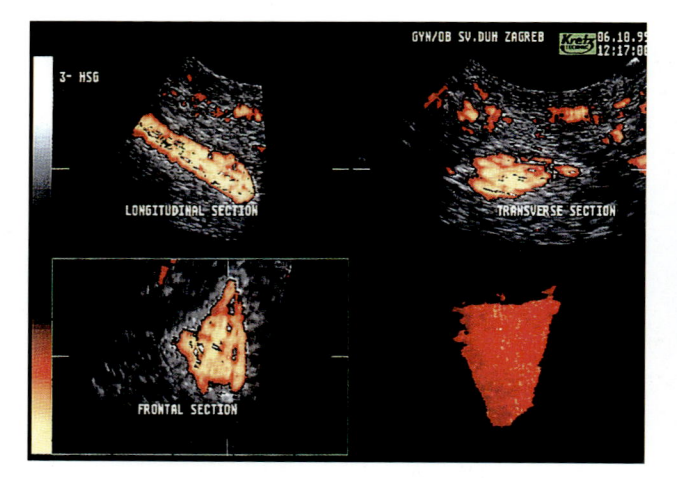

Figure 2 Three orthogonal planes of the uterus after instillation of the echogenic contrast medium, obtained by power Doppler. Note the three-dimensional power Doppler-generated image of the uterine cavity

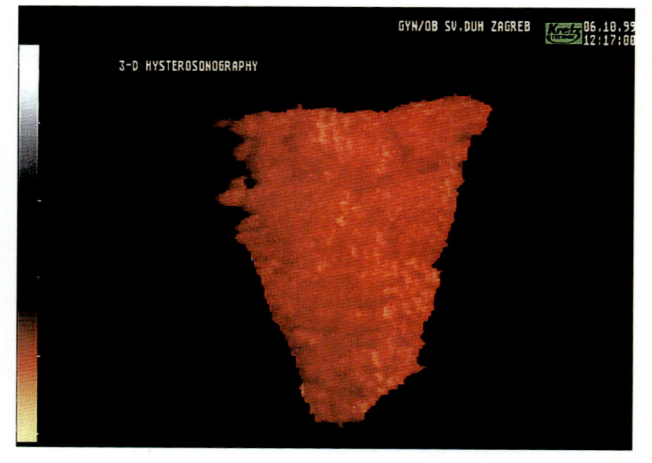

Figure 3 The same patient as in Figure 2. Power Doppler technology, sensitive to flow, facilitates visualization of the triangular uterine cavity

the left upper plane is coronal and is termed 'a', the right upper plane is sagittal and is termed 'b' and the left lower plane is transverse and is termed 'c', one can detect numerous causes of infertility.

Looking at the fundal region in 'a' it is very important not to overlook a small indentation, if it is present, in the case of septate uterus. The maximal endometrial width can be easily measured in the sagittal plane. If the transverse section shows separated uterine cornua, the finding is typical of an arcuate uterus. Clear concavity in the middle of the uterine fundus dividing the uterine cavity indicates a bicornuate uterus.

Hydrosonography is useful in the demonstration of intracavitary pathologies, such as adhesions, myomas, endometrial polyps, endometrial carcinoma, or location of intrauterine devices (IUDs). Using 3D surface rendering in the cases of intrauterine adhesions and myomas, it is possible to present the spatial orientation and the correlation of the adhesions with the surrounding uterine walls, also the round and smooth surface of the myoma, giving a feeling of depth inside the uterine cavity[47].

Hydrosonography, as well as 3D rendering, are especially important for diagnosis of an endometrial polyp. Despite the fact that the cut in the coronal plane went through the endometrial polyp, it was not demonstrated on the 'a' plane and could easily have been missed. Surprisingly, in rendering in the 'surface 58% and X-ray 42% mode', the polyp appeared on the screen. When hydrosonography was used, the polyp was easily examined in all three planes throughout the volume[47].

Fallopian tubes can be demonstrated on ultrasound only when they contain fluid (hydrosalpinx, pyosalpinx, bleeding ectopic pregnancy, or a contrast medium). In the case of hydrosalpinx, the fluid-filled Fallopian tube is demonstrated in the 'a' section, while 'b' and 'c' sections show the typical tubal epithelium. In the 'd' section, 3D rendering is shown (Figure 4). There are a number of difficulties in tubal visualization by HyCoSy[48]. Figure 5 demonstrates regular filling of the tube and free spillage from the fimbrial end as seen by 3D hysterosalpingography after injection of echogenic contrast medium. Owing to its tortuosity, the tube can rarely be seen completely in a single scanning plane and the echo-contrast medium is, therefore, observed in small sections. The position of the tube is variable, and distended bowel may prevent the visualization of the distal parts of the tubes. Therefore, usually only the tubal ostia and proximal parts of the tubes are visualized by gray-scale 2D ultrasound imaging. Free spreading of the dye is frequently difficult to visualize because the surrounding bowel can also produce strongly echogenic signals. Instead of visualizing the echo contrast with gray-scale ultrasound, Sladkevicius and colleagues[48] used 3D power Doppler technology, which is sensitive to slow flow. If the tube is patent, Doppler signals should

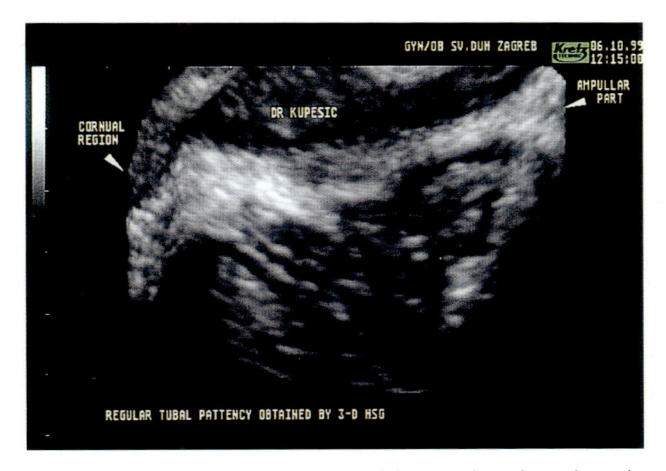

Figure 5 Three-dimensional hysterosalpingography using echogenic contrast medium. Note the regular filling of the tube, the full length of the tube and regular spillage from the fimbrial end (right)

Figure 4 Three-dimensional ultrasound scan of the fluid-filled Fallopian tube

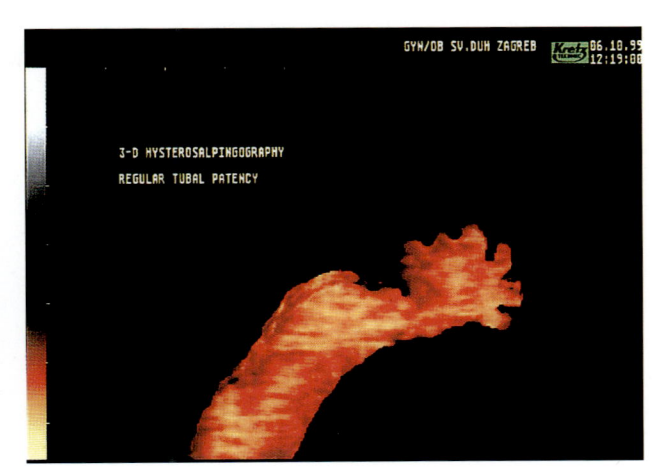

Figure 6 Power Doppler signals facilitate detection of tubal patency and evaluation of tubal morphology

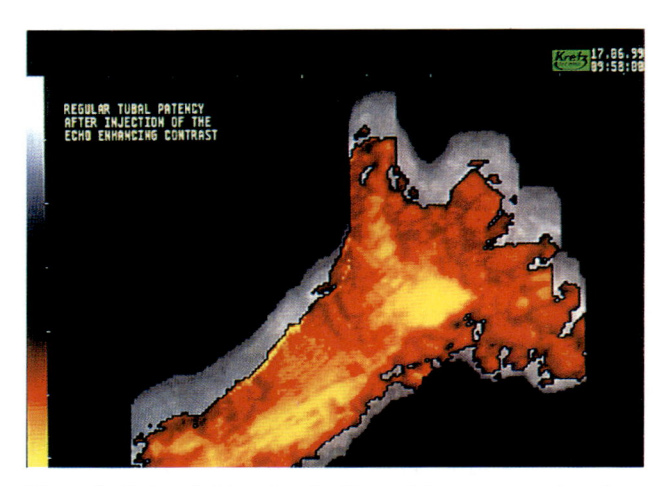

Figure 7 Entire tubal length and spillage of the contrast medium from the fimbrial end, as demonstrated by echo-enhanced three-dimensional power Doppler hysterosalpingography

be obtained from flow along the tube, and free spillage from the fimbrial end should be identified (Figure 6). Similarly, our group found that power Doppler visualization of echo-contrast flow was better than conventional imaging of the contrast media (Figure 7).

Ayida and colleagues[49] compared conventional two- and three-dimensional scanning of the uterine cavity with and without saline contrast medium. The 2D scanning suggested cavity abnormalities in four of ten women (three with fibroids; one with hyperechoic thick endometrium). The 3D scanning confirmed these and revealed one additional abnormality suggestive of a uterine septum. The 2D scanning with saline injection diagnosed abnormalities in five of ten (one with uterine septum; three with fibroids; one with endometrial polyp). The 3D contrast scanning with saline did not add any further information to the 2D contrast scanning with saline. In this pilot study, 3D scanning to assess the uterine cavity appeared to offer no advantages over conventional 2D contrast sonography.

Weinraub and colleagues[50] demonstrated the feasibility of combined 3D ultrasound and saline contrast HSG. Since volume sampling has a short pick-up time of a few seconds, the examination is over almost immediately after the uterus is reasonably distended. In this uncomfortable examination, such an advantage should not be underestimated. Evaluation of the uterine cavity at a later time allows the operator to manipulate the data at leisure and scrutinize the findings in desired planes that were not available during the initial examination. Simultaneous display of the three perpendicular planes offers a more comprehensive overview of the examined area and gives access to planes unobtainable by conventional 2D examination. Surface rendering may confirm the presence of pathological findings in equivocal cases, and characterize their appearance, size, volume and relationship to the surrounding structures. Surface rendering of polypoid structures shows echogenic masses on a pedicle protruding into the uterine cavity. Submucous fibroids appear as mixed echogenic sites bulging into the cavity. Intrauterine synechiae appear as bands of varying thickness traversing the uterine cavity. This can be useful when deciding on treatment options, such as conservative management vs. surgery, and can be a valuable tool in surgical procedures carried out under ultrasonographic guidance.

The 3D technique offers the possibility of simultaneous presentation of the uterine cavity and corresponding tube, shortening the procedure and the discomfort of the patient. Transvaginal 3D examination time is not less than that needed for 2D sonography, but some parts of the examination, such as measurements, reconstruction of the planes of interest or tomography, and surface rendering can be performed off-line. The acquired volumes of the most appropriate planes of interest can be stored on a removable hard disk for additional re-evaluations and documentation. Ultrasonic tomography can be performed using single-panel control, producing parallel sections in increments of less than 1 mm.

The ability of 3D systems to produce serial scans that can be stored for subsequent analysis, 3D reconstruction, accurate assessment of volume and a coronal plane with more detailed analysis of the uterus and endometrial cavity between uterine angles is superior to conventional 2D ultrasound.

References

1. Hill ML. Infertility and reproductive assistance. In Neiberg, DA, Hill LM, Bohm-Velez M, Mendelson EB, eds. *Transvaginal Ultrasound*. St Louis: Mosby Year Book, 1992:43–6
2. Arronet GM, Aduljie SY, O'Brien IR. A 9 year survey of Fallopian tube dysfunction in human infertility: diagnosis and therapy. *Fertil Steril* 1969;20:903–18
3. Page H. Estimation of the prevalence and incidence of infertility in a population: a pilot study. *Fertil Steril* 1969;71:571–4
4. Kerin JF, Williams DB, San Roman GA, Pearistone AC, Grundfest WS, Sucrey ES. Falloposcopic classification and treatment of Fallopian tube disease. *Fertil Steril* 1992;57:731–5
5. Thurmond AS, Rosch J. Non-surgical Fallopian tube recanalization for treatment of infertility. *Radiology* 1990;174:371–4
6. Allahbadia GN. Fallopian tube patency using color Doppler. *Int J Gynecol Obstet* 1993;40:241–4
7. Richman TS, Viscomi GN, deCherney A, Polan ML, Alcebo LO. Fallopian tubal patency assessed by ultrasound fluid injection. *Radiology* 1984;152:507–10
8. Peters JA, Coulam CB. Hysterosalpingography with color Doppler ultrasonography. *Am J Obstet Gynecol* 1991;164:1530–2
9. Stern J, Peters AJ, Coulam CB. Color Doppler ultrasonography assessment of tubal patency: a comparison study with traditional technique. *Fertil Steril* 1992;58:897–900
10. Volpi E, Zuccaro G, Patriarca A, Rustichelli S, Sismondi P. Transvaginal sonographic tubal patency testing: air and saline solution as contrast media in a routine infertility clinic setting. *Ultrasound Obstet Gynecol* 1996;7:43–8
11. Tüfekci EC, Girit S, Bayirli MD, Durmusoglu F, Yalti S. Evaluation of tubal patency by transvaginal sonosalpingography. *Fertil Steril* 1992;57:336–40
12. Kupesic S, Kurjak A. Gynecological vaginal sonographic interventional procedures – what does color add? *Gynecol Perinatol* 1994;3:57–60
13. Deichert U, Schlief R, van de Sandt M, Daume E. Transvaginal hysterosalpingo-contrast sonography for the assessment of tubal patency with gray scale imaging and the additional use of pulsed wave Doppler. *Fertil Steril* 1992;57:62–7
14. Holte J, Rasmussen C, Morris H. First clinical experience with sonicated human serum albumin (albunex) as an intrafallopian ultrasound contrast medium. *Ultrasound Obstet Gynecol* 1995;6:62
15. Rubin I. Differences between the uterus and tubes as a cause of oscillations recorded during uterotubal insufflation. *Fertil Steril* 1954;5:147–53
16. Nannini R, Chelo E, Branconi F, Tantini C, Scarselli GF. Dynamic echohysteroscopy. A new diagnostic technique in the study of female infertility. *Acta Eur Fertil* 1981;12:165–71
17. Randolph JR, Ying YK, Maier DB, Schmidt CL, Riddick CH. Comparison of real-time ultrasonography, hysterosalpingography and laparoscopy/hysteroscopy. *Fertil Steril* 1986;46:828–32
18. Deichert U, van de Sandt M, Daume E. Die vaginale Hysterokontrastsonographie – Ersatz oder Ergänzung zur Hysterosalpingographie und Chromo-Laparoskopie. *Ultraschall Klin Prax* 1987;1(suppl):48
19. Deichert U, van de Sandt M, Daume E. Vaginale Hysterokontrastsonographie zur differentialdiagnosischen Abklärung eines Pseudogestationsacks. *Ultraschall Klin Prax* 1987;2(suppl):245–8
20. Deichert U, van de Sandt M, Lauth G, Daume E. Die transvaginale Hysterokontrastsonographie (HKSG). Ein neues diagnostisches Verfahren zur Differenzierung intrauteriner und myometraler Befunde. *Geburtsh Frauenheilkd* 1988;48:835–44
21. Davison GB, Leeton J. A case of female infertility investigated by contrast-enhanced echogynecography. *J Clin Ultrasound* 1988;16:44–7
22. Allahbadia GN. Fallopian tubes and ultrasonography. The Sion experience. *Fertil Steril* 1992;58:901–7
23. Broer KH, Turanli R. Überprüfung des Tubenfaktors mitels Vaginalsonographie. *Ultraschall Klin Prax* 1992;7:50–3
24. Bonilla-Musoles F, Simón C, Sampaio M, Pellicer A. An assessment of hysterosalpingosonography (HSSG) as a diagnostic tool for uterine cavity defects and tubal patency. *J Clin Ultrasound* 1992;20:175–81
25. Deichert U, Schlief R, van de Sandt M, Junke I. Transvaginal hysterosalpingo-contrast sonography (Hy-Co-Sy) compared with conventional tubal diagnostics. *Hum Reprod* 1989;4:418–22
26. Deichert U, Schlief R, van de Sandt M, Goebel R, Daume E. Transvaginale Hysterosalpingo-Kontrastsonographie (HKSG) im B-Bild Verfahren und in der farbcodierten Dublexsonographie zur Abklärung der Tubenpassage. *Geburtsh Frauenheilkd* 1990;50:717–22
27. Timor-Tritsch IE, Rottem S. Transvaginal ultrasonographic study of the Fallopian tube. *Obstet Gynecol* 1987;70:424–8
28. Gramiak R, Shah PM. Echocardiography of the aortic root. *Invest Radiol* 1968;3:356–66
29. Meltzer RS, Tickner G, Sahines TP, Popp RL. The source of ultrasound contrast effect. *J Clin Ultrasound* 1980;8:121
30. Suren A, Puchta J, Osmers R. Fluid instillation into the uterine cavity. In Osmers R, Kurjak A, eds. *Ultrasound and The Uterus*. Carnforth, UK: Parthenon Publishing, 1995:45–51
31. Schlief R. Ultrasound contrast agents. *Radiology* 1991;3:198–207
32. Schlief R, Schürmann R, Niendorf HP. Saccharide-based ultrasound contrast media. Basic characteristics and results of clinical trials. In Katayama H, Brash RC, eds. *New Dimensions of Contrast Media*. Tokyo: Excerpta Medical, 1991:141–6
33. Schlief R, Schürmann R, Balzer T. Saccharide-based contrast agents. In Nanda NC, Schlief R, eds. *Advances in Echo Imaging Using Contrast Enhancement*. Dordrecht: Kluwer, 1993:71–96

34. McCalley M, Braunstein P, Stone S, Henderson P, Egbeat R. Radionuclide hysterosalpingography for evaluation of Fallopian tube pregnancy. *J Nucl Med* 1985;26:868–70
35. Keirse M, Wunderwellen R. A comparison of hysterosalpingography and laparoscopy in the investigation of infertility. *Obstet Gynecol* 1973;41:685–8
36. Deichert U, van de Sandt M. Transvaginal hysterosalpingo-contrast sonography (Hy-Co-Sy). The assessment of tubal patency and uterine abnormalities by contrast enhanced sonography. *Adv Echo-Contrast* 1993;2:55–8
37. Ayida G, Chamberlain P, Barlow D, Kennedy S. Uterine cavity assessment prior to *in vitro* fertilization: comparison of transvaginal scanning, saline contrast hysterosonography and hysteroscopy. *Ultrasound Obstet Gynecol* 1997;10:59–62
38. Kupesic S, Kurjak A. Evaluation of tubal patency by color Doppler hysterosalpingography. In Timor-Tritsch IE, Kurjak A, eds. *Ultrasound and the Fallopian Tube*. Carnforth, UK: Parthenon Publishing, 1995:101–10
39. Kupesic S, Kurjak A. The role of color Doppler in vaginal sonographic puncture procedures. In Kurjak A, ed. *An Atlas of Transvaginal Color Doppler*. Carnforth, UK: Parthenon Publishing, 1994:335–47
40. Peters JA, Stern JJ, Coulam CB. Color Doppler hysterosalpingography. In Jaffe R, Warsof SL, eds. *Color Doppler in Obstetrics and Gynecology*. New York: McGraw-Hill, 1992:283
41. Groff TR, Edelstein JA, Schenken RS. Hysterosalpingography in the preoperative evaluation of tubal anastomosis candidates. *Fertil Steril* 1990;53:417–20
42. Heikkinen H, Tekay A, Volpi E, Martikainen H, Jouppila P. Transvaginal salpingosonography for the assessment of tubal patency in infertile women: methodological and clinical experiences. *Fertil Steril* 1995;64:293–8
43. Battaglia C, Artini PG, D'Ambrogio G, Genazzani AD, Genazzani AR, Volpe A. Color Doppler hysterosalpingography in the diagnosis of tubal patency. *Fertil Steril* 1996;65:317–22
44. Balen FG, Allen CM, Siddle NC, Lees WR. Ultrasound contrast hysterosalpingography – evaluation as an outpatient procedure. *Br J Radiol* 1993;66:592–9
45. Raga F, Bonilla-Musoles F, Blanes J, Osborne NG. Congenital Müllerian anomalies: diagnostic accuracy of three-dimensional ultrasound. *Fertil Steril* 1996;65:523–8
46. Kyei-Mensah A, Zaidi J, Pittrof R, Shaker A, Campbell S, Tan SL. Transvaginal three-dimensional ultrasound: accuracy of follicular volume measurements. *Fertil Steril* 1996;65:371–6
47. Weinraub Z, Herman A. Three-dimensional hysterosalpingography. In Merz E, ed. *3-D Ultrasonography in Obstetrics and Gynecology*. Philadelphia: Lippincott Williams & Wilkins, 1998:57–64
48. Sladkevicius P. Three-dimensional power Doppler imaging of the Fallopian tube. *Ultrasound Obstet Gynecol* 1999;13:287
49. Ayida G, Kennedy S, Barlow D, Chamberlain P. Conventional sonography for uterine cavity assessment: a comparison of conventional two-dimensional with three-dimensional transvaginal ultrasound; a pilot study. *Fertil Steril* 1996;66:848–50
50. Weinraub Z, Maymon R, Shulman A, *et al*. Three-dimensional saline contrast hysterosonography and surface rendering of uterine cavity pathology. *Ultrasound Obstet Gynecol* 1996;8:277–82

Three-dimensional imaging of intrauterine devices

R. Bauman, S. Kupesic and A. Kurjak

The intrauterine device (IUD) is the most popular method of reversible contraception, and is used by more than 100 million women worldwide. The IUD is convenient, effective and relatively safe, with failure rates only slightly higher than those for oral contraceptives. Approximately 80% of women continue use through a full year and about 60% use it through a second year.

The IUD is a foreign body that is placed in the uterine cavity to prevent pregnancy. Devices may be either non-medicated or medicated. Medicated devices contain progesterone (Progestasert) or copper (TCu 380 A, Multiload 375, Nova T). The contraceptive action of intrauterine devices is mainly in the uterus. Devices do not affect ovulation or act abortively. It is believed that devices produce a spermicidal intrauterine environment. A non-medicated IUD produces the sterile inflammatory response to a foreign body, resulting in minor changes in the uterine cavity that are spermicidal. The copper devices release copper salts and free copper that induce morphological and biochemical changes in the endometrium. Copper also enhances local prostaglandin production and inhibits various endometrial enzymes. A progesterone-containing IUD decidualizes the endometrium and provokes atrophy of the endometrial glands. It inhibits implantation and is also spermicidal. The progestin IUD decreases blood loss and dysmenorrhea. Progestaserts are reinserted annually, and copper devices are reinserted after 8 years, when the medication is exhausted. Inert devices can be left in for longer periods if there are no complications. Contraindications to IUD use are presented in Table 1.

The role of ultrasound in control of IUD placement

Insertion is usually carried out during menses, so as not to disturb a possible pregnancy. Before the insertion it is obligatory to perform the sounding of the uterine cavity (it should be more than 6 cm and less than 9 cm in length) in order to place the IUD correctly in the fundus. Prior to the decision to insert the device, the patient should have a Papanicolaou smear in order to exclude acute or chronic infection. Ultrasonography of the pelvic organs is advisable before insertion. Transvaginal ultrasound is well known for its ability to diagnose pathological changes in the uterus and adnexa. Three-dimensional (3D) ultrasound is more reliable in detecting deformities of the cavum such as endometrial polyps, submucous leiomyomas and duplication anomalies (septate uterus, bicornuate uterus, etc.) that are contraindications for insertion of the IUD[1]. Three-dimensional power Doppler can detect malignant endometrial changes and localize the extension of the tumor in the myometrium[2]. Other contraindications to IUD use (such as adnexal masses) can also be diagnosed with ultrasound. Three-dimensional ultrasound offers a better diagnostic view of the ovary and tube, and can

Table 1 Contraindications to IUD use

Absolute
Pregnancy
Uterine abnormalities that distort the cavity
Uterine malignancy
Abnormal bleeding
Acute cervicitis
History of pelvic inflammatory disease, sexually transmitted disease, ectopic pregnancy, postpartum endometritis or infected abortion

Relative
Hypermenorrhea
Severe dysmenorrhea
Multiple sexual partners
Congenital or valvular heart disease
Nulliparity

Table 2 Complications of IUD use

Perforation of the uterus (1/1000 insertions)
Expulsion (3–12/100 women/year, usually in the first few months)
Increased risk for pelvic inflammatory disease (highest risk in the first 4 months)
Heavy bleeding
Cramping, pain
Pregnancy (pregnancy rate 1.8–2.8/100 women/year)

Table 3 Benefits of sonography prior to insertion of an IUD

Demonstration of abnormal position of the uterus (RVF, lateral position)
Demonstration of submucous leiomyoma
Demonstration of uterine congenital anomalies (bicornuate or septate uterus)
Measurement of the length of the uterus

detect benign and malignant adnexal changes. It also aids in making a more accurate distinction between tubal and ovarian lesions (sactosalpinx, hydrosalpinx and ovarian cysts)[3,4].

The presence of relative and/or absolute contraindications has been connected with complications in patients with an IUD, and these must be exluded before insertion. The complications that have arisen from IUD use are presented in Table 2.

Perforation of the uterus is a rare but serious complication of IUDs. The perforation usually occurs during traumatic insertion, but is also possible spontaneously, because of migration of the IUD[5,6]. All IUDs can be localized radiographically, but sonography is the best method to locate a lost or misplaced IUD. If the IUD is identified as perforating the myometrium or in the abdominal cavity, it should be removed by laparoscopy. If the perforating IUD is still visualized in the endometrial cavity, hysteroscopy is the best approach. Both routes may be helpful if an IUD is partially perforating. Copper in the abdominal cavity can lead to adhesion formation that makes removal necessary[7]. Because perforations commonly occur at the time of insertion, it is important to check for correct position of the IUD immediately after its insertion. In previous years this was done by identifying the string within a few weeks after insertion. Today's best means of control is transvaginal ultrasonography. The benefits of preinsertion sonography are listed in Table 3.

Ultrasound investigation of IUD malposition

The expulsion of the device can be complete or incomplete; incomplete expulsions have been connected with intrauterine pregnancies. Bernaschek and associates[8] and Meyenburg[9] showed that, in 80% of those cases of unwanted pregnancy with an IUD, the device had been placed too low. The same authors found that, in all patients with IUDs, malposition was found in 10% and 16.3%, respectively. The migration and expulsion of the device usually occurs in the first few months after insertion, so ultrasonographic control of the position of the device is advisable immediately, and 4–12 weeks after insertion. If an intrauterine pregnancy is diagnosed and the IUD string is visible, the IUD should be removed in order to prevent septic abortion. If the patient wishes to continue the pregnancy, ultrasound evaluation of the IUD is advised in order to decide whether to remove the device or not[10]. The benefits of sonography after insertion are shown in Table 4.

Currently, different types of IUD are available: plastic IUDs (Lippes-Loop), IUDs containing copper (Copper-T, Copper-7, Multiload) and IUDs containing progesterone (Progestasert-Pessar). Depending on the type of IUD and provided it is placed correctly in the cavity, the device can be visualized sonographically in the longitudinal section as a hyperechogenic stripe (Copper-T) or as five echogenic points (Lippes-Loop). In the transverse section, the Copper-T presents as a hyperechogenic point in the middle of the corpus; in the fundal area the arms of the device can be seen as a

Table 4 Benefits of sonographic examination after insertion of an IUD

Control of the position of the IUD
Diagnosis of complications (perforation, pelvic inflammatory disease)
Control of the opening of the arms of the IUD (Copper T) after insertion

hyperechogenic horizontal line. The Multiload device presents with three echogenic points lying beside one another. However, because the frontal view of the IUD may be impossible to visualize by two-dimensional (2D) ultrasound, examination of the two arms of the IUD can be very difficult. Two-dimensional ultrasound examinations have been shown to fail in the detection of a displaced IUD in about 9% of cases[11].

Three-dimensional ultrasound investigation of the IUD

Three-dimensional ultrasound is more accurate in the identification of the device that is inserted *in utero* (Figure 1). One of the main advantages of 3D ultrasound is its potential for both surface and volume rendering. Bonilla-Musoles and associates[12] found a statistically significant difference between identification of the IUD with 2D vs. 3D transvaginal sonography.

The distance between the fundal part of the uterus and the end of the device is important for assessment of whether or not the device is in the proper place. This distance can be measured by transvaginal 2D ultrasound, but better with 3D ultrasound. The distance should not be less than 2 cm[13]. However, this measurement does not count the thickness of the uterine wall, which is different in each patient. Bernaschek and associates[8] created a formula that takes into account the thickness of the anterior and the posterior wall of the uterus. The position of the device is correct if the distance between the fundus and the upper end of the device does not amount to more than four-thirds of the average thickness of the uterine wall:

Distance $\leq$ (anterior wall + posterior wall)/2 $\times$ 1.33

The arms of the device should be properly unfolded. This enables assessment of the length of the device in the longitudinal section, and also assessment of the arms of the device in the transverse section. With the use of 3D ultrasound the three perpendicular planes are visualized simultaneously, and it is much easier to locate the correct position of the device. Besides the fundus–IUD distance, the distance between the upper end of the device and the base of the endometrium seems to be a practical measurement for assessment of the correct IUD position in hyperplastic uteri. This distance should not exceed 5 mm.

Three-dimensional ultrasonography allows volume examination on the monitor simultaneously in three perpendicular planes. All three planes are located in a separate window and each of them can be rotated at 90° to each other in all three axes. After acquiring the volume, the presence of the patient is no longer needed, so the examinations last no more than 3 min[12]. The

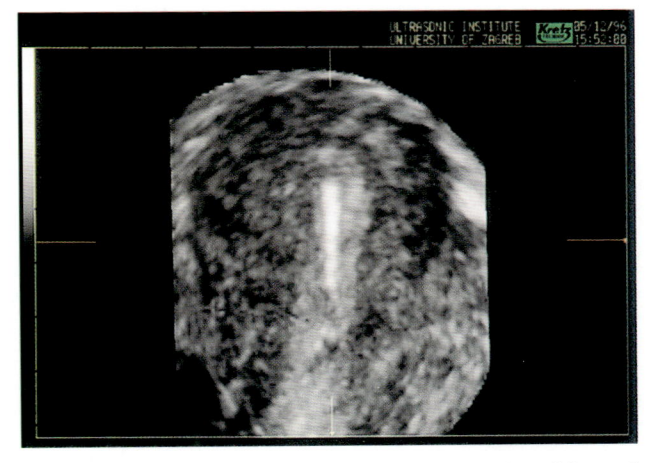

Figure 2 Frontal reformatted section of the uterus with well-inserted intrauterine device

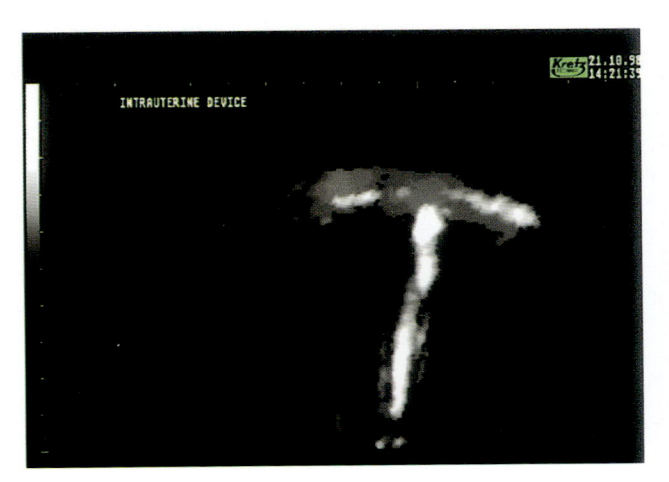

Figure 1 A uterus containing an intrauterine device in volume-rendering mode: with high-pass filtering the uterus becomes transparent and the device can be visualized in the coronal surface view

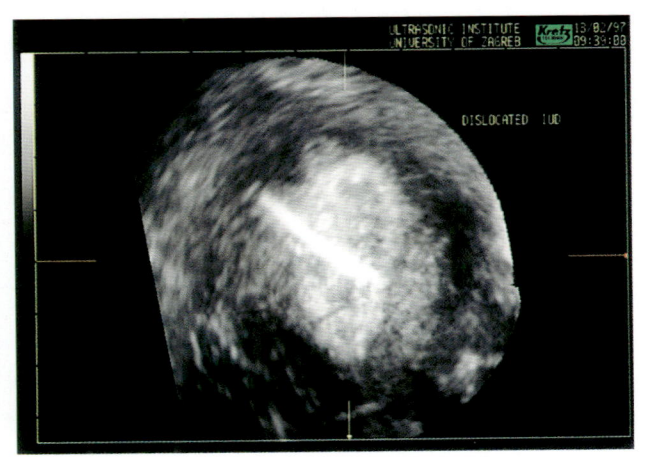

Figure 3 Displaced intrauterine device demonstrated in frontal reformatted section

volume sample of the uterus is rotated so that the three planes represent the frontal view, the sagittal view and the longitudinal view. In the three-plane mode the devices can be visualized fully only after the volumes are rotated. In a large number of patients (36%) simultaneous visualization of all parts of the IUD is not possible with the three-plane view, but all parts of the IUD can be demonstrated simultaneously by volume rendering[14].

The frontal view of the intrauterine device can rarely be presented with 2D ultrasound (Figures 2 and 3). Examination with 2D ultrasound is limited to transverse views of the shaft; the arms or other smaller parts of the IUD cannot be investigated completely.

Conclusions

Three-dimensional ultrasound is a new and promising imaging technique in obstetrics and gynecology. One of its main advantages is the ability to study a volume by stepping through it and rotating the volume in any direction[15]. Three-dimensional ultrasound allows surface and volume rendering that can produce images like a photograph. In volume rendering internal structures can be visualized by allowing the surface to become transparent. This is useful in the examination of the uterus and foreign bodies in the uterus, because structures that are not located in a single plane can be imaged simultaneously[16] (Figures 4 and 5). Three-dimensional ultrasound for investigation of IUDs provides access to the location, orientation of the shaft and also the position and orientation of the branches of the IUD. Three-dimensional ultrasound may help in the identification of unknown types of IUD. These advantages of 3D ultrasound may improve ultrasound examination in a routine follow-up of patients after insertion of an IUD.

Unfortunately, 3D ultrasound is expensive and is not available in all hospitals and family planning centers. This modality is currently reserved for diagnosis of complications related to IUD use or confirmation after doubtful 2D findings. It is believed that, in the not too distant future, 3D ultrasonographic equipment will be less expensive, which will allow its widespread application.

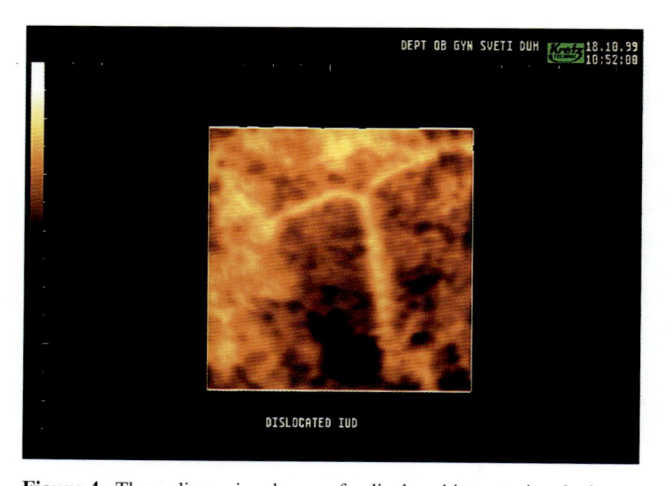

Figure 4 Three-dimensional scan of a displaced intrauterine device

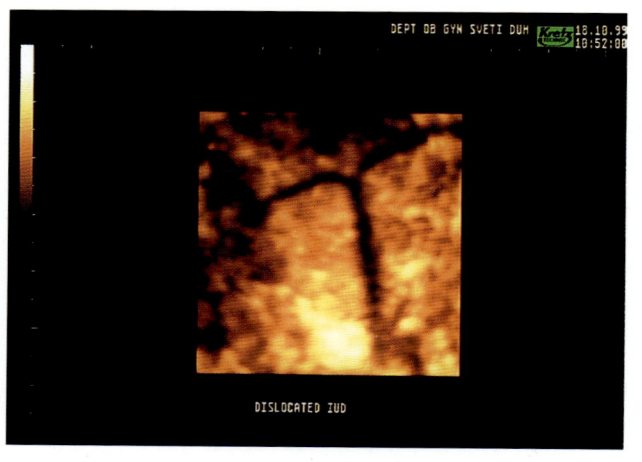

Figure 5 The same patient as in Figure 4. X-ray-like three-dimensional image of the displaced intrauterine device

References

1. Kupesic S, Kurjak A. Septate uterus: detection and prediction of obstetrical complications by different forms of ultrasonography. *J Ultrasound Med* 1998;17:631–6
2. Kupesic S, Kurjak A, Zodan T. Staging of the endometrial carcinoma by three dimensional power Doppler ultrasound. *Gynecol Perinatol* 1998;8:1–7
3. Kurjak A, Kupesic S, Jacobs I. Preoperative diagnosis of the primary Fallopian tube carcinoma by three dimensional static and power Doppler sonography. *Ultrasound Obstet Gynecol* 2000;15:1–7
4. Kurjak A, Kupesic S. Three dimensional static and power Doppler improves the diagnosis of ovarian lesions. *Gynecol Oncol* 2000;76:28–32
5. Sobrero AJ. Intrauterine devices in clinical practice. *Fam Plann Perspect* 1971;3:16–24
6. Ratnam SS, Tow SH. Translocation of the loop. In

Zatuchni GI, ed. *Postpartum Family Planning*. New York: McGraw-Hill, 1970:371–84
7. Gorsline J, Osborne N. Management of the missing intrauterine contraceptive device: report of a case. *Am J Obstet Gynecol* 1985;153:228
8. Bernaschek G, Endler M, Beck A. Zur Lagerkontrolle von intrauterinpessaren. *Geburtsh Frauenheilk* 1981;41:566–9
9. Meyenburg H. Anwendung der Ultraschall-Schnittbildtechnik zur Darstellung von Intrauterinspiralen. *Geburtsh Frauenheilk* 1978;38:950–7
10. Stubblefield PG, Fuller AF, Foster SG. Ultrasound guided intrauterine removal of intrauterine contraceptive device in pregnancy. *Am J Obstet Gynecol* 1988;72:961–4
11. Bonilla-Musoles F, Pardo G, Simon C. How accurate is ultrasonography in monitoring IUD placement? *J Clin Ultrasound* 1990;18:395–9
12. Bonilla-Musoles F, Martinez-Molina V, Blanes J, Raga F, Villalobos A. Three-dimensional ultrasound. Investigation for identification and control of intrauterine devices. In Merz E, ed. *3-D Ultrasonography in Obstetrics and Gynecology*. Philadelphia: Lippincott Williams & Wilkins, 1998;5:31–6
13. Hansmann M, Hackelöer BJ, Staudach A. *Ultraschalldiagnostik in Geburtshilfe und Gynäkologie*. Berlin: Springer, 1985
14. Lee A, Eppel W, Sam C, Kratochwil A, Deutinger J, Bernaschek G. Intrauterine device localization by three-dimensional transvaginal sonography. *Ultrasound Obstet Gynecol* 1997;10:289–92
15. Kirbach D, Wittingham TA. 3-D ultrasound: the Kretztechnik Voluson approach. *Eur J Ultrasound* 1994;1:85–9
16. Feichtinger W. Transvaginal three-dimensional imaging. *Ultrasound Obstet Gynecol* 1993;3:375–8

Three-dimensional ultrasound in urogynecology

I. Bekavac, S. Kupesic and A. Kurjak

Improved ultrasound imaging techniques have been applied to the evaluation of problems in the lower urinary tract. Examination by ultrasound is increasingly used as an alternative to radiological diagnosis. Together with history, clinical examinations and urodynamics, it improves the accuracy of the diagnosis of functional and morphological disorders.

Urinary incontinence is a common complaint of many women of all ages. It becomes more frequent and more severe with advancing age. There are two main urodynamic diagnoses: genuine stress incontinence (GSI), in which involuntary loss of urine occurs when the intravesical pressure exceeds the maximum urethral closure pressure in the absence of detrusor instability; and detrusor instability, in which the detrusor is objectively shown to contract, either spontaneously or on provocation during bladder filling[1].

Three-dimensional (3D) ultrasound allows detailed imaging of the female lower urinary tract, evaluation of the anatomy of the lower urinary tract (the urethra, urethral sphincter, pelvic floor and bladder volume) and dynamic imaging of the patients with urinary incontinence. Three-dimensional ultrasound enables an unlimited number of images to be obtained at any angle, when access is limited by the bony pelvis.

The role of two-dimensional ultrasound

Complete assessment of the incontinent patient includes history, examination and ultrasound examination in both recumbent and sitting positions. Provocative maneuvers may permit assessment of the mobility and support of the bladder neck. Passive opening of the bladder neck and proximal urethra with urinary leakage concurrent with a cough or Valsalva maneuver establishes the diagnosis of GSI. Almost invariably there is a descent of the bladder neck. The descent of more than 1 cm during straining of the bladder neck is considered diagnostic for hypermobility of the bladder neck. Therefore, it is important to monitor the changes of the anatomic location of the bladder neck during straining or coughing; the normal bladder neck should always remain retropubic. In the study of Leroy and Jeny[2], the descent or distortion of the bladder neck below the level of the symphysis was used as the endpoint to define urinary stress incontinence.

The transvaginal and perineal approaches may be used to image urinary leakage into the proximal urethra. Wise and co-workers[3] recommended the use of transperineal ultrasound for imaging of the urethra and bladder neck, not only because of the pressure applied to the urethra by the vaginal probe, but also because the probe moves on the Valsalva maneuver, making measurements of bladder neck movement difficult, particularly in women with cystocele.

In 1996 Schaer and colleagues[4] reported on the fundamentals of perineal ultrasound examination for female incontinence. In four different investigations, each involving at least 30 patients, they investigated the influence of examination position, bladder filling volume and pressure of the ultrasound probe against the perineum on the position of the bladder neck, the size of the rectovesical angle and the occurrence of funnelling.

A comparison of the results obtained in the supine and upright positions indicated that standing creates more pressure on the organs in the small pelvis, causing the meatus to lie lower, the angle to increase and funnelling to occur more often. Pressure of the probe on the perineum can cause distorted measurements, and changes in the position of the meatus internus and the angle. They found that different volumes of bladder filling did not affect numerical measurements, but influenced the detection of bladder neck funnelling and the image quality.

Unfortunately, imaging of the bladder neck and detection of urinary leakage does not enable the observer to make a diagnosis of detrusor instability, as this requires pressure measurements to record uninhibited detrusor contractions. The assessment of bladder wall thickness allows indirect measurements to be made of the detrusor muscle thickness, and this provides a potential index of detrusor activity. All the authors agreed that the bladder is best imaged transvaginally[2,3,5,6].

Kuhllar and associates[5,6] were the first to measure bladder wall thickness and relate it to urodynamic changes. In their two studies they reported the increased thickness of the bladder wall associated with detrusor instability. This was probably due to an increase in the detrusor muscle secondary to detrusor overactivity. The increase in bladder wall thickness associated with age, in the normal and detrusor instability groups, is consistent with the development of detrusor hypertrophy, secondary to increased outflow obstruction possibly due to changes in urethral elastin and collagen. No increase with age was seen in the GSI group, where there is minimal outflow obstruction.

The study of bladder wall thickness is especially interesting in postmenopausal women. Lower urinary tract symptoms are widely considered to be part of the menopause, and it has been assumed that these are dependent on sex hormones. Cardozo and colleagues[7] showed that, although estriol may produce both subjective and objective improvements in urinary symptoms, especially urgency and nocturia, it was not significantly better than placebo.

Iosif[8] showed that urogenital atrophy was completely relieved after 1 year of daily estriol treatment and that symptoms recurred with discontinuation of the therapy.

More recently, Battaglia and colleagues[9] analyzed 28 postmenopausal women with urinary symptoms before and after 1, 3 and 6 months of hormone replacement therapy. The patients underwent transvaginal ultrasound evaluation of the pelvic organs and bladder wall thickness. Hormone replacement therapy significantly increased bladder wall thickness, and this was associated with significant improvements in urinary symptoms. This was probably due to the effect of estriol on connective tissue and the large submucosal periurethral vascular plexus, which contributes to approximately one-third of urethral pressure.

Collagen, an important component of the female urethra, increases after estrogen therapy, contributing to the improvement of urethral sphincter function.

The role of three-dimensional ultrasound

Some additional information about the urethra and periurethral tissues is obtained by 3D sonography. This is mainly due to the availability of transverse planes with the transvaginal approach as well as to the possibility of demonstrating irregular surface structures three-dimensionally. Three-dimensional ultrasound allows accurate volume measurements to be made of the bladder and urethral sphincter, which are irregular structures.

A recently developed interactive system allows the examiner to access and view 3D images from memory in almost real time. Once the complete volume has been stored, the data can be accessed and re-examined at any time, even after the patient has been discharged.

Khullar and associates[10] performed a urodynamic investigation of 70 women with urinary symptoms and urethral sphincter incompetence and found significantly smaller urethral sphincter volumes compared with women with a competent urethral sphincter mechanism. The urethral sphincters were shorter and had a small maximal urethral sphincter cross-sectional area. To measure the volume of the urethral sphincter, a number of cross-sectional areas were measured along the urethral axis. The volume of the urethral sphincter[11] has been measured using 3D ultrasound and compared with the pressure measurements obtained during urethral pressure profilometry. The length of the rhabdosphincter on ultrasound was correlated with the functional urethral length. To calculate the volume of the rhabdosphincter, the central core volume was subtracted from the total urethral sphincter volume. Damage to the pudendal nerve during vaginal delivery may be the cause of atrophy of the rhabdosphincter and reduction of the sphincter volume. This is the primary and most important cause of GSI.

Three-dimensional ultrasound provides accurate volume measurements, particularly for irregularly shaped organs. Riccabona and co-workers[12] studied 50 normal volunteers. Two-dimensional (2D) volume measurements based on length, width and depth were assumed as the regular geometrical model. Three-dimensional volume measurements were based on masked slices with the voxels integrated over the entire bladder. Voided urine volumes ranged from 35 ml to 701 ml. Residual urine was present in 48% of the subjects and ranged from 1% to 14% of the voided volume. Two-dimensional volume estimates for all 50 subjects had a mean absolute value of the error of 27.5 ± 17.8%. Three-dimensional volume measurements had a mean absolute value of the error of 4.3 ± 3.7% (transverse) and 5.6 ± 3.8% (longitudinal). This makes the volume determinations obtained with the bladder scan device accurate, reliable, non-invasive and easy (Figure 1).

Athanasiou and co-workers[13] investigated the value of 3D ultrasound for imaging the anterior pelvic compartment and pelvic floor. Thirteen patients with prolapse and seven asymptomatic women were recruited into the study. The pelvic floor was visualized in the transverse plane parallel to the pubococcygeus muscle. The surface area of the levator ani hiatus was measured at rest, during maximal straining and during

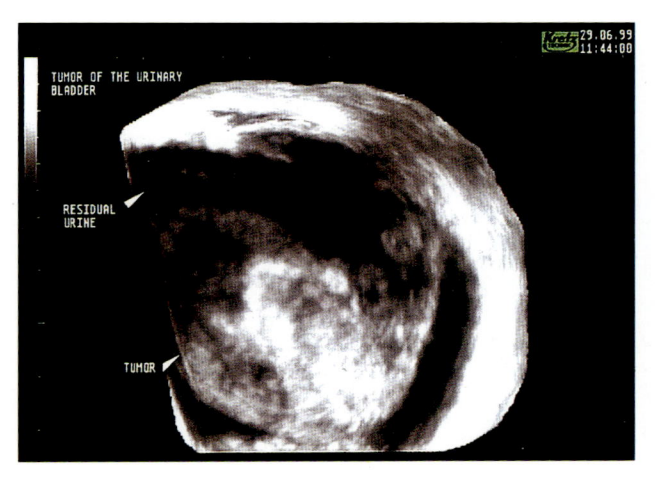

Figure 1 Three-dimensional display of a solid tumor arising from the bladder wall. Note the residual urine surrounding the lesion

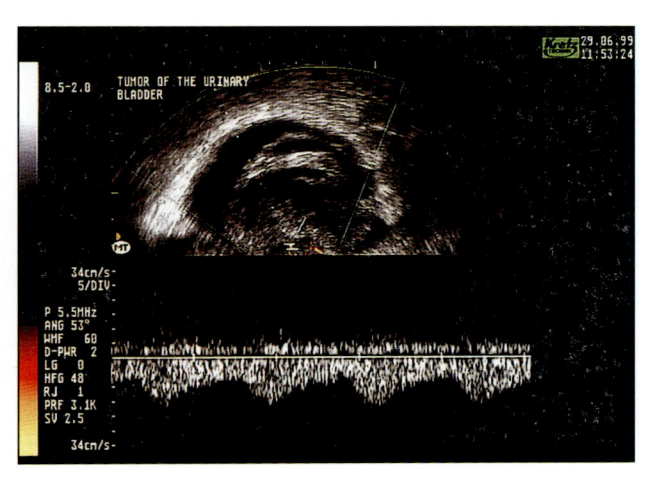

Figure 2 Transvaginal color Doppler scan of a tumor of the urinary bladder. High velocities (34 cm/s) measured in intralesional vessels are suspicious of malignancy

contraction. The surface area of the hiatus was significantly larger at rest ($p = 0.001$), during the Valsalva maneuver ($p < 0.001$) and during contraction ($p = 0.001$) in patients with prolapse. The authors showed that the surface area of the levator ani hiatus at rest, during maximal straining and during contraction was larger in women with prolapse. This measurement may be useful in predicting the development of the prolapse and evaluating the effectiveness of surgical repair.

Color Doppler and three-dimensional power Doppler

Blood flow in the lower urinary tract has been studied in normal women and women suffering from urinary incontinence. Khullar and colleagues[14] reported a reduction in the velocity of flow through the inferior vesical artery in menopausal patients. In their study, based on 38 women, they reported that the inferior vesical artery had a peak velocity of 12.4 cm/s and a mean velocity of 5.4 cm/s. There was a fall in the average peak and mean velocity of blood flow in the inferior vesical artery in women over the age of 50 not taking hormone replacement therapy (3.1 and 1.8 cm/s).

The same group of authors[15] studied blood flow in the lower urinary tract in women suffering from GSI and detrusor instability. Women with GSI had lower peak (13.8 cm/s), mean velocity (5.8 cm/s) and pulsatility index (PI; 1.43) than women with detrusor instability (peak velocity 16.7 cm/s, mean velocity 7.1 cm/s, PI 2.19). The reduced blood flow to the bladder neck in women with GSI is reduced further by increasing age.

There was no significant change in intramural blood flow in normal asymptomatic women with GSI and detrusor instability, and no decrease was noted with age. Owing to the reduction in the inferior vesical artery seen on color Doppler, estrogen replacement therapy is used to treat GSI.

Hormone replacement therapy produces significant improvements in the bladder wall vascularization and reduction of the bladder wall artery PI. Since the PI is believed to measure impedance to flow downstream from the point of sampling, and to reflect arterial tone, the reduced PI values shown following hormone replacement therapy may reflect a decrease in peripheral resistance[9].

Apart from being an appropriate technique to investigate the function of the lower urinary tract, it sometimes produces accidental findings in the lower urinary tract that may cause a diagnostic dilemma. Granberg and colleagues[16] reported on five bladder tumors in a prospective study of 400 women with postmenopausal bleeding (Figure 2).

Gynecological symptoms sometimes originate from the lower urinary tract and vice versa, and women may sometimes mistake hematuria for vaginal bleeding. Endometrioma can also be visualized, rising from the bladder wall, as well as leiomyomata.

In the diagnostic dilemma it is essential to obtain an optimum view of the interior of the bladder. In cases of bladder malignancy the depth of infiltration assessed by transvaginal or transperineal ultrasound may determine the appropriate operative treatment. Three-dimensional ultrasound is superior to conventional ultrasound in these cases for the identification of tumor spread. As tumor size is one of the prognostic factors, simultaneous display of all three orthogonal planes on the monitor provides the optimum condition for an accurate determination of tumor volume.

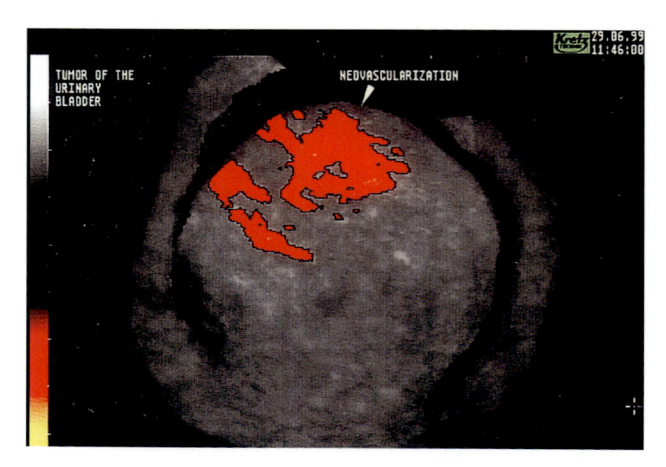

Figure 3 The same patient as in Figure 2, as seen by three-dimensional power Doppler. Randomly dispersed vessels are easily visualized within the urinary bladder tumor. Detection of aneurysm-like spaces and arteriovenous shunts is suggestive of malignancy. Histopathology revealed a malignant tumor of the urinary bladder

Three-dimensional power Doppler provides additional information in observing the neovascularization of malignant bladder neoplasms. Malignant tumor vessels are randomly dispersed, irregular, with arteriovenous shunts and aneurysm-like spaces[17] (Figure 3). Apart from evaluation of tumor vascularity by 3D power Doppler, there are new alternative measurements that provide the possibility of systematic analysis of vascularization of the entire lesion[18].

Conclusion

Three-dimensional ultrasound provides additional and new information on urogynecological structures and their relationship. It allows accurate measurements to be made of the urethral sphincter volumes and the volume of the residual urine; it also visualizes the pelvic floor and urinary bladder malignancies. Three-dimensional power Doppler provides information on the vascular network of bladder tumors and tumor-like structures and influences the treatment.

References

1. Abrams P, Blaivas JG, Stanton JT, Andersen JT. The standardisation of the terminology of lower urinary tract function. *Br J Obstet Gynaecol* 1990;6(suppl):1–16
2. Leroy B, Jeny B. Contribution of vaginal echography in urinary incontinence. *Arch Gynecol Obstet* 1988;244:530–7
3. Wise BG, Burton G, Cutner, Cardozo LD. Effect of vaginal ultrasound probe on lower urinary tract function. *Br J Urol* 1992;70:12–16
4. Schaer GN, Koechli OR, Schuessler B, Haller U. Perineal ultrasound: determination of reliable examination procedures. *Ultrasound Obstet Gynecol* 1996;7:347–52
5. Khullar V, Cardozo LD, Kelleher CJ, Abbot D, Bourne T. Transvaginal ultrasound measurements of bladder wall thickness in women. *Ultrasound Obstet Gynecol* 1993;3(suppl 2):107
6. Khullar V, Salvatore S, Cardozo LD, Bourne T, Abbot D, Kelleher CJ. A novel technique for measuring bladder wall thickness in women using transvaginal ultrasound. *Ultrasound Obstet Gynecol* 1994;4(suppl 2):220–4
7. Cardozo LD, Rekers H, Tapp A, *et al*. Oestriol in the treatment of postmenopausal urgency – a multicentre study. *Maturitas* 1993;18:47–8
8. Iosif CS. Effects of protracted administration of estriol on the lower genitourinary tract in postmenopausal women. *Arch Gynecol Obstet* 1992;251:115–20
9. Battaglia C, Salvatori S, Giuini MR, Primavera A, Gallinelli A, Volpe A. Hormonal replacement therapy and urinary problems as evaluated by ultrasound and color Doppler. *Ultrasound Obstet Gynecol* 1999;13:420–4
10. Khullar V, Salvatore S, Cardozo LD, Hill S, Kelleher CJ. Three-dimensional ultrasound of the urethra and urethral sphincter – a new diagnostic technique. *Neurol Urodyn* 1994;16:407–8
11. Khullar V, Salvatore S, Cardozo LD, Abott D, Hill S. Three-dimensional ultrasound of the urethra and urethral pressure profiles [abstract]. *Int Urogynaecol J* 1994;5:319
12. Riccabona M, Nelson TR, Pretorius DH, Davison TE. In vivo three-dimensional sonographic measurements of organ volume: validation in the urinary bladder. *J Ultrasound Med* 1996;15:627–32
13. Athanasiou S, Hill S, Cardozo LD, Khullar V, Andres K. Three-dimensional ultrasound of the urethra, periurethral tissues and pelvic floor [abstract]. *Int Urogynaecol J* 1995;6:239
14. Khullar V, Cardozo LD, Kelleher CJ, Abbot D, Bourne T. Blood flow in lower urinary tract in normal women. *Ultrasound Obstet Gynecol* 1993;(suppl 2):106
15. Khullar V, Cardozo LD, Kelleher CJ, Abbot D, Bourne TH. Blood flow in the lower urinary tract in women with genuine stress incontinence and detrusor instability. *Ultrasound Obstet Gynecol* 1993;3(suppl 2):
16. Granberg S, Wikland M, Norstrom A. Endovaginal ultrasound scanning to identify bladder tumors as the

source of vaginal bleeding in postmenopausal women. *Ultrasound Obstet Gynecol* 1991;1:63–6
17. Kurjak A, Kupesic S, Breyer B, Sparac V, Jukic S. The assessment of ovarian tumor angiogenesis: what does three-dimensional power Doppler add? *Ultrasound Obstet Gynecol* 1998;12:136–46
18. Parleitner H, Steiner H, Hasenoehrl G, Staudach A. Three-dimensional power Doppler sonography: imaging and quantifying blood flow and vascularization. *Ultrasound Obstet Gynecol* 1999;14:139–43

12

Three-dimensional sonoembryology of the first trimester

A. Kurjak, T. Zodan and S. Kupesic

Three-dimensional imaging in obstetrics

Just when it appeared that diagnostic ultrasound had reached the limits of its technical development and that further refinements would be of a minor nature, three-dimensional (3D) imaging has come on the scene, suggesting that we may still be at an early stage of this astonishing diagnostic modality[1].

At present, ultrasound technology has reached a stage where structures of only a few millimeters can be imaged *in vivo* in three dimensions. In this context, the 3D ultrasound technique will represent an important contribution to the research of the developing embryo *in vivo*.

With conventional two-dimensional (2D) ultrasonography, the assessment of the overall structural detail of the fetal hands is often difficult and time-consuming[2]. Three-dimensional ultrasonography allows visualization of fetal malformations in all three dimensions at the same time, providing an improved overview and a more clearly defined demonstration of different anatomical planes, and might be suitable for evaluation of complex fetal structures[3].

With the advent of 3D ultrasound, we are now able to review sections of the fetal face in all three mutually perpendicular (orthogonal) planes. We can also scrutinize facial features in surface-rendered and transparent views. Already, a number of investigators have effectively demonstrated that 3D ultrasound offers various advantages over conventional 2D imaging[4–10].

The use of 3D imaging can now be extended to follow pregnancy from conception to term. Although the development of this diagnostic modality started a decade ago, it was only in the 1990s that we obtained the high quality of reconstruction based on the development of advanced computer systems. This opened unexpected avenues in diagnosis in obstetrics and gynecology[11–26].

Our expanded capability for 3D imaging in normal pregnancies has focused attention on the early weeks of gestation. The embryonic period, extending from conception until 9 weeks of gestation, is extremely important. Most major anatomic structures and organ systems are formed and developed during this period. It is during this period that most major developmental anomalies originate. The sequential appearance of embryonic and fetal structures can be visualized by transvaginal ultrasonography as much as 3 weeks earlier than with the use of transabdominal ultrasound.

Recently, endoscopic uterine sonography and embryoscopy[27] have also been able to delineate embryonic structures much earlier than transvaginal sonography and with a more clearly outlined configuration. However, these two techniques are invasive procedures and neither their safety nor guidelines for their use have yet been established. Three-dimensional ultrasound is a valuable, non-invasive tool for the study of embryonic and fetal development which will replace invasive methods of investigation. Recently, Blaas and colleagues gave an excellent stage-by-stage description of brain development[28–32].

Here, we present our data on the morphological and vascular development of the embryo.

Typical embryonic features as seen by three-dimensional gray-scale imaging

Five weeks

The gestational sac can be visualized from the middle of the 5th week of amenorrhea as a small spherical anechoic structure placed inside one of the endometrial leaves. Planar mode tomograms are helpful in distinguishing the early intraendometrial gestational sac from a collection of free fluid between the endometrial leaves (pseudogestational sac). Three-dimensional sonography enables the exponentially expanding gestational sac volume to be measured precisely during the first trimester. At the beginning of the 5th week the gestational sac exceeds 8 mm[33] (Table 1). The small secondary yolk sac is visible as the earliest sign of the developing embryo. There is an increment of the yolk sac volume until 10 weeks' gestation. After reaching the maximum size it remains stable for a week and then decreases. Kupesic and co-workers[34]

CLINICAL APPLICATION OF 3D SONOGRAPHY

Table 1 Gestational sac volume determined by three-dimensional ultrasound between 5 and 12 weeks' gestation

Gestational age (weeks)	n	Gestational sac volume (cm^3) ± SD
5	18	1.62 ± 0.58
6	27	2.15 ± 1.15
7	42	8.05 ± 1.85
8	55	18.90 ± 2.50
9	48	40.02 ± 3.84
10	31	72.20 ± 7.90
11	28	120.50 ± 12.00
12	21	205.55 ± 22.05
Total	270	58.62 ± 6.48

found that 3D measurement of yolk sac volume and vascularity was predictive of pregnancy outcome. 3D ultrasound may significantly contribute to *in vivo* observations of the yolk sac, enabling scanning time to be reduced and the yolk sac's honeycomb surface pattern to be observed. Automatic volume calculation will allow us to estimate the relationship between the yolk sac and gestational sac volumes, as well as to obtain the correlation between yolk sac volume and crown–rump length (CRL) measurements.

Planar mode tomograms are useful for detecting the embryonic pole inside the gestational sac. The embryo itself can be seen 24–48 h after visualization of the yolk sac, at approximately 33 days after the last menstruation, at which it is 2–3 mm long. At this point, 3D imaging cannot show the heart of the endocardic tubes[35]. Adjacent to the yolk sac, the embryo can be seen as a small straight line when it reaches 2–3 mm in length at the end of the 5th week.

Six weeks

A rounded bulky head and thinner body characterize the 3D image of an embryo during the 6th week of pregnancy (Figure 1). The head is prominent because of the developing forebrain. Limb buds are rarely visible at this stage of pregnancy. However, the umbilical cord and vitelline duct are always clearly visible. At 6 weeks of gestation the ductus omphalomesentericus can be as much as three to four times the length of the embryo itself. The amniotic membrane is also visible, initially at the dorsal part of the embryo. A few hours later it surrounds the embryo but not the yolk sac, which remains in the extracelomic mesenchyme.

Seven weeks

During the 7th week of pregnancy, the spine gradually becomes visible, as well as the limb buds, lateral to the body. The amnion can be seen as a spherical hyperechoic membrane, still close to the embryo. The chorion frondosum can be distinguished from the chorion laeve.

Fast development of the rhombencephalon (hindbrain) takes place. This process gives even more prominence to the head. By the use of planar mode, the developing vesicles of the brain can be depicted as

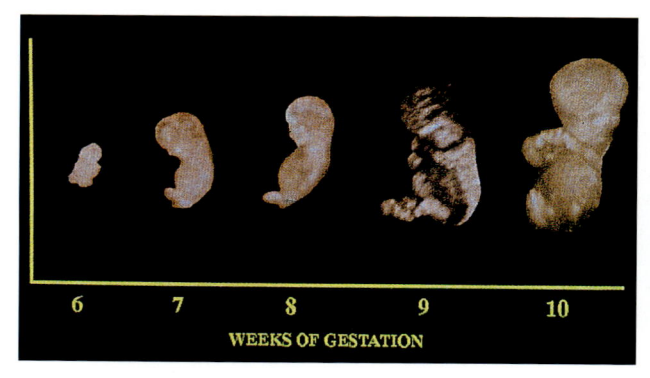

Figure 1 Embryonic and fetal development as seen by three-dimensional ultrasound during the first trimester of pregnancy

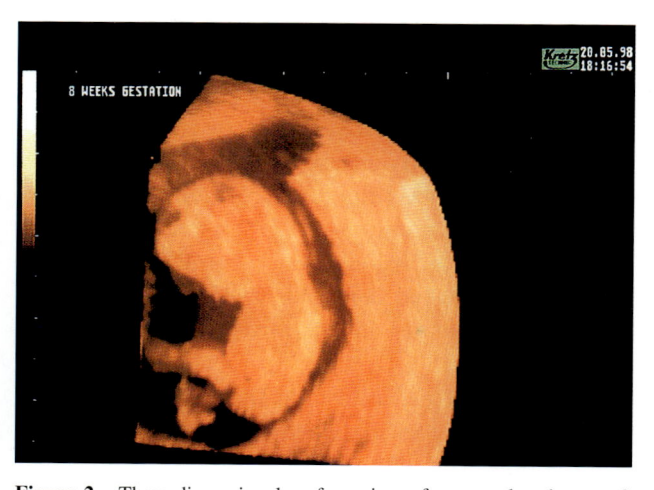

Figure 2 Three-dimensional surface view of a normal embryo at 8 weeks' gestation. Note the anterior flexion of the head, the rhombencephalon placed on the top of the head and the limb buds

anechoic structures inside the head. The largest, and usually the only visible, is the rhombencephalon on the top of the head (vertex) (Figure 2). The head is strongly flexed anteriorly, being in contact with the chest. The hypoechogenic brain cavities can be identified, including the separated cerebral hemispheres. The lateral ventricles are shaped like small round vesicles. The cavity of the diencephalon (future third ventricle) runs posteriorly. In the smallest embryos, the medial telencephalon forms a continuous cavity between the lateral ventricles. The future foramina of Monro are wide. In the sagittal plane, the height of the cavity of the diencephalon (future third ventricle) is slightly greater than that of the mesencephalon (future Sylvian aqueduct). Thus, the wide border between the cavities of the diencephalon and the mesencephalon is indicated. The curved tube-like mesencephalic cavity (future Sylvian aqueduct) lies anteriorly, its rostral part pointing caudally. It straightens considerably during the following weeks. By week 8 it is regularly identified. The rather broad and shallow rhombencephalic cavity is always visible from 7 weeks 0 days on.

Power Doppler demonstrates vascularity at the periphery of the rhombencephalic cavity at 7 weeks and 3 days of gestation, while color Doppler detects low velocity and absence of diastolic flow.

Eight weeks

The most characteristic finding is the complete visualization of the limbs, which end in thicker areas that correspond to future hands and feet. The shape of the face begins to appear but is not clearly seen. The great majority of embryos show a cranial pole flexion that makes it almost impossible to see the face. The insertion of the umbilical cord is visible on the anterior abdominal wall. During the 8th week of pregnancy there is expansion of the ventricular system of the brain (lateral, third and midbrain ventricles). Owing to these processes the head becomes erect from the anterior flexion. The vertex is now located over the position of the midbrain. Structures of the viscerocranium are not visible, because of the small size.

Blaas and co-workers[32] reported on an embryo of 7 weeks and 5 days of gestational age whose brain structures were analyzed in detail by 3D ultrasound (Figure 2). They described distinct hemispheres and how the foramina of Monro had become relatively smaller[36]. The border between the cavities of the diencephalon and the mesencephalon is not distinct at this stage, while the connection from the mesencephalon to the rhombencephalon consists of the isthmus rhombencephali. All these characteristics could be seen in the authors' 3D reconstruction.

The lateral ventricles gradually change shape from small round vesicles via thick (CRL 9.3–13.6 mm) round slices originating anterocaudally from the third ventricle (CRL 14.6–17.7 mm) into the crescent shape of the larger embryos (CRL 20.4 mm). The largest volume of the future third ventricle (11.7 mm^3) was found by Blaas and co-workers in an embryo with a CRL of 20.5 mm. The future foramina of Monro becomes distinct in embryos of 19.5 mm in CRL. The transition from the third ventricle to the mesencephalic cavity and to the lateral ventricles is wide in the early embryos. The cavity of the mesencephalon is relatively large in all embryos/fetuses. With the increasing size of the embryo/fetus, the mesencephalic cavity changes its position, and is found to be posterior in the large fetuses. The rhombencephalic cavity deepens gradually with the growth of the embryos, at the same time decreasing its length. Its position in the head changes with the increasing size of the embryo/fetus, moving posteriorly (CRL 17 mm and larger). The rhombencephalic cavity (future fourth ventricle) has a pyramid-like shape with the central deepening of the pontine flexure as the peak of the pyramid.

From 8 weeks' gestation, using conventional color Doppler, it is possible to detect blood flow signals from the internal carotid and vertebral arteries. Upon reaching the brain, the internal carotid arteries turn dorsally and alongside the diencephalon. They give off anterior, middle and posterior cerebral arteries. The internal carotid artery and its branches (middle cerebral artery, anterior cerebral artery and posterior communicating artery) mainly supply the blood flow to the cortical areas. The vertebral artery runs between the transverse processes (C2–C6) and is identified by visualizing the common carotid artery and then rotating the transducer. Arteries originating from the vertebral arteries mainly supply the cerebellum and brainstem. Within the symmetrical cerebellar hemispheres (joined by the thin and highly echogenic vermis) one can visualize the intracerebellar arteries.

Nine to ten weeks

The external ear is sometimes depicted in the 3D surface image. Merz and co-workers[37] were able to provide striking images of the fetal face at this gestational age. They reported cases in which transvaginal 3D ultrasound produced remarkably well-defined facial images as early as 9 weeks' gestation.

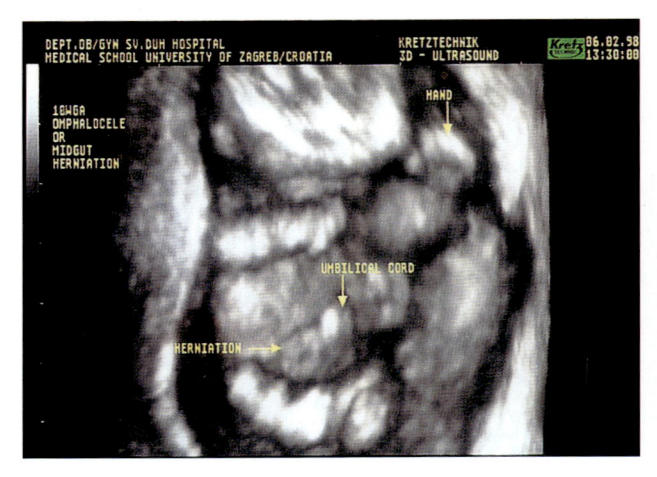

Figure 3 Surface view of the fetus at 10 weeks' gestation. The front abdominal wall should be re-evaluated in a few weeks, to differentiate mid-gut herniation and omphalocele

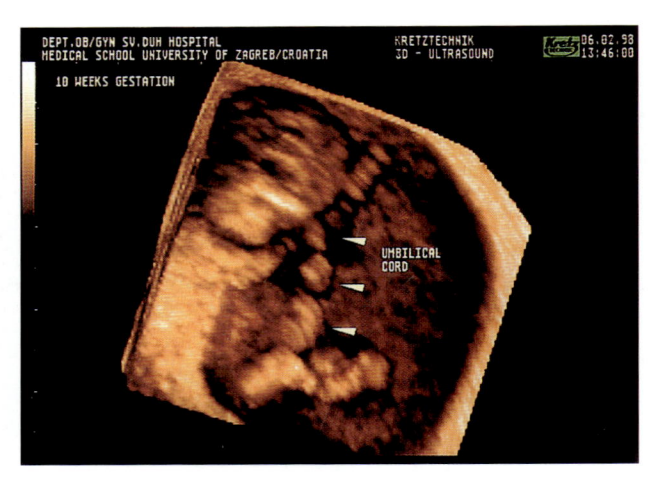

Figure 4 Surface view of the fetus at 10 weeks' gestation. The legs with knee and full length of the umbilical cord are clearly visible

Herniation of the midgut is present (Figure 3). This is a consequence of the rapid growth of the bowel and liver before closure of the abdominal wall occurs. Although this is a physiological phenomenon, sometimes it does not appear. Possibly we cannot visualize it, or else its size may vary. At 10 weeks, the bowel undergoes two turns of 170°, returning to its original position at the same time that closure and development of the abdominal wall end. The dorsal column, the early spine, can be examined in its whole length. The arms with elbow and the legs with knee are clearly visible, and the feet can be seen, approaching the midline (Figure 4).

Liang and co-workers[38] reported the first diagnosis of ectopia cordis at 10 weeks' gestation made by 2D and 3D ultrasound. Both two and three dimensions revealed a thoracoabdominal ectopia cordis and an omphalocele. The size of the lateral ventricles increases rapidly. While the third ventricle is still relatively wide at the beginning of this week, its anteromedial part narrows during this week, owing to the growth of the thalami. In the fetuses of 25 mm in CRL and more, there is a clear gap between the rhombencephalic and the mesencephalic cavity, owing to the growing cerebellum. The isthmus rhombencephali is narrow; in most cases it is not visible in its complete length. The cavity of the diencephalon decreases in the larger embryos and fetuses (CRL 25 mm), and becomes narrow, especially at its upper anterior part. The spine is still characterized by two echogenic parallel lines.

Using color and pulsed Doppler, blood flow signals from the intracerebellar arteries can be obtained from the 9th week of gestation. The posterior lateral choroidal artery is derived from the posterior cerebral artery, whereas the lateral choroidal arteries are derived from the middle cerebral artery and internal carotid artery. Blood flow signals from the choroid plexus are obtained during the 9th and 10th weeks of gestation. Blood flow signals from the internal carotid, vertebral and cerebral arteries during the 8th and 9th weeks of gestation demonstrate low-velocity flow with the absence of diastolic flow. The umbilical artery and fetal aorta show the same vascular flow features. Choroid plexus vessels can be visualized starting from the 9th week of gestation. Subtle color and pulsed Doppler signals are obtained at the inner edge of the lateral ventricle choroid plexus. The choroid plexus vascularity during the 9th and 10th weeks of gestation has two typical features: prominent venous blood flow signals and absence of diastolic flow. Thereafter, low vascular impedance (similar to that in intracerebellar arteries) is easily observed. In most of the cases, it appears that there is end-diastolic flow even earlier, but because of the wall filters (50 Hz) it is not displayed. Very low velocities are an additional reason for the end-diastolic component not being recorded before 10 weeks.

Eleven to twelve weeks

During the 11th week of pregnancy, the development of the head and neck continues. Facial details such as the nose, orbits, maxilla and mandibles are often visible (Figure 5). The herniated midgut returns into the abdominal cavity (Figure 6). Its persistence after 11 weeks of gestation is presumptive of an omphalocele. The planar mode enables detailed analysis to be undertaken of the embryonic body with visualization of the stomach and urinary bladder. The kidneys are also often visible. The arms and legs continue their development.

Hata and co-workers[39] conducted a study on visualization of fetal limbs by two and three dimensions.

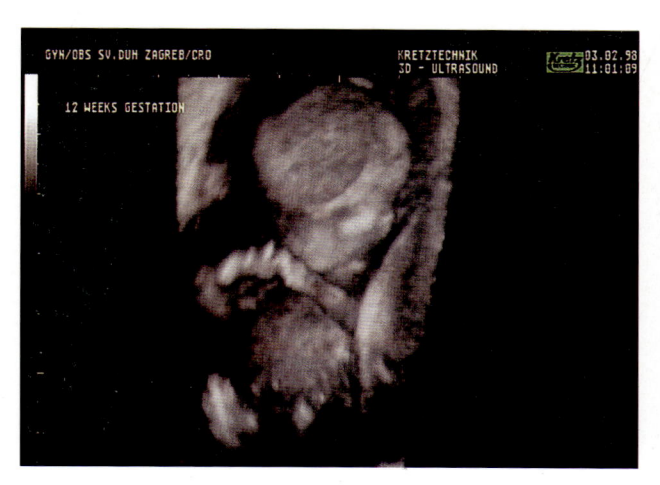

Figure 5 Three-dimensional surface image of a fetus at 12 weeks' gestation. Note the regular morphology of the fetal head, body and extremities

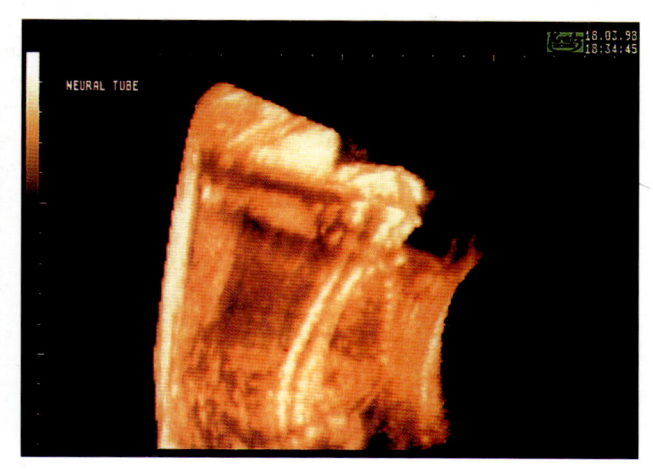

Figure 7 X-ray-like mode facilitates detailed three-dimensional analysis of the fetal spine

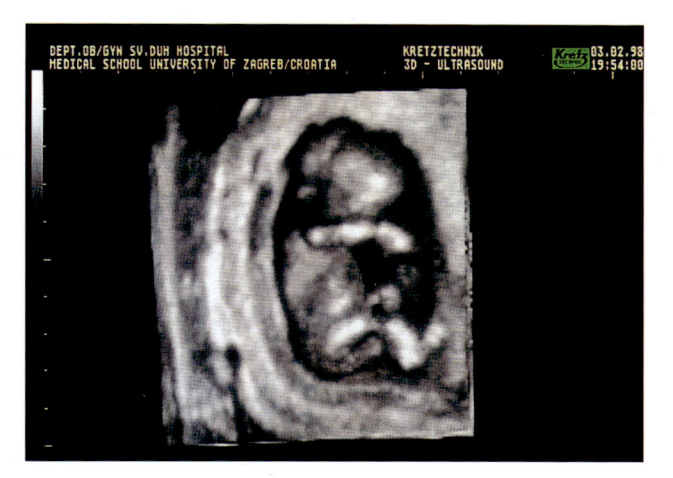

Figure 6 Surface view of the fetus at 12 weeks' gestation. Note the regularity of the front abdominal wall, since the herniated mid-gut has returned into the abdominal cavity

The ability to visualize fetal hands/fingers and feet/toes was better with 3D than with 2D ultrasonography in the late first trimester (detection rates were 65% and 41% by 3D ultrasonography for hands and feet, respectively, and 41% and 12%, respectively, by 2D ultrasonography). The long bones can be visualized as hyperechoic elongated structures inside the upper and lower extremities. Detailed 3D analysis of the fetal spine, chest and limbs is possible by using the transparent, X-ray-like mode (Figure 7). With the use of the transparent/X-ray system, starting at 13 weeks, the medullar channel, each vertebra and rib can be visualized and even the intervertebral disks can be measured. This opens unexpected possibilities for early diagnosis of skeletal malformations.

At this age, the lateral ventricles dominate the brain (in the fetus of 40 mm in CRL). The cavity of the diencephalon is too narrow to be outlined correctly on the 2D images. Both rostrally and caudally, the cavity of the mesencephalon is connected to the neighboring cavities by narrow isthmuses. The cavities of the mesencephalon and rhombencephalon are located posteriorly, while the cavities of the hemispheres occupy the anterior and superior part of the head. The 3D study shows that the thick crescent-shaped lateral ventricles fill the anterior part of the head and conceal the diencephalic cavity, which becomes smaller. The gap between the mesencephalic and the rhombencephalic cavity filled with the growing cerebellum becomes clear.

After week 11 of gestation, the lowest resistance index (RI) values are obtained from the intracerebellar and choroid plexus arteries. The Scheffe F test reveals a significantly lower RI ($p < 0.05$) for the intracerebellar artery than for the cerebral arteries and for the choroid plexus arteries than for the cerebral and carotid arteries, after the 11th week of gestation. However, the difference in RI between the carotid artery and the cerebral arteries is not statistically significant ($p > 0.05$). The difference in RI between the choroid plexus artery and the intracerebellar artery is also not statistically significant ($p > 0.05$).

There are few transvaginal color Doppler studies of cerebral blood flow in early pregnancy. In the study of Wladimiroff and colleagues[40], flow velocity waveform recordings were made in the umbilical artery, fetal descending aorta and intracerebral arteries in 30 normal pregnancies between 11 and 13 weeks of gestation. Although flow velocity waveforms in the descending aorta and umbilical artery displayed absent end-diastolic flow, flow velocity waveforms in the intracerebral arteries were characterized by forward flow throughout the cardiac cycle. These results suggest a relatively lower vascular resistance at the fetal cerebral level in early gestation. Van Zalen-Sprock and associates[41] analyzed blood flow in the fetal aorta, umbilical artery and cerebral arteries in 18 pregnant women between 6 and 16 weeks of gestation. The cerebral arteries showed positive end-diastolic velocity in all fetuses after the 10th week of gestation. In the cerebral artery, the pulsatility index (PI) showed a mild gradual decrease towards the 16th week of pregnancy. These data suggest low vascular impedance in the fetal brain, not dependent on changes in the vascular resistance of the fetal trunk or uteroplacental circulation. This apparently independent and autoregulatory mechanism thus provides an adequate blood supply to the growing fetal brain. Our data are in accordance with the results of the groups of Wladimiroff and Van Zalen-Sprock that prove that cerebral vessels are a separate hemodynamic system that is independent of the other parts of the fetal circulation from the beginning of pregnancy. Owing to this mechanism, the fetal brain is probably well protected from hypoxia even in early pregnancy.

Three-dimensional ultrasound as a tool for the measurement of fetal nuchal translucency

The decade of the 1990s has ushered in the prospect of first-trimester ultrasound screening for fetal chromosomal abnormalities. The technique of measuring nuchal translucency (NT) which gave rise to the remarkably higher detection rate of chromosomal abnormalities still has to overcome some technical difficulties. Unsuccessful NT measurements were reported in many studies[42,43]. It seems that establishment of the training regimen for NT measurement as reported by Monni and co-workers[44] and Braithwaite and Economides[45] may overcome some of these methodological problems. The study of Kurjak and co-workers[46] clearly demonstrated that 3D transvaginal ultrasound enabled the depiction of the successful mid-sagittal section of the fetus, allowing precise NT measurements to be made. This is possible, owing to the ability of 3D ultrasound to reorient the fetal position using multiplanar imaging (Figure 8).

The aim of this study was to correlate intraobserver reproducibility of the nuchal translucency measurements by 2D and 3D transvaginal ultrasound. Examinations were performed in 120 women undergoing ultrasound screening at 10–14 weeks' gestation, by two experienced ultrasonographers using both methods twice consecutively. Statistical analysis for the assessment of intraobserver reproducibility was by the paired t test.

NT measurements were obtained in 100% of cases with 3D sonography compared to only 85% with 2D sonography. Better intraobserver reproducibility was obtained for 3D than for 2D ultrasound. Three-dimensional transvaginal ultrasound improved the accuracy of NT measurement, producing an appropriate mid-sagittal section of the fetus and a clear distinction of the nuchal region from the amniotic membrane.

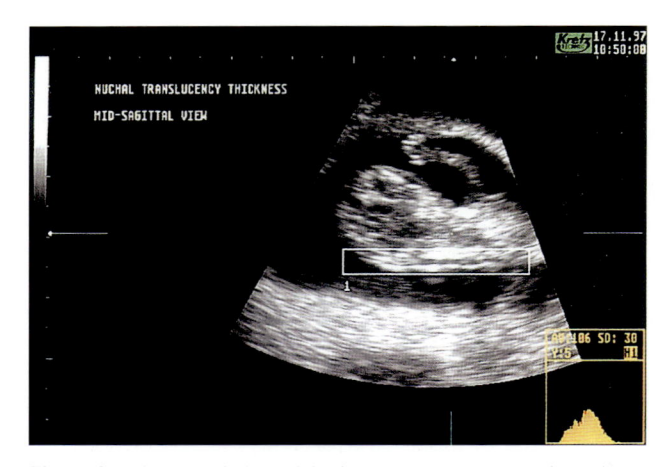

Figure 8 Mid-sagittal view of the fetus at 12 weeks' gestation. Three-dimensional ultrasound allows assessment of the mid-sagittal section in all fetuses between 12 and 14 weeks' gestation which is mandatory for accurate measurement of nuchal translucency

Three-dimensional ultrasound in the assessment of the yolk sac

The prognostic significance of the yolk sac diameter as determined by ultrasound is not clearly established. Most abnormal pregnancies have been demonstrated to have normal yolk sac measurements[47–49], whereas only a minority of abnormal early pregnancies have presented yolk sac dimensions that are either 'too small' or 'too large'[50,51]. Increased echogenicity of the yolk sac walls was reported as a sign of dystrophic changes that occur in non-viable cellular material indicating early pregnancy loss[52]. Kupesic and co-workers[34] measured gestational sac volume and yolk sac volume and vascularity in 80 women with uncomplicated pregnancy between 5 and 12 weeks of gestation. Regression analysis revealed an exponential growth of the gestational sac volume throughout the first trimester of pregnancy. Gestational sac volume measurements can be used for the estimation of gestational age in early pregnancy. An abnormal gestational sac volume measurement could potentially be used as a prognostic marker for pregnancy outcome. The yolk sac volume was found to increase from 5 to 10 weeks of gestation. However, when the yolk sac reaches its maximum volume at around 10 weeks it has already started to degenerate, which can be indirectly proved by a significant reduction in visualization rates of the yolk sac vascularity (Table 2). Therefore, the disap-

Table 2 Yolk sac volume and vascularity determined by three-dimensional ultrasound and color Doppler between 5 and 12 weeks' gestation

Gestational age (weeks)	n	Yolk sac volume (mm³) ± SD	Yolk sac vascularity visualization rates (%)
5	18	7.30 ± 1.40	0
6	27	14.20 ± 2.10	37.04
7	42	38.90 ± 4.85	83.33
8	55	51.55 ± 5.14	90.91
9	48	56.00 ± 5.35	81.25
10	31	61.60 ± 6.15	64.52
11	28	57.75 ± 5.80	25.00
12	21	52.28 ± 5.15	14.28
Total	270	42.45 ± 4.49	49.54

pearance of the yolk sac in normal pregnancies is probably the result of yolk sac degeneration rather than of a mechanical compression of the expanding amniotic cavity. These events suggest that the evaluation of the biological function of the yolk sac by measuring the diameter and/or the volume is limited. Therefore, a combination of functional and volumetric studies is necessary to identify some of the more important moments during early pregnancy.

Kurjak and colleagues[53] reported on the vascularization of the yolk sac in normal pregnancies between 6 and 10 weeks of gestation. Pulsed Doppler signals characterized by low velocity and high pulsatility were obtained in 85.71% of the yolk sacs during the 7th and 8th gestational weeks. Although the reports on the yolk sac and vitelline circulation are very exciting, it should be noted that such studies are not ethically feasible in ongoing human pregnancies, since the secondary yolk sac is a source of primary germ cells and blood stem cells[54]. Kurjak and Kupesic[55] performed research analyzing the vascularization of the yolk sac in 48 patients with missed abortions. In 18.5% of these patients three types of abnormal vascular signals were derived from the yolk sac: irregular blood flow, permanent diastolic flow and venous blood flow signals. The prognostic significance of analyzing the secondary yolk sac circulation is not clearly established, since these vessels persist inside the wall of the yolk sac up to 1 month after the cellular death of the other components[5,6]. Therefore, changes in vascular pattern as well as changes in yolk sac appearance (size, shape and echogenicity) seem to be a consequence of poor embryonic development or even embryonic death rather than a primary cause of an early pregnancy failure. Three-dimensional ultrasound may significantly contribute to *in vivo* observations of the yolk sac, enabling scanning time to be reduced and the yolk sac's honeycomb surface pattern to be observed (Figure 9). Automatic volume calculation will allow us to estimate the precise relationship between the yolk sac and gestational sac volumes, as well as to obtain the correlation between yolk sac volume and CRL measurements. Further 3D ultrasound and power Doppler will allow us to study turgescent blood vessels rising above the surface of the yolk sac (Figure 10). The same technique can be used to study the evolution from the embryo–vitelline towards the embryo–placental circulation. Since yolk sac and vitelline blood vessels are prerequisites for oxygen

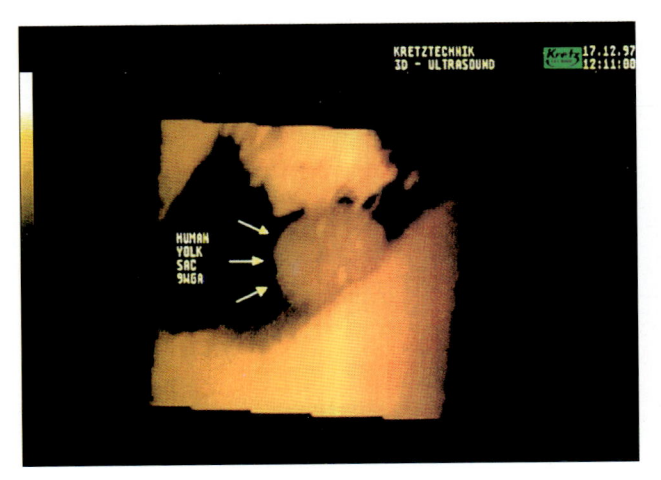

Figure 9 Three-dimensional scan of the yolk sac at 9 weeks' gestation. Note the regular echogenicity and outer contours of the yolk sac

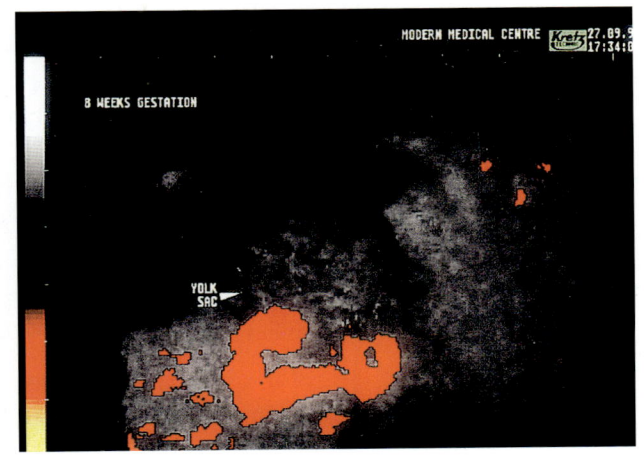

Figure 10 Three-dimensional power Doppler demonstrates visualization of the turgescent blood vessels above the surface of the yolk sac

transfer, absorption and transfer processes during the first trimester, alterations in this early circulatory system may have some prognostic value for predicting pregnancy outcome.

Three-dimensional power Doppler in the assessment of embryonic vascularity

Three-dimensional power Doppler combines two ultrasound modalities. This mode depicts the 3D continuum of the vascular network in the scanned tissue. This is a huge step ahead from the 2D images produced from the standard color and pulsed Doppler devices. In power Doppler sonography the hue and brightness of the color signal represent the total energy of the Doppler signal. This mode is more sensitive to low-velocity flow and, thus, overcomes the angle dependence and aliasing found in standard color Doppler. Owing to its capability of displaying total flow in the scanned area, images give an impression similar to that of angiography. The implementation of the 3D image integration permits the sonographer to view structures in three dimensions interactively, rather than having to assemble the sectional planar images mentally. Using this technique, improved recognition is expected of the vascular anatomy, as well as more accurate detection of heart defects.

The advantages of power Doppler can be summarized as follows:

(1) Because perfusion and not velocity is analyzed, side-by-side visualization of small and large vessels is possible in one setting without the masking effect of color Doppler;

(2) In an orthogonal plane of a vessel, color Doppler shows the mean frequency, which is near zero, and a black strip is displayed between red and blue. In power Doppler examination the information of the amplitude from both signals tends to be additive, resulting in a powerful signal. This allows an angle-independent visualization of (horizontal) vessels, which is one of the main advantages of the method, especially in prenatal diagnosis;

(3) Power Doppler has a better edge definition in displaying flow, because the signals from the vessel wall and surrounding tissue have low amplitude;

(4) In power Doppler, the color assigned to noise is uniform and is distinguishable from true flow signals, whereas in color Doppler noise is coded in the same colors as vessel flow.

All these features make this new method optimal for the 3D reconstruction of vessels[57].

Although power Doppler has several advantages over conventional color Doppler sonography, it is still a form of color Doppler imaging and, therefore, subject to some of the limitations of the conventional technique. Various parameters (e.g. pulse repetition frequency, high-pass filter, priority, power gain, color persistence, frame rate) must be optimized for 3D display, as well as for qualitative and quantitative analysis of these power Doppler data. A change in color setting may result in a radically different 3D vascular image and dissimilar quantitative results. The effects of ultrasound energy attenuation can sometimes cause a different power Doppler signal intensity and hence alter the vessel detection between the near and deep fields of the displayed image.

Kurjak and colleagues[58] used combined B-mode and power Doppler imaging in order to evaluate fetal growth and the development of the fetal circulation. Their study included 270 normally developing pregnancies. They used a fully digitized 3D device with complete storage of 3D power Doppler data (Kretz 530D, Kretz-Medison, Zipf, Austria and Seoul, Korea). Different rendering modalities were used in color-coded data processing and presentation. A minimum-intensity projection of the vascular network was used to create a translucent image, and a maximum-intensity projection was used for a surface-rendered vascular image. The former was superior in assessment of the spatial interrelationship of the vascular structures, and the latter was useful in the assessment of the morphology and outer surface of a confined vascular structure.

Five weeks

Three-dimensional power Doppler reveals intense vascular activity surrounding the chorionic shell, starting from the first sonographic evidence of the developing pregnancy during the 5th week of gestation. A hyperechoic chorionic ring is interrupted by color-coded sprouts that penetrate its borders. These are areas of the developing intervillous circulation. Future development of the 3D power Doppler program should include 3D gray-scale (anatomic) information and simultaneous power Doppler and shift spectrum information.

Six weeks

Aortic and umbilical blood flow is well depicted (Figure 11). The initial branches of the umbilical ves-

THREE-DIMENSIONAL SONOEMBRYOLOGY OF THE FIRST TRIMESTER

sels are visible at the placental umbilical insertion. Pulsed Doppler signals from the aorta and umbilical artery obtained by conventional color Doppler demonstrate absent end-diastolic flow, while umbilical vein blood flow is pulsatile.

Seven weeks

In addition to the aorta and umbilical blood flow, at the end of the 7th week, 3D power Doppler depicts features of early vascular anatomy on the base of the skull with branches evolving laterally to the mesencephalon and cephalic flexure. Pulsed Doppler analysis reveals absent end-diastolic velocities in the arteries. Apart from the embryonic circulation, 3D power Doppler can obtain blood flow signals from the intervillous space (Figure 12).

Eight weeks

Three-dimensional power Doppler imaging allows visualization of the entire fetal circulation (Figure 13). During the 8th and 9th weeks, the developing intestine is being herniated into the proximal umbilical cord (Figure 14).

Nine to ten weeks

The circle of Willis and its major branches can be depicted by 3D power Doppler (Figure 15). Continuous pan-diastolic blood flow emerges in the cerebral vessels on the base of the skull if analyzed by conventional color Doppler[59]. At that time the aorta and umbilical arteries are still characterized by absent end-diastolic blood flow.

Figure 11 Three-dimensional power Doppler image of the embryonic circulation at 7/8 weeks' gestation. The full length of the fetal aorta is well depicted. Note the color dots within the intervillous space, indicating the intervillous circulation

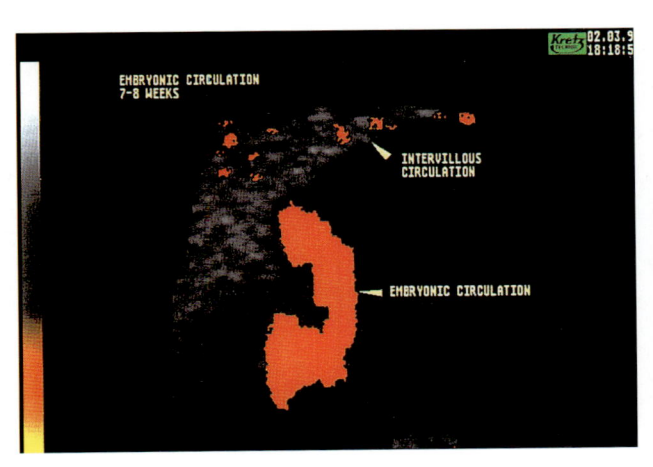

Figure 12 Three-dimensional power Doppler scan of the embryonic circulation at 7/8 weeks' gestation. Clear blood flow signals are simultaneously obtained from the intervillous space

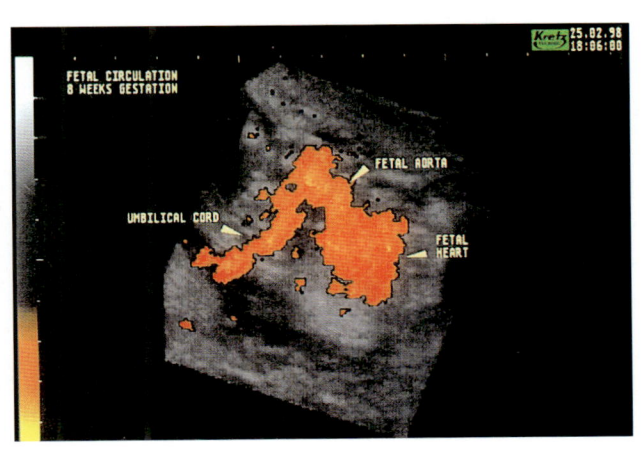

Figure 13 The fetal circulation with emphasis on the fetal heart and aorta is shown using power Doppler and gray-scale three-dimensional reconstruction

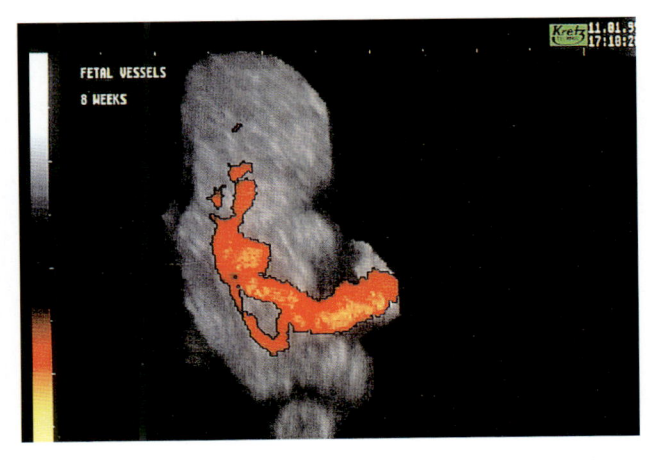

Figure 14 Three-dimensional power Doppler image of the fetal vessels at 8 weeks' gestation

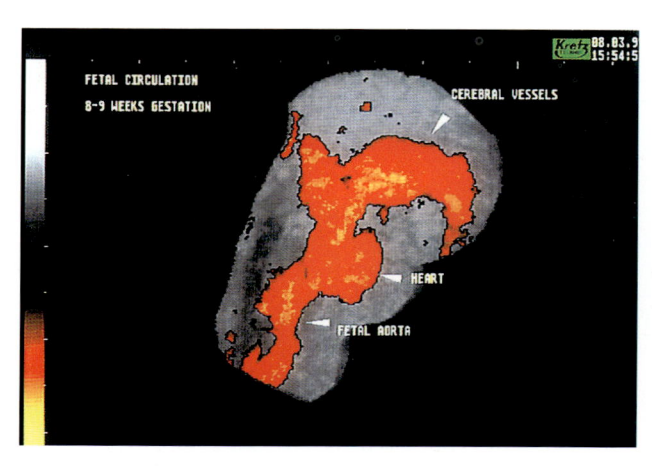

Figure 15 The fetal circulation at 8/9 weeks' gestation with emphasis on the cerebral circulation. Carotid and cerebral vessels are clearly depicted using three-dimensional power Doppler imaging

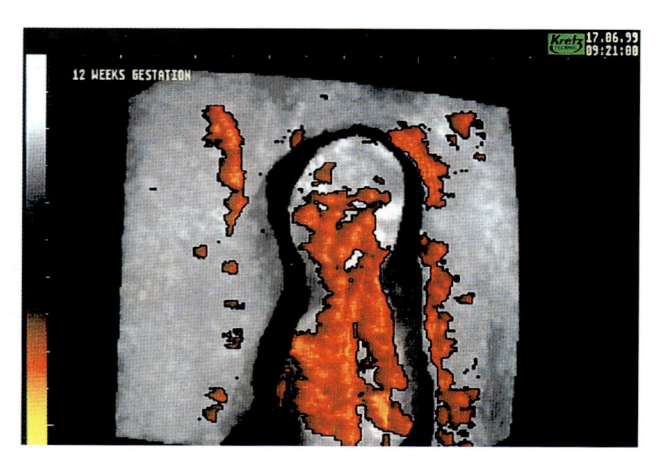

Figure 16 Three-dimensional power Doppler scan of the fetus at 12 weeks' gestation. Note the fetal aorta and its major branches: the common iliac and renal arteries. The circle of Willis and its branches are easily depicted using this modality

Eleven to twelve weeks

With the use of 3D power Doppler it is possible to depict the major branches of the aorta: the common iliac and renal arteries (Figure 16). The circle of Willis and its branches are easily visible. Pulsed Doppler analysis of the umbilical artery reveals end-diastolic velocities that gradually emerge. Continuous diastolic velocities in the fetal aorta become established a few weeks later.

Hyett and co-workers[60] conducted a morphometric analysis of the great vessels in early fetal life. They performed a pathological examination of the heart and great vessels in 61 specimens obtained after surgical termination of pregnancy for psychosocial indications at 9–18 weeks of gestation. The authors combined their results with the results of various Doppler studies. Doppler studies have demonstrated that, at 11–13 weeks, impedance in the cerebral vessels is only marginally higher than in the late second trimester. In contrast, in the descending aorta and umbilical arteries there is a major decrease in impedance during the second trimester, which is thought to be the consequence of vascular changes in the placenta[61,62]. It could be postulated that preferential blood flow to the fetal head during the first and early second trimesters of pregnancy is accomplished by the early development of low-resistance vessels in the cerebral circulation, at a stage when the resistance in other fetal parts and the placenta is high.

The authors suggested that there is an additional mechanism supporting preferential growth of the fetal head, namely relative narrowing of the aortic isthmus so that the left ventricular output is preferentially directed to the head. With advancing gestation and a decrease in peripheral resistance as well as a relative increase in the diameter of the isthmus, blood is preferentially distributed to other fetal parts, and the relative size of the fetal head to that of the rest of the body decreases.

Three-dimensional ultrasound imaging complements pathological and histological evaluation of the developing embryo, giving rise to the new term: 3D sonoembryology. We believe that studies including the combination of *in vivo* 3D power Doppler and spectral pulsed Doppler data with post-mortem histology specimens will yield new and important facts about this period of human development. Undoubtedly, rapid technological development will allow real-time 3D ultrasound to provide improved patient care on the one hand, and increased knowledge of developmental anatomy on the other.

References

1. Bonilla-Musoles F. Three-dimensional visualization of the human embryo: a potential revolution in prenatal diagnosis. *Ultrasound Obstet Gynecol* 1996;7:393–7
2. Ploeckinger-Ulm B, Ulm MR, Lee A, Kratochwil A, Bernaschek G. Antenatal depiction of fetal digit with three-dimensional ultrasonography. *Am J Obstet Gynecol* 1996;175:571–4
3. Merz E, Bahlmann F, Weber G, Macchiella D. Three-dimensional ultrasonography in prenatal diagnosis. *J Perinat Med* 1995;23:213–22
4. Nelson TR, Pretorius DH. Three-dimensional ultrasound of fetal surface features. *Ultrasound Obstet Gynecol* 1992;2:166–74
5. Lee A, Deutinger J, Bernaschek G. Voluvision: three-dimensional ultrasonography of fetal malformations. *Am J Obstet Gynecol* 1994;170:1312–14
6. Steiner H, Staudach A, Spitzer D, Schaffer H. Three-dimensional ultrasound in obstetrics and gynecology; technique, possibilities and limitations. *Hum Reprod* 1994:1773–8
7. Merz E, Bahlmann F, Weber G. Volume (3D) scanning in the evaluation of fetal malformations – a new dimension in prenatal diagnosis. *Ultrasound Obstet Gynecol* 1995;5:222–7
8. Steiner H, Merz E, Staudach A. 3D facing (video). *Hum Reprod* 1995;Update (CD-ROM)
9. Pretorius DH, House M, Nelson TR. Fetal face visualization using three-dimensional ultrasonography. *J Ultrasound Med* 1995;14:349–56
10. Merz E. Three-dimensional ultrasound in the evaluation of fetal anatomy fetal malformations. In Chervenak FA, Kurjak A, eds. *Current Perspectives on The Fetus as a Patient*. Carnforth, UK: Parthenon Publishing, 1996:75–87
11. Brinkley JF, McCallum WD, Muramatsu SK. Fetal weight estimation from length and volumes found by three-dimensional ultrasonic measurements. *J Ultrasound Med* 1984;3:162–9
12. Levaillant JM, Benoit B, Bady J, Rotten D. Ecographie tridimensionelle apport technique et clinique en ecographie obstetricale. *Reprod Hum Horm* 1995;3:341–7
13. Pretorius DH, Nelson TR. Three-dimensional use in obstetrics. In Fleischer AC, Manning FA, Jeanty P, Romero R, eds. *Principles and Practice of Ultrasonography in Obstetrics and Gynecology*, 5th edn. Norwalk, CT: Appleton Lange, 1995:119–26
14. Sohn C, Bastert G. The technical requirements of stereoscopic three-dimensional ultrasound imaging. *Sonoace Int* 1996;3:16–25
15. Kyei-Mensah A, Zaidi J, Pittrof R, Shaker A, Campbell S, Tan SL. Transvaginal three-dimensional ultrasound: accuracy of follicular volume measurements. *Fertil Steril* 1996;65:371–6
16. Fujiwaki R, Hata T, Hata K, Kitao M. Intrauterine sonographic assessments of embryonic development. *Am J Obstet Gynecol* 1995;173:1770–4
17. Bonilla-Musoles F, Raga F, Osborne N, Blanes J. The use of three-dimensional (3D) ultrasound for the study of normal and pathological morphology, of the human embryo and fetus: preliminary report. *J Ultrasound Med* 1995;14:757–65
18. Johnson DD, Pretorius DH, Budorick N. Three-dimensional ultrasound of conjoined twins. *Obstet Gynecol* 1997;90:701–2
19. Baba K, Satoh K, Sakamoto S, Okai T, Ishi S. Development of an ultrasonic system for three-dimensional reconstruction of the foetus. *J Perinat Med* 1989;17:19–24
20. Merz E, Bahlmann F, Weber G. 3D Volumensonographie in der transvaginalen Diagnostik. *Med Bild* 1994;8:43–51
21. Merz E. Volume (3D) scanning in the evaluation of fetal malformation. *Ultrasound Obstet Gynecol* 1994;4:339
22. Steiner H, Spitzer D, Weiss-Wichert PH, Graf AH, Staudach A. Three-dimensional ultrasound in prenatal diagnosis of skeletal dysplasia. *Prenat Diagn* 1995;15:373–7
23. Meyer-Wittkopf M, Cook A, McLennan A, Summers P, Sharland GK, Maxwell DJ. Evaluation of three-dimensional ultrasonography and magnetic resonance imaging in assessment of congenital heart anomalies in fetal cardiac specimens. *Ultrasound Obstet Gynecol* 1996;8:303–8
24. Brunner M, Obruca A, Bauer P, Feichtinger W. Clinical application of volume estimation based on three-dimensional ultrasonography. *Ultrasound Obstet Gynecol* 1995;6:358–7
25. King DL, King DL Jr, Shao MY. Evaluation of *in vitro* measurements: accuracy of a three-dimensional ultrasound scanner. *J Ultrasound Med* 1991;10:77–82
26. Lee A, Kratochwil A, Stuempflen I, Deutinger J, Bernaschek G. Fetal lung volume determination by three-dimensional ultrasonography. *Am J Obstet Gynecol* 1996;175:588–92
27. Merz E, Bahlmann F, Weber G. Volume scanning in the evaluation of fetal malformations – a new dimension in prenatal diagnosis. *Ultrasound Obstet Gynecol* 1995;5:222–7
28. Blaas HG, Eik-Nes SH, Kiserud T, Hellevik LR. Early development of the forebrain and midbrain: a longitudinal ultrasound study from 7 to 12 weeks of gestation. *Ultrasound Obstet Gynecol* 1994;4:183–92
29. Blaas HG, Eik-Nes SH, Kiserud T, Hellevik LR. Early development of the hindbrain: a longitudinal ultrasound study from 7 to 12 weeks of gestation. *Ultrasound Obstet Gynecol* 1995;5:151–60
30. Blaas HG, Eik-Nes SH, Kiserud T, Hellevik LR. Early development of the abdominal wall, stomach and heart from 7 to 12 weeks of gestation: a longitudinal ultrasound study. *Ultrasound Obstet Gynecol* 1995;6:240–9
31. Blaas HG, Eik-Nes SH, Bremnes JB. The growth of the human embryo. A longitudinal biometric assessment from 7 to 12 weeks of gestation. *Ultrasound Obstet Gynecol* 1998;12:346–54
32. Blaas HG, Eik-Nes SH, Kiserud T, Berg B, Angelsen B, Olstad B. Three-dimensional imaging of the brain cavi-

ties in human embryos. *Ultrasound Obstet Gynecol* 1995;5:228–32
33. Bree RL, Marn CS. Transvaginal sonography in the first trimester:embryology, anatomy, and hCG correlation. *Semin Ultrasound CT MR* 1990;12:11
34. Kupesic S, Kurjak A, Ivancic-Kosuta M. Volume and vascularity of the yolk sac studied by three-dimensional ultrasound and color Doppler. *J Perinat Med* 1999;27:91–6
35. Bonilla-Musoles F, et al. Demonstration of early pregnancy with three-dimensional ultrasound. In Merz E, ed. *3D Ultrasound in Obstetrics and Gynecology*. Philadelphia: Lippincott Williams & Wilkins, 1998:81–93
36. O'Rahilly R, Mueller F. Ventricular system and choroid plexuses of the human brain during the embryonic period proper. *Am J Anat* 1990;189:285–302
37. Merz E, Weber G, Bahlmann F, Miric-Tesanic D. Application of transvaginal and abdominal three-dimensional ultrasound for the detection or exclusion of fetal malformations of the fetal face. *Ultrasound Obstet Gynecol* 1997;9:2373
38. Liang RI, Huang SE, Chang FM. Prenatal diagnosis of ectopia cordis at 10 weeks of gestation using two-dimensional and three-dimensional ultrasonography. *Ultrasound Obstet Gynecol* 1997;10:137–9
39. Hata T, Aoki S, Akiyama M, Yanagihara T, Miyazaki K. Three-dimensional ultrasonographic assessment of fetal hands and feet. *Ultrasound Obstet Gynecol* 1998;12:235–9
40. Wladimiroff JW, Huisman TWY, Stewart PA. Intracerebral, aortic and umbilical artery flow velocity waveforms in the late-first-trimester fetus. *Am J Obstet Gynecol* 1992;166:46–9
41. Van Zalen-Sprock MM, Van Vugt JMG, Colenbrander GJ, vanGeijn HP. First-trimester uteroplacental and fetal blood flow velocity waveforms in normally developing fetuses: a longitudinal study. *Ultrasound Obstet Gynecol* 1994;4:284–8
42. Roberts LJ, Bewley S, Mackinson AM, Rodeck CH. First trimester nuchal translucency: problems with screening the general population I. *Br J Obstet Gynaecol* 1995;102:381
43. Haddow JE, Palomokie GE. Down's syndrome screening. *Lancet* 1996;347:1625
44. Monni G, Zoppi MA, Ibba RM, Floris M. Fetal nuchal translucency test for Down's syndrome. *Lancet* 1997;350:1631
45. Braithwaite JM, Economides DL. The measurement of nuchal translucency with transabdominal and transvaginal sonography – success rates, repeatability and level of agreement. *Br J Obstet Gynaecol* 1995;68:720
46. Kurjak A, Kupesic S, Ivancic-Kosuta M. Three-dimensional transvaginal ultrasound improves measurement of nuchal translucency. *J Perinat Med* 1999;27:97–102
47. Crooij MJ, Westhuis M, Schoemaker J, Exalto N. Ultrasonographic measurements of the yolk sac. *Br J Obstet Gynaecol* 1982;89:931
48. Reece EA, Sciosca AL, Pinter E, et al. Prognostic significance of the human yolk sac assessed by ultrasonography. *Am J Obstet Gynecol* 1988;159:1191
49. Goldstein SR, Kerenyi T, Scheer J, Papp C. Correlation between karyotype and ultrasound findings in patients with failed early pregnancy. *Ultrasound Obstet Gynecol* 1996;8:314
50. Jauniaux E, Jurkovic D, Henriet Y, Rodesch F, Hustin J. Development of the secondary human yolk sac. Correlation of sonographic and anatomical features. *Hum Reprod* 1991;6:1160
51. Lindsay DJ, Lyons EA, Levi CS, Zheng XH. Endovaginal appearance of the yolk sac in early pregnancy: normal growth and usefulness as a predictor of abnormal pregnancy outcome. *Radiology* 1992;83:115
52. Harris RD, Vincent LM, Askin FB. Yolk sac calcification: a sonographic finding associated with intrauterine embryonic demise in the first trimester. *Radiology* 1988;166:109
53. Kurjak A, Kupesic S, Kostovic L. Vascularization of yolk sac and vitelline duct in normal pregnancies studied by transvaginal color and pulsed Doppler. *J Perinat Med* 1994;22:443
54. Witschi E. Migration of the germ cells of human embryos from the yolk sac to the primitive gonadal folds. *Contrib Embryol Carnegie Inst* 1948;32:67
55. Kurjak A, Kupesic S. Parallel Doppler assessment of yolk sac and intervillous circulation in normal pregnancy and missed abortion. *Placenta* 1998;19:619
56. Hustin J, Jauniaux E. Implantation and the yolk sac. In Kurjak A, ed. *Textbook of Perinatal Medicine*. Carnforth, UK: Parthenon Publishing, 1998:960
57. Chaoui R, Kalache K. Three-dimensional color power imaging: principles and first experience in prenatal diagnosis. In Merz E, ed. *3D Ultrasound in Obstetrics and Gynecology*. Philadelphia: Lippincott Williams & Wilkins, 1998:135–41
58. Kurjak A, Kupesic S, Banovic I, Hafner T, Kos M. The study of morphology and circulation of early embryo by three-dimensional ultrasound and power Doppler. *J Perinat Med* 1999;27:145–57
59. Kurjak A, Kupesic S. Ultrasound of the first trimester CNS development (structure and circulation). In Levine M, ed. *Fetal and Neonatal Brain*. London: Harcourt Health Sciences, 1999
60. Hyett J, Moscoso G, Nicolaides K. Morphometric analysis of the great vessels in early fetal life. *Hum Reprod* 1995;11:3045–8
61. Wladimiroff JW, Huisman TWA, Stewart PA. Fetal cardiac flow velocities in the late first trimester of pregnancy: a transvaginal Doppler study. *J Am Coll Cardiol* 1991;17:357–9
62. Wladimiroff JW, Huisman TWA, Stewart PA. Fetal and umbilical flow velocity waveforms between 10–16 weeks' gestation: a preliminary study. *Obstet Gynecol* 1991;78:812–14

The assessment of normal fetal anatomy

B. Benoit, M. Kos and A. Kurjak

Conventional two-dimensional (2D) ultrasound provides tomographic imaging of fetal anatomy, but cannot describe it precisely. The three-dimensional (3D) technique depicts volume images, unlike 2D ultrasound. The volume scanning technique also offers a panoramic view of the fetus if the surface-rendered view is chosen. Surface images can be rendered and displayed for any object that has been stored within the volume of interest[1,2].

Sculpture-like surface-mode reconstructions represent the most recent advance in the sonographic imaging of fetal anatomy. In surface rendering, intermediate 3D geometrical data are projected on a 2D plane to obtain a solid image. It is necessary first to decide upon the direction or the viewpoint from which the 3D data are to be observed, before they are projected on the 2D plane. Shading makes the image more realistic. A viewpoint may be set arbitrarily, however. When the viewpoint and viewing direction are closer to the transmitting ultrasonic beam, clear 3D images with no defects caused by acoustic shadows should be easily obtainable[1–3]. For surface reconstruction, the volume can be rotated so that the fetus faces the examiner directly. If a region not of interest is within the scanned volume, it can be removed by 'Cartesian storage'. In this process only data from the region of interest are stored, while data outside that region are removed from the 3D calculation. All the structures within the volume can be investigated not only in surface view, but also in simultaneous image display and translucency mode[1].

Two points are essential for high-quality surface rendering with 3D ultrasound: the object of interest must be optimally displayed in the three 2D orthogonal image planes; and a sufficient volume of amniotic fluid must be present between the transducer and the surface to be rendered[1,4].

During the first trimester, 3D surface imaging is facilitated by the presence of a relatively large amount of fluid around the embryo and yolk sac[3] (Figures 1 and 2). If the probe or the fetus move during volume scanning, the volume will be distorted and the reconstruction will contain artifacts. In the second and third trimesters, the volume of amniotic fluid decreases in relation to fetal size, and it becomes increasingly diffi-

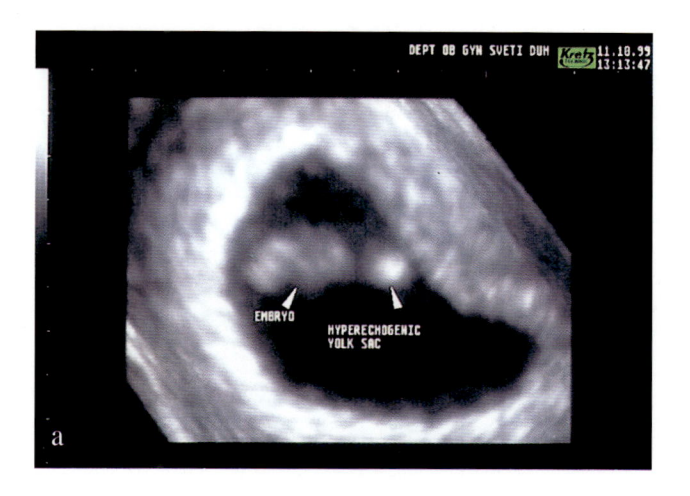

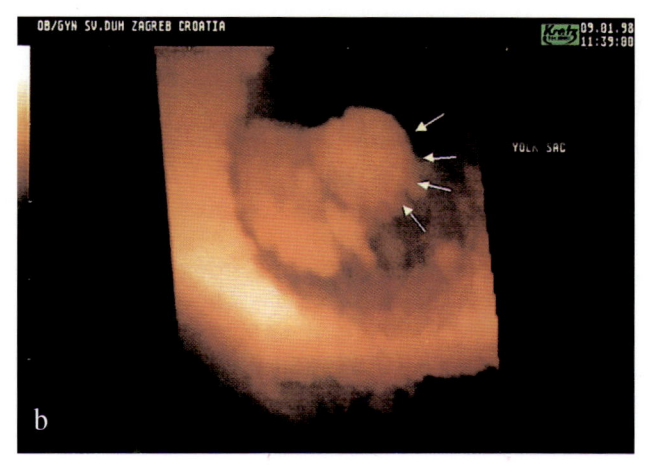

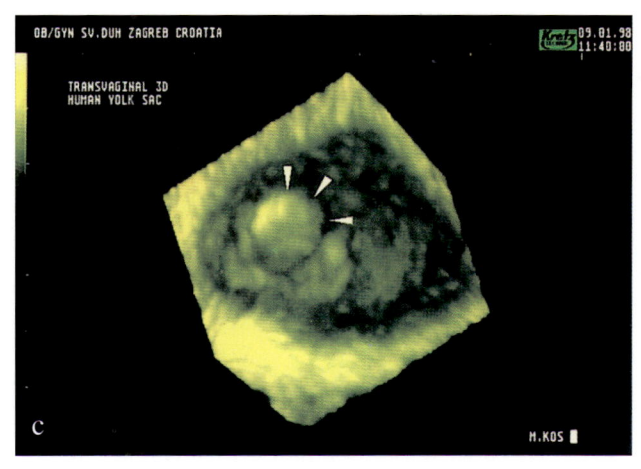

Figure 1 (a, b and c) Three-dimensional transvaginal imaging at 7–8 weeks, by surface mode. The embryo and yolk sac are depicted in various gray-scale images

CLINICAL APPLICATION OF 3D SONOGRAPHY

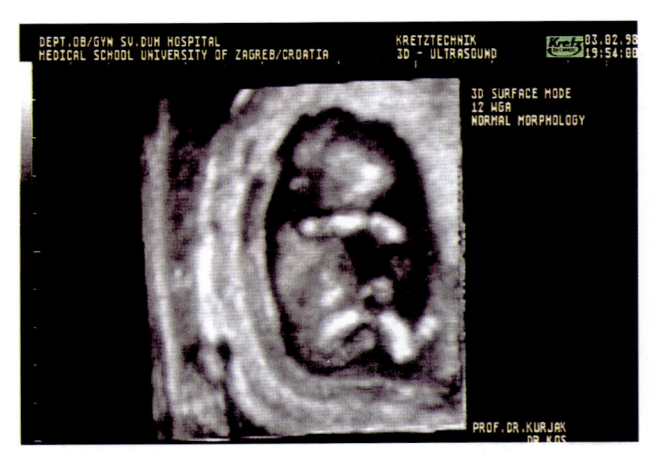

Figure 2 Normal fetal anatomy at 12 weeks, by surface mode

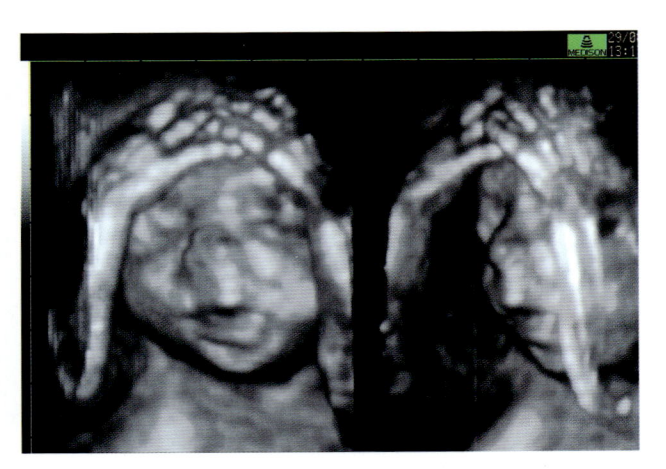

Figure 4 Fetal hands and face in the third trimester, by surface mode

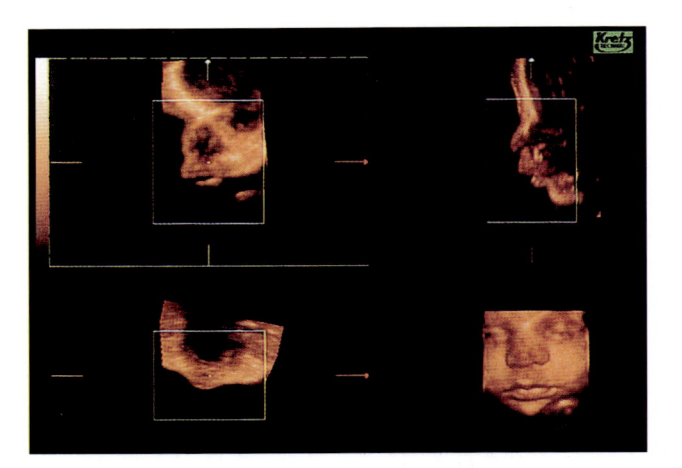

Figure 3 Three orthogonal two-dimensional images and final three-dimensional reconstruction of the fetal face

cult to obtain 3D images of the whole body of the fetus by surface rendering. If sufficient amniotic fluid is present, the object of interest is moved into a standard or 'textbook' position by rotating the three orthogonal image planes (Figure 3). The orthogonal planes are rotated again, to display the region that has been selected for surface rendering. Care is taken that the orthogonal image planes are correctly positioned so that a direct surface view is obtained. Because the stored volume can be rotated in all three planes, the standard terms of orientation, i.e. cranial, caudal, left, right, etc., pertain only to the object of interest and not to the screen, as in 2D ultrasound. Ultimately, the only view that is of interest in 3D ultrasound is the one that most clearly depicts abnormal findings. This may be in a longitudinal plane, transverse plane, or any of various oblique planes.

With an internal or integrated system, various algorithms are available for computer rendering of 3D views. The goal is to give the examiner a 3D picture of the object under study. Various rendering modes can be used alone or in combination, depending on the nature of the investigation. The surface mode is the most impressive, rendering the volume elements (voxels) that are first encountered by a virtual beam. As the name implies, this mode is used for rendering the fetal external body surface as well as the surfaces of internal structures. The surface mode is particularly useful for delineation of the fetal face and limbs[1–6] (Figure 4). Finally, 3D reconstructions, particularly surface view imaging, reassure the parents with a normal fetus, and contribute to a highly positive fetomaternal and fetopaternal relationship[2,4,6].

Unfortunately, some limitations of 3D scanning still exist. Data aquisition is possible only when the fetus is lying still. Movements during the storage process lead to recognizable motion artifacts. Oligohydramnios prevents satisfactory surface reconstruction, and overlying or adjacent structures interfere with surface rendering and must be eliminated by Cartesian storage prior to surface reconstruction[1].

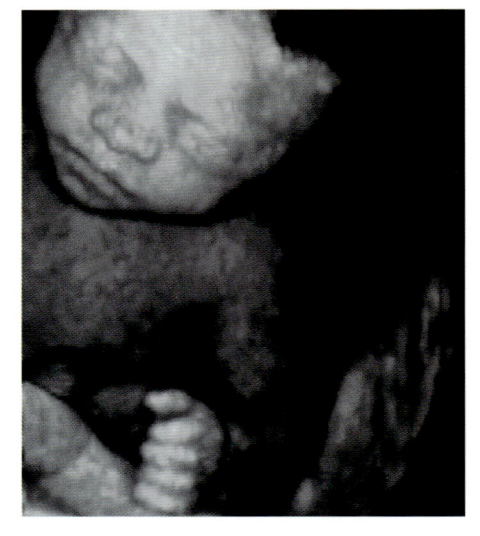

Figure 5 Fetal head, shoulders and face in the third trimester, by surface mode

THE ASSESSMENT OF NORMAL FETAL ANATOMY

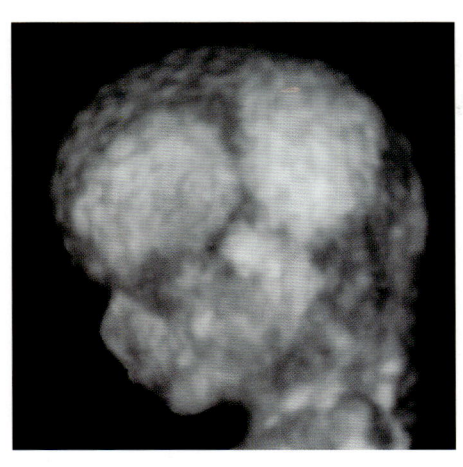

Figure 6 Cranial bones and sutures, imaged by the surface mode of 'subsurface' structures

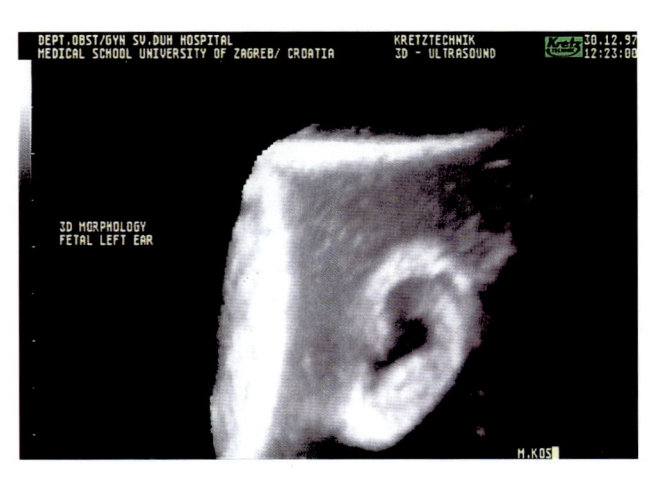

Figure 9 Normal fetal ear in the third trimester, by surface mode

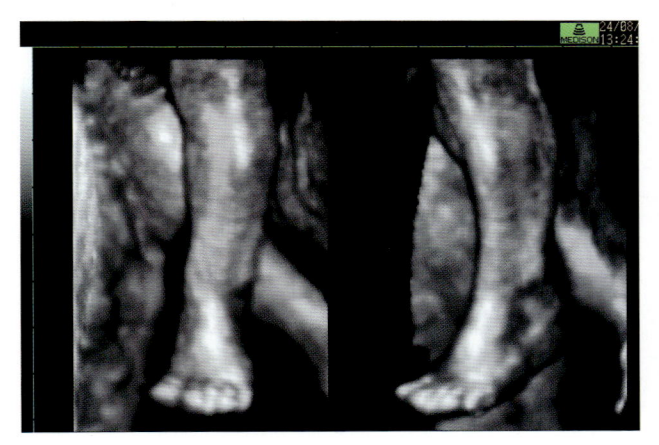

Figure 7 Fetal legs and feet at 24 weeks, by surface-rendered mode

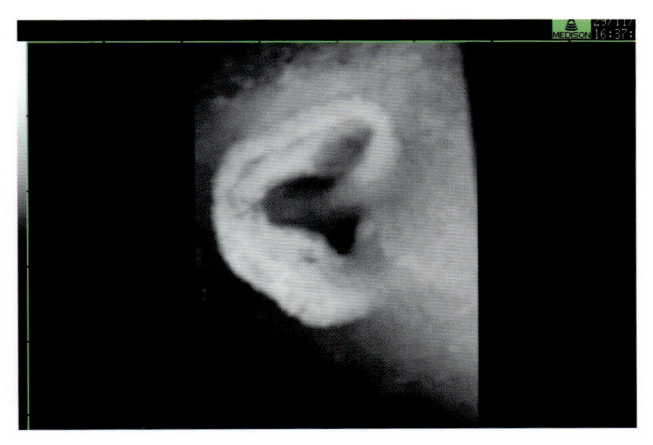

Figure 10 Normal fetal ear at 32 weeks, by surface mode

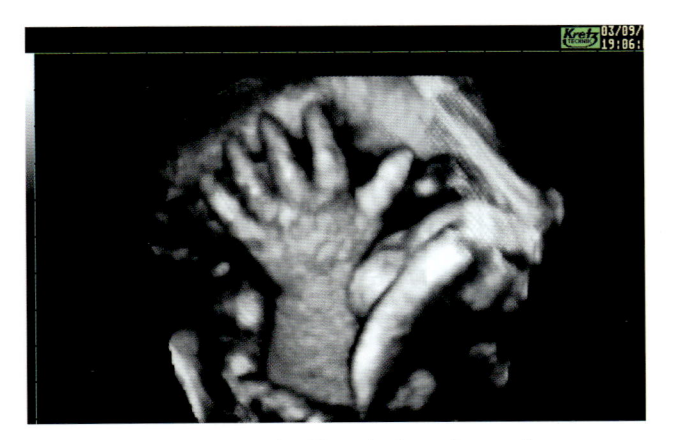

Figure 8 Opened fetal hand at 32 weeks, by surface mode

The fetal head, face and hands are the objects of greatest interest in 3D surface rendering (Figure 5). This method provides clear surface sculpture-like images from different viewing directions[1,2,4,7]. The scanning orientation for the examination of intracranial structures is either the fronto-occipital plane or the face profile. With 3D ultrasound the shape of the fetal head, cranial flat bones, orbits, ears, nose and lips can be investigated clearly, and malformations can be easily excluded[2,7–9]. The stored volume can be re-sliced in a number of viewing planes until all the morphological and topographic details are located (Figures 6–8). The ability to rotate every region of interest into an adequate position allows the examiner to investigate the fetal head from a side view as well[2,7]. For example, the location and shape of the ear can be evaluated precisely, and deviations such as a low-set or dysplastic ear can be easily demonstrated[4,8] (Figures 9 and 10).

Similarly, the 3D surface mode enables sculpture-like reconstructions to be made of the abdominal wall and the normal umbilical cord insertion[10–12]. The complete abdominal surface is 'invisible' by conventional 2D techology, with the only means of abdominal surface survey involving serial tomographic sections in sagittal and transverse planes[1]. Using the 3D surface mode, we are able to visualize the complete abdominal surface and umbilical cord insertion in a single image depicting their natural appearance (Figure 11).

123

CLINICAL APPLICATION OF 3D SONOGRAPHY

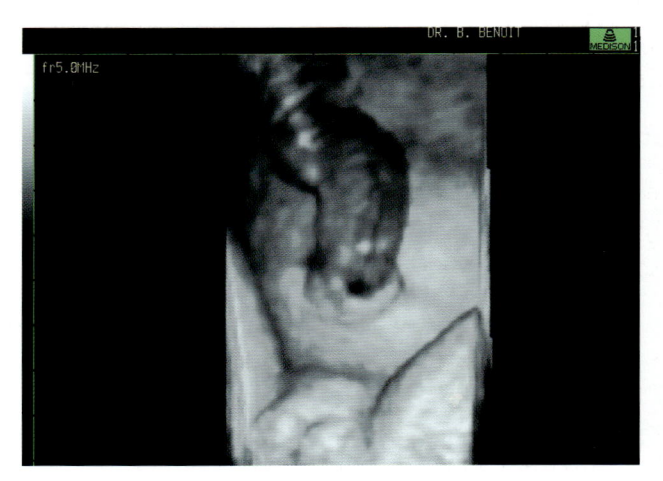

Figure 11 Anterior abdominal wall with normal umbilical cord insertion in the second trimester, by surface mode

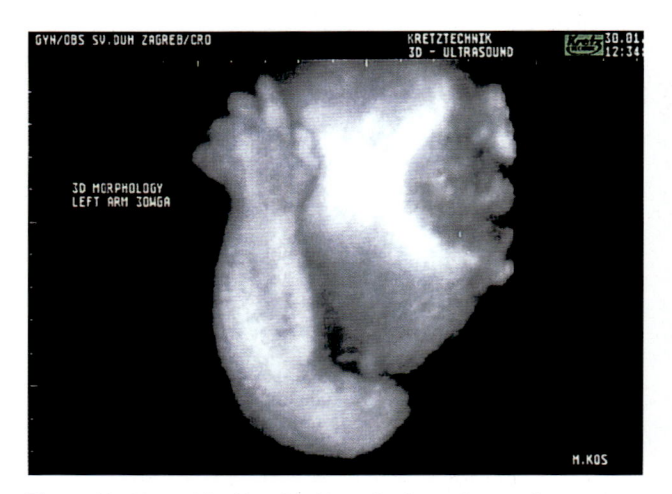

Figure 12 Normal fetal hand at 30 weeks, by surface mode

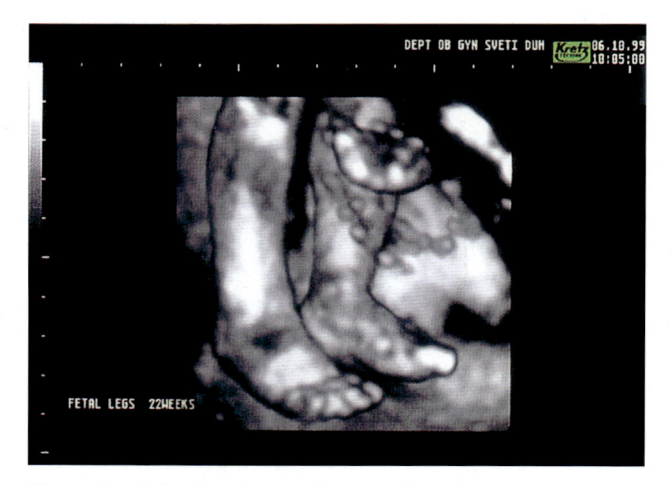

Figure 13 Normal fetal legs at 22 weeks, by surface mode

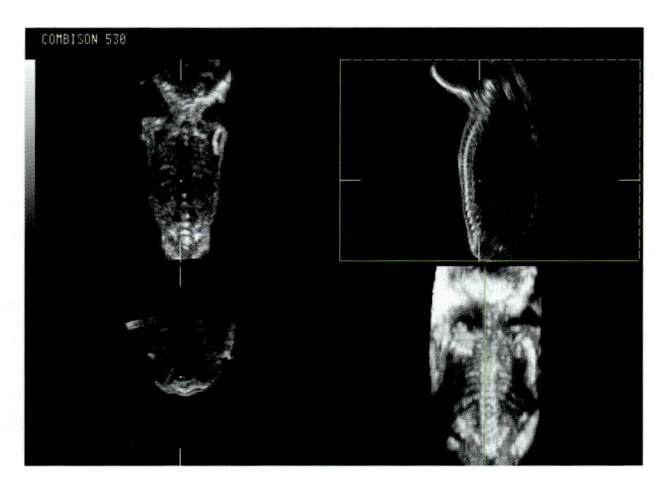

Figure 14 Three orthogonal images of the fetal skeleton and final three-dimensional reconstruction, by transparent view

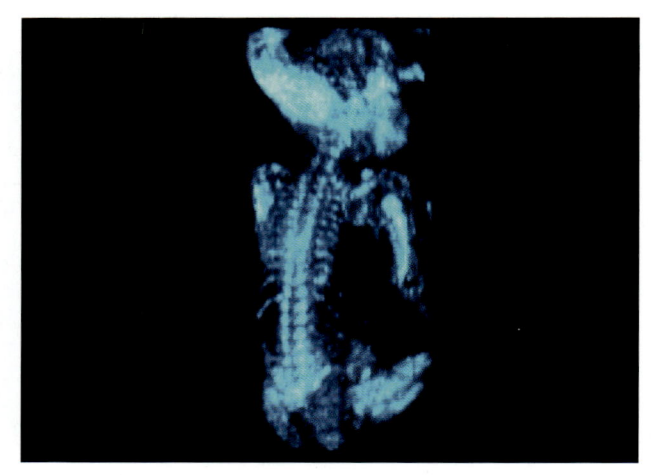

Figure 15 Normal skeleton, by transparent-mode reconstruction

Abdominal wall defects, such as omphalocele or gastroschisis, can be easily excluded. The same principle is acceptable in surface examination of the fetal back, confirming the normal skin integrity over the neural tube[13,14].

Examination of fetal extremities in surface mode enables us to present clear displays of all segments of the limbs and deviations from the normal anatomical axis (Figures 12 and 13). Pathological angulations and morphological anomalies of the limbs, hands, feet and digits should be looked for in screening for chromosomal disorders[2,4,15–17]. As fingers and toes are clearly visible in the surface mode, this technique is very useful in demonstrating the normal morphology of these structures.

Unfortunately, abnormalities of bony structures of the fetal skeleton can be depicted only in the transparent or translucency mode, providing an image of the structures only with high echogenicity (Figures 14 and 15). Bony structures of the fetus can be visualized also in X-ray-like images. These techniques enable detailed analysis to be made of the normal skeletal anatomy and the detection of structural and topographic abnormalities[4–6].

External genitalia can be clearly recognized by surface rendering, and complex malformations or developmental anomalies should be diagnosed easily and

THE ASSESSMENT OF NORMAL FETAL ANATOMY

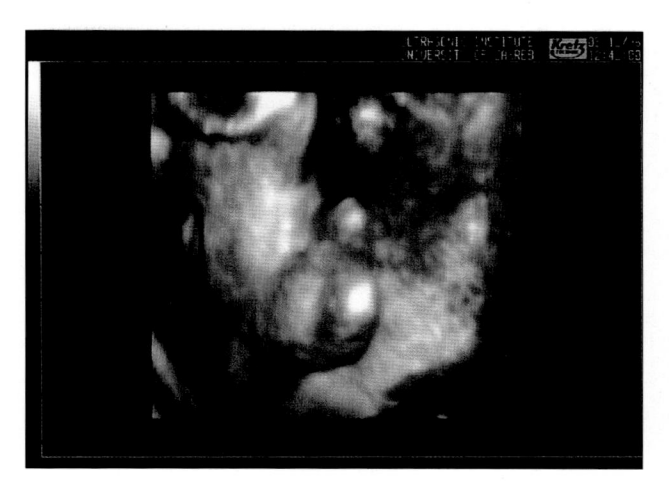

Figure 16 Male external genitalia, by surface mode

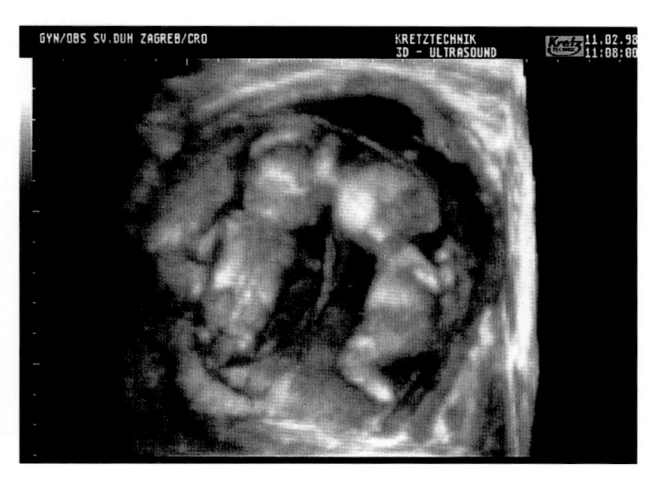

Figure 18 Dichorionic/diamniotic twins at 13 weeks. Dividing membranes and two placentas are visible by transvaginal surface-mode reconstruction

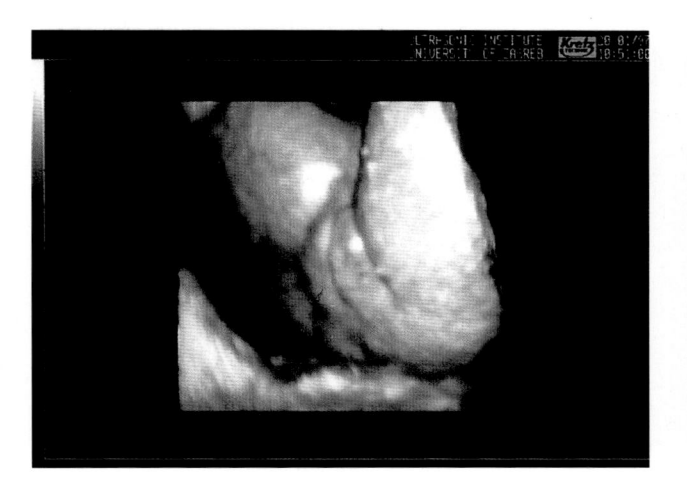

Figure 17 Female external genitalia, by surface mode

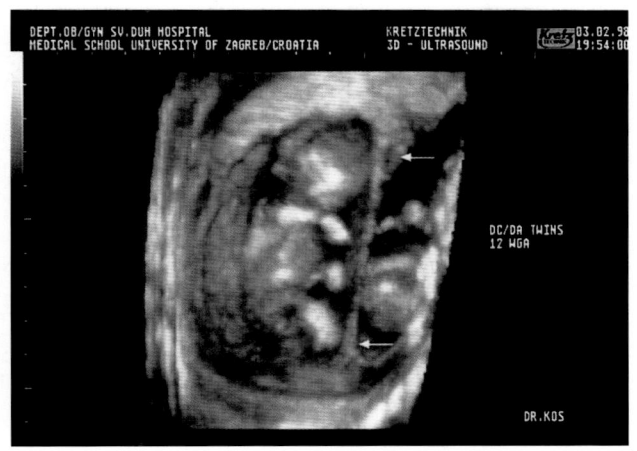

Figure 19 Dichorionic/diamniotic twins at 12 weeks. The 'twin peak' or 'lambda sign' (arrow) is shown on transvaginal surface-mode reconstruction

much earlier than was previously possible[2,12] (Figures 16 and 17).

Determining chorionicity and amnionicity during the early second trimester may be much easier by 3D surface rendering (Figures 18 and 19). All of the relevant criteria can be used. These include: counting the number of placentas; determining whether each fetus is within its own amniotic sac; describing the appearance of the dividing membrane; and looking for the presence of a triangular projection of placental tissue beyond the chorionic surfaces (lambda or twin-peak sign)[2,4,12].

Surface-rendered images, the most attractive images in 3D ultrasonography, are still greatly influenced by amniotic fluid volume, fetal movements and the pathway of the ultrasonic beam. Unfortunately, clinically useful and representative images cannot be obtained in every patient. In cases of oligohydramnios, severe obesity and/or intense fetal movements, 3D imaging can be compromised. Current problems with 3D imaging may be resolved in the near future. New processors may reduce calculation time for image rendering, and storage capacity may be enhanced. Three-dimensional real-time ultrasound has recently been developed to solve some of these technical problems[1,5]. The introduction of real-time 3D equipment is also starting to enable 3D ultrasound imaging of the fetal heart[18–20].

125

References

1. Baba K, Okai T. Basis and principles of three dimensional ultrasound. In Baba K, Jurkovic D, eds. *Three-dimensional Ultrasound in Obstetrics and Gynecology*. Carnforth, UK: Parthenon Publishing, 1997:1–20
2. Benoit B. Three dimensional surface mode for demonstration of normal fetal anatomy in the second and third trimester. In Merz E, ed. *3D Ultrasound in Obstetrics and Gynecology*. Philadelphia: Lippincott Williams and Wilkins, 1998:95–100
3. Feichtinger W. Transvaginal three-dimensional imaging. *Ultrasound Obstet Gynecol* 1993;3:375–8
4. Kurjak A, Kos M. Three dimensional ultrasonograhy in prenatal diagnosis. In Chervenak FA, Kurjak A, eds. *Fetal Medicine*. Carnforth, UK: Parthenon Publishing, 1999:102–8
5. Merz E. Three dimensional ultrasound in the evaluation of the fetal malformations. In Baba K, Jurkovic D, eds. *Three-dimensional Ultrasound in Obstetrics and Gynecology*. Carnforth, UK: Parthenon Publishing, 1997:37–44
6. Merz E, Bahlaman F, Weber G, Macchiella D. Three dimensional ultrasonography in prenatal diagnosis. *J Perinat Med* 1995;23:213–22
7. Pretorius DH, Nelson TR. Three dimensional ultrasound of fetal surface features. *Ultrasound Obstet Gynecol* 1992;2:166–202
8. Shih JC, et al. Antenatal depiction of fetal ear with three-dimensional ultrasonography. *Obstet Gynecol* 1998;91:500–5
9. Pretorius DH, House M, Nelson TR, et al. Evaluation of normal and abnormal lips in fetuses: comparison between three- and two-dimensional sonography. *Am J Roentgenol* 1995;165:1233–7
10. Hata T, et al. Three-dimensional ultrasonographic assessment of umbilical cord during the 2nd and 3rd trimesters of pregnancy. *Gynecol Obstet Invest* 1998;159–64
11. Merz E. Three-dimensional ultrasound in prenatal medicine. In Kurjak A, ed. *Textbook of Perinatal Medicine*. Carnforth, UK: Parthenon Publishing, 1998:346–51
12. Kurjak A, Kupesic S. *Slide Atlas of Three-dimensional Sonography in Gynecology and Obstetrics*. Carnforth, UK: Parthenon Publishing, 1998
13. Johnson DD, Pretorius DH, Riccabona M, Budirock NE, Nelson TR. Three dimensional ultrasound of fetal spine. *Obstet Gynecol* 1997;89:434–8
14. Riccabona M, Johnson D, Pretorius DH, Nelson TR. Three dimensional ultrasound: display modalities in the fetal spine and thorax. *Eur J Radiol* 1996;22:41–5
15. Shimizu T, Salvador L, Hughes-Benziee R, Dawson L, Nimrod C, Allanson J. The role of reduced ear size in the prenatal detection of chromosomal abnormalities. *Prenat Diagn* 1997;17:545–9
16. Kurjak A, Kupesic S, Di Renzo GC, Pooh R, Kos M, Hafner T. Recent advances in perinatal sonography. *Prenat Neonat Med* 1998;3:194–207
17. Ploeckinger-Ulm B, Ulm MR, Lee A, Kratochwil A, Bernaschek G. Antenatal depiction of fetal digits with three dimensional ultrasonography. *Am J Obstet Gynecol* 1996;175:571–4
18. Nelson T, Sklansky M, Pretorius DH. Fetal heart assessment using three dimensional ultrasound. In Merz E, ed. *3D Ultrasound in Obstetrics and Gynecology*. Philadelphia: Lippincott Williams and Wilkins, 1998:125–33
19. Nelson TR, Pretorius DH, Sklansky M, Hagen-Ansert S. Three dimensional echocardiographic evaluation of fetal heart anatomy and function: acquisition, analysis and display. *J Ultrasound Med* 1996;15:1–9
20. Leventhal M, Pretorius DH, Sklansky MS, Budorick NE, Nelson TR, Lou K. Three-dimensional ultrasound of the normal fetal heart: a comparison with two dimensional imaging. *J Ultrasound Med* 1998;17:341–8

The normal and abnormal fetal face   14

B. Benoit, M. Kos and A. Kurjak

Introduction

We can state with certainty that the sculpture-like, plastic visualization of the fetal face is the most spectacular product of three-dimensional (3D) ultrasonography (Figures 1–4). None of the modalities of ultrasound visualization and examination have changed our way of visual perception of the fetal face as much as 3D ultrasound, for two main reasons. First, the technical possibilities of 3D ultrasonography have solved the problems that arise when the fetal face is examined with conventional two-dimensional (2D) ultrasound. The fetal face is a convex, surface structure, for whose visualization an optimal frontocoronal section must be obtained. Usually, this is one of the most difficult sections to obtain, and the transvaginal access has been only a partial help in obtaining it.

Second, the 3D portrait-like reconstructions and the 'Live-3D' technique are enabling us to accept the fetal face as the most objective element of real fetal individuality. Visualization of the fetal face provides not only a window to the developing fetus, but also an ethical challenge as the first contact with a new 'person'. The psychological and emotional effect upon the examiner, and especially upon the parents, represents a completely new moment, as important as, and

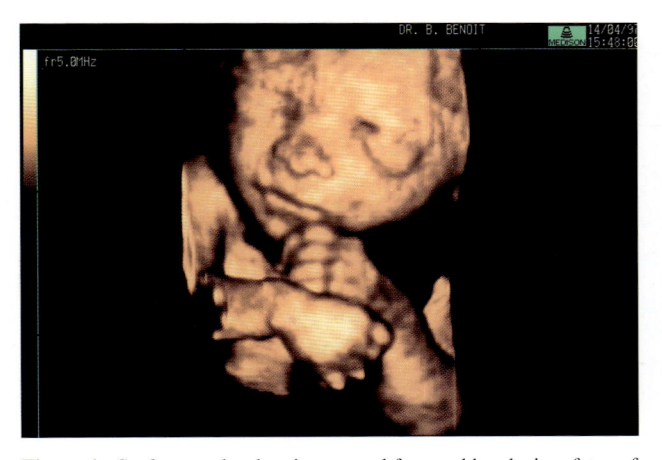

Figure 1 Surface mode, showing normal face and hands, in a fetus of 22 weeks' gestation

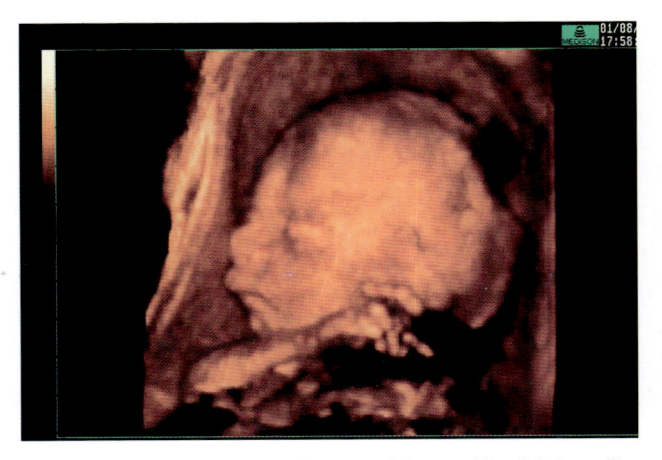

Figure 2 Surface mode, showing normal face and head, left profile, in a fetus of 22 weeks' gestation

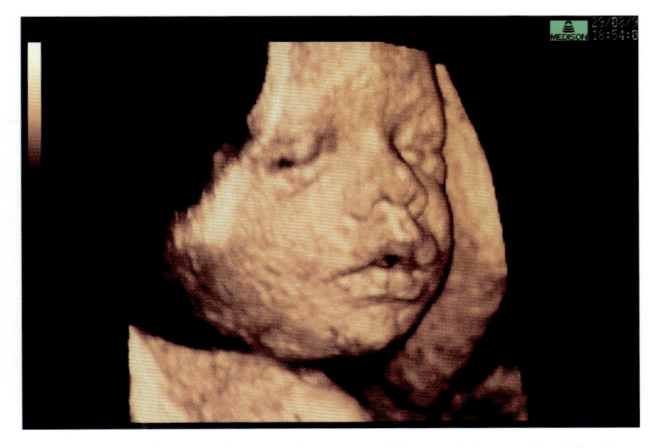

Figure 3 Surface mode, showing normal face, right semiprofile, in a fetus of 30 weeks' gestation

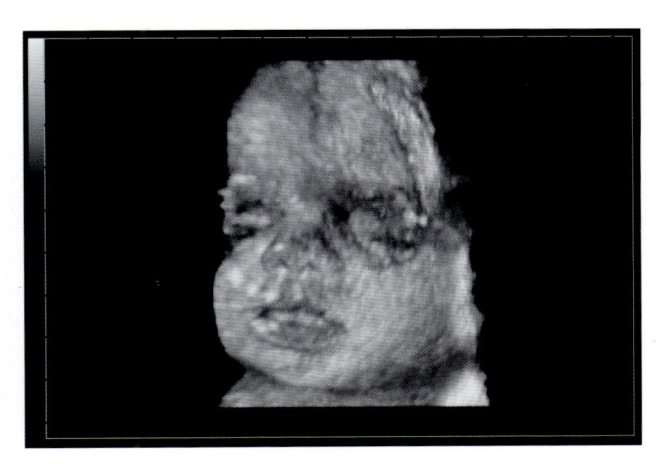

Figure 4 Normal face of a fetus in the third trimester

perhaps even more important than, the first visualization of the fetal heart action at the beginning of pregnancy.

The commercial, i.e. economic, effect resulting from the above-mentioned possibilities inficts upon us the imperative of achieving better and better machines and much more sophisticated software packages for the visualization and image processing, affecting thus the faster technical improvement of 3D ultrasound itself.

Evaluation of normal and abnormal anatomy

Examination of the fetal face is the basic part of ultrasonic examination for low-risk and high-risk pregnancies, but it can be analyzed only to a limited extent by conventional 2D sonography. The fetal face represents an object of the greatest interest in 2D and 3D sonography, but until this decade it was impossible to perform a detailed sonographic investigation, primarily because of a few technical disabilities. It was very difficult to obtain the coronal sections of the fetal head using a transabdominal probe during the second trimester. Moreover, imaging resolution of the transabdominal probes was sometimes not suitable for depicting important details of facial morphology. With the introducion of transvaginal sonography, it became possible to examine the fetal head and face much earlier in pregnancy, using a higher resolution of imaging. However, some basic problems, related primarily to the limits of probe manipulation and the use of inappropriate frontal and coronal sections, have remained. Even under optimal conditions, the physiological curvature of the face makes it impossible to obtain an image of the entire face in a single scan.

The second-trimester examination of the face should include a complete impression of the head, face and profile, followed by identification of normal frontal bones and forehead, orbits, eyelids, nose, filtrum, upper and lower lip, chin and cheeks. Facial dysmorphism associated with developmental and biometrical disorders of normal structures represent important markers of chromosomal abnormalities, and 3D ultrasonography may be useful for effective screening.

Three-dimensional surface mode provides clear imaging of all structures previously mentioned, particularly if associated with an appropriate amount of amniotic fluid in front of the fetal face[1-3]. The surface mode renders the volume elements (voxels) that are first encountered by a virtual beam. As the name implies, this mode is used for rendering fetal surfaces:

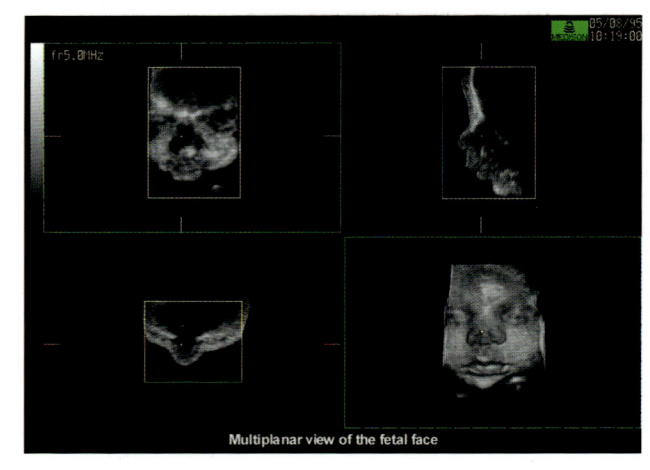

Figure 5 Multiplanar view of the normal fetal face in the third trimester. Three orthogonal planes are visible: frontal, sagittal (profile) and transverse (axial)

face, external body surfaces and the surfaces of internal structures[4]. The presence of amniotic fluid is the most important physical prerequisite for high-quality images. Moreover, to obtain the best surface-mode rendering, a larger amount of amniotic fluid must be present over the facial surface; the face has to be turned towards the probe and the pocket of amniotic fluid should be located just between the probe and the surface of the face. Following these conditions it will be possible to prepare an optimal 2D multiplanar image of the fetal face (frontal, profile and transverse planes; Figure 5). These three orthogonal, 2D images are representatives of the rendered volume, which is a data bank for successful 3D surface reconstruction. Initial review of facial volume data involves rotating the volume to an optimal position so that images are produced corresponding to the frontal, profile and transverse planes. All images are extracted from a single volume data set. Subsequently, the examiner is able to scroll through the volume and evaluate image planes parallel to the frontal, profile or transverse planes. An advantage of 3D volume acquisition, compared to 2D scanning, is that it is not necessary to acquire the volume in a conventional orientation. Any orientation is acceptable, because the volume can be rotated after the data are acquired. One of the most important aspects of assessing the fetal face with 3D imaging is that the fetal face can be rotated into various anatomic orientations. Rendered surfaces of the fetal face can be used to assess the overall facial anatomy and provide the most realistic visualization. These methods allow evaluation of different projections of the face in a rapid and reproducible fashion from the earliest stage of pregnancy[5]. If the probe or the head or the mother move during the volume scanning, the entire volume will be deformed and low-

THE NORMAL AND ABNORMAL FETAL FACE

quality surface reconstruction with movement artifacts will be obtained. Following the basic principles of orientation and in the presence of an appropriate amount of amniotic fluid it should be possible to collect a highly representative atlas of fetal facial images, including normal and abnormal facial anatomy[3]. Moreover, some of these images can depict specific mimic movements of the face and can be interpreted as a reflection of the fetal behavioral state during pregnancy (Figures 6 and 7).

By combining surface-mode imaging and transparent-mode imaging within the rendered volume, even the structures underlying the facial surface should be recognizable. Particular attention should be targeted to the visualization of cranial flat bones, to exclude the craniosynostoses (Figure 8). Owing to the facilitated orientation within multiplanar reconstruction, even the fetal tooth germs and palate can be evaluated as parameters of normal development[6,7]. The possibility of plastic reconstruction and detailed differentiation between normal, physiological variations and pathological forms of the fetal profile have to be particularly stressed. Some of these forms could be either an expression of normalcy or an expression of inherited systemic disease (Figure 9).

Despite the great diagnostic potential of 2D sonography, in some special cases limitations still exist. An unfavorable fetal position can make it impossible to visualize small structures such as the face and fingers. Three-dimensional ultrasonography has the strong potential for improved visualization and morphological evaluation of the fetal face (Figure 10). Producing a clear and quick visualization of the fetal face sometimes represents a practical problem and challenge

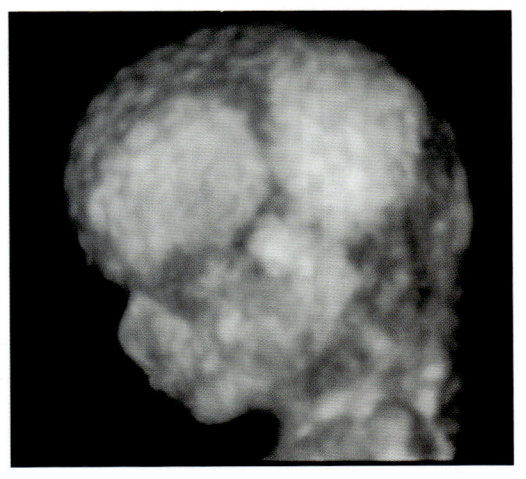

Figure 8 Surface imaging of fetal cranial flat bones, sutures and fontanelles

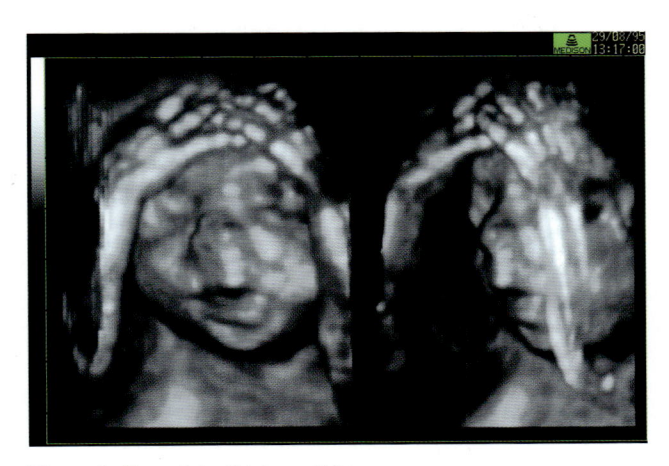

Figure 6 Face of the 'frightened' fetus

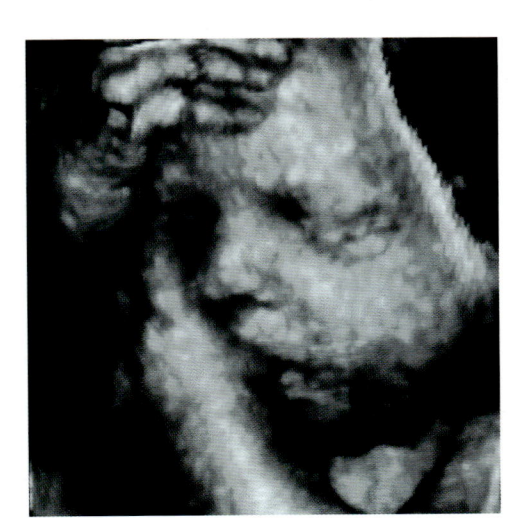

Figure 7 Fetal head and face. The fetus is sucking its thumb

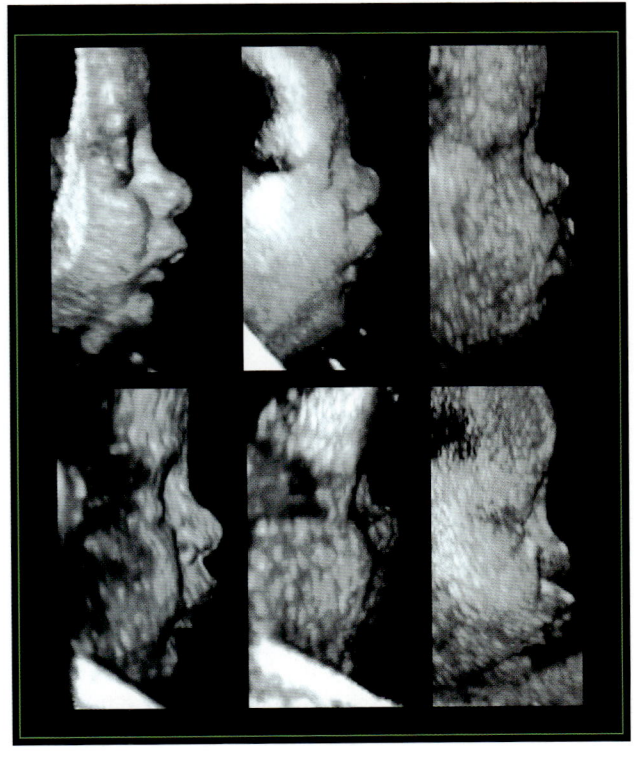

Figure 9 Six normal variants of fetal profiles

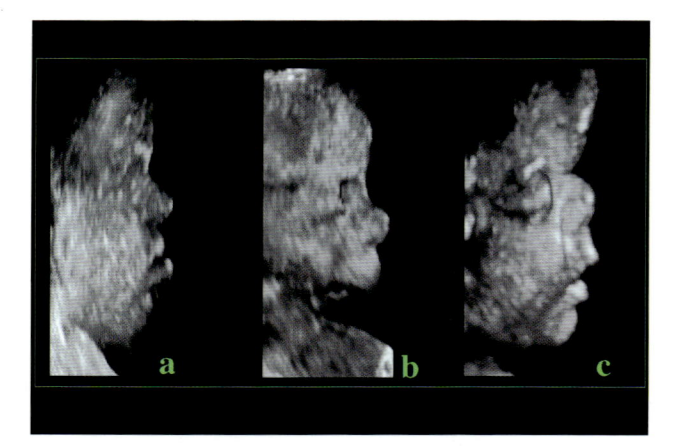

Figure 10 Three abnormal profiles: (a) Down's syndrome; (b) micrognathia; (c) Apert's syndrome. Clear differentiation is possible, following the main anatomical landmarks: frontal bossing, nasal bridge, nose flattening, prognathia or micrognathia and general facial dysmorphism

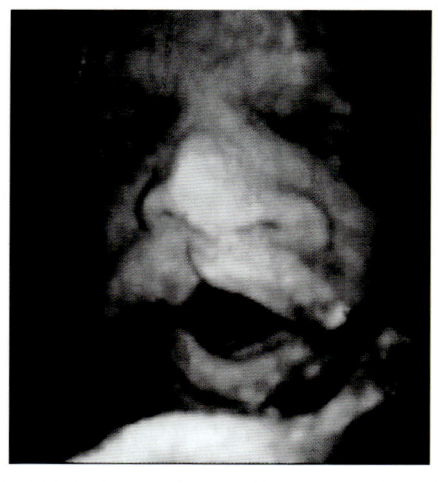

Figure 11 Third-trimester fetus, with open mouth and unilateral upper cleft lip

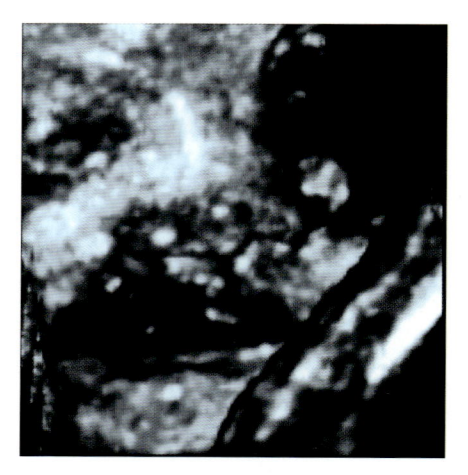

Figure 12 Third-trimester fetus, with right-sided cleft lip

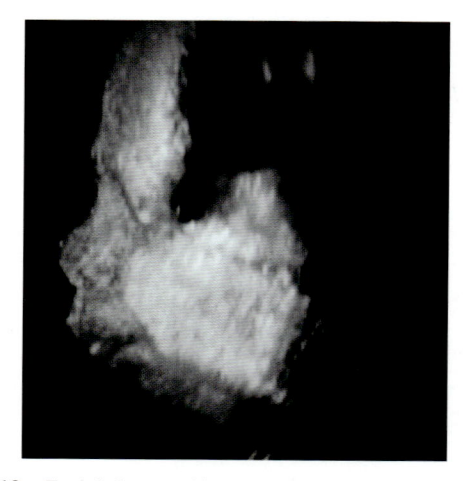

Figure 13 Facial dysmorphism with micrognathia in a second-trimester fetus

area of fetal diagnosis, which is particularly important as congenital anomalies of the face can be an expression of chromosomal abnormalities and some inherited diseases[1,8,9]. The main difficulties in correct recognition of anatomical details and minor malformations are related to the curvature of the face and limitations of probe manipulation. Three-dimensional sonography may help to solve these problems by allowing the free choice of any possible viewing section. Pretorius and Nelson[1] were able to obtain satisfactory images of the fetal face in 24 of 27 fetuses studied. They stressed that scanning after 19 weeks produced images of higher quality than scans obtained earlier, possibly due to the limits in sonographic resolution and anatomic definition of detailed structures. Merz and colleagues[10] performed 3D ultrasound examinations in more than 200 patients with fetal malformations found by conventional 2D ultrasound. Facial dysmorphisms and facial clefts were better seen with 3D ultrasound (Figures 11–15). A great difference is found between the transvaginal and transabdominal depiction and recognition of facial anomalies, and 3D ultrasound consistently displays facial abnormalities with greater accuracy and clarity than conventional 2D imaging. This particularly applies to chromosomal disorders and syndromes associated with subtle facial abnormalities requiring a detailed evaluation[11]. Rare morphological anomalies such as single nostril, flat nose, proboscis, cyclopia and hyper- or hypotelorism can be easily depicted and diagnosed using all of the modalities within the 3D imaging techniques[1,8,10–14].

However, the main dilemma still remains[13,14]: in which cases can we expect the higher quality of imaging and detection compared to the 2D ultrasound technique?

(1) Fetal cleft lip and palate, easily recognizable following instruction for use of the optimal scanning technique;

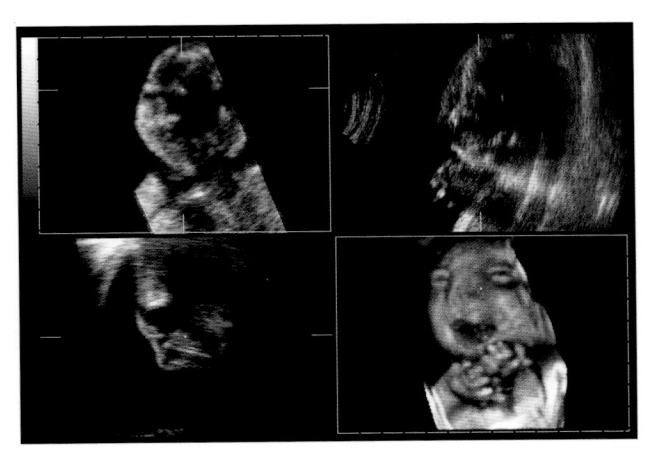

Figure 14 Facial dysmorphism in fetal pterygium syndrome. The typical appearance of the face is called 'bird face'

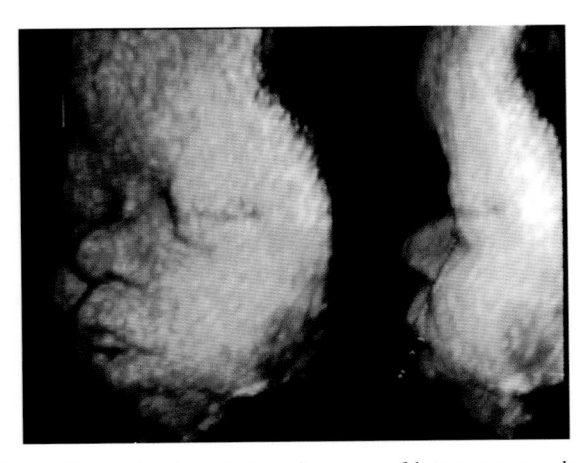

Figure 15 Facial dysmorphism in a case of heterozygous achondroplasia. Frontal bossing, depressed nasal bridge and prognathia are clearly recognizable

(2) Recognition of the curvature of the fetal face in a profile reconstruction (normal or abnormal);

(3) Minor defects of the face related to chromosomal disorders (cleft lip and palate);

(4) Fetal face/profile dysmorphism related to systemic or metabolic disorders (pterygium syndrome, skeletal dysplasias);

(5) Facial profile investigation (micrognathia, absent nose, frontal bossing, nasal bridge);

(6) Fetal tooth germ investigations (oligodentia or anodentia).

Additional studies will be necessary to evaluate the efficacy of 3D ultrasonography. It is evident that 3D ultrasonography improves the visualization of the normal and abnormal fetal face, giving clear, plastic information about the extent of defects. This is useful not only to obstetricians, but also to pediatricians and pediatric surgeons.

References

1. Pretorius DH, Nelson TR. Fetal face visualization using three-dimensional ultrasonography. *J Ultrasound Med* 1995;14:349–56
2. Baba K, Okai T. Clinical applications of three-dimensional ultrasound in obstetrics. In Baba K, Jurkovic D, eds. *Three-dimensional Ultrasound in Obstetrics and Gynecology*. Carnforth, UK: Parthenon Pubilishing, 1997:29–44
3. Benoit B. Three dimensional surface mode for demonstration of normal fetal anatomy in the second and third trimester. In Merz E, ed. *3D Ultrasound in Obstetrics and Gynecology*. Philadelphia: Lippincott Williams and Wilkins, 1998:95–100
4. Merz E, Bahlaman F, Weber G, et al. Fetal malformations – assessment by three-dimensional ultrasound in surface mode. In Merz E, ed. *3D Ultrasound in Obstetrics and Gynecology*. Philadelphia: Lippincott Williams and Wilkins, 1998:109–20
5. Kurjak A, Kos M. Three-dimensional ultrasonography in prenatal diagnosis. In Chervenak FA, Kurjak A, eds. *Fetal Medicine*. Carnforth, UK: Parthenon Publishing, 1999:102–8
6. Ulm MR, Kratochwill A, Ulm B, Solar P, Aro G, Bernaschek G. Three-dimensional ultrasound evaluation of fetal tooth germs. *Ultrasound Obstet Gynecol* 1998; 12:240–3
7. Johnson DD, Pretorius DH, Budorick NE, et al. Three-dimensional ultrasound of the fetal lip and primary palate. *Radiology* 2000;in press
8. Lee A, Deutinger J, Bernaschek G. Three-dimensional ultrasound: abnormalities of the fetal face in surface and volume rendering mode. *Br J Obstet Gynaecol* 1995;102:302–6
9. Nicolaides K, Shawwa L, Brizot M, Snijders R. Ultrasonographically detectable markers of fetal chromosomal defects. *Ultrasound Obstet Gynecol* 1993;3: 56–69
10. Merz E, Bahlaman F, Weber G. Volume scanning in the evaluation of fetal malformations: a new dimension in prenatal diagnosis. *Ultrasound Obstet Gynecol* 1995;5: 222–7
11. Merz E, Weber G, Bohlaman F, Miric-Tesanic D. Application of transvaginal and abdominal three-dimensional ultrasound for the detection or exclusion of mal-

formations of the fetal face. *Ultrasound Obstet Gynecol* 1997;9:237–43
12. Pretorius DH, House MH, Nelson TR, Hollenbach KA. Three-dimensional ultrasound of fetal lip anatomy: a preliminary clinical investigation. *Am J Roentgenol* 1995;165:1233–7
13. Hull AD, Pretorius DH. Fetal face: what we can see using 2-dimensional and 3-dimensional ultrasound imaging. *Semin Roentgenol* 1998;33:369–74
14. Pretorius D. The fetal face: 3D ultrasound. Presented at the *2nd World Congress on 3D Ultrasound in Obstetrics and Gynecology (syllabus)*. Las Vegas, NV, 1999

The assessment of abnormal fetal anatomy

A. Kurjak, M. Kos, B. Benoit and S. Kupesic

Introduction

The first generation of three-dimensional (3D) technology, during the early 1980s, provided a pseudo-3D image by the simultaneous display of three orthogonal planes. This offered some advantages over conventional two-dimensional (2D) imaging[1,2]. Modern systems are capable of generating surface and transparent views depicting the sculpture-like reconstruction of fetal surface structures or the transparent images of fetal inner anatomy. These are the most impressive products within modern 3D ultrasound imaging. The main advantages of 3D technology in perinatal medicine and antenatal diagnosis include scanning in the coronal plane, improved assessment of complex anatomic structures, surface analysis of minor defects, volumetric measuring of organs, 'plastic' transparent imaging of the fetal skeleton, spatial presentation of blood flow arborization and storage of scanned volumes and images[3-8]. With arbitrary sectional display in 3D ultrasonography, the orientation of tomograms is unlimited, despite the limits of probe manipulation or the unfavorable position of fetal structures. These facts are extremely important in the first trimester of pregnancy, when the manipulation of the vaginal probe is restricted and obtainable ultrasound sections are limited[9]. Additional progress has been made, owing to the permanent possibility of repeated analysis of previously saved 3D volumes and Cartesian elimination of surrounding structures and artifacts[3,10,11]. Three-dimensional reconstruction of a stored image is the most impressive benefit of 3D scanning. The region of interest is first identified and manually delineated; this is followed by an automatic process of echo extraction. The surface of the organ of interest is thus displayed in three dimensions. The transparent mode is another way of showing ultrasound images in three dimensions. In this mode, only the strongest and lowest signals are displayed, so that the internal structure of the organ of interest can be analyzed[12]. A comparison of two-dimensional (2D) and 3D techniques shows that the 3D method provides a diagnostic gain in a large percentage of cases, owing to the possibility of surface and transparent-mode imaging. The accurate topographic depiction of the desired image plane is much easier[3,13,14].

First-trimester applications

Three-dimensional ultrasonography is a relatively new diagnostic imaging technique undergoing rapid advances, particularly in the field of obstetrics and prenatal diagnosis. Three-dimensional scanning offers advantages in assessing embryonic morphology in the first trimester, owing to the ability to obtain multiplanar images through endovaginal volume acquisition. Limitations due to transducer movements prohibit

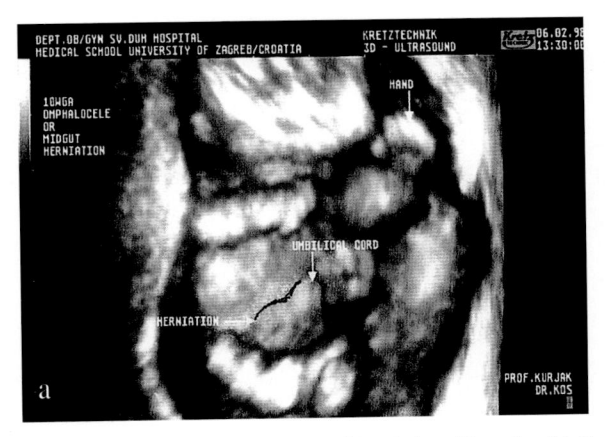

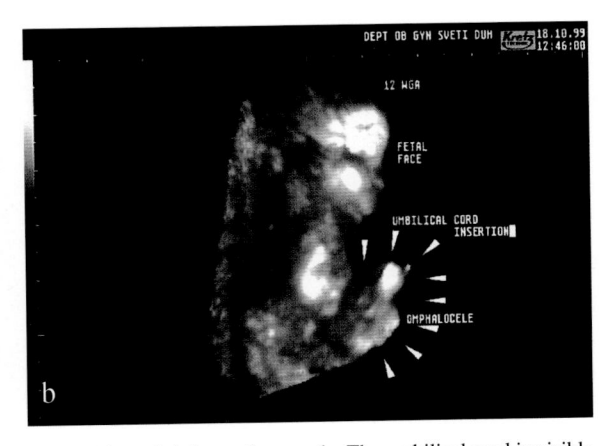

Figure 1 (a) Physiological umbilical herniation, 10 weeks. (b) Omphalocele (12 weeks), by surface mode. The umbilical cord is visible on the top of the sac

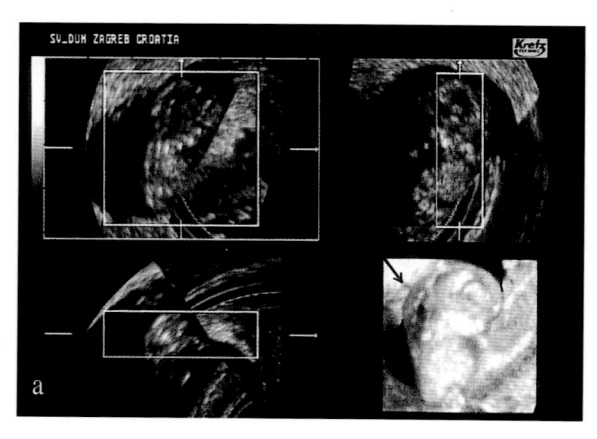

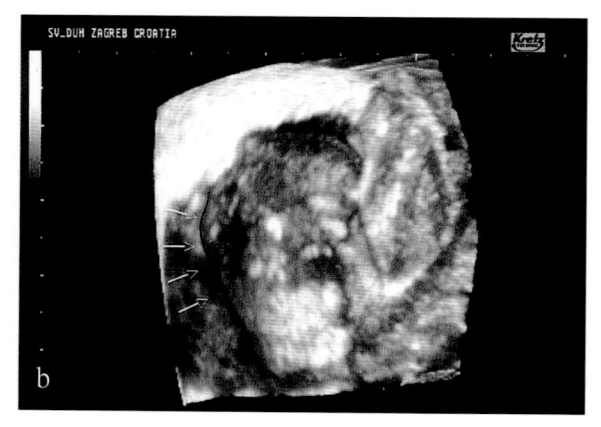

Figure 2 (a) Multiplanar scan of nuchal translucency (11 weeks) and three-dimensional reconstruction (arrow). (b) Surface-mode reconstruction, with visible nuchal collection of fluid (arrows)

obtaining many images on conventional 2D scanning. The 3D possibility of rotation of the scanned object and close analysis of the scanned volume has allowed a more systematic review of embryonic and extraembryonic anatomy.

Our experience confirms that transvaginal 3D ultrasonography during the first trimester provides significant visualization benefit, particularly because of an additional possibility for 3D morphological and power Doppler analysis of embryonic and extraembryonic 'static' structures, such as the gestational sac and yolk sac. Embryonic developmental disorders related to chromosomal abnormalities are of great interest within modern sonography[3,10,12]. During the first trimester, 3D surface and sculpture-like imaging includes excellent morphological recognition and follow-up of the physiological midgut herniation process, with consequtive abdominal anterior wall visualization (Figure 1). Three-dimensional depiction of retarded resolution of the umbilical herniation and development of omphalocele is possible during the 11th and 12th weeks of gestation. Following the possibilities of 3D transparent mode imaging, the morphology related to nuchal translucency and cystic hygroma can be recognized earlier than the development of biometrically detectable nuchal thickening (Figure 2). Moreover, case reports such as that by Liang and co-workers[15], which identified ectopia cordis at 10 weeks of gestation, are very encouraging.

Second- and third-trimester evaluation

Various studies have shown that the 3D ultrasound can detect or exclude not only major anomalies, but particularly subtle abnormalities. Besides impressive demonstration of normal fetal structures, 3D ultrasonography is adding a new window to the diagnosis of fetal malformations. During the second and third trimesters, 3D sonography provides a completely new method of visual perception of an unborn baby. Reconstructions and sculpture-like images, generated from the surface rendering mode, are the most impressive presentations. Three-dimensional imaging of the fetal surface greatly refines and expands our capabilities in the evaluation of normal anatomy and in the detection of fetal anomalies[16-21]. Fetal surface abnormalities can be selectively visualized, and the extent of a defect can be determined in all spatial dimensions.

Head and neck malformations

The fetal head is an essential part of routine sonographic examination. Even under optimal conditions, the position of the fetal head makes it difficult to obtain adequate images by 2D ultrasonography, and many cross-sectional images are required to imagine the complete impression of normal structure. Volume-rendered 3D images of the fetal head are easily recognizable by both families and physicians. One of the most important aspects of assessing the fetal head by 3D imaging is that the fetal face can be depicted in sculpture-like appearance. The complete head can be rotated into various spatial positions. This allows evaluation of different projections of the head and face in a rapid and reproducible fashion from the earliest stage of pregnancy.

In evaluations of the fetal head, scanning with a 3D probe can clearly demonstrate major anomalies, such as anencephaly or hydrocephaly[21,22]. It can also define the extent of an encephalocele[19,21]. The dysmorphic appearance of fetal anencephalia and acrania can be much better understood by presenting the fetal head

THE ASSESSMENT OF ABNORMAL FETAL ANATOMY

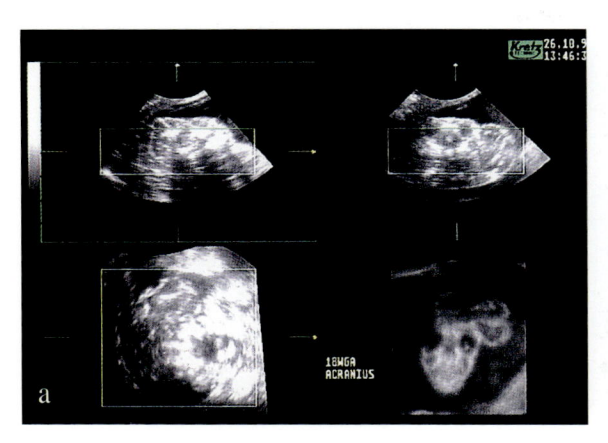

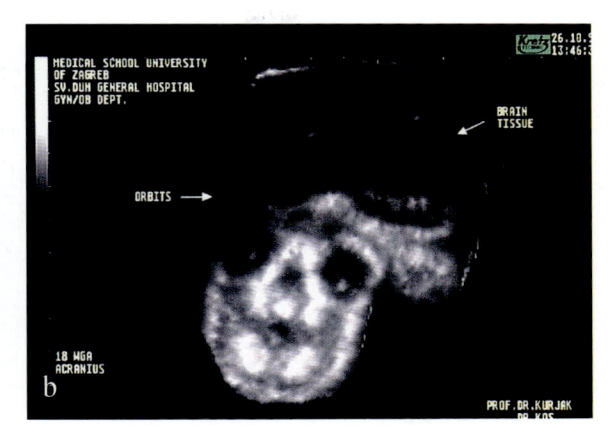

Figure 3 (a) Multiplanar scan of acrania (18 weeks) and three-dimensional reconstruction. (b) Three-dimensional reconstruction of acrania. The dysplastic brain is visible as a cerebrovascular area covering the base of the skull

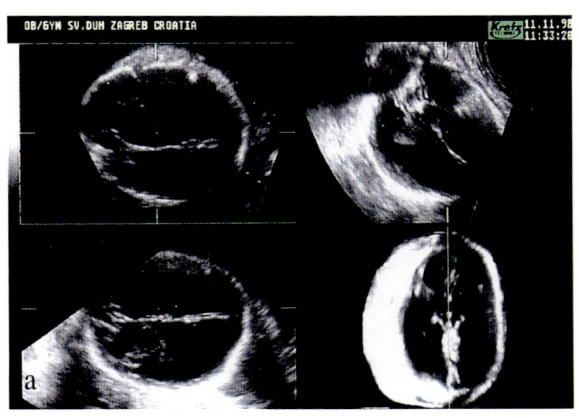

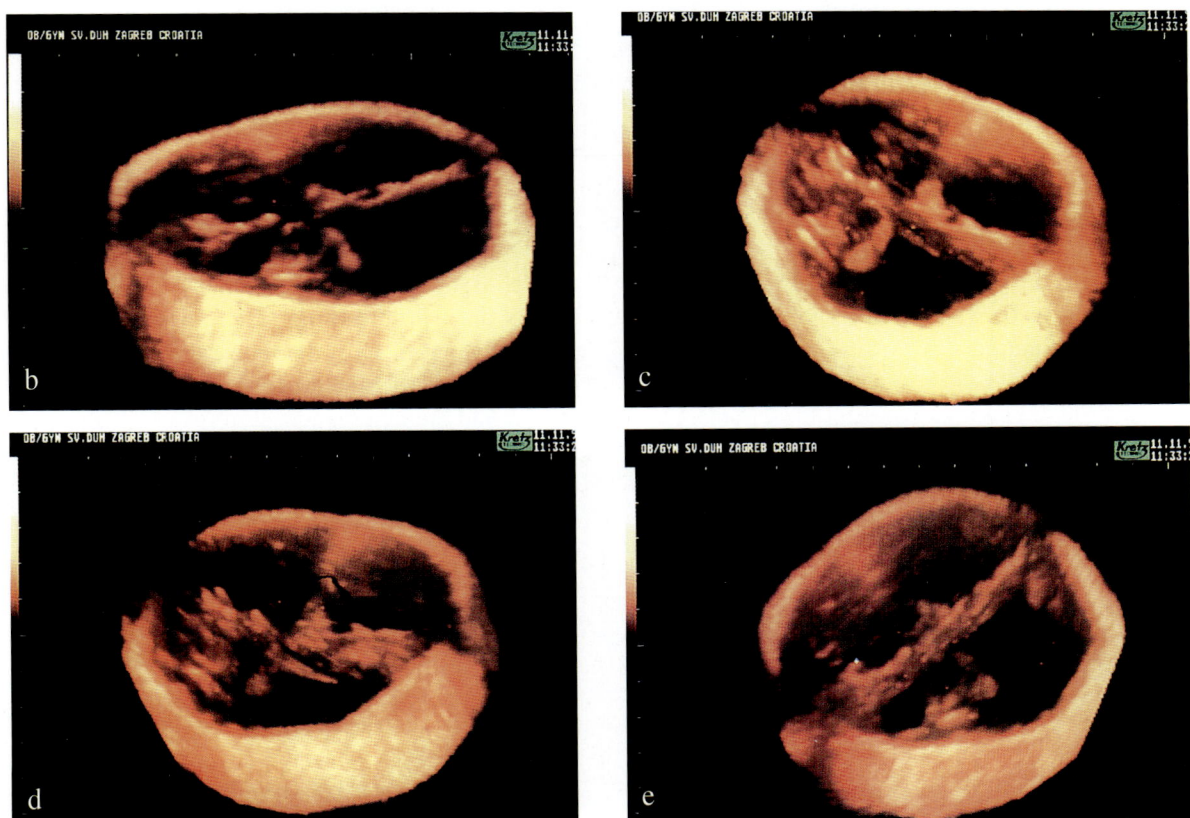

Figure 4 (a) Hydranencephaly (20 weeks), by multiplanar view and three-dimensional reconstruction. Brain tissue is completely reduced. (b–e) Surface-rendered views of abnormal intracranial anatomy. The midline echo and choroid plexus are normal; brain tissue is significantly reduced

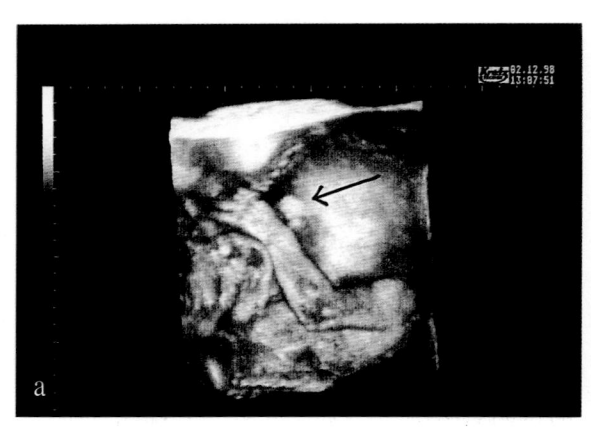

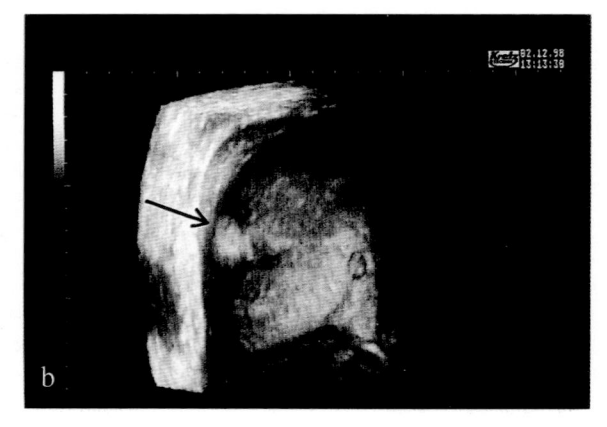

Figure 5 (a) Dysmorphic fetal face (21 weeks) and proboscis (arrow) were associated with trisomy 18. (b) The proboscis is marked by an arrow. The fetal face is dysmorphic, without normal orbits and nose. On the top of the mandibular arch, a dysplastic ear is visible

and neck in 3D volume scanning (Figure 3). The dysplastic fetal brain is recognized as an area of cerebrovasculosa covering the skull base, and orbits are recognizable as protuberances on the top of the dysmorphic head[22]. Fetal hydrocephaly is one of the most common malformations detected by ultrasonography, and is also assessed by 3D ultrasonography[22]. Spatial reconstruction of intracranial contents offers plastic anatomic and topographic data on ventricle enlargement and consequent brain tissue damage (Figure 4). If hydrocephalus or holoprosencephaly are present, 3D surface images of central nervous system (CNS) structures can be obtained by electronically eliminating the calvaria from the image. The extent and structure of intracranial tumors can also be evaluated[19,21].

Some defects, such as cleft lip, facial dysmorphia, anophthalmia and proboscis are easier to depict with 3D surface mode (Figure 5)[20,23,24]. Facial changes such as profile abnormalities and facial tumors can be specifically detected or excluded as early as 24 weeks of gestation (Figure 6). These facial and head deformities are important markers of chromosomal abnormalities, and 3D technology may be useful for increasing the selectivity of ultrasound screening and confirming normal anatomy[20,25,26]. Three-dimensional ultrasound can demonstrate all of the above-mentioned abnormalities and the operator can rotate the image to gain an impression of the depth of the defect. A simple cleft lip, for example, can be reliably differentiated from a more severe cleft involving the lip, maxilla and palate. Volume-rendered data offer a real benefit for analysis of some subsurface structures inside the head. It is possible to obtain three orthogonal slices of palate, pharynx and soft tissues regardless of intrauterine head position (Figure 7). On the other hand, surface structures of face and head become visible despite significant shadowings or malpresentation from overlying structures.

Lateral head abnormalities such as auricular deformities and low-set ears can also be detected[20-22,25]. It is generally agreed that anomalous shape or size of fetal ears is associated with a number of known morphological and chromosomal syndromes. To recognize a congenital anomaly of the fetal ear *in utero* is generally difficult, possibly owing to the complex shape of the ear and the inherent characteristics of conventional 2D ultrasound. Three-dimensional surface imaging of the fetal ear offers complete analysis of the details related to the phenotypic expression of some inherited syndromes[26]. Through the clues of the anomalous ear obtained from 3D imaging, we can diagnose some other, more subtle fetal anomaly that may be overlooked in a simple, 2D ultrasound scan.

In the neck region, 3D transvaginal sonography can clearly demonstrate early changes, such as early nuchal translucency (Figure 2) Transabdominal scanning can detect later changes: larger cystic hygromas, occipital cephalocele, thyroid tumors, etc.[27,28]

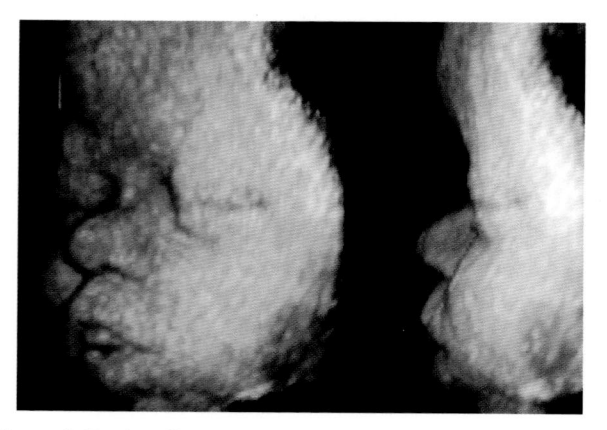

Figure 6 Fetal profile (31 weeks) in a case of achondroplasia. Frontal bossing and depressed nasal bridge are clearly visible

THE ASSESSMENT OF ABNORMAL FETAL ANATOMY

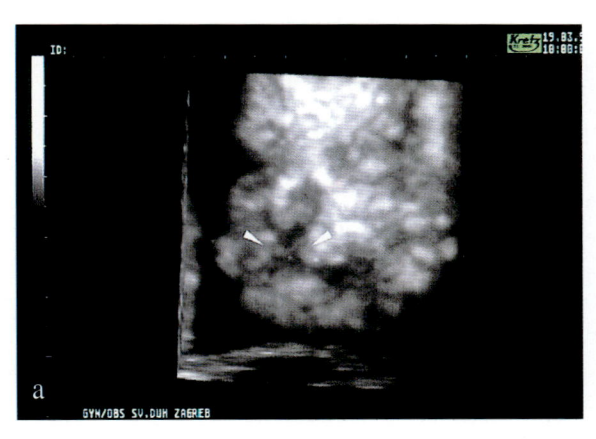

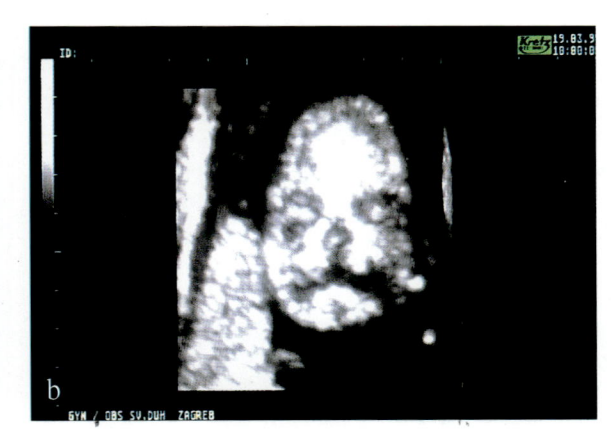

Figure 7 (a) Surface-rendered fetal face with cleft lip. (b) Changing to transparent mode, and moving to the internal coronal plane, the palate cleft is recognizable

Abdomen and thorax

Three-dimensional surface rendering in fetuses with dorsal cleft anomalies permits an accurate surface analysis to be performed that can clearly differentiate the level and extent of a protruding lesion[16,21]. Complete rachischysis, isolated spina bifida, myelomeningocele and some other defects of the spinal column can be easily depicted (Figure 8). In a case of myelomeningocele, the sac can be 'electronically resected' to demonstrate the actual surface defect, even if the orifice is quite small. The transparent mode is more useful for detecting abnormalities of the fetal thorax, but in some conditions, such as a very narrow thorax, the surface mode technique could be of great clinical importance. The animated rotating display is particularly useful for detecting significant thoracic disproportion relative to the abdomen.

In fetuses with ventral body clefts, 3D ultrasound offers new capabilities for visualization of the defect

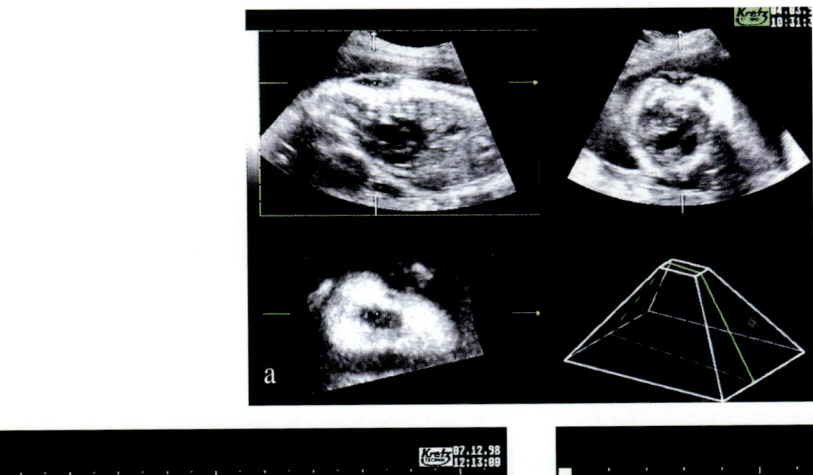

Figure 8 (a) Multiplanar view of lumbar myelomeningocele. The surface of the fetal skin and opened neural tube defect are depicted. (b) Surface mode of myelomeningocele (23 weeks). (c) Transparent mode reconstruction of severe rachischysis (23 weeks)

137

and prolapsed organs[16,19,21]. Although most of these defects are large and are well depicted by 2D sonograms, the rotating display enables the defect to be viewed from multiple angles and often provides a better impression of the severity of the anomaly. The surface mode enables sculpture-like reconstructions of abdominal defects such as omphalocele or gastroschisis. Using this modality, the type and extension of the defect are precisely demonstrated, depicting the size of the defect, the involved organs, the umbilical cord position and the amnioperitoneal coverage[29]. Even the structural changes of the fetal skin surface can be evaluated, emphasizing the possibilities of visual demonstration of congenital ichthyosis[30].

Postprocessing offers the possibility of surface imaging of intra-abdominal structures. It is possible to construct any slice nearly parallel to the mothers abdominal wall in an arbitrary section or orthogonal triple-section display, thus making it possible to observe the esophageal–gastric junction and pylorus. The electronic pen or electronic eraser are used to 'cut out' the overlying body segments, producing either a longitudinal or a transverse section. Once this has been done, a pathological organ can be evaluated separately (Figure 9) Three-dimensional ultrasound confirms a suspected multicystic dysplastic kidney as well as renal agenesis, and the pelvis-ureter junction and ureterovesical junctions are easily observable[31].

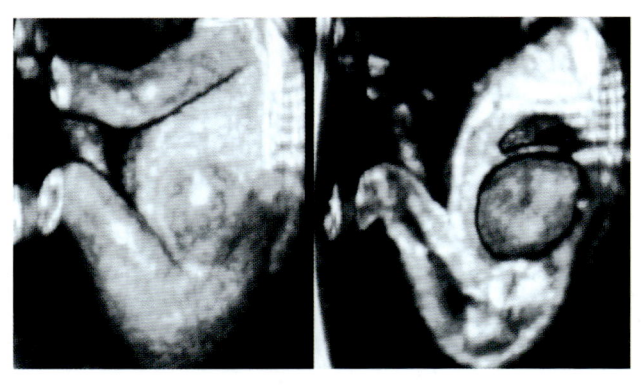

Figure 9 (a) Intra-abdominal tumor reconstructed in the 28th week. (b) Using the technique of surface mode for internal structures, an ovarian cyst or renal cyst was suspected

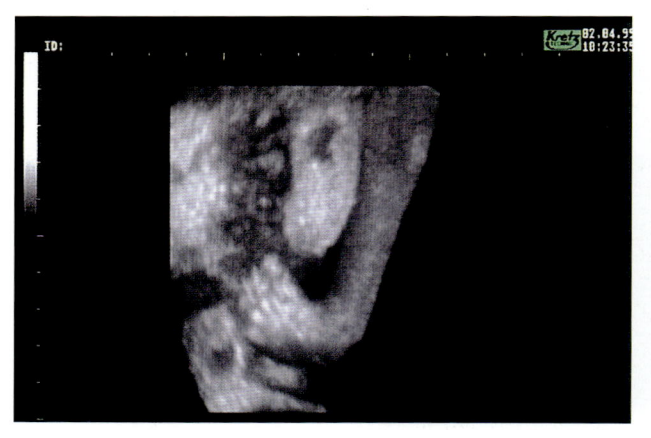

Figure 10 Clubfoot (26 weeks), by surface mode

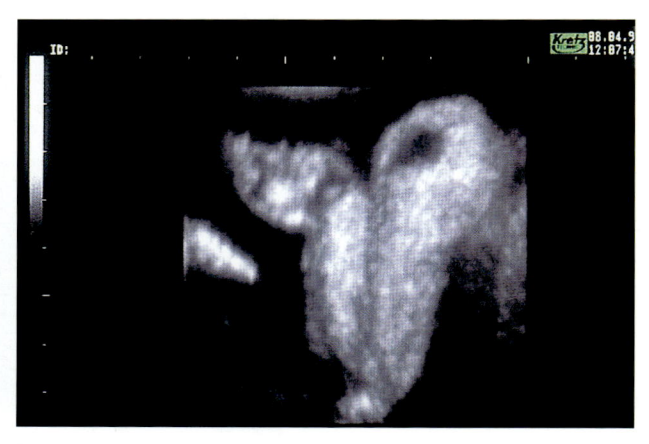

Figure 11 Left arm (23 weeks). Flexion contractures of all three segments of the upper limb visualized in a case of congenital arthrogryposis

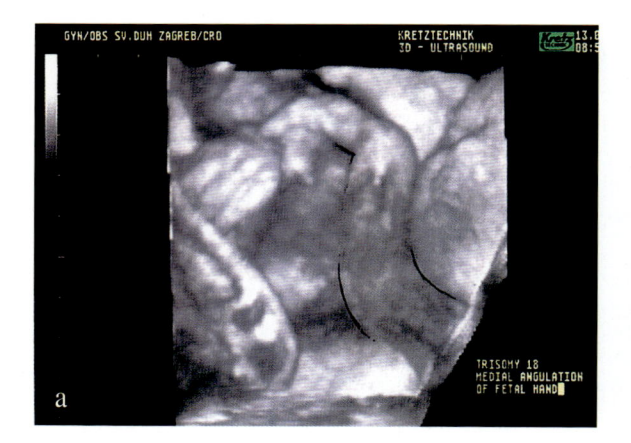

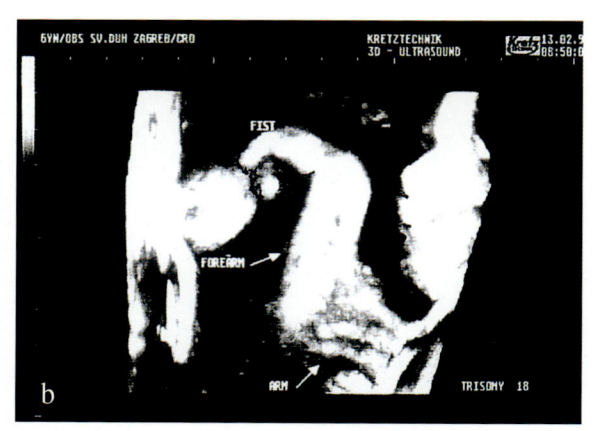

Figure 12 (a) Surface mode of the fetal face and left arm. A flexion contracture of the left hand (wrist) is visible. (b) Maximum mode presents normal bones, but angulations between the arm and forearm, as well as between the forearm and hand, are abnormal

Extremities and the skeleton

Surface rendering in 3D ultrasonography gives a clear display of normal and abnormal extremities[16,21,32–34]. Using these techniques it is possible to assess malformations and deformations of fetal extremities and related skeletal structures (Figures 10, 11 and 12). Surface-rendered images in 3D ultrasound give clear displays of distortions of the normal anatomical axis. With 3D ultrasound, two orthogonal sections can be displayed together. The section at the exact midpoint of the limb can thus be obtained with good reproducibility. Clubfoot, reversible or irreversible pathological angulation of the normal anatomical axis and other limb abnormalities are easy to define using the available orientation[21]. Three-dimensional imaging is helpful in assessing the precise topographic relationship between all three segments of each limb, but also of the wrist, hand and fingers. Congenital deformities and contractures of limbs and joints, related either to the fetal position or to primary neurological damage, are recognizable synchronously in three orthogonal planes depicting their spatial relationship. It is important to note that there will be some fetuses in which it is not possible to scan adequate volumes of the hands and feet, owing to the rapid movements of the extremities. Significant disproportion and reduction of extremities associated with skeletal dysplasias can be clearly appreciated in the rotating volume display[35]. With 3D ultrasound, fingers are also very well observed. It is thus useful for detecting polydactyly, syndactyly and overlapping fingers (Figures 13 and 14). Anomalies of the hands and feet should be looked for in screening for chromosomal defects.

Particular importance is related to the visualization of malformations and deformations of the fetal skeleton by volume rendering using the transparent mode, maximum mode and X-ray-like imaging[36]. This technique includes the volume-rendered imaging possibilities of the minimum–maximum intensity method. The transparent mode of 3D ultrasonography allows imaging of the fetal skeleton, depicting its malformation in spatial orientation. The vertebral column is originally curved anteroposteriorly. If it is pathologically curved laterally, it is impossible to display the whole vertebral column in one 2D tomogram. The advantage of 3D ultrasound is the ability to visualize both curvatures at the same time. Anomalies such as scoliosis, kyphosis, lordosis and spina bifida may be overlooked by 2D ultrasound, but are easy to recognize using the 3D maximum mode (Figure 15). Congenital malformations of the fetal spine and ribs can be identified easier using 3D surface imaging and transparent mode reconstruction together. Specific vertebral body level may be accurately identified by simultaneous evaluating of axial planes of the spine within a volume rendered image or within the coronal plane image. It is difficult to acquire the entire spine in a single volume and thus multiple volumes are often necessary to evaluate the spine completely. The impressive transparent

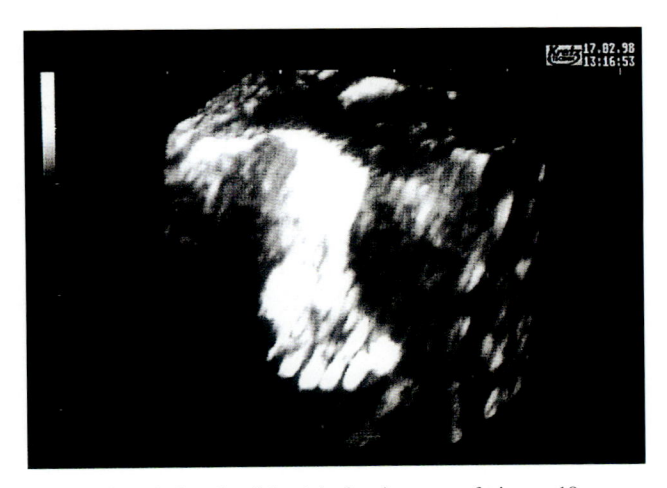

Figure 13 Polydactyly of the right foot in a case of trisomy 18

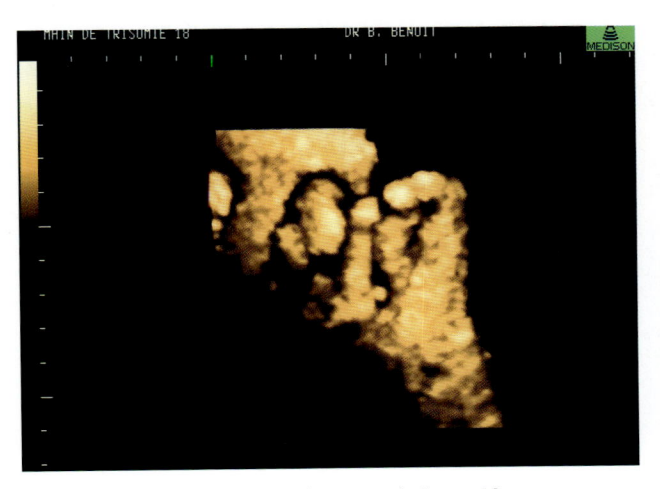

Figure 14 Overlapping fingers in a case of trisomy 18

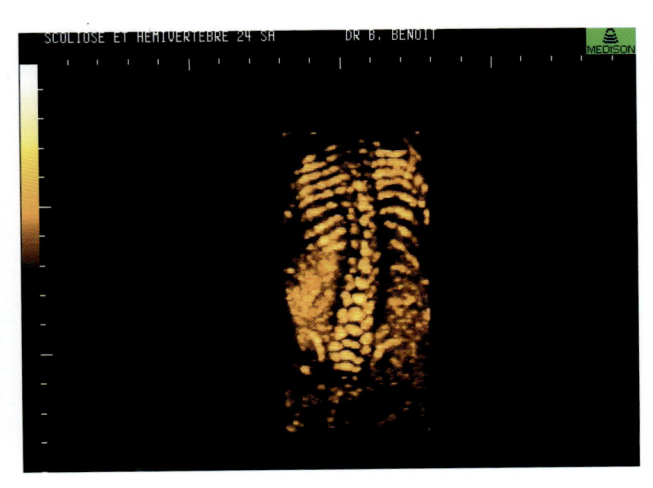

Figure 15 Fetal scoliosis, at 24 weeks, by maximum mode

mode reconstruction will result in a complete skeletal 'babygram'[20,21,36].

Cardiovascular system

The heart is poorly displayed by 3D ultrasound, owing to its motion. However, there are some reports of its use in the fetal cardiovascular system[37,38]. Kuo and colleagues noted the heart, valves and running of the great vessels to be easily understood on simultaneous orthogonal triple-section display, by scrolling the sections vertical to those corresponding to the four-chamber, five-chamber or short-axis views of the great vessels. Jurkovic and co-workers observed the intracardiac anatomy by transparency display and obtained good cardiac images at 20 weeks' gestation[37]. In 3D ultrasound examination of the adult heart with regular rhythm, 3D data are generally acquired over a period of many heart beats, monitored by an electrocardiogram (ECG). A 3D image at each part of the cardiac cycle is constructed using data for only that particular part. For a fetus, an ECG for synchronization is not possible. Nelson and colleagues[38] solved this problem by using the movement of a heart wall/valve instead of the ECG, and constructed 3D images of the fetal heart without distortion due to beating[37,39–41]. A four-dimensional (3D + movement) display of the fetal heart was possible by constructing many 3D images at many parts of the cardiac cycle and displaying them in sequence. These authors also measured the cardiac output based on volume change in the lumen of the heart. However, much time was required to obtain 3D data and fetal movements were a significant problem. Smith and associates developed a 2D array probe for obtaining 3D data in real time and applied it to the fetal heart and real-time 3D ultrasound with simultaneous multisection display[37]. The resolution is poor, but a real-time 3D probe with high resolution should become possible with new techniques such as sparse array.

Fetal tumors

One of the most impressive patterns of 3D ultrasonography is the surface rendering of fetal tumors. Fetal tumors alone represent a rare group of morphological disorders, and ultrasound diagnosis is always a great challenge for the operator. Three-dimensional ultrasonography provides accurate and quick detection, associated with instructive visual imaging (Figures 16 and 17). Cystic hygroma and sacrococcygeal teratoma are the most frequent fetal tumors, easily recognizable by 3D surface mode[19,21,22].

Parents with malformed fetuses are provided with clear 'photographic' images of the baby, the sonographer can evaluate the malformation at the different angles, giving a clear 'plastic' impression of the shape and severity of the defect to the parents[42].

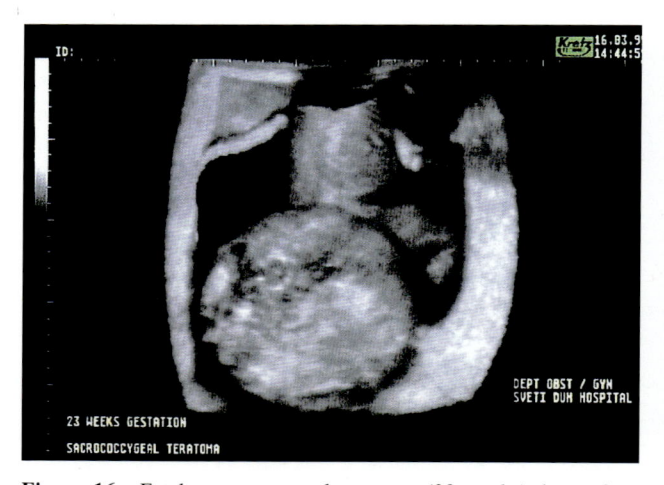

Figure 16 Fetal sacrococcygeal teratoma (23 weeks), by surface mode

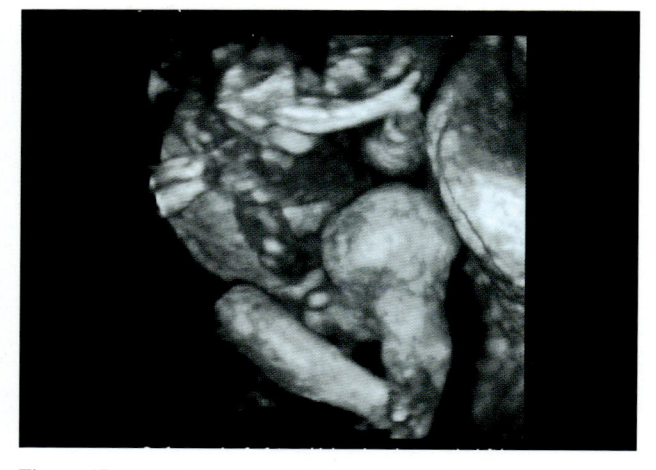

Figure 17 Lymphangioma of the fetal knee (27 weeks), by surface mode

References

1. Baba K, Satch K, Sakamoto S, Okal T, Shiego I. Development of an ultrasonic system for three dimensional reconstruction of the fetus. *J Perinat Med* 1989;17:19–24
2. Fredfelt KE, Holm HH, Pedersen JF. Three dimensional ultrasonic scanning. *Acta Radiol Diagn* 1984;25:237–40
3. Merz E, Bahlaman F, Weber G, Macchiella D. Three dimensional ultrasonography in prenatal diagnosis. *J Perinat Med* 1995;23:213–22
4. Gregg A, Steiner H, Staudach A, Weiner CP. Accuracy of 3D sonographic volume measurements. *Am J Obstet Gynecol* 1993;168:348–55
5. Kossoff G, Griffiths KA, Warren PS, et al. Three-dimensional volume imaging in obstetrics. *Ultrasound Obstet Gynecol* 1994;4:196–200
6. Kou HC, Chang FM, Wu CH, Yao BL, Liu CH. The primary application of three dimensional ultrasonography in obstetrics. *Am J Obstet Gynecol* 1992;166:880–6
7. Merz A, Macchiela D, Bahlamann F, Weber G. Three dimensional ultrasound for the diagnosis of fetal malformations. *Ultrasound Obstet Gynecol* 1992;2:137–45
8. Chiba Y, Hayashi K, Yamazaki S, Takamizawa K, Sasaki H. New techniques of ultrasound, thick slicing 3D imaging and the clinical aspects in the perinatal field. *Ultrasound Obstet Gynecol* 1994;4:195–8
9. Feichtinger W. Transvaginal three-dimensional imaging. *Ultrasound Obstet Gynecol* 1993;3:375–8
10. Baba K, Okai T. Clinical applications of three dimensional ultrasound in obstetrics. In Baba K, Jurkovic D, eds. *Three-dimensional Ultrasound in Obstetrics and Gynecology*. Carnforth, UK: Parthenon Publishing, 1997:29–44
11. Kirbach D, Whittingham TA. 3D ultrasound – the Kretz Voluson approach. *Eur J Ultrasound* 1994;1:85–9
12. Jurkovic D, Jauniaux E, Campbell S. Three dimensional ultrasound in obstetrics and gynecology. In Kurjak A, Chervenak F, eds. *The Fetus as a Patient*. Carnforth, UK: Parthenon Publishing, 1994:135–40
13. Merz E, Weber G, Bahlmann F, Mirić-Tešanić D. Application of transvaginal and transabdominal three-dimensional ultrasound for the detection or exclusion of malformations of the fetal face. *Ultrasound Obstet Gynecol* 1997;9:237–43
14. Merz E, Bahlmann F, Weber G. Volume 3D scanning in the evaluation of fetal malformations – a new dimension in prenatal diagnosis. *Ultrasound Obstet Gynecol* 1995;5:222–7
15. Liang RI, Huang SE, Chang FM. Prenatal diagnosis of ectopia cordis at 10 weeks of gestation using two-dimensional and three-dimensional ultrasonography. *Ultrasound Obstet Gynecol* 1997;10:137–9
16. Pretorius DH, Nelson TR. Fetal face visualisation using three dimensional ultrasonography. *J Ultrasound Med* 1995;14:349–56
17. Merz E. Update technical application of 3-D sonography in gynaecology and obstetrics. *Ultraschall Med* 1997;18:190–5
18. Blaas HG, Eik-Nes SH, Kiserund T, Berg S, Angelsen B, Olstad B. Three-dimensional imaging of the brain cavities in human embryos. *Ultrasound Obstet Gynecol* 1995;5:228–32
19. Merz E. Three-dimensional ultrasound in the evaluation of fetal malformations. In Baba K, Jurkovic D, eds. *Three-dimensional Ultrasound in Obstetrics and Gynecology*. Carnforth, UK: Parthenon Publishing, 1997;37–44
20. Benoit B. Three dimensional surface mode for demonstration of normal fetal anatomy in the second and third trimester. In Merz E, ed. *3D Ultrasound in Obstetrics and Gynecology*. Philadelphia: Lippincott Williams and Wilkins, 1998:95–100
21. Merz E, Bahlaman F, Weber G, et al. Fetal malformations – assessment by three dimensional ultrasound in surface mode. In Merz E, ed. *3D Ultrasound in Obstetrics and Gynecology*. Philadelphia: Lippincott Williams and Wilkins, 1998:109–20
22. Kurjak A, Kos M. Three-dimensional ultrasonograhy in prenatal diagnosis. In Chervenak FA, Kurjak A, eds. *Fetal Medicine*. Carnforth, UK: Parthenon Publishing, 1999:102–8
23. Pretorius DH, Nelson RT. Fetal face visualization using three dimensional ultrasonography. *J Ultrasound Med* 1995;14:349–56
24. Lee A, Deutinger J, Bernaschek G. Three dimensional ultrasound: abnormalities of the fetal face in surface and volume rendering mode. *Br J Obstet Gynaecol* 1995;102:40–4
25. Shih JC, et al. Antenatal depiction of fetal ear with three-dimensional ultrasonography. *Obstet Gynecol* 1998;91:500–5
26. Kurjak A, Kupesic S, Di Renzo GC, Pooh R, Kos M, Hafner T. Recent advances in perinatal sonography. *Prenat Neonat Med* 1998;3:194–207
27. Bonilla-Musoles F, et al. First-trimester neck abnormalities: three-dimensional evaluation. *J Ultrasound Med* 1998;17:419–25
28. Kurjak A, et al. Three-dimensional transvaginal ultrasound improves measurement of nuchal translucency. *J Perinat Med* 1999;27:97–102
29. Hata T, et al. Three-dimensional ultrasonographic assessment of umbilical cord during the 2nd and 3rd trimesters of pregnancy. *Gynecol Obstet Invest* 1998:159–64
30. Benoit B. Three dimensional ultrasonography of congenital ichthyosis. *Ultrasound Obstet Gynecol* 1999;13:380–3
31. Candiani F. The latest in ultrasound: three-dimensional imaging. *Eur J Radiol* 1998;27(suppl 2):179–82
32. Hata T, et al. Three-dimensional ultrasonographic assessment of fetal hands and feet. *Ultrasound Obstet Gynecol* 1998;12:235–9
33. Budorick NE, et al. Three-dimensional ultrasound examination of fetal hands: normal and abnormal. *Ultrasound Obstet Gynecol* 1998;12:227–34
34. Linney AD, et al. Three-dimensional morphometry in ultrasound-review. *Proc Inst Mech Eng* 1999;213:235–45

35. Lee A. Kratochwil A, Deutinger J, Bernaschek G. Three-dimensional ultrasound in diagnosing phocomelia. *Ultrasound Obstet Gynecol* 1995;5:238–40
36. Lee A. Visualization of malformations of the fetal skeleton by volume rendering in three dimensional ultrasound. In Merz E, ed. *3D Ultrasound in Obstetrics and Gynecology.* Philadelphia: Lippincott Williams and Wilkins, 1998:121–4
37. Zosmer N, Gruboeck K, Jurkovic D. Three-dimensional fetal cardiac imaging. In Baba K, Jurkovic D, eds. *Three-dimensional Ultrasound in Obstetrics and Gynecology.* Carnforth, UK: Parthenon Publishing, 1997:45–53
38. Nelson T, Sklansky M, Pretorius DH. Fetal heart assessment using three dimensional ultrasound. In Merz E, ed. *3D Ultrasound in Obstetrics and Gynecology.* Philadelphia: Lippincott Williams and Wilkins, 1998:125–33
39. Nelson TR, Pretorius DH, Sklansky M, Hagen-Ansert S. Three dimensional echocardiographic evaluation of fetal heart anatomy and function: acquisition, analysis and display. *J Ultrasound Med* 1996;15:1–9
40. Sklansky M. Three dimensional fetal echocardiography: gated versus non-gated techniques. *J Ultrasound Med* 1998;17:451–7
41. Nelson TR. Three dimensional fetal echocardiography. *Prog Biophys Mol Biol* 1998;69:257–72
42. Maier B, Steiner H, Weinerroither F, Standach A. The psychological impact of three dimensional fetal imaging on the fetomaternal relationship. In Baba K, Jurkovic D, eds. *Three-dimensional Ultrasound in Obstetrics and Gynecology.* Carnforth, UK: Parthenon Publishing, 1997:67–73

Three-dimensional ultrasound markers of chromosomal anomalies

A. Kurjak and R. Matijevic

Introduction

In 1968 the first antenatal diagnosis of Down's syndrome was made, and screening on the basis of selecting women of advanced maternal age for amniocentesis was gradually introduced into medical practice. In 1983 it was shown that low maternal serum α-fetoprotein (MSAFP) was associated with Down's syndrome. Later, raised maternal serum human chorionic gonadotropin hCG and low unconjugated estriol were found to be markers of Down's syndrome. In 1988 these three biochemical markers were used together with maternal age as a method of screening, and this has been widely adopted[1]. However, the sensitivity and specificity of both age-related screening and screening based on biochemical testing did not fit the criteria for screening in the general population.

Methods of screening need to be fully evaluated before being introduced into routine clinical practice. This includes choosing markers for which there is sufficient scientific evidence of efficacy; quantifying performance in terms of detection and false-positive rates; and establishing methods of monitoring performance. Some of the chromosomal markers detected by ultrasound fit these criteria. These include nuchal fold thickness, cardiac abnormalities, duodenal atresia, choroid plexus cysts, femur length, humerus length, pyelectasis and hyperechogenic bowel. Until recently, all these markers have been assessed by two-dimensional (2D) real-time ultrasound. With the advent and evolution of three-dimensional (3D) ultrasound technologies during the past 5 years, we now stand at a new threshold in non-invasive diagnosis. There is no question that 3D ultrasound offers new diagnostic modalities in modern obstetrics. The technique was found to be superior to 2D ultrasound in some segments of prenatal diagnosis. The aim of 3D ultrasound is to create a volume, unlike in 2D ultrasound, whose aim is to create section planes. We do not claim that 3D ultrasound will replace 2D ultrasound; however, it does offer tremendous potential in the investigation of complex structures and may help examiners experienced in conventional ultrasound to detect and evaluate some abnormalities. In this chapter, we assess its potential use in the screening program for detection of chromosomal abnormalities based on the determination of ultrasound markers.

Hyperechogenic bowel

The diagnostic potential of hyperechogenic fetal bowel to act as a hallmark for prenatal cystic fibrosis screening in the general population has been known for a number of years. It is currently routine practice in Western countries for cystic fibrosis screening to be offered to families in which fetal hyperechogenic bowel is diagnosed at routine ultrasound examination[2]. The association between second-trimester hyperechogenic bowel and Down's syndrome has been well established in the literature. Hyperechogenic bowel does not need to be present during the whole course of pregnancy to act as a chromosomal marker. It is commonly present in the late first and early second trimesters; however, if it is present only in the third trimester it could be a late manifestation of Down's syndrome[3]. Together with cystic fibrosis and chromosomal anomalies, increased bowel echogenicity is related to unfavorable obstetric outcome, especially if it is combined with increased MSAFP[4].

Fetal bowel hyperechogenicity found in women with elevated second-trimester MSAFP levels is associated with poor fetal outcome, particularly fetal growth restriction resulting in fetal and neonatal death, and should be considered an ominous prenatal finding. The presence of hyperechogenic bowel on ultrasound examination in the early second trimester increases the background risk for chromosomal anomalies 5.5 times, representing one of the most important markers for chromosomal anomalies. These include trisomies 13, 18 and 21 and triploidies. The prevalence of these chromosomal abnormalities seems to be greatest in fetuses exhibiting the most extreme levels of abnormal echogenicity. However, despite alarming reports, increased abdominal echogenicity should be interpreted with caution, since many fetuses with such a finding are normal. One of the problems with the diagnosis of fetal echogenic bowel is its subjectiveness, as there is no measurable criterion in the discrmination between normal and abnormal.

Using the 3D ultrasound technique, there is a possible improvement in the detection and determination of the bowel echogenicity of the fetus, with the use of the minimum–maximum mode. However, this method is new, hence the experience is limited.

Echogenic foci in the fetal heart

Preliminary data indicate that the presence of an intraventricular echogenic cardiac focus in the fetal heart carries an increased risk of fetal aneuploidy[5]. In the same study, among 149 women with an intraventricular echogenic focus found while they were undergoing fetal karyotype analysis, 15 had an abnormal karyotype, resulting in a relative risk of 3.30 of aneuploidy when compared to fetuses without echogenic cardiac foci. Some other studies do not agree with this, making the diagnosis and counselling more difficult. In a recent study, echogenic fetal heart foci were detected in three out of 15 706 fetuses (prevalence 0.019%), being located in the right atrium. Normal chromosomes and negative TORCH titers were observed in all affected cases, and all fetuses demonstrated adequate intrauterine growth and had normal neonatal outcome[6]. We believe that women carrying fetuses with intracardiac echogenic foci should be informed of the statistical association with trisomy 21. In a high-risk obstetric population, the association between fetal intracardiac echogenic foci and trisomy 21 was statistically significant. The sensitivity, specificity, positive predictive values, and negative predictive values for intracardiac echogenic foci in predicting trisomy 21 were 18%, 98%, 13% and 98%, respectively[7].

Detection of intracardiac echogenic foci is relatively easy using 2D ultrasound. They present as small, round structures with bone-like echogenicity in different parts of the fetal heart. They move together with heart action, hence the limitation for the use of 3D ultrasound. As 3D echocardiographic efforts are focused on the adult and pediatric patient, fetal cardiac imaging remains an important and challenging area.

Conventional 3D ultrasound imaging equipment can produce a static volume of the heart that has shown some promise in imaging of the great vessels and relatively non-moving areas. Critical areas of cardiac anatomy, including echogenic foci, are generally poorly visualized because of motion and small size[8,9].

Fetal long-bone biometry

The efficacy of second-trimester fetal long-bone biometry (femur, humerus, tibia and fibula length) acting as an ultrasound marker for chromosomal defects has been known for a number of years. Second-trimester fetal long-bone biometry is useful in detecting trisomy 21 and may be used to adjust the background risk of both high- and low-risk women[10]. Isolated short femur is the commonest marker used, and it increases the background risk based on maternal age and gestation 2.5 times if below the 5th centile for measured gestational age. Rarely it may present the signs of dwarfism. As well as a short femur, the finding of a shortened humerus (observed/expected ratio < 0.90) alone and/or combined with other markers had high sensitivity for Down's syndrome detection. A short humerus combined with a small abdominal circumference (observed/expected ratio < 0.92), or an anatomic defect had a sensitivity of 46.7% for any significant chromosome defect[11]. A normal ultrasound finding including normal length of the long bones substantially reduces the risk of Down's syndrome and any chromosome abnormality. With a normal ultrasound finding the risk of Down's syndrome in the baby of a 39-year-old woman falls from 1 : 100 to < 1 : 292. This information is useful in counselling women who decline amniocentesis on the basis of maternal age.

For a number of years, B-mode real time 2D ultrasound was used in the measurement of the long bones. However, with the use of conventional 2D ultrasound, the fetal skeleton can pose obstacles to the examiner. This is most prominent in early pregnancy, especially

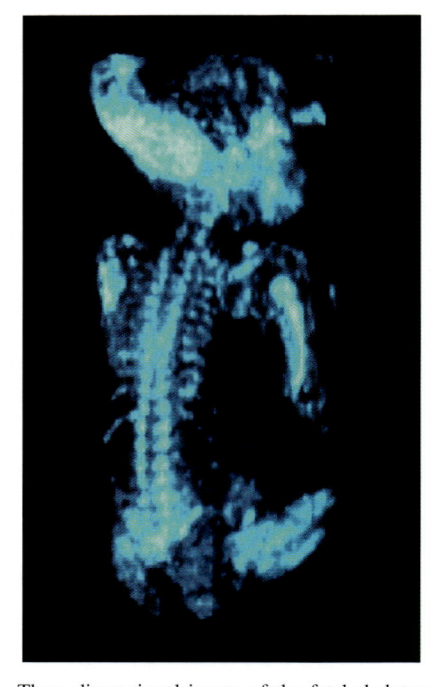

Figure 1 Three-dimensional image of the fetal skeleton. The long-bone biometry can be performed precisely, and the patients can be counselled on the risk of chromosomal defects on the basis of such measurements

in the correct determination of the end of the bone, when the process of ossification is not completed. Three-dimensional ultrasound provides a significant improvement in this field. With 3D ultrasound in the volume rendering mode, a significant improvement was found in detecting malformations of the fetal skeleton. This mode is helpful in the measurement of the long bones and may help in the correct assessment and better counselling of patients at risk for chromosomal defects (Figure 1). The correct measurements may be made earlier using 3D ultrasound, hence the risk can be estimated at a more appropriate time for counselling to undertake further diagnostic tests[12].

Renal pyelectasis

Renal pyelectasis alone or in combination with other conditions is still one of the leading soft tissue markers for chromosomal anomalies. Pyelectasis is more frequently detected by high-resolution transvaginal sonography in the first half of pregnancy than in the second half. There are several reasons for this, the most common being its transitory appearance. When detected in early pregnancy, it may be associated with an increased risk of abnormal fetal karyotypes. The incidence of abnormal fetal karyotype related to the presence of pyelectasis is still doubtful. In a recent study[13], the importance and evolution of isolated, mild fetal pyelectasis, detected in early pregnancy by high-resolution transvaginal sonography, was analyzed. Transvaginal scanning was performed at 11–16 weeks' gestation and combined with transabdominal ultrasound examinations at the time of amniocentesis (16–18 weeks) in 1093 pregnant women undergoing genetic amniocentesis because of advanced maternal age. Each patient was screened for fetal pyelectasis, defined as an increase in anteroposterior renal pelvic diameter, using cut-off values related to various stages of pregnancy. Isolated fetal pyelectasis was detected at the first ultrasound examination in 5.1% of women in early pregnancy. This number declined to 2.9% at the time of amniocentesis, and remained constant until 24 weeks' gestation. However, only two fetuses in this series demonstrated abnormal karyotypes at amniocentesis.

In general, pyelectasis increases the background risk for Down's syndrome 1.5 times. The most important problem is in the high false-positive rate. Because a considerable overlap of sonographic markers exists among trisomy 21 fetuses, use of those that are not independent predictors leads to an increase in the false-positive rate without a gain in sensitivity[14].

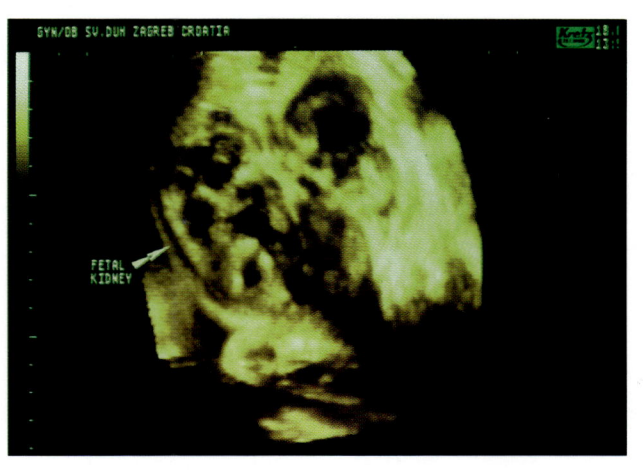

Figure 2 Three-dimensional image of the fetal kidney. Using such an approach, pyelectasis can accurately be measured in all diameters as the image may be rotated in all three directions

Currently, pylectases are diagnosed using 2D B-mode real-time ultrasound. With this technique, only 2D measurement of renal structures is possible, and in some circumstances it may become very difficult and inaccurate, owing to the fetal position. Together with the nature of the marker, this also may lead to the high false-positive rate in prediction of abnormal karyotype. Three-dimensional ultrasound allows better visualization of pelvic dilatation and, by image rotation, all three diameters of the kidney can be visualized (Figure 2). Consequently, volumetric studies can be performed, improving the diagnostic accuracy and positive predictive value in the diagnosis. As well as in the initial diagnosis, 3D ultrasound examination may be of benefit for the evaluation and follow-up of mild pyelectasis. Follow-up scanning prior to delivery may be considered, to identify those fetuses who will require postpartum intervention; 3D ultrasound may present pelvic dilatation more precisely[15].

Choroid plexus cysts

Isolated fetal choroid plexus cysts detected in early pregnancy by either transabdominal or transvaginal ultrasound examination carries an increased genetic risk and is associated with abnormal fetal karyotype[16]. There has been conflicting information regarding the incidence of chromosomopathies in the presence of chorioid plexus cysts. A prospective study performed in 1692 pregnant women (aged > 37 years) who underwent transvaginal scanning at 11–16 weeks' gestation before genetic amniocentesis, indicated the prevalence of isolated choroid plexus cyst in our population of 1.48%, detecting an abnormal fetal karyotype in only one case[17]. Recent studies suggest that further diagnostic tests are necessary only if choroid plexus cysts are combined with other anomalies or increased risk on serum screening. Therefore, if the triple-screen result is abnormal, and additional anomalies (i.e choroid plexus cysts) are seen on ultrasonography, or the mother is aged over 35 years, then fetal karyotyping is recommended[18].

Fetal choroid plexus cysts can be visualized by 2D ultrasound. They are located in the lateral ventricles with a small amount in the roof of the third ventricle. In most of the cases 3D ultrasound can present intracranial structures more precisely, making the diagnosis of normal anatomy easier (Figure 3). Choroid plexus cysts need to be distinguished from normal corpus striatum, which can produce a similar appearance. Three-dimensional imaging can clearly diagnose corpus striatum at its anatomical position, making impression of lower portion of the lateral ventricles (Figure 4). Consequently, assessment of isolated choroid plexus cysts can be easier, and measurements obtained with better accuracy (Figure 5).

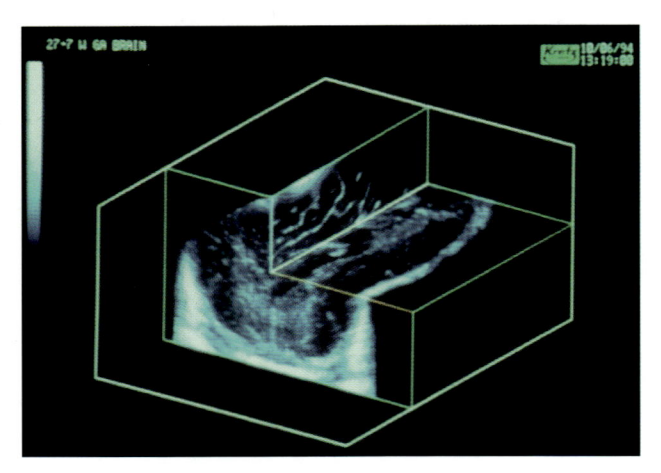

Figure 3 Three-dimensional image of the fetal brain. All structures can be analyzed by an expert on the image stored earlier by ultrasonographers

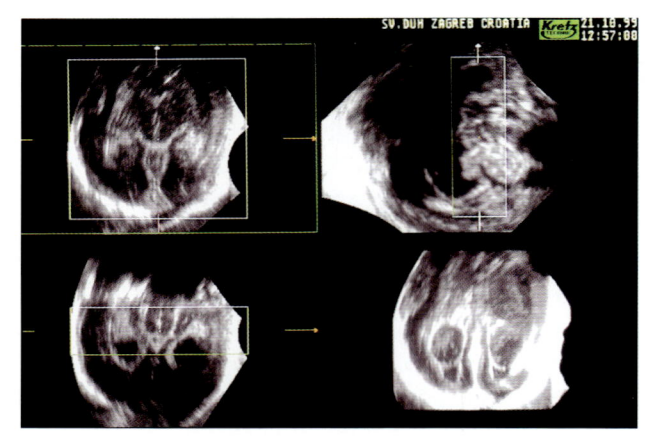

Figure 4 Three-dimensional image of a fetal choroid plexus cyst in three perpendicular planes

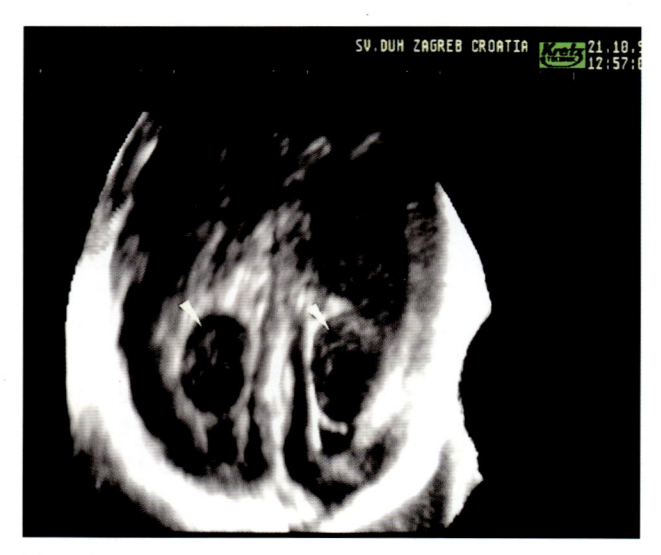

Figure 5 Three-dimensional reconstruction of the fetal choroid cyst

Nuchal translucency

Nuchal translucency (NT) is skin edema in the fetal neck region. It may be visualized by ultrasound in early pregnancy (between 10 and 14 weeks) and represents a common expression of trisomies (13, 18 and commonly 21), structural defects and genetic syndromes. The heterogeneity in conditions associated with increased NT suggests that there may not be a single underlying mechanism for the fluid collection in the skin of the fetal neck. Possible mechanisms include cardiac failure in association with abnormalities of the heart and great vessels, abnormal or delayed development of the lymphatic system, altered composition of the subcutaneous connective tissue and venous congestion in the head and neck in association with superior mediastinal compression. Cardiac failure is the commonly used explanation for the increased NT and is based on the mechanism of abnormal venous return and consequently fetal edema being most prominent in the neck region.

Regarding the lymphatic vessel hypoplasia hypothesis, a possible mechanism for increased NT is based on dilatation of the jugular lymphatic sacs because of developmental delay in the connection with the venous system, or a primary abnormal dilatation or proliferation of the lymphatic channels, interfering with normal flow between the lymphatic and venous systems[19]. Another possible cause may be underlying hypoproteinemia (this is named the osmotic hypothesis). Hypoproteinemia is a recognized cause of fetal hydrops. Trisomy 21 is associated with a reduced concentration of MSAFP. Albumin and MSAFP are two high molecular weight plasma proteins with a high degree of homology. Fetuses with Turner's syndrome were found to have various degrees of hypoalbuminemia. Deficit of the two above-mentioned proteins suggests that, in addition to lymphatic hypoplasia, osmotic mechanisms may contribute to increased NT[20]. The altered composition of the extracellular matrix presents another hypothesis for increased NT. In trisomy 21 the composition and consequently the properties of collagen type IV are altered, leading to the accumulation of interstitial fluid. It may be possible that, in the heart of the trisomy 21 fetuses, the expression of the genes COL6A1 and 2 is increased in relation to the COL6A3 gene, resulting in the production of heterotrimeric collagen type IV and consequent impairment in heart contractility[21]. Since many of the component proteins of the extracellular matrix are encoded on chromosomes 21, 18 and 13, the increased skin thickness in trisomic fetuses could be a consequence of gene dosage effect. The last possible mechanism associates diaphragmatic hernia and increased nuchal translucency. In diaphragmatic hernia, intrathoracic compression may be the underlying mechanism for increased NT, owing to venous congestion in the head and neck caused by mediastinal compression and impaired venous return.

The first published reports about NT measurement date from the early 1990s. In the study of Nicolaides and colleagues[22], fetal nuchal translucency of 3 mm and more was found to be a useful first-trimester marker for fetal chromosomal abnormalities. The authors found that, in the 6% of fetuses screened in the general low-risk population with nuchal translucency of 3–8 mm, the incidence of chromosomal defects was 35%. In contrast, only ten of the remaining 776 (1%) fetuses with NT less than 3 mm were chromosomally abnormal. In a prospective study of screening for fetal abnormalities and chromosomal defects carried out by ultrasound examination at 13–15 weeks of gestation and 20–22 weeks, based on NT measurements, similar results were obtained several years later[23]. Among 3514 fetuses examined, 21 were chromosomally abnormal, including ten cases of trisomy 21. Comparison of all markers analyzed found increased NT thickness (4 mm and more) at the 13–15-week scan to be the most effective. It was present in seven of the ten fetuses with trisomy 21 and in six of the 11 cases with other chromosomal abnormalities. The problem with NT assessment is in the reproducibility of the measurements and consequently the diagnostic accuracy. It is now generally agreed that screening for increased NT in a low-risk population requires established guidelines, updated ultrasound equipment capable of measuring distances of 0.1 mm and adequate training[24,25].

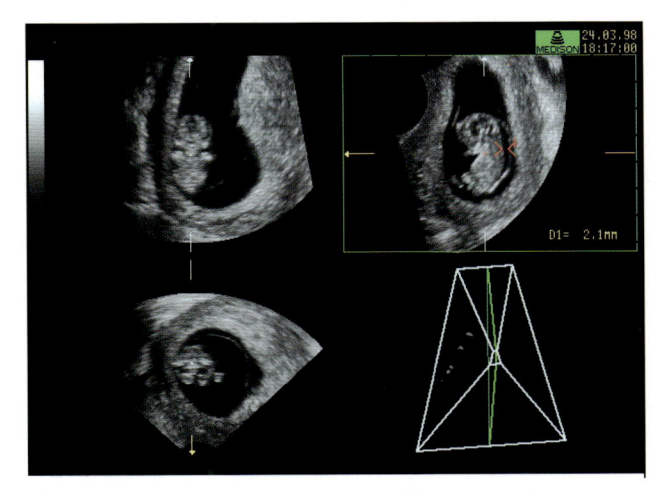

Figure 6 A fetus at 12 weeks' gestation. Three perpendicular planes: plane A allows a frontal view of the fetal nuchal region; plane B gives an ideal mid-sagittal view of the fetus; plane C gives a symmetrical transverse section of the fetus. These planes make measurement of nuchal translucency much easier and more accurate

Obvious limitations of NT measurements by 2D ultrasound include suboptimal fetal position, observation of inappropriate median sagittal section of the fetus, attachment of the nuchal region to the amniotic membrane and the small size of the structure to be measured[26]. All these factors have led to the high failure rate and poor reproducibility of the measurements[27]. However, it seems that the reported limitations may be overcome by using 3D ultrasound (Figure 6).

By 3D ultrasound, after storing the volume data on a memory medium, volume scanning and assessment of the nuchal region may be repeated from all directions. These include:

(1) Three perpendicular reformatted sections simultaneously displayed on the screen, enabling rotation and observation of the mid-sagittal view of the fetus. The examiner must clearly distinguish the fetal skin from amnion.

(2) Three-axial center of rotation, which may be fixed to the central part of the fetal nuchal region on plane A (Figure 4), followed by the same procedure for the symmetrical transverse view on plane C. The most representative mid-sagittal view of the fetus appears in plane C, allowing precise measurement of the NT.

In our recent study[26], 120 women undergoing ultrasound screening at 10–14 weeks' gestation were examined by both 2D and 3D transvaginal ultrasound. The aim of the study was to evaluate and correlate visualization rates of NT, and to assess the intraobserver reproducibility of the measurements by two techniques. After a proper sagittal view of the fetus was depicted by 2D ultrasound, NT was measured between the skin and the soft tissue overlying the cervical spine, as described[22]. The image was considered satisfactory when the fetus was occupying three-quarters of the screen on the regular size image and the amniotic membrane was clearly separated from the nuchal region. Callipers were positioned to the inner sides of the skin and soft tissue in the measured region. This was followed by 3D studies of NT using a B-mode ultrasound machine, which monitors spatial orientation of images, and stores them as a volume set in the computer memory. At the moment when the fetal nuchal region was visualized by the conventional 2D method, the ultrasound probe was kept still and the volume mode was turned on. Three-dimensional volume was generated by automatic rotation through 360°. After storage of the volume in the memory, volume scanning was repeated from all directions. In the same study, 3D sagittal views of the fetus were obtained in all 120 women included (Figure 7)(Table 1). These measurements were much better than the 15% of unsuccessful measurements using conventional 2D ultrasound. Mean NT measurement obtained by 3D transvaginal ultrasound was found to be of greater accuracy than that of 2D ultrasound. Using 3D ultrasound, repeated NT measurements on the same subject were not statistically different from subsequent measurements, as was the case using 2D measurements (Table 2). Therefore, the intraoperator reproducibility is superior in 3D measurements compared to 2D measurements. The time required for NT examination is an important parameter. Kormman and associated[28] proposed that NT measurements should not be conducted during routine ultrasound examination but rather under special quality-assured conditions. Technological advances in the form of 3D ultrasound may help to overcome these concerns, as stored volumes may be analyzed later by a more experienced ultrasonographer. Similar results were obtained by a group of Korean authors (unpublished results). In their recent study they measured NT in 616 pregnant women between 10 and 14 weeks of gestation. Eight out of 15 fetuses with abnormal NT measurement

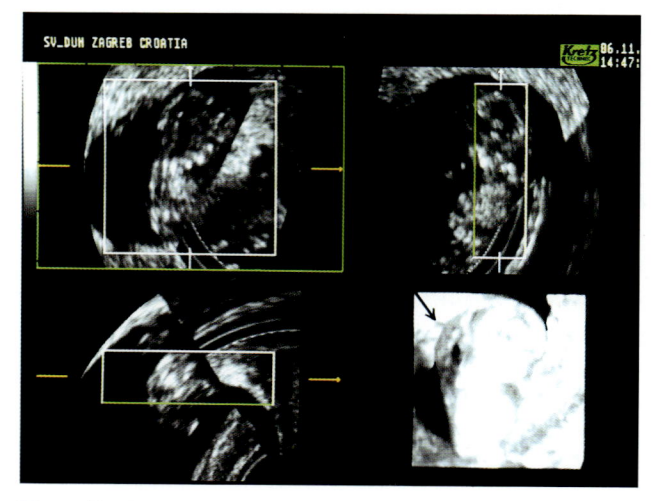

Figure 7 Three-dimensional image of a fetus in three perpendicular planes. The arrow points to the area of nuchal translucency

Table 1 Data on nuchal translucency visualization rates between 10 and 14 weeks of gestation by two-dimensional (2D) and three-dimensional (3D) transvaginal sonography (TVS). From reference 26, with permission

		\multicolumn{4}{c}{Nuchal translucency visualization rates}
Gestational age (weeks)	No. of cases	\multicolumn{2}{c}{2D TVS}	\multicolumn{2}{c}{3D TVS}
		n	%	n	%
10–11	9	8	88.9	9	100
11–12	21	18	85.7	21	100
12–13	48	42	87.5	48	100
13–14	33	25	75.8	33	100
14–14+5	9	9	100.0	9	100
Total	120	102	85.0	120	100

Table 2 Mean nuchal translucency (NT) thickness obtained by two measurements using two-dimensional (2D) and three-dimensional (3D) transvaginal ultrasound. From reference 26, with permission

	2D transvaginal ultrasound		3D transvaginal ultrasound	
	Mean NT ± SD (mm)	p Value	Mean NT ± SD (mm)	p Value
First measurement	1.64 ± 0.71	p < 0.05	1.75 ± 0.53	p > 0.05
Second measurement	1.73 ± 0.68		1.78 ± 0.51	

underwent fetal karyotyping. Two cases of Down's syndrome and two of Turner's syndrome were detected; among other fetuses with normal karyotype, two were found to have serious malformations on the 20-week ultrasound scan. The same group reported excellent reproducibility, without significant intra- and interobserver variations in 3D NT measurement, which was much better compared to 2D measurements.

Our experience supports 3D ultrasound measurements of NT in the first trimester[26]. Using the 3D ultrasound technique, the mid-sagittal section of the fetus can be visualized with a 100% success rate. Furthermore, the initial scan may be performed by a less experienced ultrasonographer, and stored volumes analyzed by an expert, in settled conditions. Three-dimensional ultrasound improves the accuracy of NT measurement, producing an appropriate mid-sagittal section of the fetus and making a clear distinction of the nuchal region from the amniotic membrane. Also, 3D ultrasound measurements of NT present better intraobserver reproducibility than that in conventional 2D ultrasound, increasing the effectiveness of screening programs.

References

1. Wald NJ, Kennard A, Hackshaw A, McGuire A. Antenatal screening for Down's syndrome. *J Med Screen* 1997;4:181–6
2. Muller F, Dommergues M, Simon-Bouy B, et al. Cystic fibrosis screening: a fetus with hyperechogenic bowel may be the index case. *J Med Genet* 1998;35:657–60
3. Sepulveda W, Bower S, Fisk NM. Third-trimester hyperechogenic bowel in Down syndrome. *Am J Obstet Gynecol* 1995;172:210–11
4. Achiron R, Seidman DS, Horowitz A, Mashiach S, Goldman B, Lipitz S. Hyperechogenic fetal bowel and elevated serum alpha-fetoprotein: a poor fetal prognosis. *Obstet Gynecol* 1996;88:368–71
5. Vibhakar NI, Budorick NE, Scioscia AL, Harby LD, Mullen ML, Sklansky MS. Prevalence of aneuploidy with a cardiac intraventricular echogenic focus in an at-risk patient population. *J Ultrasound Med* 1999;18:265–8;269–70
6. Petrikovsky B, Klein V, Herrera M. Prenatal diagnosis of intra-atrial cardiac echogenic foci. *Prenat Diagn* 1998;18:968–70
7. Manning JE, Ragavendra N, Sayre J, et al. Significance of fetal intracardiac echogenic foci in relation to trisomy 21: a prospective sonographic study of high-risk pregnant women. *Am J Roentgenol* 1998;170:1083–4
8. Zosmer N, Jurkovic D, Jauniaux E, Gruboeck K, Lees C, Campbell S. Selection and identification of standard cardiac views from three-dimensional volume scans of the fetal thorax. *J Ultrasound Med* 1996;15:25–32
9. Mertz E, Bahlmann F, Weber G. Volume scanning in the evaluation of fetal malformations: a new dimension in prenatal diagnosis. *Ultrasound Obstet Gynecol* 1995;5:222–7
10. Vintzileos AM, Egan JF, Smulian JC, Campbell WA, Guzman ER, Rodis JF. Adjusting the risk for trisomy 21 by a simple ultrasound method using fetal long-bone biometry. *Obstet Gynecol* 1996;87:953–8
11. Bahado-Singh RO, Deren O, Tan A, et al. Ultrasonographically adjusted midtrimester risk of trisomy 21 and significant chromosomal defects in advanced maternal age. *Am J Obstet Gynecol* 1996;175:1563–8
12. Dorin S, Dufour P, Valat AS, et al. Ultrasonographic signs of chromosome aberrations. *J Gynecol Obstet Biol Reprod (Paris)* 1998;27:290–7
13. Guariglia L, Rosati P. Isolated mild fetal pyelectasis detected by transvaginal sonography in advanced maternal age. *Obstet Gynecol* 1998;92:833–6
14. Vergani P, Locatelli A, Piccoli MG, et al. Best second trimester sonographic markers for the detection of trisomy 21. *J Ultrasound Med* 1999;18:469–73
15. Bobrowski RA, Levin RB, Lauria MR, Treadwell MC, Gonik B, Bottoms SF. In utero progression of isolated renal pelvis dilation. *Am J Perinatol* 1997;14:423–6
16. Whitlow BJ, Lazanakis ML, Kadir RA, Chatzipapas I, Economides DL. The significance of choroid plexus cysts, echogenic heart foci and renal pyelectasis in the first trimester. *Ultrasound Obstet Gynecol* 1998;12:385–90
17. Guariglia L, Rosati P. Prevalence and significance of isolated fetal choroid plexus cysts detected in early pregnancy by transvaginal sonography in women of advanced maternal age. *Prenat Diagn* 1999;19:128–31
18. Sullivan A, Giudice T, Vavelidis F, Thiagarajah S. Choroid plexus cysts: is biochemical testing a valuable adjunct to targeted ultrasonography? *Am J Obstet Gynecol* 1999;181:260–5
19. van der Putte SCJ. Lymphatic malformation in human fetuses. *Virchows Arch* 1988;376:233–46
20. Nicolaides KH, Warenski JC, Rodeck CH. The relationship of fetal plasma protein concentration and hemoglobin level to the development of hydrops in rhesus isoimmunisation. *Am J Obstet Gynecol* 1985;152:341–4
21. Duff K, Williamson R, Richards SJ. Expression of

genes encoding two chains of the collagen type VI molecule during human fetal heart development. *Intern J Cardiol* 1990;27:128–9
22. Nicolaides KH, Azar G, Byrne D, Mansur C, Marks K. Fetal nuchal translucency: ultrasound screening for chromosomal defects in first trimester of pregnancy. *Br Med J* 1992;304:867–9
23. D' Ottavio G, Meir YJ, Rustico MA, *et al.* Screening for fetal anomalies by ultrasound at 14 and 21 weeks. *Ultrasound Obstet Gynecol* 1997;10:375–80
24. Monni G, Zoppi MA, Ibba RM, Loris M. Fetal nuchal translucency test for Down syndrome. *Lancet* 1997;350:754
25. Seeds JW. Ultrasonographic screening for aneuploidy. *N Engl J Med* 1997;337:381
26. Kurjak A, Kupesic S, Kosuta-Ivancevic M. Three-dimensional transvaginal ultrasound improves measurement of nuchal translucency. *J Perinat Med* 1999;27:97–102
27. Haddow JE, Palomokie GE. Down's syndrome screening. *Lancet* 1996;374:1625
28. Kormman LH, Morssink LP, Beekhius JR, DeWolf BT, Herringa MP, Mantingh A. Nuchal translucency cannot be used as a screening test for chromosomal abnormalities in the first trimester of pregnancy in a routine ultrasound practice. *Prenat Diagn* 1997;17:785–8

Three-dimensional ultrasound for nuchal translucency measurement at 10–14 weeks of gestation

B. L. Chung, Y. P. Kim and M. H. Nam

Background

Increased nuchal translucency is a common feature of major chromosomal defects. In the first trimester of pregnancy, a high nuchal translucency measurement gives an increased risk not only for chromosomal defects but also for cardiac abnormalities and several genetic syndromes[1–3].

Nuchal translucency has been measured by ultrasound examination since the early 1990s[4]. Although numerous centers have reported variable sensitivities of the test, none has questioned the validity of the association between increased nuchal translucency and fetal aneuploidy[5].

The conventional method for the measurement by two-dimensional (2D) ultrasound has some limitations: suboptimal fetal position and difficulty in distinguishing nuchal skin from amnion. These inevitably result in prolonged examination time or failure of the measurement, causing variable results[6–9].

Compared with 2D ultrasound scanning for the measurement, three-dimensional (3D) volume scanning acquires 3D volume data of the fetal neck. A satisfactory mid-sagittal view of the fetal neck can be obtained from these 3D data and we can utilize this saved volume for review even when the patient is absent. Besides these advantages, tomographic examination of the sagittal view is convenient for distinguishing nuchal skin from amnion. We have therefore applied 3D ultrasound to fetal nuchal translucency measurement.

The aims of this prospective study were to calculate the success rate in measuring fetal nuchal translucency and to assess intra- and interoperator variabilities of the measurement using 3D ultrasound.

Subjects and methods

A total of 616 women with singleton pregnancy visiting St Luke's Obstetrics and Gynecology Clinic (Seoul, Korea) from November 1997 to June 1999 were included in this prospective study. Fetal nuchal translucency was measured at 10–14 weeks of gestation in an unselected population. All women had shown regular menstrual cycles before pregnancy. The measurements were expressed as millimeters according to gestational days, based on crown–rump length (Dr Hansmann's data). All the patients consented to participate in this study.

In all cases, 3D transvaginal sonography was performed with an empty bladder. The equipment used was a Voluson 530D machine with type S-VDW 5–8 MHz transvaginal probe (Medison Kretztechnik).

When the fetus presented its nuchal region on the 2D image, the volume acquisition was started. The volume scan was automatically performed by a slow tilting movement of the 2D scanning mechanics. The maximum sweep angle of the transducer was 95°.

After the volume data had been saved on a removable hard disk, another volume acquisition was also performed at a different view of the same fetus. Measurement of the thickness was made from all the saved volume data by reorienting the fetal position using multiplanar imaging[10] (Figure 1). Diagrams demonstrating the advantage of 3D ultrasound in gen-

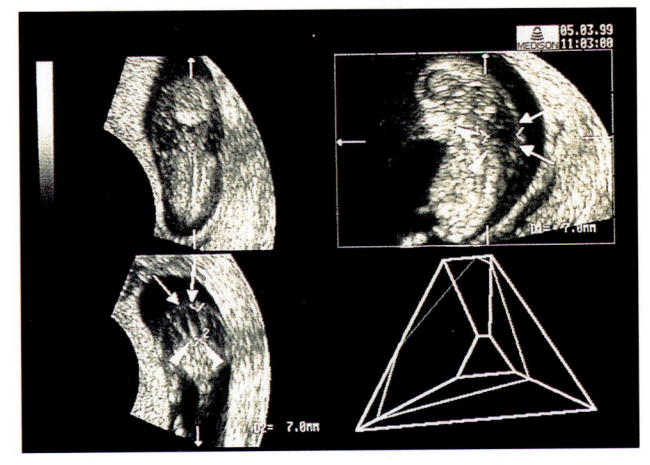

Figure 1 Display of three perpendicular planar reformatted images in a case of trisomy 21 at 10 weeks plus 5 days' gestation. A satisfactory mid-sagittal view of the fetus is shown in the B plane (upper right). The translucency thickness can be seen on both the B and the C plane. The results of dual measurements are the same (7.0 mm)

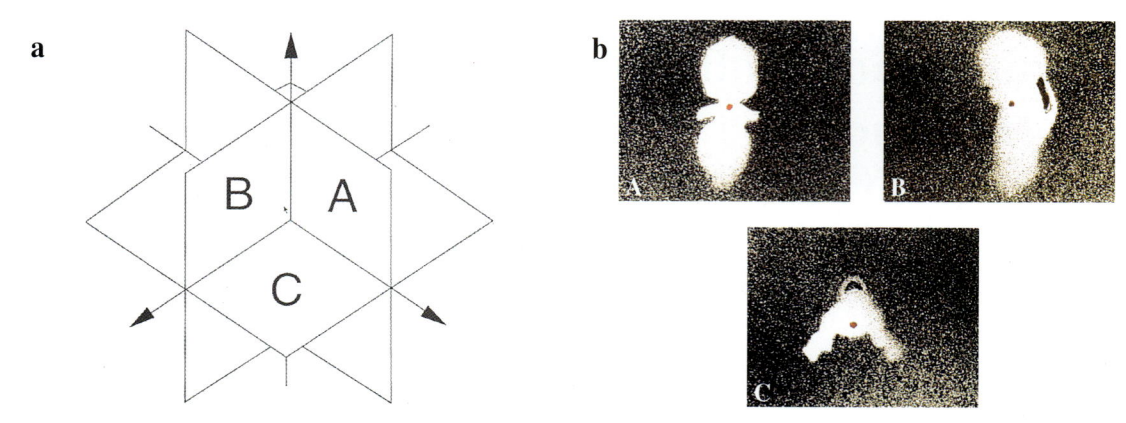

Figure 2 Three sectional planes of three-dimensional ultrasound (a). These three planes are to be perpendicularly crossed with one another at the three-axial center of rotation. Display of A, B, and C planes (b). The center of rotation is fixed on the mid-line of the fetal neck on the A plane (upper left). When a symmetrical frontal view of the fetus on the A plane and a symmetrical transverse view of the fetal neck on the C plane (lower left) are manipulated, the satisfactory mid-sagittal view consequently appears on the B plane (upper right). The translucency thickness can be detected on both B and C planes

erating a satisfactory mid-sagittal view of the fetus are shown in Figure 2.

In general, guidelines for the measurement described by Snijders and Nicolaides[1] have been observed. Tomographic examination of the sagittal view was especially helpful for distinguishing nuchal skin from amnion.

Other volume data were also reviewed with the same procedure. We chose the better of these two images and saved it on the disk as the initial position, which automatically appeared after volume acquisition. Measurement of the thickness was made twice on each fetus with the selected optimal image. The larger thickness was used as the nuchal translucency value of the measurement.

To assess intraoperator variability, the measurement was blindly repeated by the same operator with the previously selected optimal image in the first 86 out of 616 women. The measurement was made twice in each fetus, and the larger was used as the second value of the measurement.

In 86 randomized fetuses out of the 616, interoperator variability was examined by comparing measurements of two operators (A and B), A having experience of about 500 cases and B having experience of about 100 cases. The volume acquisition, saving and measurement were carried out by operator B, using the same procedure performed by operator A. The two operators were blinded to each other's results.

The paired t test was used to detect operator variability. The degree of association and consistency of two measurements by the same operator or different operators was also examined by using correlation analysis and the regression model. In analyzing regression, we used the model of simple linear regression with no intercept, and tested whether the coefficient of the slope was unity or not. All analyses were performed with the use of SAS software (release 6.12), and statistical tests were two-tailed. The p value of 0.05 was used as the level of significance.

Results

The mean maternal age was 29 years. The distribution of nuchal translucency thickness in 616 fetuses is shown in Figure 3. Out of 616 fetuses, 15 were classified as screen-positive, having increased nuchal translucency thickness of $\geq$ 3 mm. The outcome of fetuses with increased nuchal translucency thickness is shown in Table 1. Eight out of 15 fetuses underwent karyotyping. Two cases were confirmed as Down's syndrome and two as Turner's syndrome. Two fetuses with a chromosomally normal karyotype had severe abnormal sonographic findings at 20 and 22 weeks of gestation. Two others were spontaneously aborted before invasive testing. We were able to obtain good sagittal views of fetuses and to measure the thickness in all cases. There was no failure of the measurement.

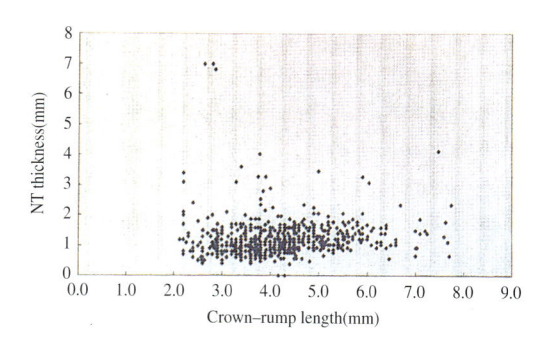

Figure 3 Distribution of nuchal translucency (NT) thickness according to crown–rump length

Table 1 Outcome of 15 fetuses with increased nuchal translucency (NT) thickness

Case no.	Maternal age (years)	NT thickness (mm)	Karyotype	Outcome
1	39	3.5	*	*
2	31	3.6	not done	spontaneous abortion
3	29	6.5	not done	spontaneous abortion
4	40	7.0	47,XX+21	termination
5	32	3.3	not done	healthy birth
6	26	4.4	45,X	termination
7	32	4.3	46,XX	ventriculomegaly; both hydronephrotic
8	29	3.7	*	*
9	26	3.1	46,XY	healthy birth
10	29	3.4	46,XX	healthy birth
11	43	6.6	47,XX+21	termination
12	24	3.1	45,X	termination
13	29	3.1	*	*
14	37	3.0	46,XY	dysplastic kidneys (both)
15	34	3.5	*	*

* Lost to follow-up

Table 2 Comparison of nuchal translucency thickness at first and second measurements

	Mean ±SD (mm)	p Value*
First measurement (n = 86)	1.514 ± 0.568	0.862
Second measurement (n = 86)	1.516 ± 0.546	
Difference	0.002 ± 0.124	

* By paired t test (t = 0.174, df = 85)

The mean thickness of nuchal translucency at the first measurement was not significantly different ($p = 0.862$) from the second measurement (Table 2). The association between the first and second measurements was highly significant ($r = 0.976$, $p = 0.0001$), as shown in Figure 4.

The mean thickness of nuchal translucency measured by operator A was not statistically different ($p = 0.931$) from that of operator B (Table 3). The strong association between the data of operator A and B ($r = 0.977$, $p = 0.0001$) is shown in Figure 5. All these results showed good intra- and interoperator variabilities.

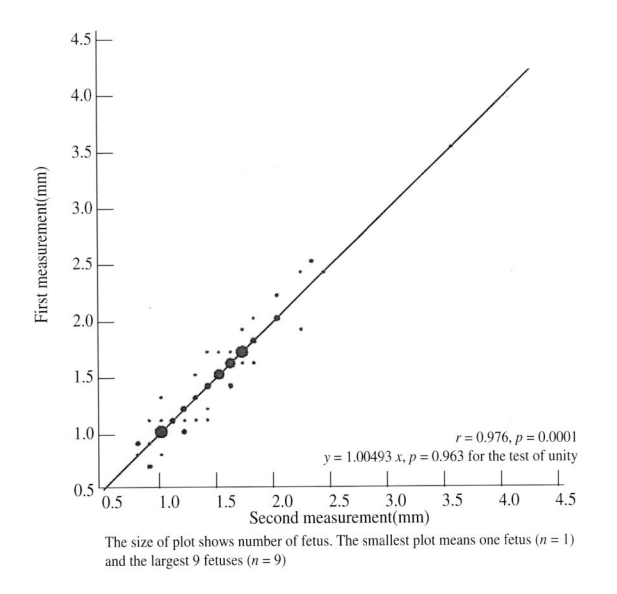

Figure 4 Correlation and regression analysis for intraoperator variability. The size of each symbol reflects the number of fetuses (smallest, one fetus; largest, nine fetuses)

Discussion

Measuring fetal nuchal translucency by 2D ultrasound is not technically easy. Roberts and colleagues[6] report-

Table 3 Comparison of nuchal translucency thickness measured by operators A and B

	Cases (n)	Mean ±SD (mm)	p Value*
Operator A	86	1.515 ± 0.571	0.931
Operator B	86	1.516 ± 0.546	
Difference		0.001 ± 0.025	

* By paired t test (t = 0.087, df = 85)

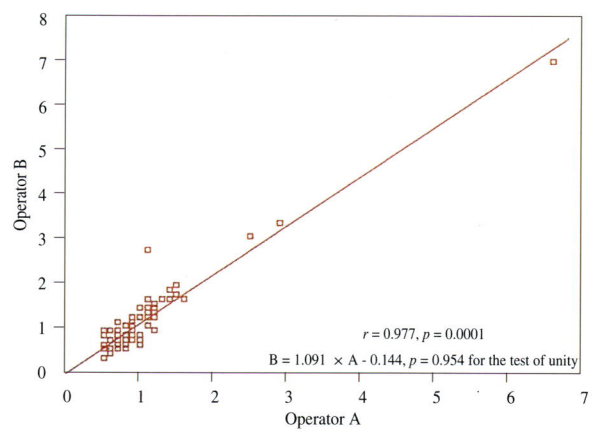

Figure 5 Correlation and regression analysis for interoperator variability

ed unsuccessful measurements in 18% of all their cases, as did Haddow and Palomaki[7]. Hermann and colleagues[8] proposed an image-scoring method, in which almost one-third of their cases were troublesome for the measurement. A recent paper[9] comparing measurements by both 2D and 3D ultrasound showed unsuccessful measurements in 15% of the patients undergoing 2D ultrasound examination. Also, poor reproducibility of the measurement was reported by Roberts and colleagues[6].

Our study demonstrated a success rate of the measurement of 100%. The same result was obtained by Kurjak and associates[9] with the use of 3D ultrasound versus a success rate of 85% by 2D ultrasound. Our results also showed good intra- and interoperator variabilities.

In addition, patients felt negligible discomfort, because of the short examination time, and operators could easily perform the measurement, owing to established procedures.

In conclusion, 3D transvaginal ultrasound improves fetal nuchal translucency measurement at 10–14 weeks of gestation. However, its advantages may need further evaluation.

References

1. Snijders RJM, Nicolaides KH. In *Ultrasound Markers for Fetal Chromosomal Defects*. Carnforth, UK: Parthenon Publishing, 1996;2:122,128
2. Suka AP, Snijders RJM, Novakov A, Soares W, Nicolaides KH. Defects and syndromes in chromsomally normal fetuses with increased nuchal translucency thickness at 10–14 weeks of gestation. *Ultrasound Obstet Gynecol* 1998;6:391–400
3. Hyatt JA, Perdu M, Shaland JK, Snijders RJM, Nicolaides KH. Increased nuchal translucency at 10–14 weeks of gestation as a marker for major cardiac defects. *Ultrasound Obstet Gynecol* 1997;10:242–6
4. Szabo J, Gellen J. Nuchal fluid accumulation in trisomy 21 detected by vaginosonography in first trimester. *Lancet* 1990;8:1133
5. Fleischer AC, Manning FA, Jeanty P, Romero R. Prenatal diagnosis during the first trimester. In *Sonography in Obstetrics and Gynecology* 5th edn. Appleton & Lange, 1996:368–9
6. Roberts LJ, Bewley S, Mackinson AM, Rodeck CH. First trimester nuchal translucency: problems with screening the general population 1. *Br J Obstet Gynaecol* 1995; 102:381–5
7. Haddow JE, Palomaki GE. Down's syndrome screening. *Lancet* 1996;347b:1625
8. Hermann A, Maymon R, Dreazen E, *et al.* Nuchal translucency audit: a novel image-scoring method. *Ultrasound Obstet Gynecol* 1998;12:398–403
9. Kurjak A, Kupesic S, Mirjana IK. Three-dimensional transvaginal ultrasound improves measurement of nuchal translucency. *J Perinat Med* 1999;27:97–102
10. Chung BL, Kim HJ, Lee KH. The application of three-dimensional ultrasound to nuchal translucency measurement in early pregnancy (10–14 weeks): preliminary study. *Ultrasound Obstet Gynecol* 2000;15:122–5

Three-dimensional color and power imaging: experience in prenatal diagnosis

R. Matijevic and A. Kurjak

Introduction

Compared to imaging in all other fields of medicine, the examination of the pregnant woman and fetus is highly dependent on ultrasound. After development of high-resolution real-time B-mode imaging, the transvaginal approach, color, pulsed and power Doppler, the improvement in computer technology with fast central processors enabled the development of three-dimensional (3D) ultrasound machines, providing a logical continuation in the development of ultrasound in obstetrics. The first 3D ultrasound machines produced gray-scale visualization of the fetus with acceptable acquisition time and image rendering. However, in recent years, 3D visualization of blood vessels has become a reality, improving the diagnostic potential of the technique in fetal medicine[1,2].

Compared to the conventional color Doppler technique used in two-dimensional (2D) imaging, 3D color imaging is based on power rather than on the color Doppler technique, as color power was found more suitable for 3D reconstruction[3] (Figure 1). At first, the vessels of interest are optimally visualized by the 2D technique superimposed by color power mode. With the freehand technique, the probe is tilted to obtain a scan volume. This is followed by the choice of specific settings for image rendering and on-line 3D reconstruction of the vascular network.

Unfortunately, the 3D image of the vascular network does not contain gray-scale information. This image is visualized on the ultrasound screen and the rotation over the determined axis produces a 3D impression. The data may be stored and processed retrospectively to two dimensions, to choose other slice thicknesses, image views or color maps (Figure 2). This technique is still new, but it is a growing field and is promising for further research.

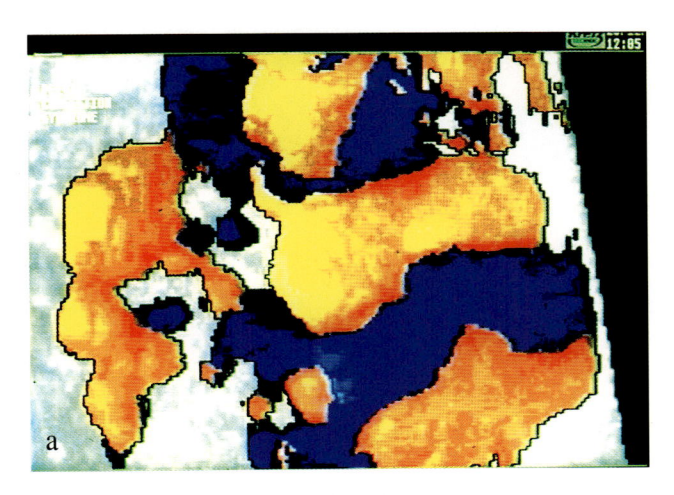

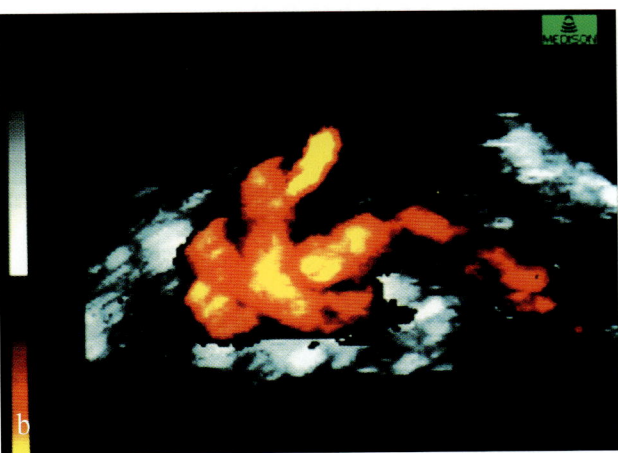

Figure 1 Features of color Doppler (a) and power Doppler (b), showing the advantages of power Doppler for three-dimensional reconstruction. The blood flow visualized by power can be seen despite the orthogonal approach and is rendered in uniform color. It is identically rendered in the arteries and vein, as it is not related to the velocity. The neighboring structures are sharp and clear

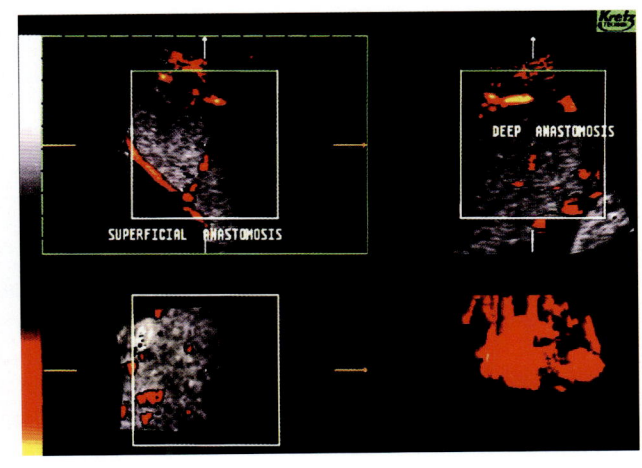

Figure 2 Principles of three-dimensional color power angiography

Potential clinical application of three-dimensional color power imaging

Power Doppler imaging has many synonyms, such as amplitude mode Doppler or power Doppler energy. In all of them, both color and power Doppler are used to present the flow in blood vessels. Because of this, the technique is also named power Doppler angiography. Using power Doppler ultrasound, the acquired information from Doppler signals in three dimensions is not analyzed by frequency assessment but by employing the amplitude of the signal. Consequently, the method is up to five times more sensitive than the conventional color Doppler system[4]. The advantages of color power Doppler for 3D reconstruction are presented in Table 1.

The potential clinical application of power Doppler angiography is summarized in the work of Chaoui and Kalache[5] (Table 2). In the assessment of the fetal placenta there are numerous advantages offered by the use of power Doppler angiography. Three-dimensional color and power Doppler can clearly demonstrate placental vessels (Figure 3) in their anatomical position and can help in the detection of placenta previa, demonstrating vessels overlapping the internal cervical os (Figure 4). The placental vessel anatomy will be better understood by means of the 3D power Doppler mode, by visualization of the crossing of the vessels, with easy analysis of their size, course and shape. In the twin-twin transfusion syndrome (TTTS), power Doppler angiography can clearly present the placental vascular tree of both monochorionic twins, together with the deep placental anastomosis responsible for exchange transfusion between the twins (Figure 5). This is helpful in determination of the risk in monochorionic twin pregnancy, as visualization of the deep anastomosis may be used as a predictive factor for TTTS, necessitating close surveillance of such preg-

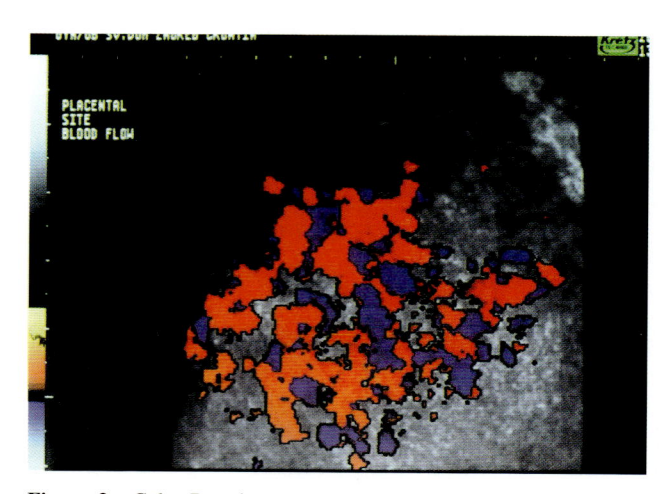

Figure 3 Color Doppler presentation of placenta previa displaying numerous placental blood vessels covering the internal cervical os

Table 1 The advantages of color power Doppler for three-dimensional reconstruction

Blood flow can be noted despite the vertical approach (at 90°)
Flow is identically rendered in both arteries and veins, as it is independent of velocity and related to the density of the blood
The edge definition of surrounding structures is better and gives an impression of the third dimension
As the signal obtained analyzes perfusion and not velocity, it is possible to analyze small and large blood vessels side by side in one setting
Color assigned to noise is uniform and is distinguishable from true flow signals

Table 2 Potential applications of three-dimensional power Doppler in prenatal diagnosis. From reference 5

Region	Application
Placenta	placental vessels, placenta previa, placental tumors, communication of the placentae in twin-twin transfusion syndrome
Uteroplacental vessels	spiral arteries
Umbilical cord	insertion, vasa previa, nuchal cord, abnormalities of vessels (single umbilical artery), abnormalities of insertion
Fetal abdominal vessels	abnormal umbilical vein, torsion of fetal abdominal vessels
Kidneys	agenesis of kidneys, renal arteries, horseshoe kidney, pelvic kidney, possible abnormal vessel course in cystic renal malformation
Lung	vessel architecture in cystic lung malformation, congenital diaphragmatic hernia, bronchopulmonary sequestration
Brain	galen aneurysm, cerebral malformations and vascular anatomy (see Figure 11), corpus callosum agenesis, encephalocele
Heart	atrioventricular connections
Great vessels	spatial distribution of great vessels in transposition
Tumors	chorangioma, teratoma, hygroma, lung sequestration, acrania

THREE-DIMENSIONAL COLOR AND POWER IMAGING

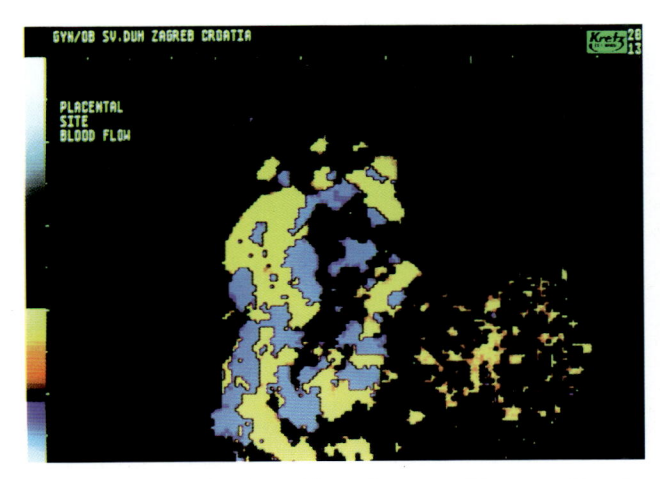

Figure 4 Similar situation to Figure 3, presented by power Doppler sonography

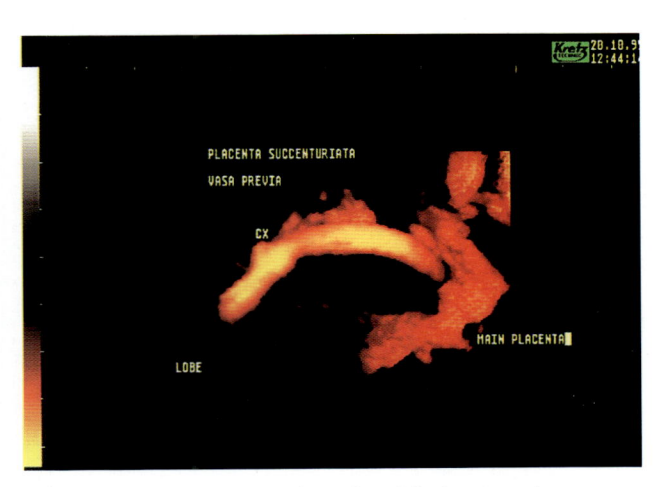

Figure 6 Color Doppler angiography of the lower uterine segment with placenta succenturiata and communicating vessels overlying the internal cervical os (vasa previa). The placenta was found on the anterior uterine wall in the lower uterine segment, while the succenturiate lobe was located on the posterior uterine wall

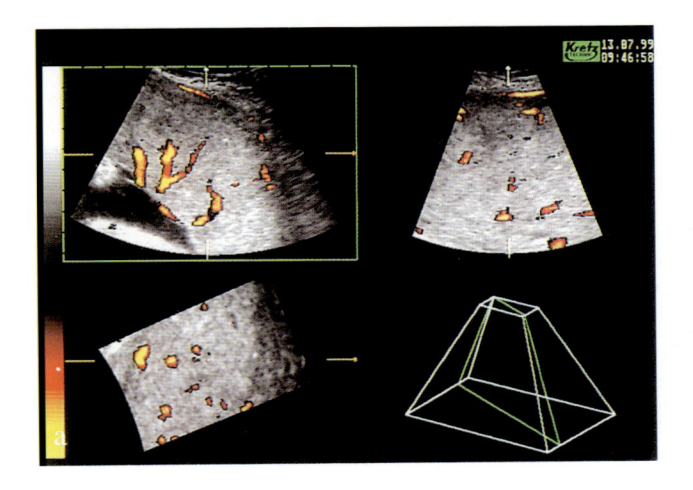

Figure 7 Three-dimensional power Doppler image of the uteroplacental vessels

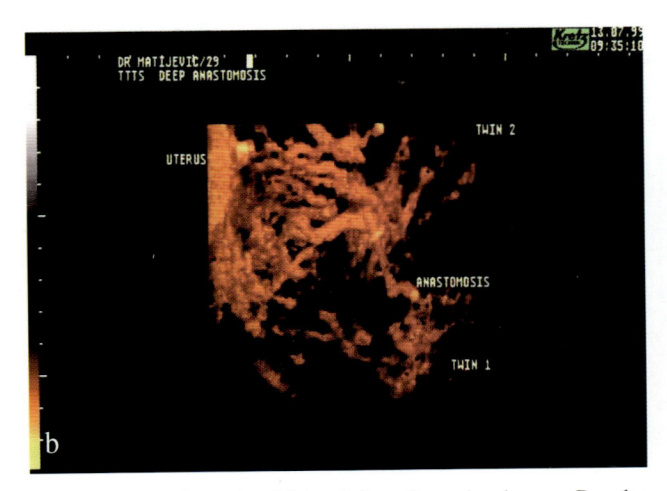

Figure 5 Two-dimensional (a) and three-dimensional power Doppler reconstruction (b) of the placenta in twin–twin transfusion syndrome. In (a), despite all three planes being analyzed, only the superficial anastomosis can be seen. In (b), the vascular tree of each monochorionic twin is clearly displayed, with the connecting blood vessel representing the deep placental anastomosis responsible for interfetal transfusion

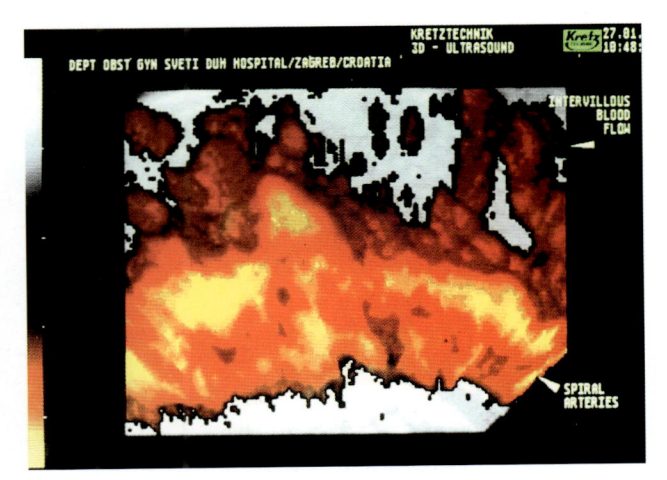

Figure 8 Three-dimensional power Doppler presentation of the maternal spiral arteries and intervillous space

157

CLINICAL APPLICATION OF 3D SONOGRAPHY

nancies. In cases of placenta succenturiata and/or vasa previa, color power angiography can present the vessels overlying the internal cervical os (Figure 6).

Regarding the uteroplacental vessels, color Doppler angiography was found to be superior in the visualization of the distal branches of the uterine artery (i.e. the arcuate, radial and spiral arteries) (Figure 7) and intervillous blood flow (Figure 8) compared to 2D color Doppler imaging. Studies of spiral artery blood flow and intervillous blood flow have produced promising results, which might be used in a screening program for pregnancy-induced hypertension and intrauterine growth restriction.

In the assessment of the umbilical cord, 3D power Doppler angiography was found to be very useful in the detection of the nuchal cord (Figure 9). This is of

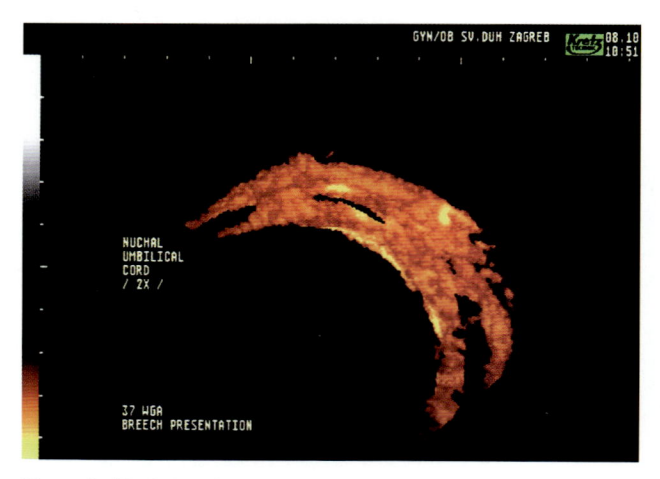

Figure 9 Nuchal cord as presented by power Doppler angiography

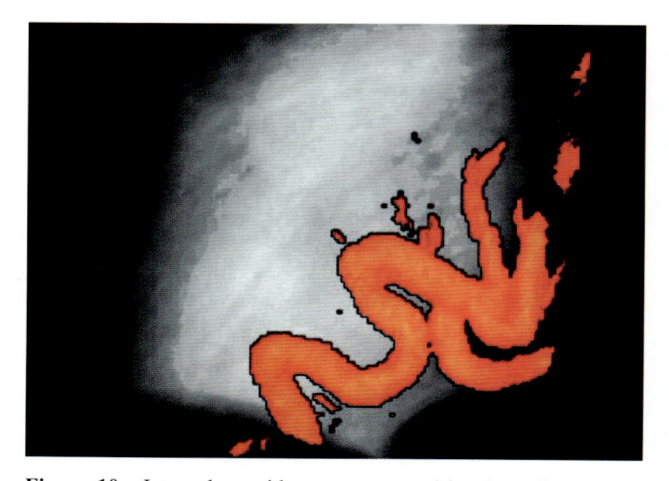

Figure 10 Internal carotid artery presented by three-dimensional power angiography

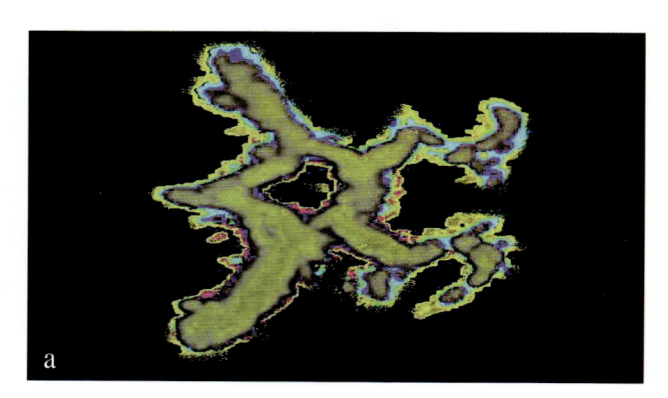

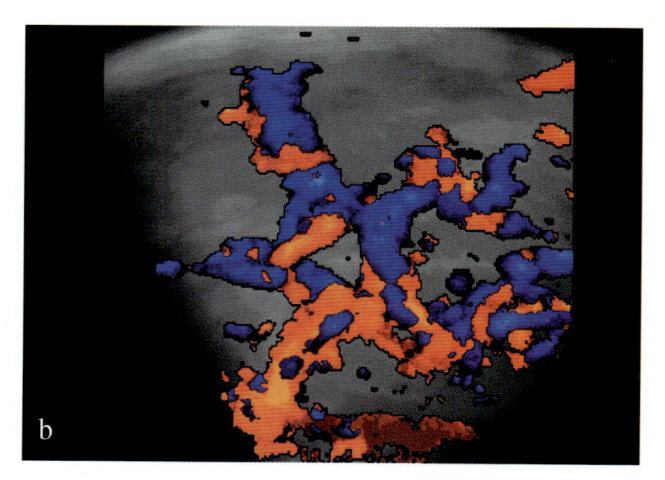

Figure 11 (a) and (b) Three-dimensional color power angiography of the circle of Willis in a transverse plane

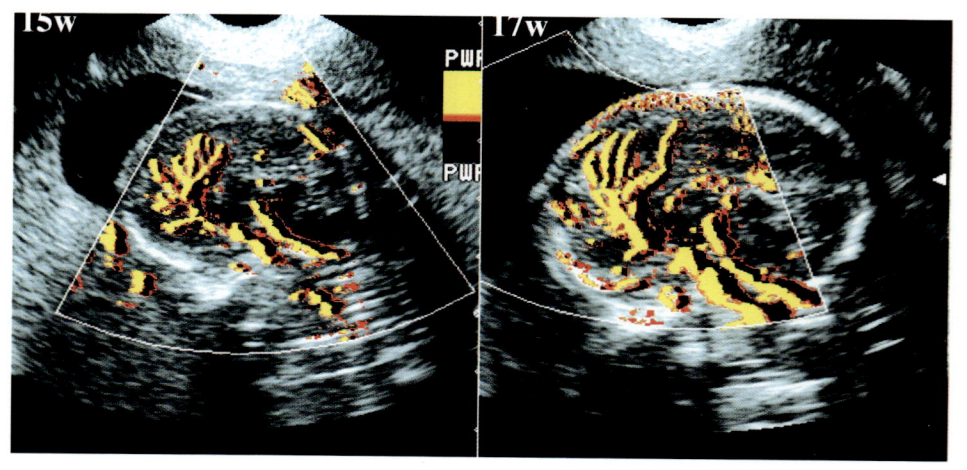

Figure 12 Three-dimensional power Doppler angiography of the sagittal plane of the fetal brain

importance in the management of labor in fetuses with breech presentation. In such cases, especially if the condition is combined with oligohydramnios, power Doppler can help diagnose loops of the umbilical cord around the fetal neck, indicating the need for Cesarean section. The same technique may present other fetal vessels in their anatomical position with clearer visualization of their relationship to surrounding structures (Figure 10). Using this technique the vessel anatomy can easily be understood (its size, course and shape). Because of the movements of the fetal heart during data acquisition, 2D power Doppler angiography of this organ is still not possible.

The power Doppler blood flow assessment of cerebral vessels shows the vascular tree of the circle of Willis (Figure 11). Depending on the approach, two different vascular regions may be detected by using 3D color power angiography: the transverse plane (Figure 11) and the sagittal plane (Figure 12). In the sagittal plane, the pericallosal arteries can be visualized to their ramification. In the assessment of fetal tumors, as in sacrococcygeal teratoma (Figure 13), visualization of the intratumoral vessels is of importance for the diagnosis. In such tumors, 3D power Doppler angiography can detect normal and aberrant vessels (Figure 13).

Settings and possible problems

Despite obvious benefits, 3D power Doppler imaging has its limitations. They arise from the system used and from the prenatal approach. To obtain the best possible image it is important to consider some optimal settings of the color power angiography mode in acquiring a 3D image[5]. Pulse repetition frequency (PRF) should be set at 700 or 1000 Hz in order to assess small vessels. If a selective visualization of arteries with a higher flow is preferred, a higher PRF should be chosen. The gain is set between 60 and 70%, with the tendency to use a lower gain than generally necessary to acquire the color power angiographic image. The wall filter should be set on medium and the dynamic motion differentiation should be set to avoid signals appearing as background noise on 3D sonography. Priority should be set on high, while sensitivity is set on medium. These setting are listed as a guide only and they may differ according to the model and manufacturer of the machine used.

The main limitations of 3D power Doppler imaging are the same as for the 3D approach in general. Fetal movements are well known to prevent the obtaining of a good-quality 3D gray-scale image. Unfortunately, in prenatal diagnosis we are dealing with small regions where information is needed, and the smallest movement of the probe will result in serious artifacts. The gain should be reduced to the minimal value to obtain a better spatial impression. Also, the PRF should be adjusted according to the investigated vessels. To detect vascular branching, the PRF should be set to the lower values; and for clear visualization of the main branch of the vessel, the investigator should chose a high PRF.

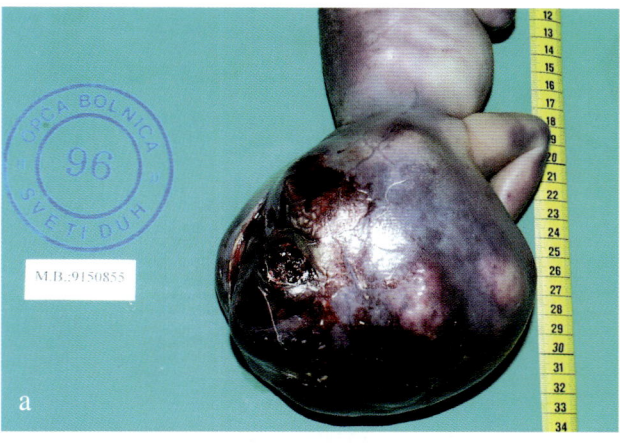

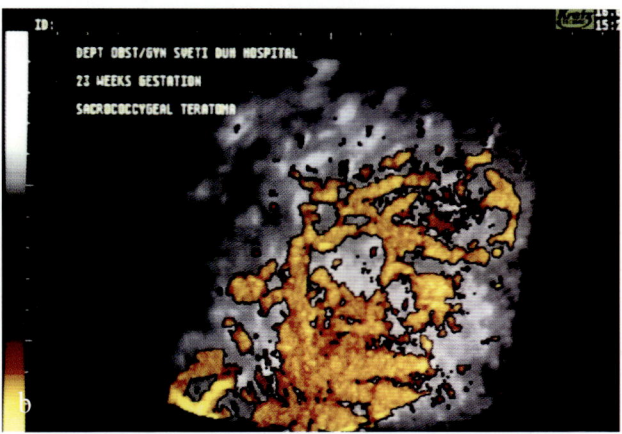

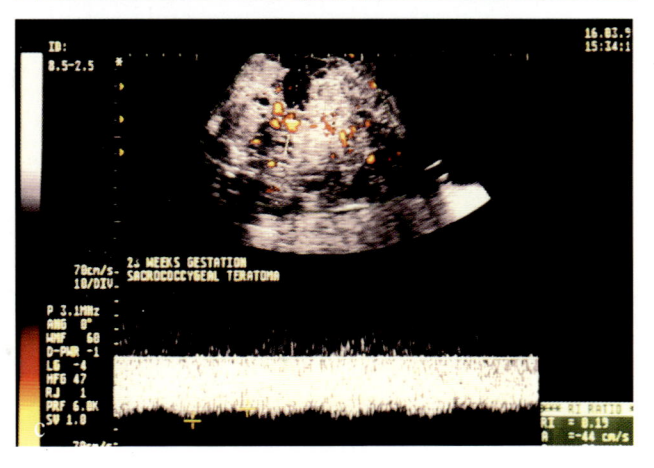

Figure 13 (a) A sacrococcygeal teratoma detected at 25 weeks of pregnancy. (b) Three-dimensional color power angiography presenting the rich vascularization and clearer spatial distribution of the vessels. (c) Pulsed Doppler assessment of the intratumoral blood flow

Conclusion

The 3D power Doppler mode is a new diagnostic tool in prenatal diagnosis. It should be used only by examiners experienced in color Doppler and gray-scale 3D imaging. In the second and third trimesters of pregnancy, rendering in the power Doppler mode has potential benefits. However, investigations are still in the early stages, and intensive research is needed before final conclusions are drawn.

References

1. Miyagi Y, Masaoka H, Akamatsu N, Sekiba K. Development of a three-dimensional color Doppler system. *Med Prog Techol* 1992;18:201–8
2. Downey DB, Fenster A. Vascular imaging with a three dimensional power Doppler system. *Am J Roentgenol* 1995;165:665–8
3. Ritchie CJ, Edwards WS, Mack LA, Cyr DR, Kim Y. Three dimensional ultrasonic angiography using power mode Doppler. *Ultrasound Med Biol* 1996;22:277–86
4. Fortunato SJ. The use of power Doppler and color power angiography in fetal imaging. *Am J Obstet Gynecol* 1996;174:1828–31
5. Chaoui R, Kalache K. Three-dimensional color power imaging: principles and first experience in prenatal diagnosis. In Merz E, ed. *3D Ultrasound in Obstetrics and Gynecology*. Philadelphia: Lippincott Wiliams & Wilkins, 1998:135–41

Three-dimensional fetal echocardiography

G. Bega and K. Kuhlman

Introduction

Congenital cardiac malformation is the most common major birth defect, with an incidence of approximately 8.8 in 1000 live births[1]. Although great progress has been achieved in our understanding and detection of congenital heart defects, especially with two-dimensional (2D) fetal echocardiography techniques, the fetal heart is a complex dynamic organ often difficult to image. The standard ultrasound screening of the fetal heart is largely based on the four-chamber view of the fetal heart[2], which detects approximately one-third of major cardiac defects[3]. More than 90% of congenital heart diseases (CHDs) occur in the low risk population. Despite efforts to obtain additional cardiac views that would improve the detection of CHD[4], there are a number of limiting factors that influence fetal heart imaging, such as experience of the operator, position of the fetus, maternal body habitus and gestational age. The Radius trial demonstrated that the detection rate of CHD in the second trimester was very low, only 18% in tertiary centers and 0% in non-tertiary centers[5,6].

In three-dimensional (3D) ultrasound a volume of ultrasound data is acquired and stored, allowing the subsequent extraction of an infinite number of scan planes[7]. With 3D ultrasound the fetal heart can be encompassed in a volume of ultrasound data, which can be sliced to obtain many 2D ultrasound heart views, including the four-chamber view, outflow tracts and great vessels, which might not be readily obtained by 2D ultrasound. These technical features of 3D ultrasound facilitate both the acquisition of heart views and our 3D understanding of the heart, which in standard 2D ultrasound requires the mental construction of the heart anatomy from 2D images.

Technical considerations

Acquisition

There are two related methods of acquiring volumes of fetal heart data with 3D ultrasound imaging. In both methods a conventional 2D ultrasound examination of the fetal heart is initially obtained.

External positioning systems

Otherwise called the freehand method, this technique utilizes a position sensor mounted on a conventional transducer, providing position and orientation information of the captured 2D images, as the probe is manually swept through the fetal chest. There are several different kinds of position sensor used: articulated arms, acoustic, optical, etc. The most commonly used is the electromagnetic position sensor. The area between the source and the sensor should be free of metallic objects that could distort the sensing field. The advantages of these systems are in their ability to scan larger volumes and thus larger anatomic areas using conventional high-resolution 2D transducers with freehand techniques. The main disadvantages are artifacts produced during the acquisition of images with the freehand method, creating positional distortions. Therefore, volume calculations are not accurate with this method. There is a delay in the display of data acquired with these systems because of the calibration calculations necessary to co-ordinate position data with the acquired images.

Integrated positioning systems

In a dedicated 3D ultrasound system, a position sensor is integrated inside a mechanical or electronic transducer assembly, which automatically sweeps through the region of interest digitally, recording a stack of 2D images. During the acquisition the transducer is fixed over the region of interest, and the volumes acquired have the shape of a truncated pyramid. The transducer is hosted in a box sufficiently large to allow the sweep. Therefore, these transducers are larger than the conventional transducers, but light enough to allow normal use. The advantages of these systems derive from their ability to acquire artifact-free volumes along with scaling information, allowing accurate measurements to be made of volumes and distances.

An attempt is made to acquire heart volumes in a relatively quiet fetal state to avoid fetal motion artifacts. In integrated systems the patient is asked to remain still for a period of 3–5 s, in order to avoid motion artifacts from breathing movements. Once in the desired acquisition plane, a volume box (similar to a color box) is placed in the region of interest (e.g. four-chamber view). The smallest possible volume box is used, to achieve the shortest possible acquisition time. In the Voluson 530D system from Medison, USA, there are three acquisition speeds available on the equipment (low, normal, high) and the normal acquisition speed is selected for most of the acquisitions.

In systems using a freehand technique the probe is moved manually over the region of interest, and the acquisition time is usually longer, typically 20–30 s, depending on the sample rate (scanned images per second) or the number of frames per cardiac cycle.

Visualization of fetal heart volume data

Both methods rely on specialized 3D software, which allows processing of the acquired volumes either on-line, through a built-in computer, or off-line, on a workstation. Volume data of the fetal heart can be displayed in a variety of ways. The digitally stored volume data can be displayed in a multiplanar array which simultaneously shows three perpendicular planes through the volume: the axial, sagittal and the reconstructed coronal views. The planes in the multiplanar display can be explored as desired by scrolling through parallel planes in any of the three views or rotating the planes in order to view the structures of interest interactively and optimally. In the multiplanar display of the heart, 2D heart views, which might not be readily obtained by conventional 2D ultrasound, can be visualized.

Heart volumes can also be rendered. At the time of writing, the rendered heart chamber data do not show a particular advantage over the multiplanar display. Rendering of the color or power Doppler information of the great vessels is an interesting feature but still lacks the clarity and dynamic information obtained with 2D ultrasound.

Cardiac gating

An important aspect of fetal heart screening is the real time assessment of heart function. In 3D ultrasound, contractility, valve movement and blood flow information can be studied in relation to the cardiac cycle if a synchronization method is utilized. In adult 3D cardiac imaging, electrocardiographic data provide the gating signal for synchronization. In the fetus, owing to the weak electrical activity compared to the maternal electrocardiogram, conventional gating is not yet possible with this technique[8,9]. Fetal motion, a very difficult variable to control, is another factor that limits gating of the fetal heart. Alternative methods, using temporal Fourier analysis[10] or M-mode[8] have been used for gating. At this time, these gating options can be used only with the freehand method of acquisition, using external position sensors. Systems with faster acquisition speeds may potentially obviate the need for gating and overcome the fetal motion problem.

Clinical studies

There have been several studies of the feasibility of 3D fetal echocardiography. Studies using the freehand method have all utilized gating techniques, while those utilizing integrated position sensors have studied the non-gated use of this modality.

In a recent study in our institution, non-gated 3D ultrasound was used to acquire and reformat volumes of fetal heart data at 16–24 weeks of gestation[11]. Each patient had a standard 2D ultrasound examination, of up to 10 min in duration, obtaining the following views: four-chamber view; left outflow tract; right outflow tract; aortic arch; ductal arch; pulmonary artery and branches; and the inferior (IVC) and superior vena cava (SVC). A 3D ultrasound examination using a dedicated system (Voluson 530D) was then performed with a duration of up to 10 min, obtaining fetal heart volumes from three acquisition planes: a transverse plane at the level of the four-chamber view; a longitudinal (para-sagittal) plane to the left outflow tract; and a non-standard view in transverse or sagittal

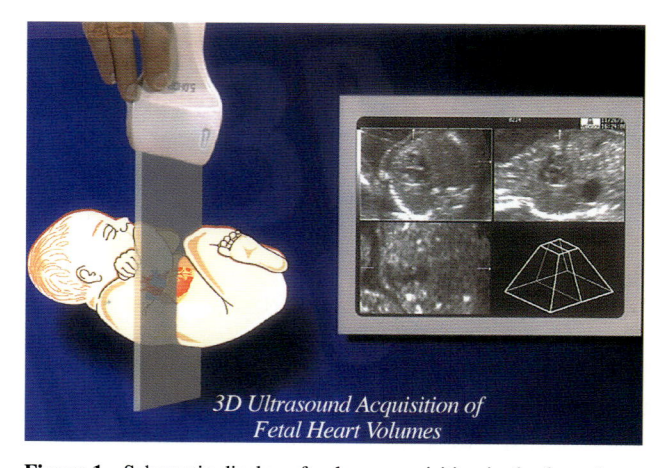

Figure 1 Schematic display of volume acquisition in the four-chamber view of the fetal heart and the corresponding three orthogonal views in the multiplanar display

plane whenever a non-conventional, but clear view of some intracardiac anatomy could be obtained (Figure 1). The mean time for extraction of standard heart views from the stored volumes was 14 min.

A reproducible method for obtaining additional screening views out of the four-chamber acquisition plane was developed. After the fetal heart volume is obtained from the four-chamber view, the planes are manipulated so that the fetal spine is rotated to the 6 o'clock position. The center-point (plane intersection point in each multiplanar window) is placed in the ascending aorta. At a plane 90° perpendicular, the ductal arch is displayed in another multiplanar window (Figure 2). The ductal arch is at approximately 35° to the aortic arch, so that rotating the plane of the four-chamber view through this angle brings the aortic arch into view (Figure 2). The IVC/SVC is almost parallel to the ductal arch, moving rightward towards the atrium (Figure 3). The planar rotations to obtain all great vessels from the four-chamber view acquisition plane are summarized in Figure 4.

The outflow tracts (right and left) may be obtained when the four-chamber view and the ductal arch are displayed (Figure 5). The left outflow tract is obtained by moving the center-point upward from the four-chamber view 3–4 mm and rotating the plane approximately 35° towards the right side of the fetus. The right outflow tract is obtained when the center-point is moved up 5–6 mm and the plane rotated approximately 30–35° towards the left side of the fetus (Figures 6 and 7). This method may prove to be very useful in reformatting fetal heart volumes when 3D ultrasound is carried out in real time and gated.

The four-chamber acquisition plane, with the spine down or lateral, generated more heart views than any other acquisition planes. Volumes acquired from a four-chamber plane generated additional screening views more than the other acquisition planes. The right outflow tract, aortic arch and ductal arch were obtained more frequently in 3D-derived views obtained from a four-chamber acquisition plane than in 2D ultrasound (Table 1). Two acquisition planes,

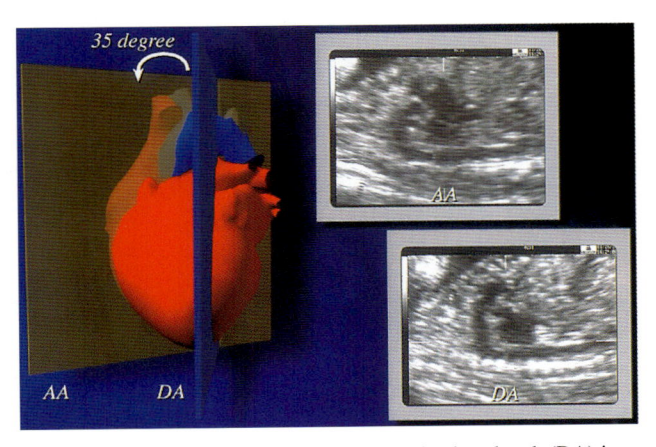

Figure 2 Sagittal planes of the fetal heart. The ductal arch (DA) is at an angle of approximately 35° to the aortic arch (AA)

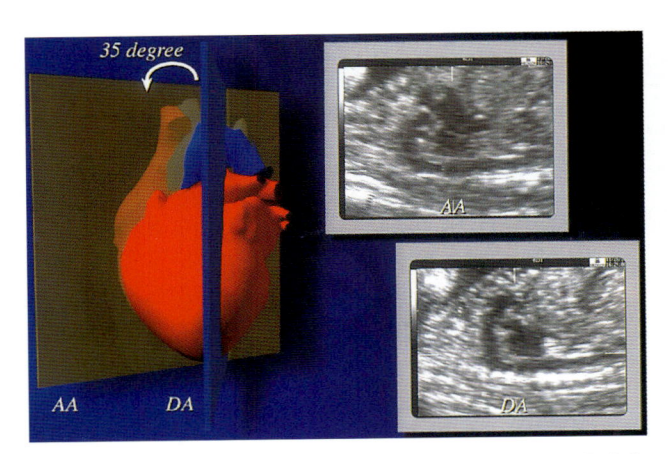

Figure 3 Sagittal planes of the fetal heart. The ductal arch (DA) is parallel to the inferior vena cava/superior vena cava (IVC/SVC)

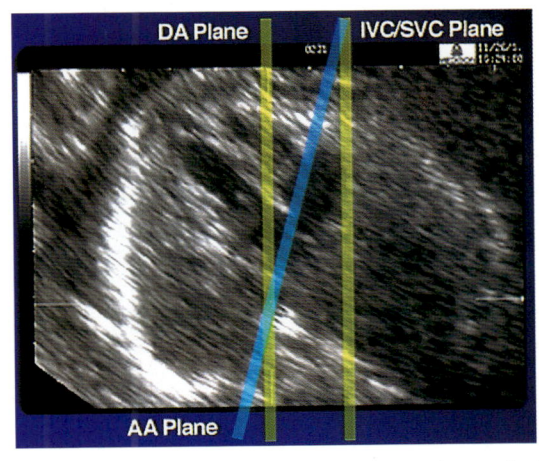

Figure 4 Sagittal planes of the fetal heart in relation to the four-chamber view. The ductal arch (DA) is parallel to the inferior vena cava/superior vena cava (IVC/SVC) and at an approximately 35° angle to the aortic arch (AA)

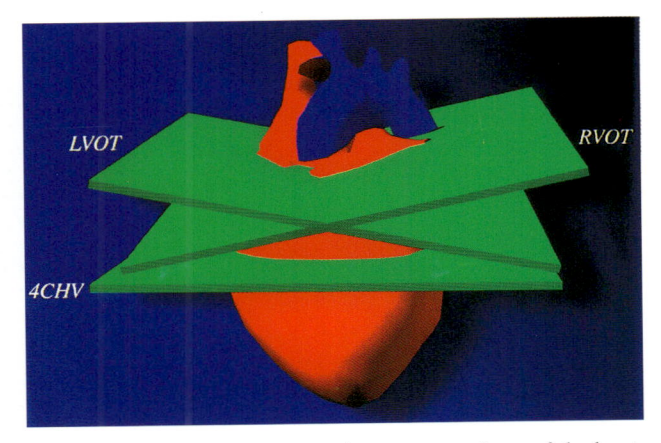

Figure 5 Relationships between the transverse planes of the heart. The left (LVOT) and right outflow tract (RVOT) planes are not quite parallel to the four-chamber view (4CHV) but at an angle of 30–35° at each side

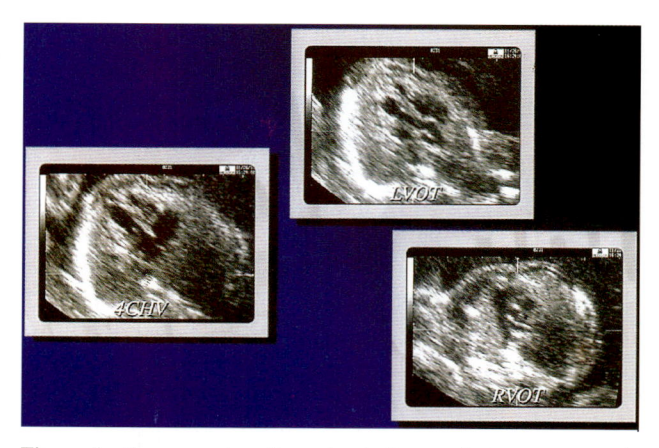

Figure 6 Transverse two-dimensional ultrasound views corresponding to transverse planes. LVOT, left outflow tract; RVOT, right outflow tract; 4CHV, four-chamber view

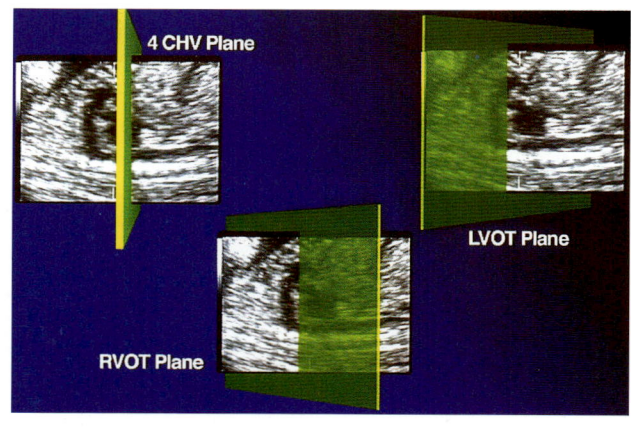

Figure 7 Transverse planes in relationship to the ductus arteriosus. 4CHV, four-chamber view; LVOT, left outflow tract; RVOT, right outflow tract

the four-chamber view and the para-sagittal view, were necessary for a complete heart study, since the para-sagittal plane provided the left outflow tract in all cases (Table 2). The quality of the heart views involving the center of the heart, such as the right and left outflow tracts, were adversely affected by fetal heart movements, generating motion artifacts. The IVC, SVC, aortic arch and ductal arch views were the least affected by fetal heart movements.

Although many heart views were obtained in a majority of cases by manipulating one or two acquisition planes, image quality would have been improved with gating. In some cases there were problems with shadowing from the fetal ribs during volume acquisition, as the beam swept through the fetal thorax. The computer-reconstructed coronal plane, a plane that is much utilized postnatally, demonstrated less than optimal resolution and was not used in our analysis.

Screening of CHD thus can be based on one or two acquisition views, obtaining cardiac views not readily obtained in 2D ultrasound, owing to fetal position. Even non-standard fetal heart acquisition planes may provide valuable information on heart anatomy.

Zosmer and colleagues[12] studied the feasibility of

Table 1 Comparison of the heart views obtained with two-dimensional versus three-dimensional ultrasound

	Two-dimensional (n=16)		Three-dimensional (n=16)	
	n	%	n	%
Four-chamber view	15	93	15	93
Left outflow tract	11	68	14	87
Right outflow tract	11	68	16	100
Aortic arch	2	12	14	87
Ductal arch	3	18	16	100
Pulmonary artery and branches	2	12	10	62
Inferior and superior vena cava	4	25	14	87

Table 2 Comparison of the three-dimensional ultrasound-derived heart views from three acquisition planes

	Three-dimensional ultrasound							
	Four-chamber view (n=15)		Para-sagittal view (n=7)		Transverse view (n=13)		Sagittal view (n=3)	
	n	%	n	%	n	%	n	%
Four-chamber view	15	100	3	42	8	61	1	33
Left outflow tract	7	46	7	100	7	53	2	66
Right outflow tract	13	86	5	71	9	69	2	66
Aortic arch	10	66	4	57	9	69	1	33
Ductal arch	13	86	5	71	11	84	2	66
Pulmonary artery and branches	8	53	2	28	3	23	1	33
Inferior and superior vena cava	12	80	6	85	5	38	2	66

3D ultrasound in fetal echocardiography in 54 healthy pregnant women. Two volumes were obtained and analyzed in a four-chamber acquisition plane (apical and lateral), analyzing only volumes with a clear four-chamber view. In this study the aortic arch was very difficult to identify, so it was excluded from the study. Their best results were obtained between 22 and 27 weeks, when the four-chamber view and left outflow tract was visualized in 93% of cases. The lateral volumes were less successful than apical ones. They concluded that the method could improve screening for fetal cardiac anomalies. Our data regarding the views obtained from the four-chamber plane are similar, but in our study we included volumes acquired not only in the four-chamber plane alone but also in the parasagittal and incidental planes. Although we limited the scanning period to 10 min, we were able satisfactorily to identify the aortic arch in a significant number of patients.

Another study compared 2D and 3D ultrasound in imaging the standard heart views and concluded that 3D reconstructed non-cardiac-gated sonography yielded inadequate image quality for basic echocardiography views[13]. In this study, there was a significant difference among the interpreters of 3D ultrasound-derived heart views ranging from 10 to 71%; this may have resulted from differences in the fetal heart reformatting method or the ability to work with reformatted volume data.

Gated techniques of 3D ultrasonography of the fetal heart have also been studied[14,15]. Nine fetuses were scanned using a 2D system with an electromagnetic position sensor mounted to the transducer. The data were analyzed off-line using a computer graphics workstation. The volumes were acquired with free-hand sweeps through the fetal heart in transverse or sagittal orientation. Cardiac gating was performed off-line using a temporal Fourier transform. Two-dimensional imaging provided fairly complete imaging of the fetal heart. Non-gated 3D ultrasound provided visualization of some structures not demonstrated with 2D ultrasound. Gated 3D ultrasound provided better visualization and comprehension of 3D anatomy, derived from the ability to view cardiac motion. Although gated 3D ultrasound shows great potential, the technique is not yet commercially available. The gating method used is still time-consuming, performed off-line in a graphics workstation, and requires information from two transducers, one for the volume acquisition and one for gating. Hopefully this crucial issue will be solved in the near future by special software and transducer design.

Real-time 3D ultrasound has demonstrated fewer artifacts compared to the conventional 3D reconstruction methods. Recently, some preliminary work with real-time 3D fetal echocardiography has been reported[16]. Ten fetuses, four of which had congenital heart defects, were scanned with a real-time 3D ultrasound system (Volumetric Medical Imaging, Durham, NC) using a 2D phased array probe, scanning a pyramidal volume at 20 volumes/s. High acquisition speed permits assessment of the dynamic behavior of the contractility and valve motion. Cardiac motion could be slowed, stopped or viewed at its original speed. This approach seems to overcome some of the problems encountered with conventional 2D and 3D ultrasound systems with respect to gating and random movements while preserving the benefits of volume scanning, which allows selection of planes.

Although there remain difficulties with the 3D ultrasound technique, we believe that this is a useful method for screening fetal heart views and that it assists in training for fetal echocardiography. Improvements in resolution, faster acquisition times and gating will be necessary to improve the study of the fetal heart. It remains to be shown whether multi-planar 3D ultrasound, when applied in large-scale fetal heart screening, would provide the same or higher confidence and accuracy in the detection of fetal heart malformations than conventional 2D ultrasound.

Networking

Interpretation of fetal echocardiography examinations often requires expertise not available at the primary clinical site. A potential benefit of 3D ultrasound lies in ultrasound documentation, storage and networking. Volumes of heart data can be readily copied, transferred and stored in digital format in removable cartridges or directly in the hard disk of central workstations through DICOM connections. These volume data can be analyzed interactively after the patient has been discharged. Volume data can be compressed, encrypted for security and sent over the Internet through different formats (still images as tiff or jpeg files, a sequence of surface-rendered images in motion as an AVI file, or as compressed volume data.)

Research is needed to determine the advantages and limitations of fetal heart volume data transfer across networks and off-line interpretation. The role of 3D fetal echocardiography is not yet firmly established, but there is no doubt that it will have a substantial impact on the way fetal echocardiography is performed. Through this technology, primary clinical sites in remote areas may have access to expert consultation and off-line interpretation, enabling high quality and cost-effective medical care. The digitally stored heart volumes can be accessed and analyzed, also facilitating training in fetal echocardiography.

Conclusion

With its ability to reconstruct power or color information in 3D display, this technology has great applications in studying the fetal cardiovascular system. In several 3D ultrasound systems, great efforts are being made towards faster acquisition periods with the goal of real-time gray scale and color scanning, which would further improve fetal heart imaging[17].

Three-dimensional ultrasound information is based on compilation and manipulation of conventional 2D ultrasound data. As with 2D ultrasound, factors affecting resolution must be considered. The coronal planes (which are computer-reconstructed planes) have weaker lateral resolution. Volumes are still prone to motion artifacts due to maternal respiration, fetal respiration and fetal movements. Despite recent improvements in faster volume acquisition, lighter probes, electronic scalpelling, etc., there is a need for higher resolution, better software performance and automatic volume measurements. Although this new modality is a great technological improvement in medical imaging, it will not make up for poor scanning technique, poor resolution due to maternal body habitus, or oligohydramnios. In order to be able to acquire clinically useful information and work with fetal heart volume ultrasound data displayed in a multiplanar format, additional training and experience is required. The acquisition of the heart volumes should be in specific anatomic planes, preferably in the four-chamber view, in order to yield the maximum information with optimal resolution. Research is still ongoing to establish techniques for optimal acquisition and planar reformatting of volume data in standard anatomic planes, as well as its application for general heart screening.

References

1. Hoffman JIE, Christianson R. Congenital heart disease in a cohort of 19,502 births with long-term follow up. *Am J Cardiol* 1978;42:641
2. American Institute of Ultrasound in Medicine. *Guidelines for Obstetrical Scans.* Bethesda, MD: American Institute of Ultrasound in Medicine, 1991
3. Sharlan GK, Allan LD. Screening for congenital heart disease prenatally. Results of 2½ year study in the South-East Region. *Br J Obstet Gynaecol* 1992;99:220
4. DeVore G. The aortic and pulmonary outflow tract screening examination in the fetus. *J Ultrasound Med* 1992;11:345
5. Ewingman BG, Crane JP, Frigoletto FD, LeFevre ML, Bain RP, McNellis D. Effect of prenatal ultrasound on perinatal outcome. *N Engl J Med* 1993;329:821–7
6. Crane JP, LeFevre ML, Winborn RC, et al. Randomized trial of prenatal ultrasound screening: impact on detection, management and outcome of anomalous fetuses. *Am J Obstet Gynecol* 1994;171:392–9
7. Merz E, Bahlmann F, Weber G. Volume scanning in the evaluation of fetal malformations: a new dimension in prenatal diagnosis. *Ultrasound Obstet Gynecol* 1995;5:222–7
8. Deng J, Gardener JE, Rodeck CH, Lees WR. Fetal echocardiography in three and four dimensions. *Ultrasound Med Biol* 1996;22:979–86
9. Kwon J, Shaffer E, Shandas R, et al. Acquisition of three-dimensional fetal echocardiograms using an external trigger source. *J Am Soc Echocardiogr* 1996;9:389
10. Nelson TR, Pretorius DH, Sklansky M, Hagen-Ansert S. Three-dimensional echocardiographic evaluation of fetal heart anatomy and function: acquisition, analysis, and display. *J Ultrasound Med* 1996;15:1–9
11. Bega G, Kuhlman K, Lev-Toaff A, Kurtz A. Fetal heart screening by three dimensional multiplanar ultrasound. Proceedings of Annual Meeting of the American Institute of Ultrasound in Medicine, San Antonio, Texas, March 1999. *J Ultrasound Med* 1999;18:S132
12. Zosmer N, Jurkovic D, Jauniaux E, Gruboeck K, Lees C, Campbell S. Selection and identification of standard cardiac views from three-dimensional volume scans of the fetal thorax. *J Ultrasound Med* 1996;15:25–32
13. Leventhal M, Pretorius D, Budorick N, et al. Three-dimensional ultrasonography of the normal fetal heart: comparison with two-dimensional imaging. *J Ultrasound Med* 1998;17:341–8
14. Sklansky MS, Nelson TR, Pretorius DH. Three-dimensional fetal echocardiography: gated versus nongated techniques. *J Ultrasound Med* 1995;17:451–7
15. Sklansky MS, Nelson TR, Pretorius DH. Usefulness of gated three-dimensional fetal echocardiography to reconstruct and display structures not visualized with two-dimensional imaging. *Am J Cardiol* 1997;80:665–8
16. Sklansky MS, Nelson TR, Strachan M, Pretorius DH. Real-time three-dimensional fetal echocardiography: initial feasibility study. *J Ultrasound Med* 1999;18:745–52
17. Belohlavek M, Foley DA, Gerber TC, et al. Three- and four-dimensional cardiovascular ultrasound imaging: a new era for echocardiography. *Mayo Clin Proc* 1993;68:221–40

Three-dimensional power Doppler in the study of placental and umbilical cord abnormalities

A. D. Hull and D. H. Pretorius

Three-dimensional (3D) ultrasound is beginning to enter everyday practice in a variety of settings. As yet, there is no large body of scientific evidence supporting its general superiority over conventional two-dimensional (2D) scanning. Nonetheless, there are some specific areas in which 3D ultrasound has clear advantages over 2D ultrasound, such as imaging of the fetal face[1] and spine[2]. One area in which 3D ultrasound seems to afford advantages over 2D ultrasound is in the imaging of abnormalities of the placenta and cord. This is especially true when the multiplanar capability of 3D ultrasound is combined with dynamic assessment of blood flow using power or color flow Doppler. We have recently had considerable success using 3D ultrasound coupled with power Doppler in the imaging of patients with invasive placentation[3], abnormal placental cord insertion and vasa previa.

Placental invasion

Invasive placentation (placenta accreta, increta and percreta) has become a much more common entity in North American practice in the past decade[4]. The reasons for this are unclear, although an increased Cesarean section rate coupled with changes in surgical technique for uterine closure are possible factors. The well-known association between prior uterine scarring, placenta previa and invasive placentation, has been well explored[5]. There is as yet no 'gold standard' for the diagnosis of invasive placentation, although suggestive sonographic features have been identified (Table 1). The diagnostic role of alternative imaging techniques such as magnetic resonance imaging (MRI) is unclear[6].

We have recently reported a case in which 3D ultrasound coupled with color Doppler imaging allowed a more accurate diagnosis of placenta percreta to be made prior to surgery[3]. We have since seen several patients in whom the use of 3D ultrasound with color flow and power Doppler imaging allowed refinement of the diagnosis of placental invasion, correctly predicting placenta percreta with bladder invasion. Figure 1 shows one of these patients imaged at 33 weeks' gestation. Power Doppler showed an abnormal pattern of blood flow in the area between the base of the bladder and the placenta, with flow bridging the placental substance. Surgery confirmed bladder invasion. A similar case is shown in Figure 2, here imaged at 26 weeks' gestation. Again, there is no recognizable tissue plane between the bladder and the placenta, and power Doppler shows a markedly increased and chaotic pattern of blood flow in the area between the base of the bladder and the placenta. The degree of

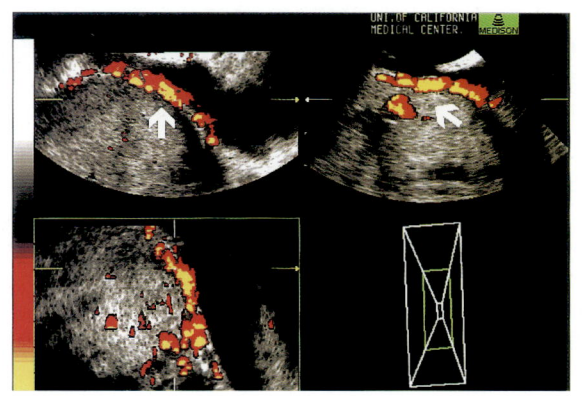

Figure 1 Placenta percreta involving the bladder. Multiplanar images of the placenta and bladder at 33 weeks' gestation obtained by transvaginal scanning. Three perpendicular planes are shown in the upper left, upper right and lower left images. There is loss of normal tissue margins between the placenta and bladder. Power Doppler shows a markedly increased and chaotic pattern of blood flow in the area between the base of the bladder and the placenta. Flow is seen to bridge the placental substance (arrows)

Table 1 Gray-scale sonographic criteria for suspicion of placental invasion

Loss of the retroplacental hypoechoic myometrial zone
Presence of numerous vascular lacunae within the placental substance
Thinning or disruption of the linear hyperechoic boundary echo,
  representing the uterine serosa and its interface with the posterior wall of the bladder
Focal nodular projections beyond the expected plane of the uterine margin

CLINICAL APPLICATION OF 3D SONOGRAPHY

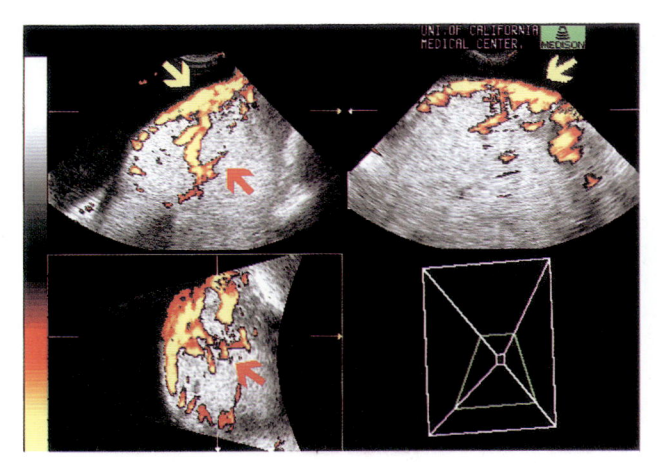

Figure 2 Placenta percreta involving the bladder. Multiplanar images of the placenta and bladder at 26 weeks' gestation obtained by transvaginal scanning. Three perpendicular planes are shown in the upper left, upper right and lower left images. There is no recognizable tissue plane between the bladder and the placenta. Power Doppler shows a markedly increased and chaotic pattern of blood flow in the area between the base of the bladder and the placenta. This is most notable in the area marked by the yellow arrows; the placenta was found to be deeply invasive at this site at Cesarean hysterectomy. An abnormal pattern of bridging flow is again seen (red arrows)

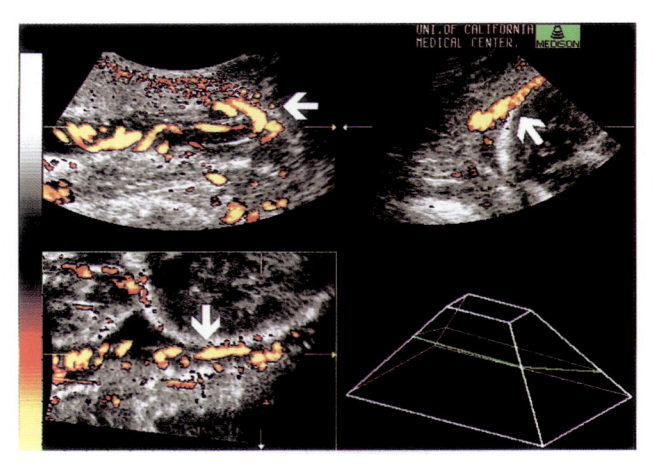

Figure 3 Velamentous placental cord insertion. Multiplanar images of the placenta and cord at 30 weeks' gestation obtained transabdominally. Three perpendicular planes are shown in the upper left, upper right and lower left images. Power Doppler shows that the umbilical cord ramifies through the membranes before becoming inserted into the placental margin (arrows)

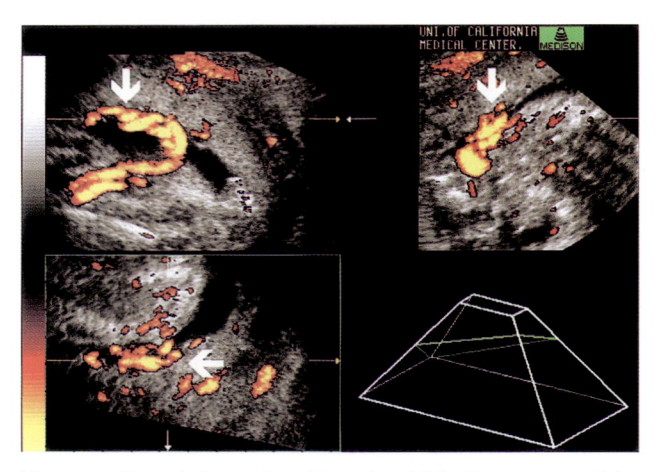

Figure 4 Normal placental cord insertion. Multiplanar images of the placenta and cord at 23 weeks' gestation obtained transabdominally. Three perpendicular planes are shown in the upper left, upper right and lower left images. Power Doppler shows that the umbilical cord is inserted at least 3 cm from the placental margin (arrows)

bladder invasion found at surgery in this case necessitated a partial cystectomy. It is important to recognize that the first suspicion of placental invasion in both these cases arose from conventional 2D gray-scale imaging. Subsequent color and power Doppler studies further refined the diagnosis; however, 3D ultrasound with power Doppler provided convincing evidence of the degree of placental invasion. We feel that the multiplanar capability of 3D ultrasound imaging, which allows structures to be visualized from multiple viewpoints simultaneously, is the key to its utility. One is able to 'step through' the placenta and adjacent structures in a series of slices, to view those sections from sagittal, coronal and transverse planes at the same time and thereby gain a more coherent view of the degree of placental invasion present. Since the mortality and morbidity associated with invasive placentation increases significantly with the degree of invasion present, correct diagnosis is central to appropriate management and surgical planning.

Placental cord insertion

Velamentous cord insertion is associated with fetal growth restriction[7,8], an increased risk of congenital defects[9] and preterm delivery[8]. Because of this we have made it part of our routine practice to identify placental cord insertion in all patients undergoing routine obstetric ultrasound examination. Since marginal cord insertions (where the placental cord insertion site is less than 2 cm from the placental edge) are at risk of evolving into velamentous insertions[10], they are also identified and followed. The sensitivity of identification of abnormal placental cord insertion with conventional 2D ultrasound, with and without color or power Doppler imaging, has been reported to range from 42%[10] to 69%[11], although the specificity in the same studies was high (95% and 100%, respectively). We have found 3D ultrasound coupled with power Doppler imaging useful in the clarification of abnormalities suspected using conventional imaging.

Figure 3 shows an example of a velamentous cord insertion at 30 weeks' gestation. The use of multiplanar imaging makes it easy to track the cord as it ramifies through the membranes prior to its insertion into the placenta. This is difficult to show in a static image

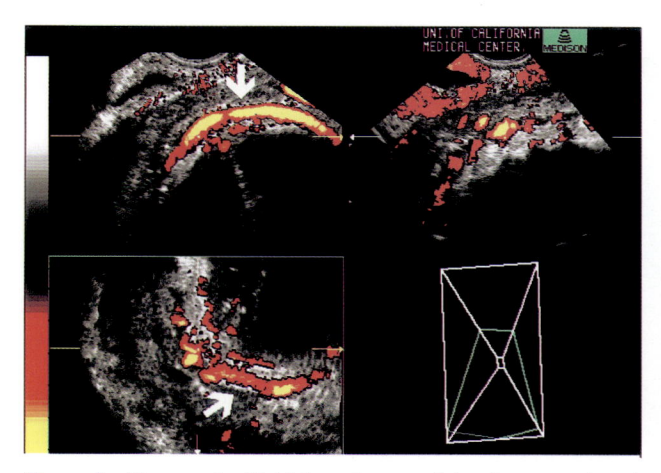

Figure 5 Vasa previa. Multiplanar images of the placenta and cord vessels at 30 weeks' gestation obtained transvaginally. Three perpendicular planes are shown in the upper left, upper right and lower left images. Power Doppler clearly demonstrates cord vessels running through the membranes below the fetal head (arrows)

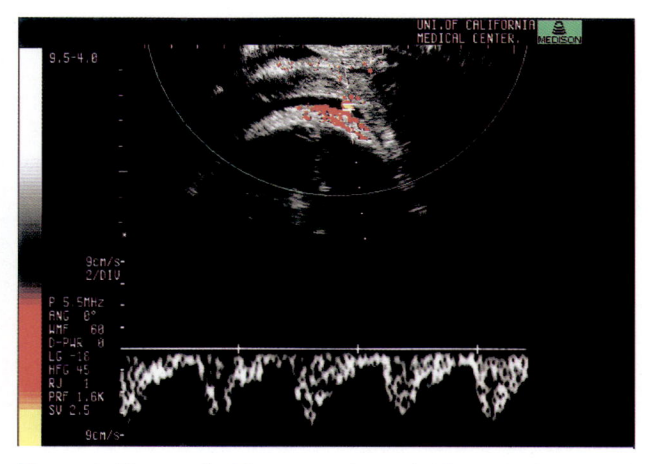

Figure 6 Vasa previa. The same patient as in Figure 5, also scanned transvaginally. Simultaneous power Doppler and spectral Doppler imaging of fetal vessels running through membranes below the fetal head. The characteristic umbilical artery waveform is clearly seen

but is an easy task to accomplish if one scrolls through the saved volume data. In contrast, Figure 4 shows a normal cord insertion in a patient previously identifed as having a marginal cord insertion on a 12-week scan. This emphasizes the need to follow up abnormalities suspected on early studies.

Vasa previa

Perhaps one of the most tragic causes of fetal loss is fetal hemorrhage secondary to vasa previa. At least 75% of cases of vasa previa are associated with placenta bipartita or a succinturiate lobe. Therefore, simply identifying a normal placental cord insertion site does not guarantee that a vasa previa is not present. A high level of suspicion is needed in order to make a prenatal diagnosis of vasa previa. It has been suggested that all patients at high risk of vasa previa (those with bipartite, low-lying and succinturiate-lobed placentae, *in vitro* fertilization (IVF) pregnancies, velamentous cord insertions and multiple gestations) should be aggressively screened for vasa previa[12]. The literature contains several cases of vasa previa identified antenatally, most commonly by transvaginal sonography with color Doppler. A recent prospective study[13] points to the utility of this approach with all three cases of vasa previa correctly identified in a population of 45 women at risk.

We have taken the opportunity of performing 3D ultrasound studies with power Doppler in several recent patients thought to have vasa previa from examination with standard 2D ultrasound and color flow Doppler imaging. One such study is shown in Figures 5 and 6. This was a patient at 30 weeks' gestation with a normal placental cord insertion and a succinturiate lobe identified on routine scanning. Subsequent transvaginal ultrasound examination suggested vasa previa, which was confirmed with 3D ultrasound and power Doppler. Although the diagnosis was readily made using conventional imaging, 3D ultrasound enabled full evaluation of the extent of the vasa previa to be made with ease. The multiplanar capability of 3D ultrasound is extremely useful in such cases.

Clearly, the combination of 3D ultrasound and power Doppler constitutes a powerful diagnostic tool. Its place in the evaluation of the placenta and umbilical cord will become settled as greater experience is gained.

References

1. Hull AD, Pretorius DH. Fetal face: what we can see using two-dimensional and three-dimensional ultrasound imaging. *Semin Roentgenol* 1998;33:369–74
2. Johnson DD, *et al*. Three-dimensional ultrasound of the fetal spine. *Obstet Gynecol* 1997;89:434–8
3. Hull AD, *et al*. Three-dimensional ultrasonography and diagnosis of placenta percreta with bladder involvement. *J Ultrasound Med* 1999;18:853–6
4. Miller DA, Chollet JA, Goodwin TM. Clinical risk factors for placenta previa–placenta accreta. *Am J Obstet Gynecol* 1997;177:210–4
5. Clark SL, Koonings PP, Phelan JP. Placenta previa/accreta and prior cesarean section. *Obstet Gynecol* 1985;66:89–92
6. Levine D, *et al*. Placenta accreta: evaluation with color Doppler US, power Doppler US, and MR imaging. *Radiology* 1997;205:773–6
7. Eddleman KA. *et al*. Clinical significance and sonographic diagnosis of velamentous umbilical cord insertion. *Am J Perinatol* 1992;9:123–6
8. Heinonen S, *et al*. Perinatal diagnostic evaluation of velamentous umbilical cord insertion: clinical, Doppler, and ultrasonic findings. *Obstet Gynecol* 1996;87:112–17
9. Robinson LK, Jones KL, Benirschke K. The nature of structural defects associated with velamentous and marginal insertion of the umbilical cord. *Am J Obstet Gynecol* 1983;146:191–3
10. Pretorius DH, *et al*. Placental cord insertion visualization with prenatal ultrasonography. *J Ultrasound Med*, 1996;15:585–93
11. Di Salvo DN, *et al*. Sonographic evaluation of the placental cord insertion site. *Am J Roentgenol* 1998;170:1295–8
12. Oyelese KO, *et al*. Vasa previa: an avoidable obstetric tragedy. *Obstet Gynecol Surv* 1999;54:138–45
13. Mâegier P, Gorin V, Desroches A. Ultrasonography of placenta previa at the third trimester of research for signs of placenta accreta/percreta and vasa previa. Prospective color and pulsed Doppler ultrasonography study of 45. *J Gynecol Obstet Biol Reprod* 1999;28:239–44

Fetal brain assessment by three-dimensional ultrasound

R. K. Pooh

Introduction

The fetal central nervous system (CNS) dramatically changes its appearance during pregnancy[1], and its three-dimensional (3D) form should be understood in the basic sagittal, coronal and axial planes. In postnatal life, magnetic resonance imaging (MRI) and computed tomography (CT) have been commonly used for assessment of CNS 3D morphology and circulation (Figure 1). The 3D method should be adopted in antenatal evaluation of the fetal CNS for comprehending the anatomical orientation and for easy identification of lesions.

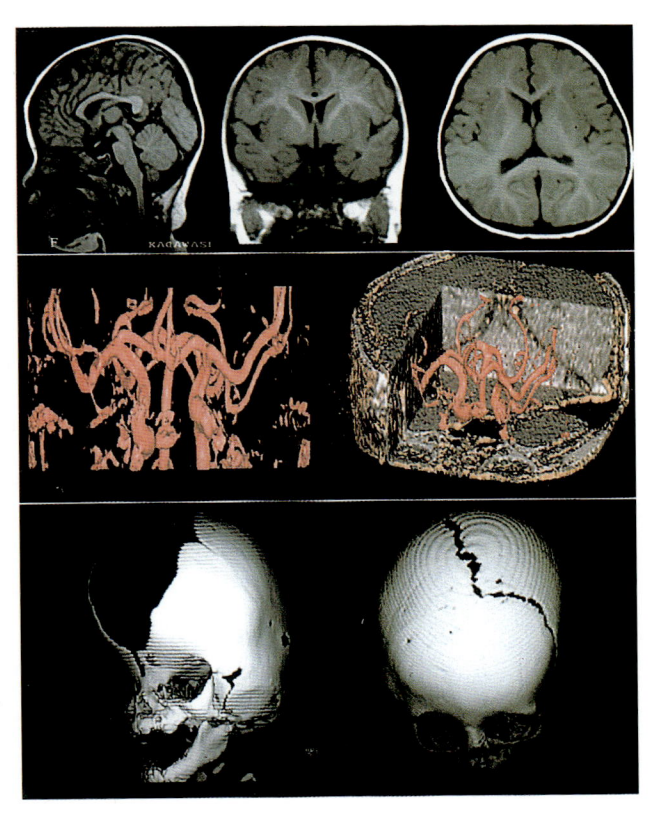

Figure 1 Postnatal assessment of the brain and head. Magnetic resonance imaging (upper panel) demonstrates sagittal, coronal and axial sections of a normal infant brain. Intracranial structures can be assessed by parallel sections of those basic three planes. Recent three-dimensional (3D) computed tomography (CT) angiography (middle panel) shows a clear image of the 3D brain circulatory system. Three-dimensional reconstructed CT of the skull (lower panel) demonstrates fusions of the cranial sutures

Fetal calvarial structure by two- and three-dimensional ultrasound

The frontal, parietal and occipital bones of the skull are separated from each other by the sutures and fontanelles. Some previous reports on anatomical and embryonic studies showed the early development of the calvaria and sutures. The calvaria and its major sutures develop at 12–18 weeks of fetal life by the dura's guiding tissue in the morphogenesis of the skull. Overlying the central zones between the dural reflections, ossification takes place, whereas none occurs over the reflections of the dura, these being the suture sites[2]. The assessment of calvarial development is important, because many congenital craniofacial abnormalities exist, such as craniosynostosis, and embryonic studies have not established the crucial period of cranial fusion[3].

Cranial formation is detectable in some cases at 10 and 11 weeks' gestation, and in most cases from 12 weeks. The sagittal suture is first recognized at 13 weeks as a short, wide space between parietal bones. At 12 weeks, the metopic suture is recognizable as a very short space between the bilateral orbits, and the wide anterior fontanelle occupies most of the cranium from the top of the head to the forehead. Between 13 and 17 weeks of gestation, the metopic suture is rapidly formed as a linear suture with development of the bilateral frontal bones. The calvarial formation, observed by two-dimensional (2D) ultrasound with a tangential approach to the fetal skull[4], is shown in Figure 2. The fetal cranial bone formation can be objectively and intelligibly demonstrated by 3D ultrasound with surface rendering[5] (Figure 3).

Cranial sutures and fontanelles play an important role as ultrasound windows for fetal brain observation. Considering the width and anatomical location of sutures and fontanelles, the sagittal suture and anterior/posterior fontanelle are the most appropriate ultrasound windows for sonographic assessment of the fetal intracranial structure[5]. Therefore, the transvaginal approach to the fetal brain via those windows from the fetal parietal direction is the most reasonable for fetal CNS assessment.

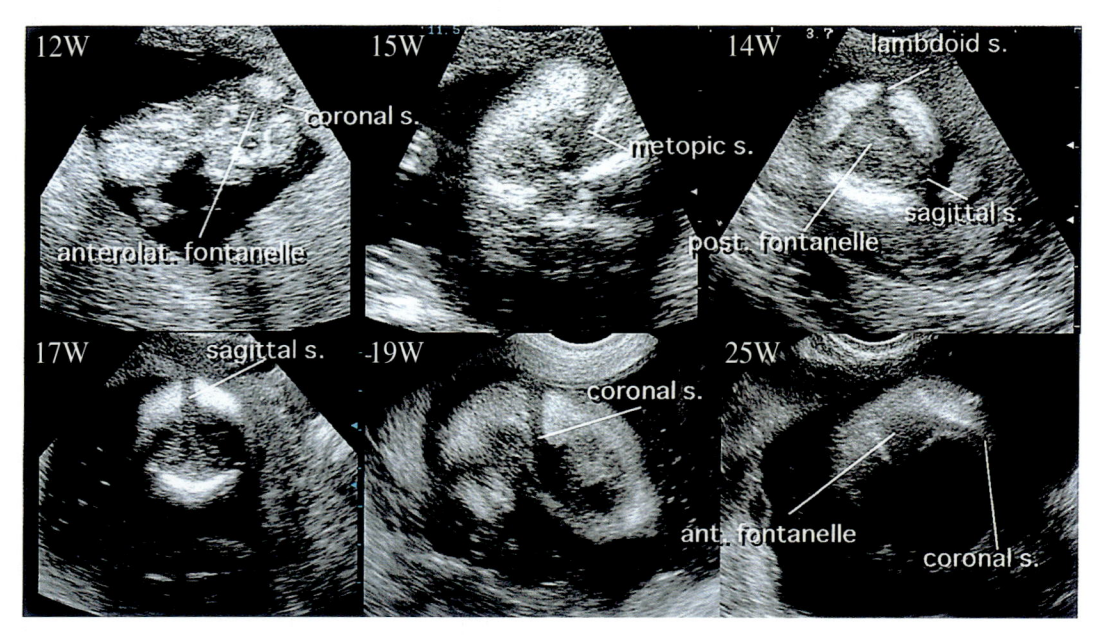

Figure 2 Fetal calvarial structure detected by two-dimensional (2D) ultrasound. Tangential planes of the fetal skull by 2D ultrasound demonstrate the sagittal, coronal, metopic and lambdoid sutures, and the anterior, posterior and anterolateral fontanelles in the first and second trimesters

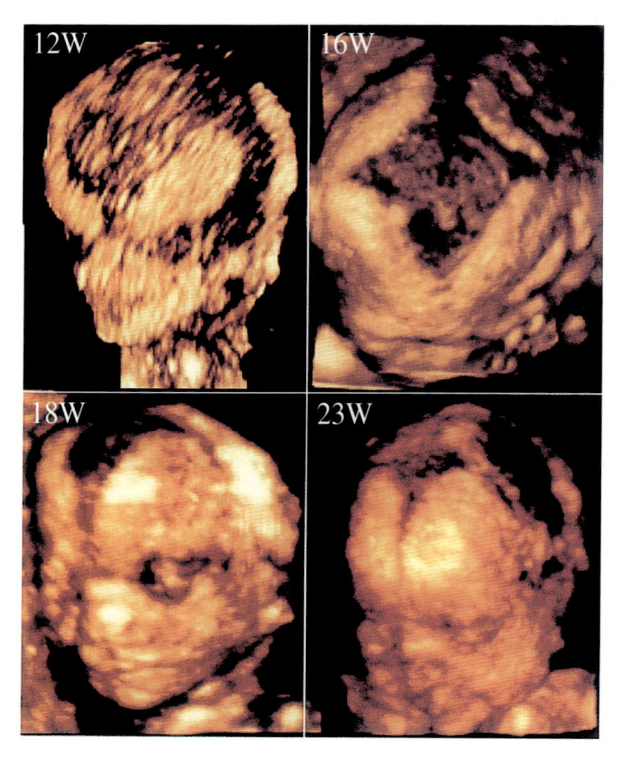

Figure 3 Fetal calvarial formation demonstrated by three-dimensional (3D) ultrasound. Surface mode of 3D ultrasound objectively and intelligibly demonstrates the skull development during pregnancy. The appearance of calvarial sutures and fontanelles changes according to cranial bone development

Fetal brain assessment by transvaginal two-dimensional sonography

The introduction of the high-frequency transvaginal transducer has established the new field of sonoembryology[6]. Detailed sonographic appearances of the developing fetal CNS in early pregnancy have been studied[7–9]. In 1989, the first case of intracranial abnormality diagnosed by the vaginal transducer in the second trimester was reported[10]. As the first practical application of 3D CNS assessment, the transvaginal approach to the normal fetal brain during the second and third trimesters was introduced in the beginning of the 1990s[11]. Transvaginal observation of the fetal brain can produce the sagittal and coronal views of the brain from the fetal parietal direction[12–16], and sonographic images through the fontanelles and/or the sagittal suture demonstrate the detailed structure (Figure 4). This method has contributed to the establishment of the new field of neurosonography[14]. The prenatal sonographic assessment of not only congenital CNS anomalies but also acquired brain damage *in utero* has progressed remarkably (Figure 5), compared with the capabilities of the conventional transabdominal method.

FETAL BRAIN ASSESSMENT BY THREE-DIMENSIONAL ULTRASOUND

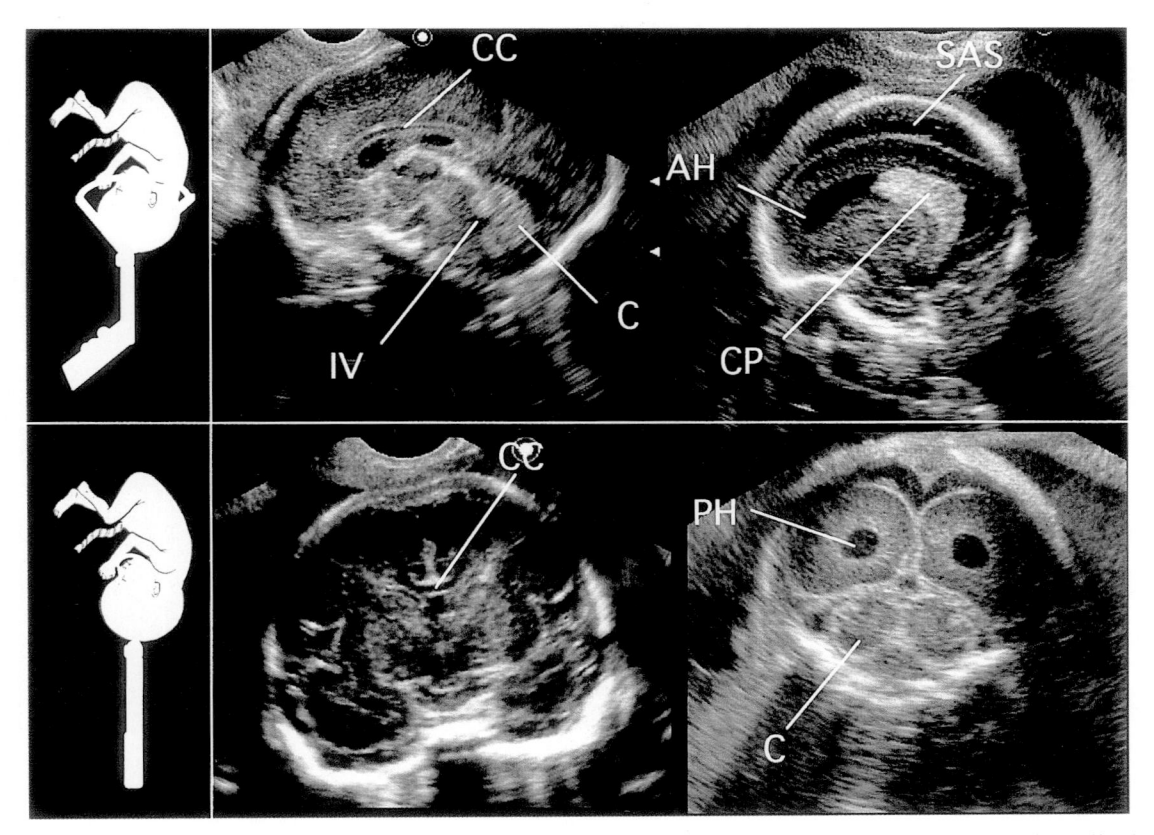

Figure 4 Normal fetal brain structure (transvaginal two-dimensional sonography). Sonographic images through the fontanelles and/or the sagittal suture demonstrate detailed brain structure. CC, corpus callosum; IV, forth ventricle; C, cerebellum; AH, anterior horn of lateral ventricle; CP, choroid plexus of lateral ventricle; SAS, subarachnoid space; PH, posterior horn of lateral ventricle

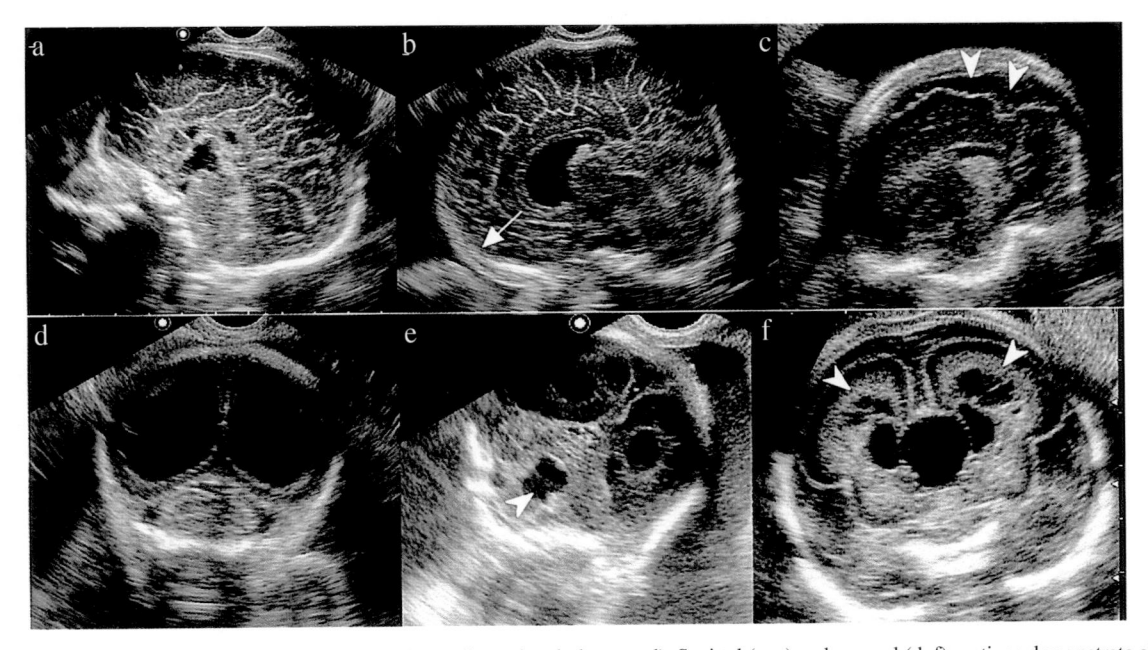

Figure 5 Abnormal fetal brain structure (transvaginal two-dimensional ultrasound). Sagittal (a–c) and coronal (d–f) sections demonstrate abnormal morphology of the fetal brain. (a) Agenesis of the corpus callosum (37 weeks); radiated formation of cerebral sulci associated with absence of the corpus callosum. (b) Intracranial structure in a case of craniosynostosis (35 weeks); deviation of the whole brain structure towards the forehead (arrow). (c) Brain atrophy after severe ischemia (27 weeks); atrophic cerebrum (arrowheads). (d) Symmetrical hydrocephalus (35 weeks); disappearance of the subarachnoid space associated with enlarged ventricles and compressed brain. (e) Defect of the cerebellar vermis (28 weeks) in a case of Dandy–Walker malformation. (f) Fetal periventricular leukomalacia (27 weeks); cystic formation (arrowheads) within a hyperechoic lesion

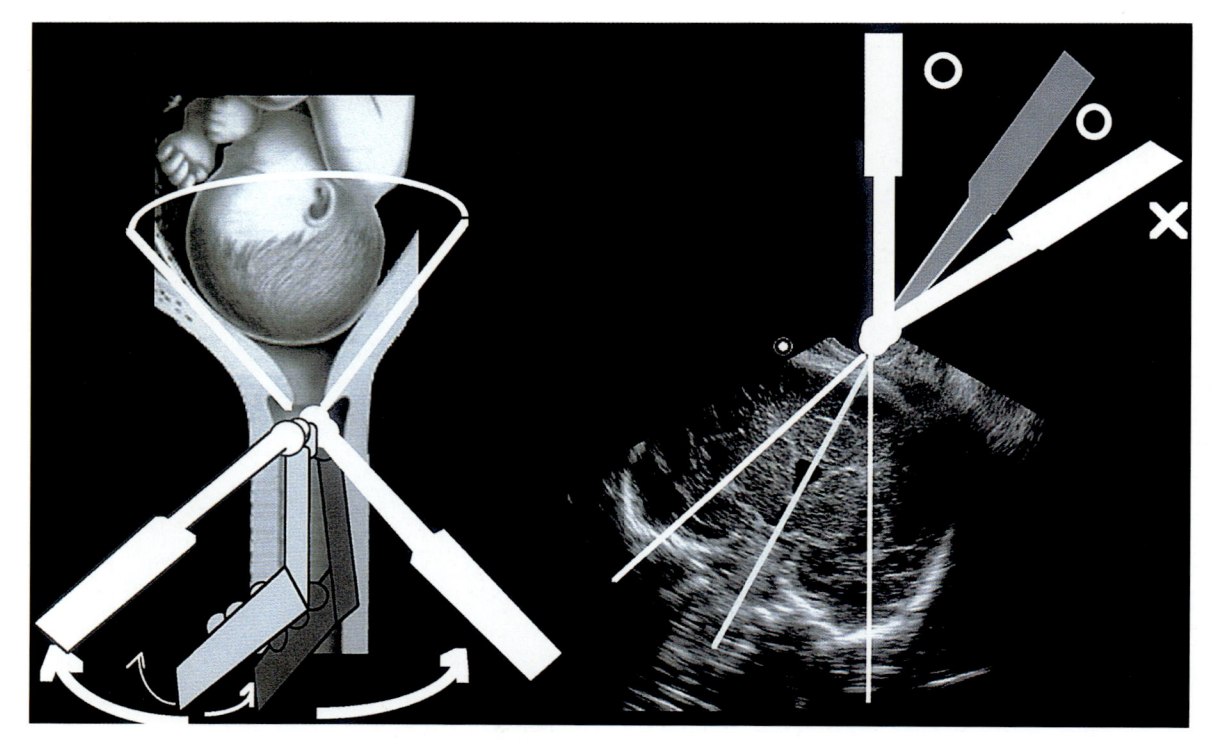

Figure 6 The limits of transvaginal two-dimensional assessment of the fetal brain in motion of the transducer shaft due to the narrow space of the vagina (left); and when the fetal head is located in the oblique position to the vaginal transducer (right), when it is sometimes impossible to obtain information on the whole brain

The limits of transvaginal two-dimensional assessment

In the practical evaluation of the fetal brain by transvaginal scanning, it is impossible to demonstrate parallel planes in the coronal and sagittal sections, which are usually used in CT and MRI. Transvaginal imaging of the fetal brain produces serial oblique sections[14] from the same ultrasound window, by shifting and changing the angle of the transducer. However, transvaginal 2D sonography has a limitation in the motion of the transducer shaft, owing to the narrow space of the vagina. It is sometimes impossible to obtain information on the whole brain when the fetal head is located in the oblique position to the vaginal transducer (Figure 6). For the accurate identification of brain structure and data storage, this method also requires considerable scanning time, well-trained technique and occasionally mothers' discomfort.

New CNS assessment method by transvaginal three-dimensional ultrasound

Recent advanced 3D ultrasound[17] has remarkably improved not only surface rendering but also multiplanar analysis of internal structures. Automatic scanning requires a few seconds for data acquisition without shifting of the transducer. Parallel slicing and rotating of serial scanning planes after automatic data acquisition can be used for objective visualization of internal morphology. The combination of both 3D ultrasound and the transvaginal approach to the fetal brain seems to solve the problems of 2D ultrasound mentioned above.

Before volume data acquisition, the fetal brain is observed in the 2D coronal or sagittal section via the cranial suture or fontanelles for localization. The region of interest for volume acquisition is set surrounding the brain structure. After setting up the transducer at the middle position of the fetal brain, automatic volume acquisition of the brain can be performed. This technology produces the volume data of the whole brain structure without shifting and/or changing the angle of the transducer. After scanning of the brain, it is possible to demonstrate not only the sagittal and coronal sections but also the axial sections of the brain, which cannot be demonstrated from the parietal direction in conventional 2D transvaginal sonography (Figure 7). Table 1 shows the acquisition time for the whole brain volume data from 15 to 40 weeks of gestation.

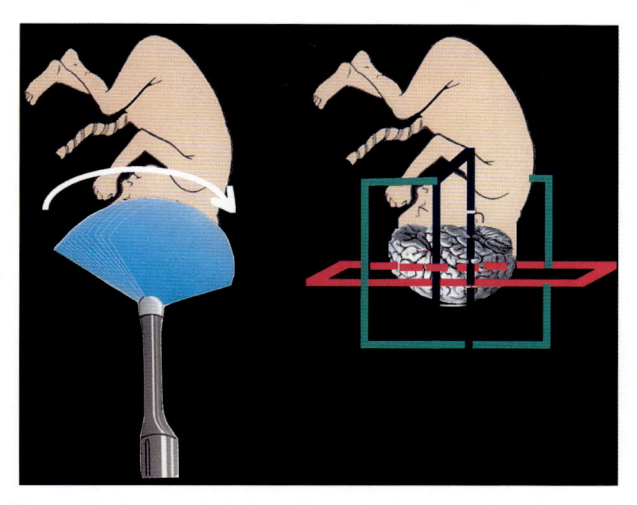

Figure 7 Transvaginal three-dimensional sonography of the fetal brain. After setting up the transducer at the middle position of the fetal brain, automatic volume acquisition of the brain is performed without shifting or angle-changing of the transducer (left). After the scanning of the brain, it is possible to demonstrate not only the sagittal and coronal sections but also the axial sections, which cannot be demonstrated from the parietal direction in a conventional two-dimensional transvaginal sonogram (right)

Table 1 Acquisition time for fetal brain volume

Gestational weeks	Acquisition time (s)
15	1.84
20	3.30
30	4.76
40	6.07

Advantages of transvaginal three-dimensional ultrasound

Transvaginal 3D sonography of the fetal brain enables us not only to obtain information on the whole brain, despite the short duration, but also to analyze the multiplanar brain structure off-line. Rotation of volume data is helpful in understanding the brain anatomy. Multiplanar image analysis (Figure 8) allows us to observe the brain in the parallel sagittal, coronal and axial sections in a similar way to MRI. Figure 9 shows multiplanar brain images in a case with congenital CNS abnormality.

Until 20 weeks of gestation, the fetal head is not always located in an appropriate position for brain

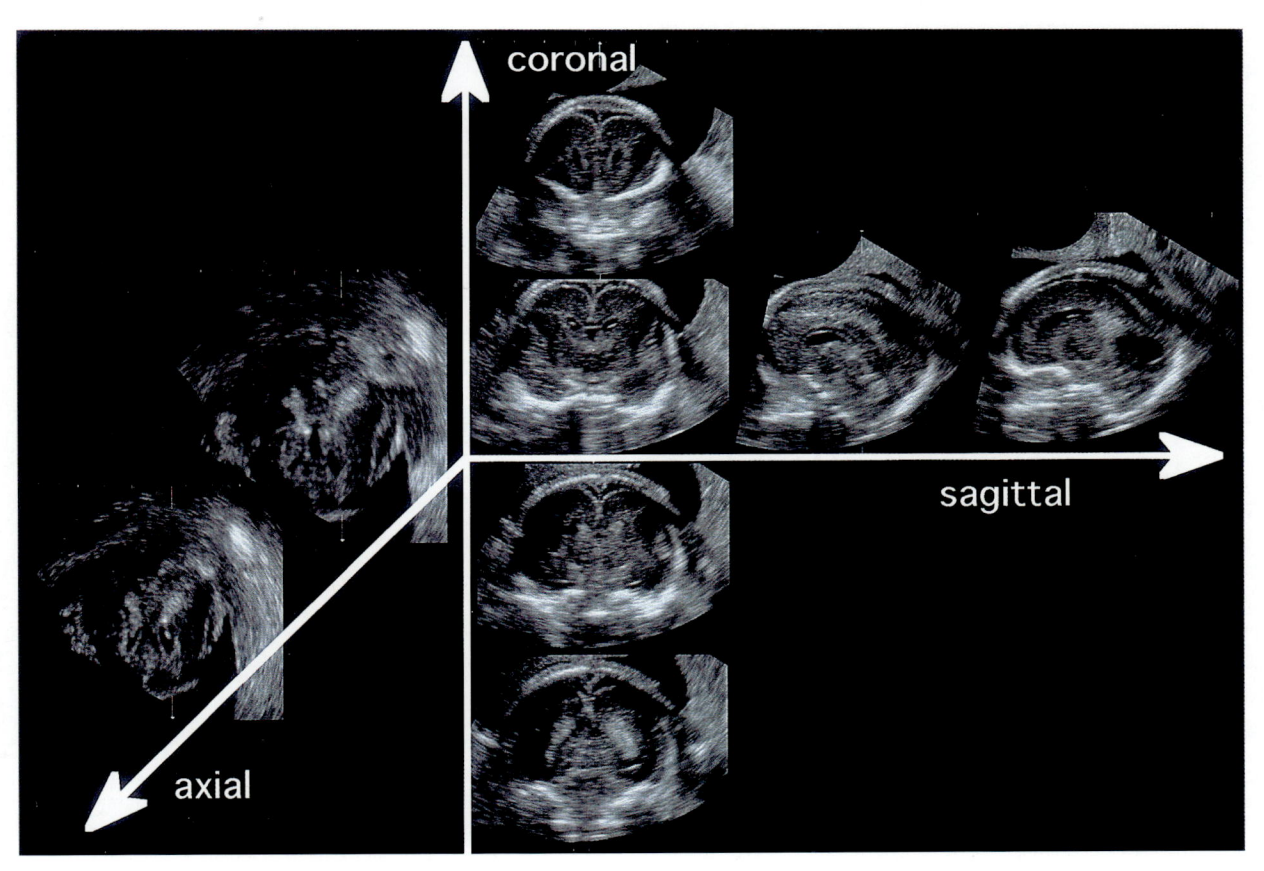

Figure 8 Multiplanar image analysis allows us to observe the normal brain in the parallel sections of the sagittal, coronal and axial planes in a similar way to magnetic resonance imaging

175

CLINICAL APPLICATION OF 3D SONOGRAPHY

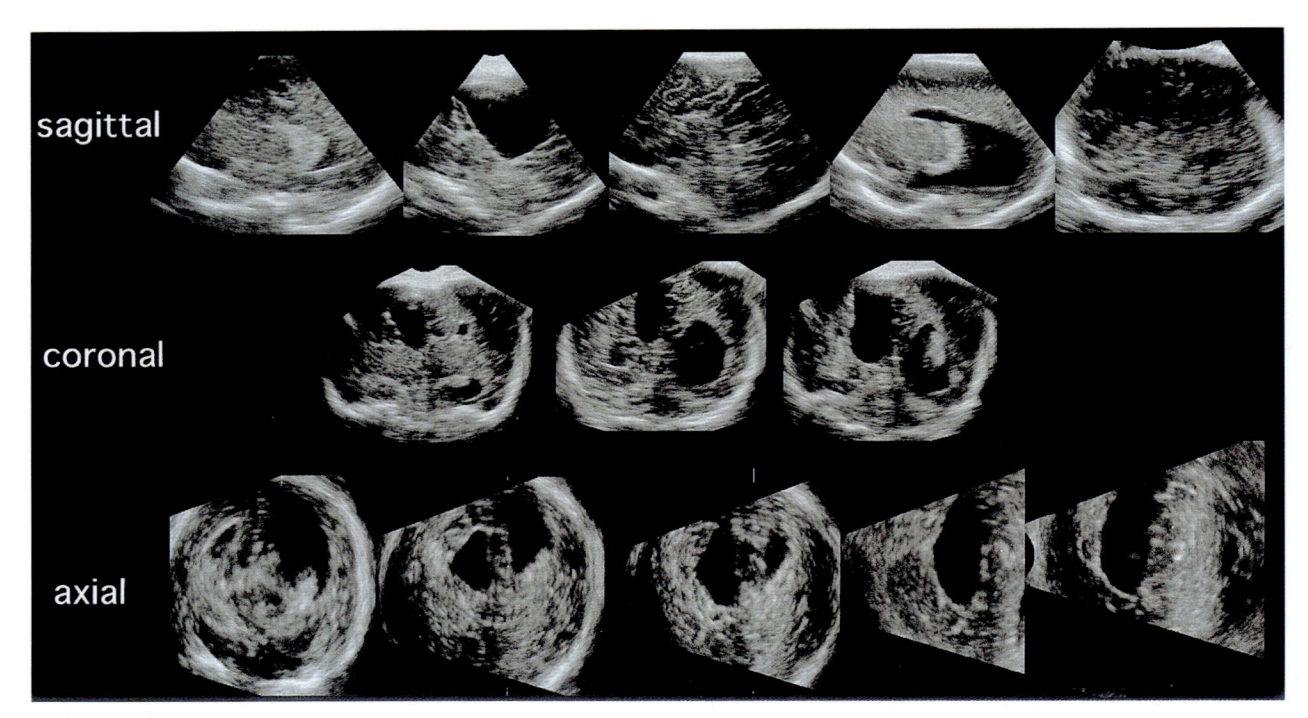

Figure 9 Multiplanar image analysis of congenital CNS abnormalities. Asymmetrical ventriculomegaly (colpocephaly) and interhemispheric cyst, associated with agenesis of the corpus callosum, are demonstrated in serial sections of sagittal, coronal and axial planes. The scanning time was approximately 5 s

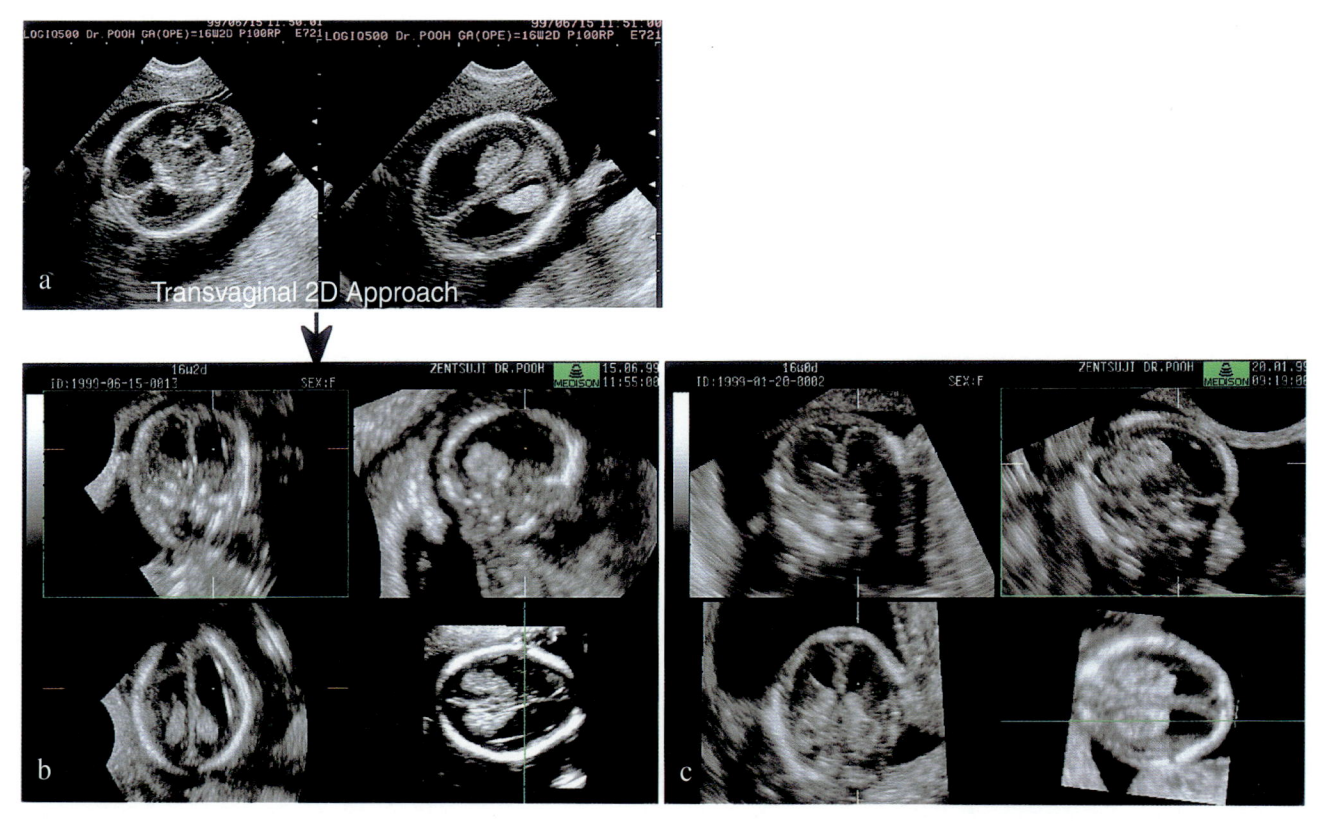

Figure 10 The usefulness of transvaginal three-dimensional (3D) ultrasound in the early second trimester. Even when only the axial plane can be observed by the two-dimensional (2D) transvaginal approach, owing to the fetal head position (a), rotating the brain after 3D volume acquisition produces the coronal and sagittal images (b). In this case, mild ventriculomegaly was suspected. Those images were compared with a normal image (c) in exactly the same section. Mild ventriculomegaly at the anterior horn and mild posterior deviation of the choroid plexus were confirmed

assessment from the parietal direction, because of fetal size and fetal active motion. Even when only the axial plane can be observed by the 2D transvaginal approach, owing to the fetal head position, rotating the brain after 3D volume acquisition produces the coronal and sagittal images (Figure 10). Furthermore, an abnormal brain image can be compared with a normal image in exactly the same section.

Pendulous examination by swinging the brain image demonstrates similar images to those of transfontanelle sonography in neonates (Figure 11). Without transvaginal probe shifting while scanning, brain structures can be observed in serial oblique sections.

Thus, this new method provides intelligible information despite a short scanning time, less complex technique and less discomfort for the mother. Furthermore, storage/extraction of volume data sets is quick and easy. Therefore, consultation with neurospecialists by using 3D volume data may be more objective than with conventional 2D images.

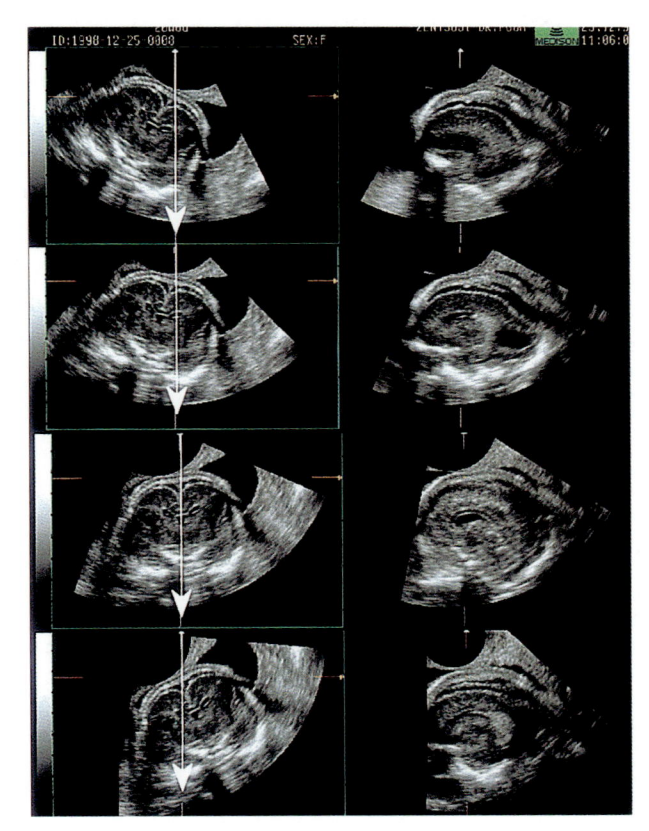

Figure 11 Off-line pendulous examination of the brain. By swinging the brain image, similar images to those of transfontanelle sonography can be obtained in fetuses and neonates. Without shifting of the transvaginal probe while scanning, the brain structure can be observed in serial oblique sections

Brain circulatory assessment by transvaginal three-dimensional ultrasound

Intracranial Doppler studies of the human fetus have been performed mainly by observation of the middle cerebral arteries, which can be easily depicted in the transabdominal axial section. However, according to the anatomical location of the brain vessels, the circle of Willis, the source of the cerebral arteries and the transverse sinus can be demonstrated in the axial section, but many of the brain vessels must be demonstrated in the sagittal and coronal sections. Therefore, the transvaginal approach to the fetal brain also plays an important role in brain circulatory assessment. The combination of both the transvaginal approach to the fetal brain and color/power Doppler technology produces information on the intracranial circulatory system[18,19] as well as the transfontanelle approach to the neonatal brain. Transvaginal 2D angiography of the brain circulation gives us the presence of the cerebral vessels and their location. However, it is difficult to demonstrate the complex 3D structure of the brain vessels in a single 2D plane. For instance, the main stream and branches of the middle cerebral artery run in a different direction, and both main line and branches cannot be detected in the same coronal section.

Three-dimensional ultrasound with color/power Doppler has recently been introduced in prenatal diagnosis[20–22]. The neonatal brain circulation has also been elucidated by transfontanelle 3D power Doppler[23]. The combination of both transvaginal color/power Doppler and 3D ultrasound may contribute to fetal brain circulatory assessment.

The method of obtaining volume data of the brain circulation is almost the same as gray-scale volume acquisition. The automatic data acquisition of 3D color/power Doppler is performed by holding the transvaginal transducer at the middle position of the fetal head. The data acquisition time of the Doppler mode takes 15–25 s, which is much longer than the B-mode volume scan. Therefore, fetal head movement occasionally obstructs the smooth scanning of the Doppler volume data. After obtaining the vascular volume data, the brain vessels can be identified on the gray-scale brain structure by using multiplanar images, and 3D reconstruction images of color/power volume data show the well-oriented 3D brain vessels[24] (Figure 12). Since the 3D vascular image can be rotated in any direction, the vessels can be observed from the frontal, occipital, lateral, oblique, parietal or basilar part of the brain.

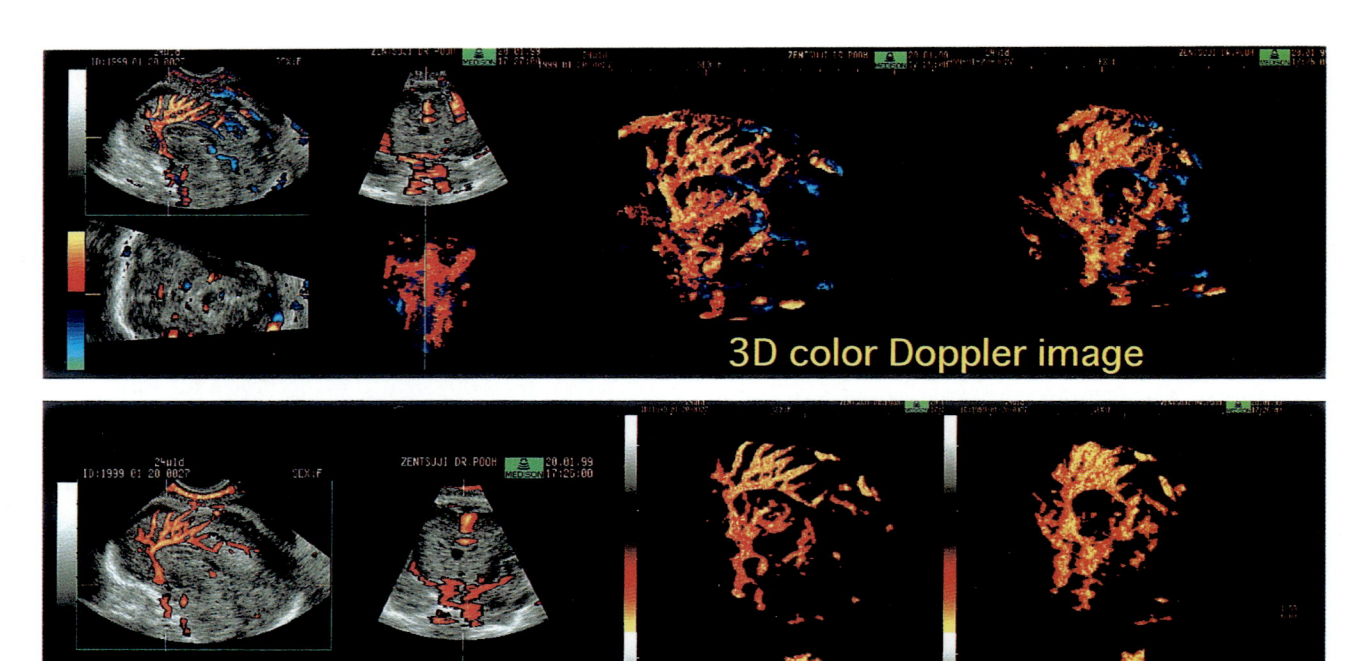

Figure 12 Three-dimensional (3D) color/power Doppler images of the fetal brain circulation. Brain vessels identified on the gray-scale brain structure by multiplanar images (left); 3D reconstruction of color/power volume data showing well-oriented 3D brain vessels (right)

Conclusions

Transvaginal 3D sonography is an easy, non-invasive and reproducible method with less required technique and a short scanning duration, and produces comprehensible and objective information. This method is suited to fetal brain screening. Longitudinal volume data storage of the fetal brain morphology will contribute to *in vivo* investigation of the natural history of congenital anomalies and acquired brain damage in the field of fetal neurology.

References

1. Monteagudo A. Fetal neurosonography: should it be routine? Should it be detailed? *Ultrasound Obstet Gynecol* 1998;12:1–5
2. Smith DW, Tondury G. Origin of the calvaria and its sutures. *Am J Dis Child* 1978;132:662–6
3. Pooh RK, Nakagawa Y, Pooh KH, Nakagawa Y, Nagamachi N. Fetal craniofacial structure and intracranial morphology in a case of Apert syndrome. *Ultrasound Obstet Gynecol* 1999;13:274–80
4. Pooh RK, Maeda K, Pooh KH, Kurjak A. Sonographic assessment of the fetal brain morphology. *Prenat Neonat Med* 1999;4:18–38
5. Pooh RK. Fetal cranial bone formation: sonographic assessment. *9th World Congress on Ultrasound in Obstetrics and Gynecology* Bologna: Monduzzi Editore, 1999
6. Timor-Tritsch IE, Peisner DB, Raju S. Sonoembryology: an organ-oriented approach using a high-frequency vaginal probe. *J Clin Ultrasound* 1990;18:286–98
7. Timor-Tritsch IE, Monteagudo A, Warren WB. Transvaginal ultrasonographic definition of the central nervous system in the first and early second trimesters. *Am J Obstet Gynecol* 1991;164:497–503
8. Blaas H-G, Eik-Nes SH, Kiserud T, Hellevik LR. Early development of the forebrain and midbrain: a longitudinal ultrasound study from 7 to 12 weeks of gestation. *Ultrasound Obstet Gynecol* 1994;4:183–92

9. Blaas H-G, Eik-Nes SH, Kiserud T, Hellevik LR. Early development of the hindbrain: a longitudinal ultrasound study from 7 to 12 weeks of gestation. *Ultrasound Obstet Gynecol* 1995;5:151–60
10. Benacerraf BR, Estroff JA. Transvaginal sonographic imaging of the low fetal head in the second trimester. *J Ultrasound Med* 1989;8:325–8
11. Monteagudo A, Reuss ML, Timor-Tritsch IE. Imaging the fetal brain in the second and third trimesters using transvaginal sonography. *Obstet Gynecol* 1991;77:27–32
12. Monteagudo A, Timor-Tritsch IE, Moomjy M. In utero detection of ventriculomegaly during the second and third trimesters by transvaginal sonography. *Ultrasound Obstet Gynecol* 1994;4:193–8
13. Pooh RK, Aono T. Fetal brain assessment using transvaginal sonography and power Doppler mapping. In Kurjak A, Di Renzo GC eds. *Modern Methods of the Assessment of Fetal and Neonatal Brain.* Rome: CIC Edizioni Internazionali, 1997:156–63
14. Timor-Tritsch IE, Monteagudo A. Transvaginal fetal neurosonography: standardization of the planes and sections by anatomic landmarks. *Ultrasound Obstet Gynecol* 1996;8:42–7
15. Pooh RK, Nakagawa Y, Nagamachi N, et al. Transvaginal sonography of the fetal brain: detection of abnormal morphology and circulation. *Croat Med J* 1998;39:147–57
16. Monteagudo A, Timor-Tritsch IE. Development of fetal gyri, sulci and fissures: a transvaginal sonographic study. *Ultrasound Obstet Gynecol* 1997;9: 222–8
17. Kurjak A, Kupesic S, Di Renzo GC, Pooh R, Kos M, Hafner T. Recent advances in perinatal sonography. *Prenat Neonat Med* 1998;3:194–207
18. Pooh RK, Aono T. Transvaginal power Doppler angiography of fetal brain. *Ultrasound Obstet Gynecol* 1996;8:417–21
19. Pooh RK, Pooh KH, Nakagawa Y, Maeda K, Fukui R, Aono T. Transvaginal Doppler assessment of fetal intracranial venous flow. *Obstet Gynecol* 1999;93: 697–701
20. Bonilla-Musoles F, Raga F, Bonilla F Jr, Blanes J, Osborne NG. Early diagnosis of conjoined twins using two-dimensional color Doppler and three-dimensional ultrasound. *J Natl Med Assoc* 1998;90:552–6
21. Pretorius DH, Nelson TR, Baergen RN, Pai E, Cantrell C. Imaging of placental vasculature using three-dimensional ultrasound and color power Doppler: a preliminary study. *Ultrasound Obstet Gynecol* 1998:12;45–9
22. Liang RI, Wang P, Chang FM, Chang CH, Yu CH. Prenatal sonographic characteristics and Doppler blood flow study in a case of a large fetal mediastinal teratoma. *Ultrasound Obstet Gynecol* 1998;11:214–18
23. Hayashi T, Ichiyama T, Nishikawa M, Kaneko J, Nakashima K, Furukawa S. Three-dimensional reconstruction of the power flow Doppler imaging of intracranial vascular structures in the neonate. *J Neuro Imaging* 1998;8:94–6
24. Pooh RK. Transvaginal 2D and 3D Doppler angiography of the fetal brain circulation. In Kurjak A, Nelson T, eds. *3D Power Doppler in Obstetrics and Gynecology.* Carnforth, UK: Parthenon Publishing, 1999:105–11

Three-dimensional neonatal neurosonography

G. Thieme, M. L. Manco-Johnson and D. Cioffi-Ragan

Ultrasound imaging of the neonatal brain (neurosonography) is a well-established diagnostic tool that has been used since the early 1980s to diagnose the presence and extent of intracranial hemorrhage (ICH) in the premature infant, to diagnose the presence, degree and cause of hydrocephalus and to evaluate suspected neonatal brain malformations[1-20].

It is possible to obtain excellent images of the neonatal brain through the open anterior fontanelle until that acoustic window closes at about 6 months of age. These premature babies have a high incidence of ICH and are often severely ill, unstable and in isolettes. Performance of standard two-dimensional (2D) sonography often requires 15–30 min, exposing the sick neonate to potentially significant stress.

The Medison Voluson 530D color system was used, with a specially designed, high-resolution (5–8 MHz) neonatal head three-dimensional (3D) probe (supplied by a grant through Medison America, Inc., Pleasanton, CA, USA). It was hoped that rapid, 3D volume acquisitions would supply adequate diagnostic information and significantly decrease the examination time, thus exposing the neonate to less stress. We have found that 3D volume acquisitions can yield diagnostic information similar to that from conventional 2D study and that the examination time can be less than 5 min. For some diagnostic problems, the 3D technique provides even more information than the standard 2D technique[21] (also submitted by the present authors for publication).

Conventional 2D imaging of the neonatal brain is accomplished by real-time scanning with a hand-held transducer. As the operator orients the transducer in coronal planes and sagittal planes through the anterior fontanelle, a series of representative images at selected locations of the brain anatomy are captured for electronic or film archiving. Interpretation and reporting are based upon this selected set of images. If questions arise with regard to the diagnostic content of the examination, another session is needed to provide the additional views. The conventional 2D imaging technique is dependent upon the operator recognizing normal and abnormal anatomy during the examination and documenting the findings with a sufficiently large set of images to convey the diagnostic information to the sonologist.

Technique of three-dimensional neurosonography

Three-dimensional volumetric imaging of the neonatal brain is accomplished by using a specialized transducer that mechanically sweeps the image plane through a predetermined angle (e.g. 90°) and digitally records images at fixed angular increments (e.g. every 2°). The spatial relationships among the individual image planes of the 3D volume data set constitute a comprehensive representation of the sonographic features of the brain. The 3D method minimizes operator-dependent gaps in the information set. To maximize image detail, the high-resolution mode is used. The digital data set is saved, so that it can be recalled, examined and interpreted off-line. Using specialized software, the sonologist can generate orthogonal sets of images in any desired plane throughout the 3D volume. In addition to the standard sagittal and coronal planes that are traditionally obtained through the anterior fontanelle, the brain can be viewed in axial planes and oblique planes, which cannot be obtained by conventional 2D imaging through the anterior fontanelle. The 3D method allows the sonologist to review the examination at a convenient time and generate as many views as are needed for the diagnosis.

Similarly to conventional 2D imaging, proper labelling of the right side, the left side, the anterior direction and the posterior direction of images that are displayed from the 3D volume data set is important for accurate description of anatomy and pathology. The rendering software must change the labelling automatically as new viewing planes are generated from the 3D data set. In other words, the orientation labels must follow the anatomy as the orthogonal image planes are rotated. For the Medison Voluson imaging system, an algorithm performs this function after the operator has established the orientation of the originally acquired orthogonal image set.

The 3D ultrasound technique is extremely important. The following procedure is specific to the

Medison Voluson 530D equipment. The neonatal probe (S-VNA 5-8) is used in the Program 1 setting. The transducer is held so that the groove on the probe is towards the right side of the baby's head when placed in a coronal plane in the anterior fontanelle. Image size is adjusted with the B-Mag magnification control, so that the entire brain is included in the cranial–caudal field of view. The focal zones should be evenly spaced within this field of view. Resolution mode is selected. While imaging the region of the third ventricle, the TCG and gain are set for optimal resolution and appearance. After selecting Volume Mode, the Volume-Angle (sweep angle) is set to the largest setting, so that the full anterior–posterior depth of the brain is imaged. The B-Angle Volume-Box size (angle) and position are adjusted so that the entire width of the brain is included in the coronal field of view and is centered in the image display. The Slow acquisition time (speed) is used to maximize the image plane density during the acquisition phase and to optimize the spatial resolution during off-line processing. While the transducer is held still in the neonate's anterior fontanelle, the Volume-Start button or the Freeze button is pressed to begin the volume mode sweep. Once the volume data are acquired, the multiplanar images are scrolled through from anterior to posterior and left to right, to determine whether all of the brain is imaged.

The most important aspect of the technique is the labelling of the scan orientation so that the right and left markers and the anterior and posterior markers will track appropriately during off-line image processing. This step is essential when describing the location of an abnormality or structure in the brain, as the orientation of the image planes will change when the multiplanar projections are manipulated. To label the scan orientation when a volume acquisition is performed in the coronal plane, the Plane ID section is accessed and the Cranial key is selected. Only that key should be highlighted. The Anterior key is the default selection and should be turned off. The Rotate knob is then turned to R (Right); this is correct only if the groove is facing the right side of the neonate's head. The image will have correct orientation at all times after the above information is entered.

When a volume acquisition is performed in the sagittal plane, the transducer should be held so that the groove is pointing towards the front of the head (anterior) in the fontanelle. The steps are similar to those outlined above for the volume acquisition in the coronal plane. However, labelling of the scan orientation is different. The Plane ID window is accessed and the Cranial key is selected. Only that key should be highlighted; the default Anterior key is turned off. The Rotate knob is then turned to A (Anterior) as the transducer groove is now facing anteriorly on the baby. All images will have the correct orientation labels as the multiplanar projections are manipulated.

Although the 3D method minimizes dependence upon the operator recognizing the pathology and obtaining the needed views at the time of the examination, performance of the 3D examination still requires a level of technical skill that is similar to that needed for the conventional 2D examination. The acquisition time for the 3D examination is brief (typically 5 s or less), when compared to a conventional 2D examination. The operator can immediately view the 3D data set at the ultrasound system console and determine whether the data set is technically adequate. For the conventional 2D examination, the time required to obtain a complete image set may range from 5 to 20 min; individual images must be recorded as the examination progresses and are not reviewed on-line. In addition, the sagittal plane requires a second acquisition with re-positioning of the baby and transducer. An axial plane acquisition requires even more time and the scan must be performed through the side of the head, through the temporal bone.

The interpretation time for a 3D examination at a diagnostic workstation can be similar to or shorter than that of a conventional 2D examination if the volume set is surveyed for pathology in the multiplanar mode and key views are saved in a digital DICOM archive. A complete set of 2D images (similar to a conventional examination) can be obtained from the 3D set during the interpretation phase by selecting the coronal view box and then photographing or storing each image as the brain is scrolled through from front to back. Similarly, by selecting the sagittal view box, one can photograph or store images of important structures as one scrolls through the brain from left to right. This process can be performed in the axial view, starting at the top of the brain and moving down through the ventricles to the base of the brain. In the axial view, the image is oriented so that the anterior part of the brain is at the top of the image. At times, reviewing the 3D volume set may take longer, however, since there are so many interesting structures that are seen in one plane and then are located in the other orthogonal planes.

In theory, spatial resolution for the displayed 2D images is optimal only for the original plane used to acquire the 3D volume set. Because other imaging planes must be interpolated from lateral beam width and slice thickness information, degraded spatial resolution is expected for those planes. When imaging through the anterior fontanelle during neonatal brain sonography, only coronal-plane and sagittal-plane imaging is possible. Theoretically, images displayed in the coronal plane will have the best resolution when acquired in the coronal plane; images displayed in the sagittal plane from coronally acquired data will have slightly degraded resolution. Similarly, images displayed in the sagittal plane will have the best resolution when acquired in the sagittal plane; images displayed in the coronal plane from sagittally acquired data will have slightly degraded resolution. However, with respect to practical experience, the authors have not noted any significant difference in resolution in the sagittal and coronal images. This is not true in the axial plane (C-plane), which is perpendicular to the original beam axis and is heavily interpolated from slice thickness information. As expected, the authors have observed significantly degraded spatial resolution for axial images, especially for the near field and the far field depths (outside the focal zone).

The applications of 3D volume ultrasound imaging are similar to those of conventional 2D ultrasound imaging. These include assessing the extent of ICH, detecting periventricular leukomalacia, assessing the degree and cause of ventriculomegaly and evaluating congenital malformations of the brain. The 3D technique can provide a shorter acquisition time and can improve understanding of the pathology through better depiction of 3D relationships between structures. Diagnostic accuracy has been shown to improve also, since the complete data set, rather than a limited set of images, is available for the sonologist's review.

Normal brain anatomy

The relationship of the cavum septi pellucidi and cavum vergae with respect to the corpus callosum, lateral ventricles, caudate nuclei and thalami is shown in Figure 1. The point of rotation for each set of orthogonal images is marked by a white dot. Figure 1A is the originally acquired coronal image through the interhemispheric fissure (mid-line), demonstrating the small lateral ventricles on either side of the central fluid-filled cavum septi pellucidi (white dot). The top of the head or cranial aspect (Cr) is towards the top of the image and the right (R) side of the brain is on the left of the image. Figure 1B is the sagittal display of the coronally acquired data set at the point of the white dot (vertical black arrows on Figure 1A). The frontal or anterior part of the brain is on the left of the image. Now, the full length of the cavum septi pellucidi and cavum vergae is seen (white dot), with the corpus callosum being the thin curved band of tissue that drapes over the cavum from front to back. Figure 1C is the displayed axial plane at the level of the white

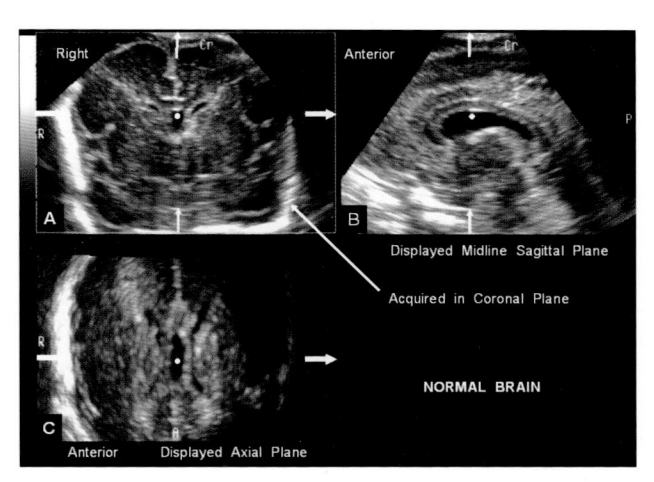

Figure 1 This multiplanar image set shows normal brain anatomy that is centered on the cavum septi pellucidi. The three-dimensional volume data are acquired in the coronal plane (A). The sagittal image (B) and the axial image (C) are reconstructed at right angles to the coronal plane. The white dot marks the center of rotation for the orthogonal set of images and represents the common point of intersection of these planes. For the sagittal view, the anterior and posterior directions conform to standard convention. For the axial view, the convention is reversed, so that the posterior end is at the top and the anterior end is at the bottom

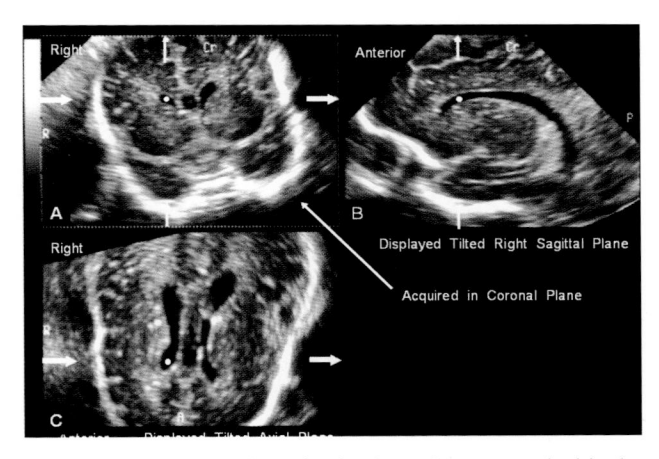

Figure 2 These three-dimensional volume data are acquired in the coronal plane (A). The center of rotation (white dot) is moved into the frontal horn of the right lateral ventricle; the coronal image is rotated counter-clockwise around the point of rotation until the length of the right lateral ventricle is brought into view in its entirety in the sagittal reconstruction (B). The axial plane (C) tilts so that the body of the left lateral ventricle is elongated, compared to the right lateral ventricle. The common point of reference is the point of rotation represented by the white dot

dot and horizontal white arrows in Figure 1A. In this projection, the front of the infant's head (anterior) is on the bottom of the image. This shows the full length of the left lateral ventricle and a small amount of the right left ventricle. By tilting the coronal image plane in Figure 1A and moving the point of rotation (white dot) over to the right lateral ventricle, the multiplanar image set in Figure 2 is obtained. This allows the right lateral ventricle to be seen in a sagittal plane (Figure 2B) and both lateral ventricles to be seen in axial view

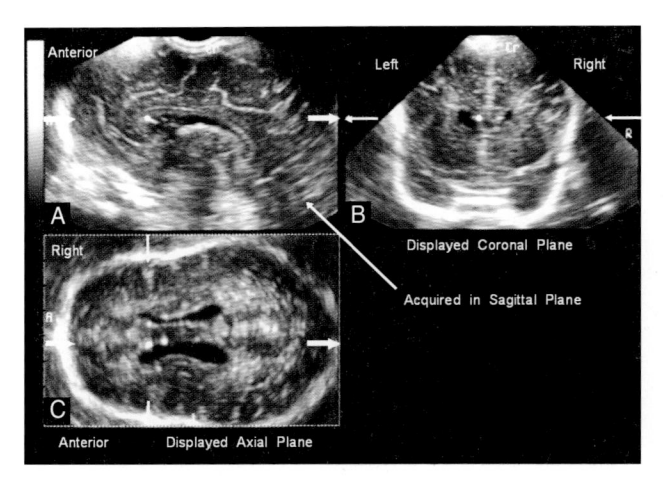

Figure 3 These three-dimensional volume data are acquired in the sagittal plane. The coronal image (B) and the axial image (C) are reconstructed at right angles to the sagittal plane. The white dot marks the center of rotation for the orthogonal set of images and represents the common point of intersection of these planes through the genu of the corpus callosum on the left. The left and right sides of the coronal view are reversed from the standard right–left convention, as this data set was acquired in the sagittal plane. The axial view (C) is turned on its side with the right side of the head towards the top of the image and the anterior (frontal) aspect of the head to the left of the image

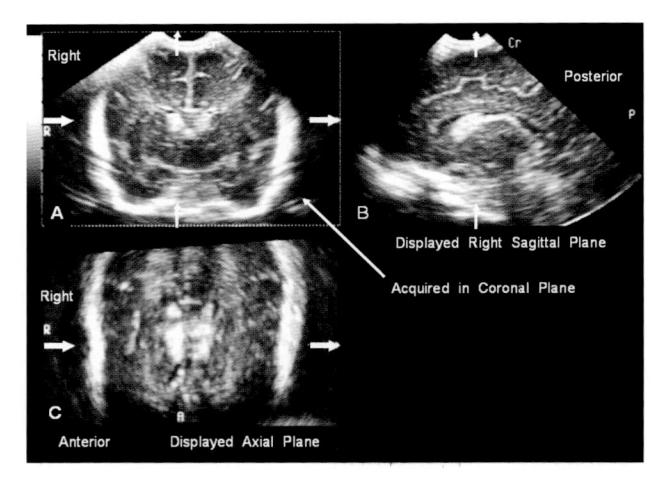

Figure 4 The multiplanar image set is centered on the right germinal matrix hemorrhage in this premature infant with Grade I intracranial hemorrhage. Orthogonal views demonstrate the relationship of the hemorrhage to the surrounding normal brain anatomy, as seen in the coronal (A), sagittal (B) and axial (C) planes. The three-dimensional volume data are acquired in the coronal plane

(Figure 2C). These coronal and displayed sagittal images follow the normal 2D imaging convention. For the displayed axial plane, the anterior and posterior ends are flipped. When the 3D volume data are acquired in the sagittal plane, the sagittal image is viewed in the standard orientation (Figure 3A) and the right and left sides of the coronally displayed image are flipped (Figure 3B). Also, the displayed axial view is now positioned on its side (Figure 3C) so that we are looking down on the head from above. Because the proper labelling of the acquired volume has been performed, the anatomic relationships are correctly labelled on the displayed views. The importance of proper labelling of the data set at the time of the examination cannot be overemphasized.

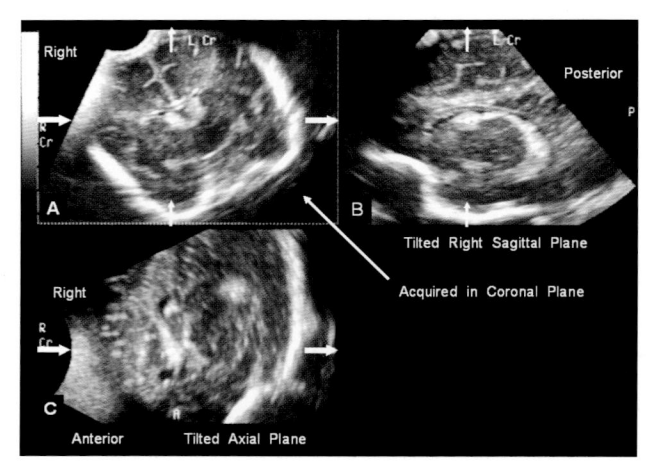

Figure 5 This is the same three-dimensional volume data that are shown in Figure 4. The point of rotation is still centered on the right germinal matrix hemorrhage, but the coronal image (A) is rotated counter-clockwise around the white dot until the length of the right lateral ventricle is seen in the sagittal view (B). The relationship of the choroid plexus to the germinal matrix hemorrhage is clearly demonstrated. The axial plane (C) is not diagnostically significant because of the angular tilt

Intracranial hemorrhage

Intracranial hemorrhage occurs frequently in premature infants below 32 weeks' gestational age[3,7,13,15–18] and usually starts in the germinal matrix in the subependymal area near the base of the lateral ventricles. There are four grades of ICH, indicating the increasing severity of the bleed, starting with Grade I, in which the bleed is confined to the germinal matrix. Grade II is present when the bleed extends into the lateral ventricle, but no ventriculomegaly has occurred. Because hemorrhage into the ventricle causes ventriculitis, the ventricles often enlarge; when hydrocephalus is present, it is considered Grade III. If the bleed extends into the brain parenchyma, it is considered Grade IV. Acutely, hemorrhage is echogenic on ultrasound; within a few weeks it becomes cystic, as the clot is removed by macrophages. This appears as an area of porencephaly within the brain.

Grade I

The 3D ultrasound examination (Figure 4) shows bilateral Grade I germinal matrix hemorrhages in the brain of this premature infant. The orthogonal image planes (Figure 4A, B and C) are centered on the right

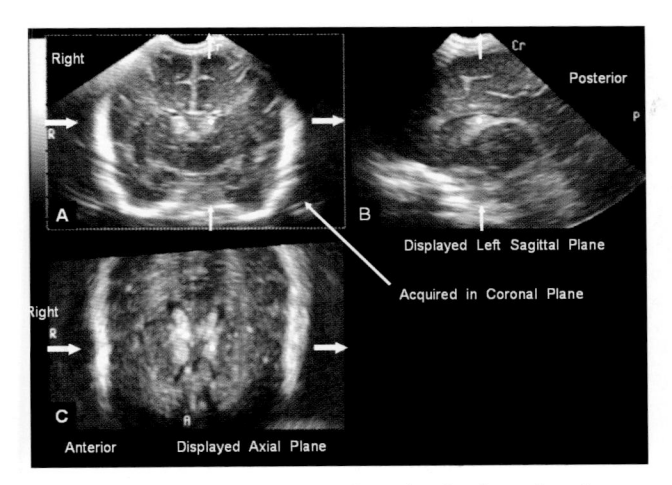

Figure 6 This is the same three-dimensional volume data that are shown in Figure 4. The center of rotation (white dot) is moved to a new location that overlies the left germinal matrix hemorrhage. The multiplanar image set shows the relationship of the hemorrhage to the surrounding normal brain anatomy, as seen in the coronal (A), sagittal (B) and axial (C) planes

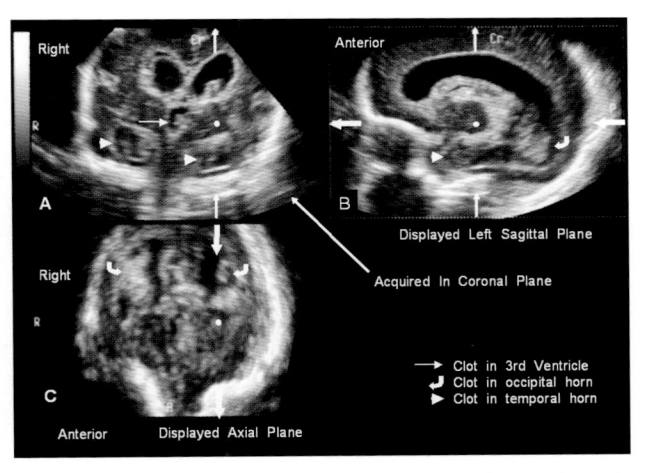

Figure 8 The same three-dimensional volume data that are shown in Figure 7. The center of rotation (white dot) is moved to a new location that overlies the left thalamus. The multiplanar image set changes to show the clots in the left lateral ventricle, as seen in the coronal (A), sagittal (B) and axial (C) planes

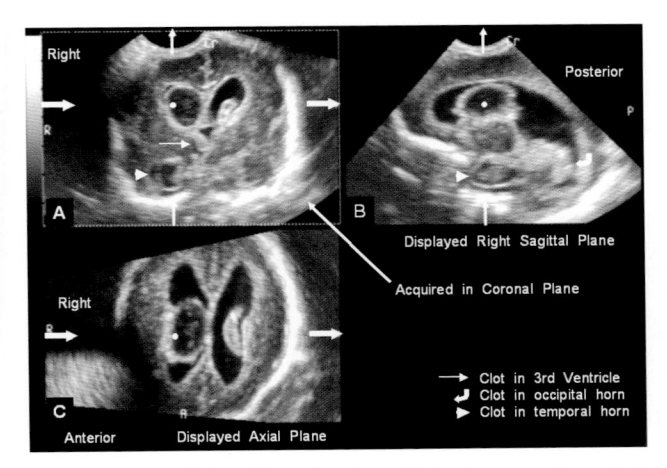

Figure 7 Coronal three-dimensional acquisition in a premature infant with Grade III intracranial hemorrhage. The point of rotation (white dot) of the multiplanar image set is centered on the partially lysed clot in the right lateral ventricle. Orthogonal views demonstrate the relationship of the hemorrhage to the surrounding brain anatomy, as seen in the coronal (A), sagittal (B) and axial (C) planes. Arrows point to the clots within the third ventricle (straight arrow), the occipital horn of the lateral ventricle (curved arrow) and temporal horn of the lateral ventricle (arrowhead)

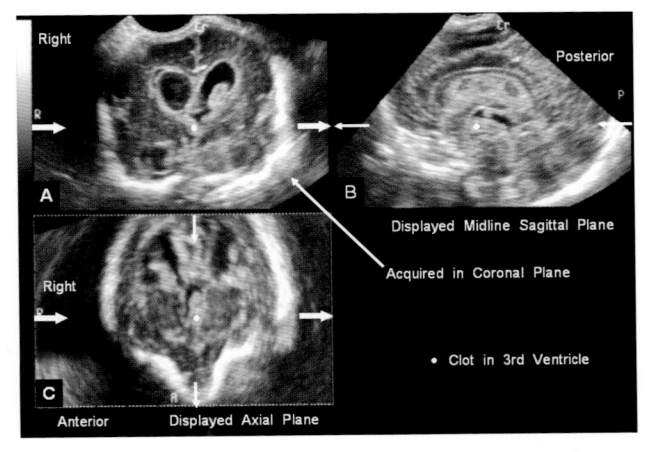

Figure 9 The same three-dimensional (3D) volume data that are shown in Figure 7. The center of rotation (white dot) is moved to a new location that overlies the clot within the third ventricle. Coronal (A), sagittal (B) and axial (C) planes demonstrate the anatomic relationships. All of the different images in Figures 7–9 came from one 3D acquisition and this is only a small illustration of the power of this technique

subependymal hemorrhage (white dot). With the point of rotation (white dot) over the right hemorrhage, the coronal plane is tilted (Figure 5A) to produce an oblique sagittal plane that is angled through the right lateral ventricle (Figure 5B), which allows visualization of the full length of the right lateral ventricle and echogenic choroid plexus. The point of rotation (white dot) is then shifted to the left germinal matrix hemorrhage (Figure 6A) in the coronal image; the corresponding sagittal image of the left ICH is displayed (Figure 6B). The axial image (Figure 6C) is unchanged, except for the location of the point of rotation (white dot). The arrows in Figure 6A mark the locations of the corresponding multiplanar reconstructions. Although the diagnosis can be made just as easily from conventional 2D images, the multi-planar relationships of the coronal and sagittal planes are unknown; also, there is no axial view[21].

Grade III

The 3D ultrasound examination shows a Grade III intracranial hemorrhage in the brain of this premature infant. The orthogonal views show the spatial relationships of the partially lysed clot within the dilated right lateral ventricle (white dot in Figure 7A, B and C), the hyperechoic clot within the occipital horn (curved arrow, Figure 7B) and the isoechoic clot within the temporal horn (arrowhead, Figure 7A and B). Also, clot is present within the dilated third ventricle (thin horizontal arrow, Figure 7A). By moving the point of rotation over the left thalamus (Figure 8A), the clot in the body, atrium, occipital horn and temporal horn of the left lateral ventricle are shown (Figure 8A, B and C). The clot within the dilated third ventricle is demonstrated in all three orthogonal planes by placing the point of rotation within the third ventricle (Figure 9).

Grade IV

Orthogonal views generated from the 3D volume data set show the extent of the large Grade IV hemorrhage in this premature newborn (Figure 10). The bleed (echogenic material) into the parenchyma of the right frontal lobe and right parietal lobe can be appreciated on all three planes. The mid-line shift to the left that results from the large right intraparenchymal hemorrhage and right intraventricular clot is best seen in the displayed axial view. By moving the point of rotation (white dot) to the left (Figure 11), the clot that forms a cast within the dilated left lateral ventricle is shown (Figure 11B). By selecting the coronal box and expanding that image to fill the screen, one can move the point of rotation from anterior to posterior and generate a series of conventional coronal views from the 3D volume data set (Figure 12). When compared to conventional 2D imaging, viewing of the 3D volume data enhances understanding of the relationships of this complex case of ICH.

Periventricular leukomalacia

Periventricular leukomalacia is infarction and necrosis of the periventricular white matter in premature infants. This is usually due to hypotension, severe hypoxia and ischemia[4,14,17–20]. Although periventricular leukomalacia is less common than ICH, it is a much more significant abnormality with nearly universally poor prognosis. In babies with periventricular leukomalacia, spastic diplegia or quadriplegia is almost always a late sequela and cortical blindness and developmental delays are often seen.

The location of periventricular leukomalacia is usually in the arterial border zones of the white matter at the level of the trigone of the lateral ventricle and in the frontal cerebral white matter. Initially, the ultrasound examination in periventricular leukomalacia may be negative. However, within 7 to 14 days the periventricular region becomes very echogenic and then, 2–4 weeks following the initial insult, multiple cystic areas will develop. The cystic pattern is usually bilateral and often symmetric.

The extent and severity of the periventricular leukomalacia in this neonatal brain is shown in the following sequence of images that were generated using a surface-rendering technique. These views were obtained by looking down on the plane represented by the dotted line. The first image set (Figure 13) is a standard coronal plane. The second image set (Figure

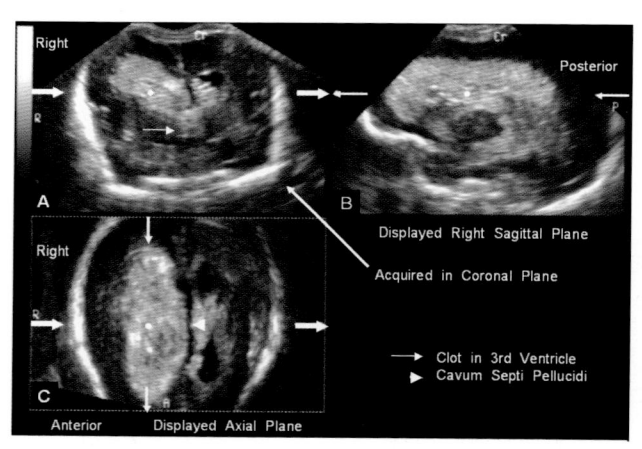

Figure 10 These three-dimensional (3D) volume data show features of a Grade IV intracranial hemorrhage. The point of rotation (white dot) of the orthogonal image set is centered on the intraparenchymal hemorrhage within the right frontal lobe and parietal lobe, as seen in the coronal (A), sagittal (B) and axial (C) planes. The displayed axial plane shows a significant mid-line shift that results from the mass effect of the large intraparenchymal hemorrhage and the large intraventricular clot within the right lateral ventricle, bulging into the cavum septi pellucidi (arrowhead). The clot totally fills the ventricle and there is no evidence of free cerebrospinal fluid (CSF). The 3D volume data were acquired in the coronal plane

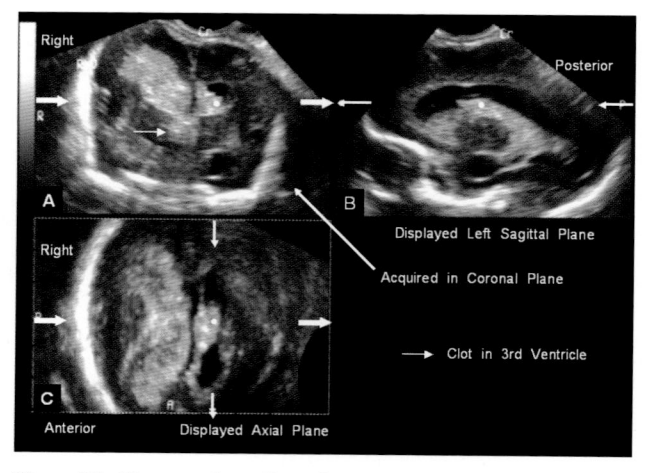

Figure 11 The same three-dimensional volume data that are shown in Figure 10. The center of rotation (white dot) is moved to a new location that overlies the left subependymal hemorrhage, thus allowing visualization of the left lateral ventricle. The multi-planar image set shows the clot within the dilated left lateral ventricle, as seen in the coronal (A), sagittal (B) and axial (C) planes. Cerebrospinal fluid, however, is seen within the mildly dilated ventricle

14) is a standard sagittal plane. The third image set (Figure 15) is an axial plane that cannot be obtained using the conventional 2D technique when the brain is scanned through the anterior fontanelle. Multiple cystic lesions are seen adjacent to the lateral ventricles on the coronal and sagittal views and above the lateral ventricle in the axial view.

Other intracranial abnormalities

During conventional 2D imaging of a premature neonate for evaluation of possible intracranial hemorrhage, a hyperechoic peripheral mass was discovered near the frontal–parietal junction in the left cerebral hemisphere (Figure 16). Power Doppler imaging showed a vessel at the lateral margin of the mass. The initial differential diagnosis included focal hemorrhage, neoplasm and vascular malformation. A magnetic resonance imaging exam showed normal anatomy. Surface-rendered images (Figure 17) in the axial plane showed that the mass lay within a sulcus in the

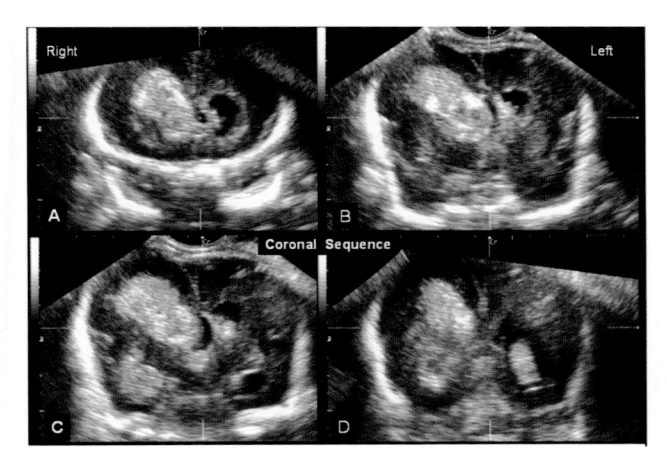

Figure 12 The same three-dimensional volume data that are shown in Figure 10. To produce this series of images, the coronal box was selected and the image was expanded to fill the screen. Then, the point of rotation (white dot) was scrolled from anterior to posterior. Key images that demonstrate the extent of the Grade IV intracranial hemorrhage were selected for storage in the still-frame digital archive, from the frontal region over the orbits (A), to a cut showing the intraparenchymal hemorrhage displacing the cavum septi pellucidi to the left (B). C is a slightly more posterior slice through the third ventricle (filled with blood) and the temporal horns, where the right temporal horn is filled with blood and the left temporal horn is filled with cerebrospinal fluid. The last selected image (D) is a coronal view through the trigone region that shows the posterior extent of the right intraparenchymal hemorrhage. The left choroid plexus in the trigone appears uninvolved

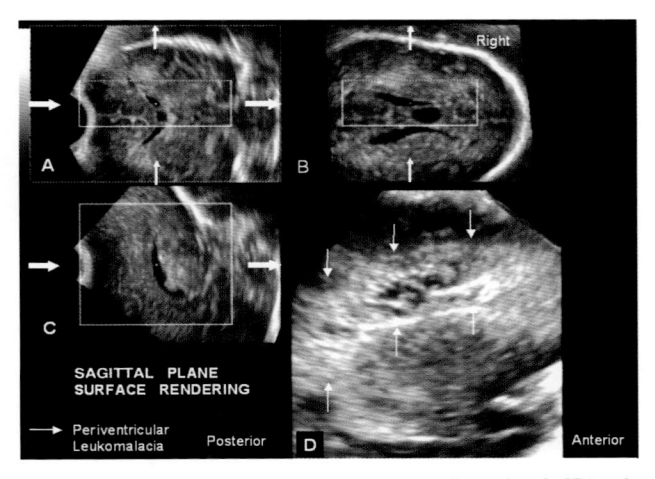

Figure 14 The orthogonal images of the three-dimensional (3D) volume data set have been rotated to produce a surface-rendered image of the periventricular leukomalacia in a sagittal plane (D). The 3D relief effect is generated using a surface-rendering technique where the viewer looks down on the plane represented by the dotted-line side of the rectangular box in the coronal image (A) and axial image (B)

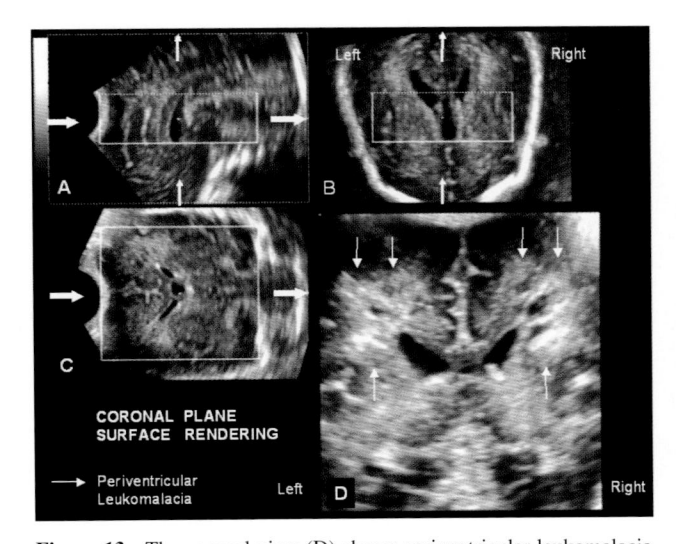

Figure 13 The coronal view (D) shows periventricular leukomalacia features (arrows) in this neonatal brain. Small cysts are seen within the hyperechoic periventricular tissues. The three-dimensional relief effect is generated using a surface-rendering technique where the viewer looks down on the plane represented by the dotted-line side of the rectangular box shown in the sagittal image (A) and axial image (B)

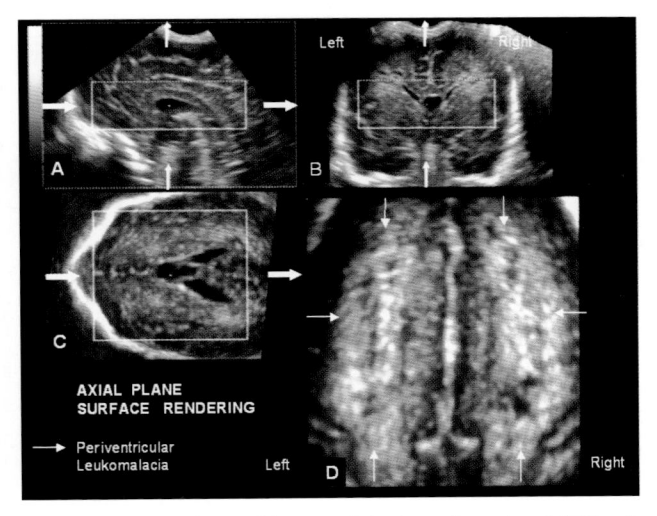

Figure 15 The orthogonal images of the three-dimensional (3D) volume data have been rotated to produce a surface-rendered image of the periventricular leukomalacia in an axial plane (D). The 3D relief effect is generated using a surface-rendering technique where the viewer looks down on the plane represented by the dotted-line side of the rectangular box in the sagittal image (A) and coronal image (B)

left hemisphere and that the mass was symmetrically positioned with respect to a normal density within the corresponding sulcus of the right hemisphere. These gyri and sulci features are seen only in the axial plane, which can be obtained only by rendering from the 3D volume data set. When serial examinations showed no change with time, it was concluded that the density was simply benign subarachnoid tissue occupying space between opposing gyri.

Congenital malformations of the neonatal brain can be visualized beautifully by 2D ultrasound[2,3,7,8,10–12] and even more so with 3D neurosonography. The scope of this chapter does not allow a full discussion of the range of pathological conditions that can be detected and differentiated by 3D ultrasound. In general, when an abnormality is seen on standard 2D neonatal neurosonography, it is visualized even better with the 3D technique. Because of the multiplanar capability it is possible to work out the relationships of the enlarged ventricles and to determine with certainty the presence or absence of the corpus callosum, the interhemispheric fissure and the vermis of the cerebellum. By moving the point of rotation to an area of interest in the 3D volume data set, it is possible to refer to these anatomic structures in all three orthogonal planes with a degree of precision that is not possible with conventional 2D imaging.

The images in Figures 18, 19 and 20 illustrate how the 3D technique helps the sonologist to understand the relationships of the mid-line brain anatomy in this newborn with agenesis of the corpus callosum and ventriculomegaly. Absence of the corpus callosum is easily appreciated in the coronal views. The anatomy of the third ventricle in axial views and coronal views is much easier to comprehend when it can be related to corresponding locations seen in sagittal views. Initially, the point of rotation is placed in the third ventricle at the level of the foramen of Monro, just anterior to the massa intermedia (Figure 18). Next, the location of the massa intermedia is identified (Figure 19) in all three planes. Finally, the point of rotation is moved into the posterior aspect of the dilated third ventricle (Figure 20).

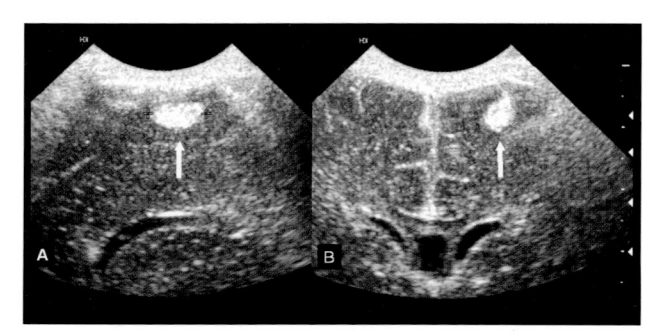

Figure 16 Conventional two-dimensional images of the brain show a solid hyperechoic mass near the frontal–parietal junction in the left cerebral hemisphere (Figure 17). An arrow points to the mass in the sagittal image (A) and the coronal image (B)

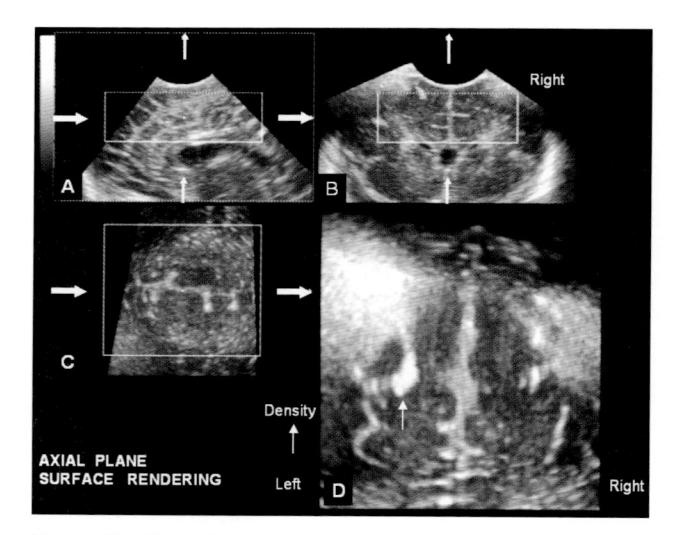

Figure 17 The surface-rendered image (D) in the axial plane shows that the mass lies within a sulcus in the left hemisphere and that the mass is symmetrically positioned with respect to a normal density within the corresponding sulcus of the right hemisphere. These gyri and sulci features are seen only in the axial plane, which can be obtained only by reconstructing from the three-dimensional volume data set

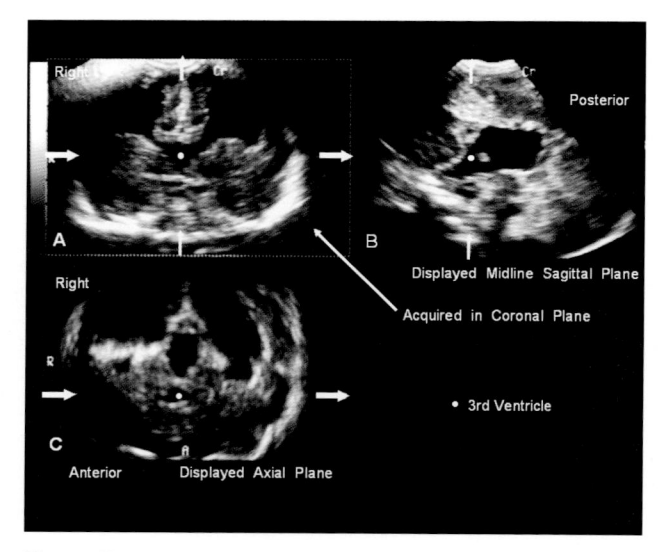

Figure 18 This orthogonal image set shows sonographic features of agenesis of the corpus callosum and ventriculomegaly. The anatomy of the third ventricle in axial (C) views and coronal (A) views is much easier to comprehend when it can be related to corresponding locations seen in sagittal views. Initially, the point of rotation (white dot) is placed in the third ventricle at the level of the foramen of Monro, just anterior to the massa intermedia. The open foramen between the lateral ventricle and the third ventricle is well seen in (A). The interhemispheric fissure is seen above the center point (A), but the normal corpus callosum is absent in the axial (A) and sagittal (B) views. (Compare with Figure 1)

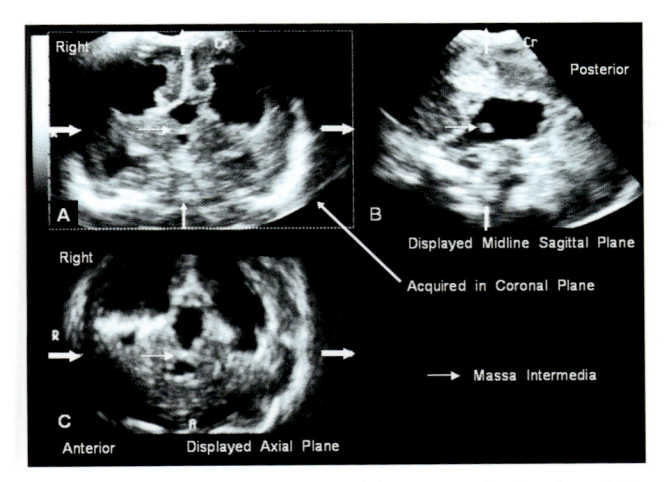

Figure 19 For the same orthogonal image set, the location of the massa intermedia (arrow) is identified in all three planes by moving the point of reference over the massa intermedia. This is most easily achieved in the sagittal view

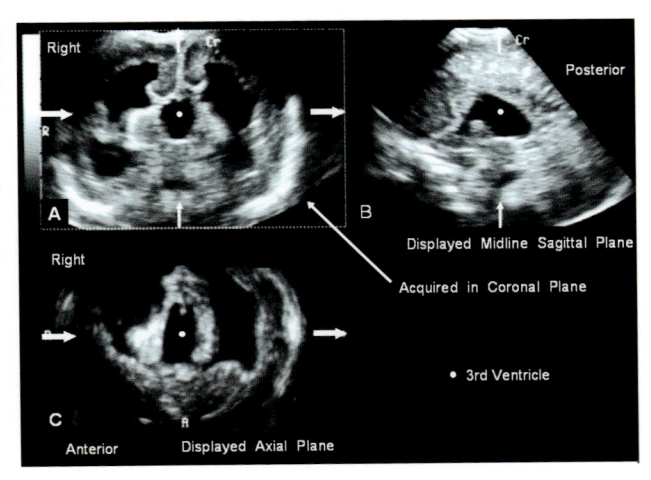

Figure 20 For the same orthogonal image set, the point of rotation is moved to the posterior aspect of the dilated third ventricle. Absence of the corpus callosum is apparent

Conclusion

The major diagnostic advantage of 3D volume imaging is the ability to view three orthogonal image planes centered at any selected anatomic location. This 3D relationship can be approximated in conventional 2D imaging only by careful, conscious localization of the sagittal and coronal planes at the selected sites of pathology (or interest) during real-time scanning. Viewing the axial plane relationships is not possible with the conventional 2D technique. Furthermore, the conventional 2D image set is a composition of selected representative images that may not necessarily depict the pathology accurately, especially if the pathology was not recognized at the time of the examination. The additional step of videotaping the 2D examination can potentially fill the information gap. However, videotape review is time consuming and still-frame image documentation from videotape requires specialized video equipment. With the 3D system, the sonologist can send DICOM images from the workstation to the digital storage system (or DICOM printer), as the examination is interpreted. Each recorded image set can include the three-view orientation image, which shows the relationship of the chosen orthogonal image planes, and selected enlarged images of any one of the multiplanar slices. In addition, the acquisition of the data is faster and the exposure to the neonate is less with 3D ultrasound.

We believe this new and exciting technique will become the primary imaging tool in the neonatal brain.

References

1. Johnson ML, Mack LA, Rumack CM, et al. B-mode echoencephalography in the normal and high risk infant. *Am J Roentgenol* 1979;133:375–81
2. Johnson ML, Rumack CM. Ultrasonic evaluation of the neonatal brain. *Radiol Clin North Am* 1980;18:117–31
3. Rumack CM, Johnson ML. *Perinatal and Infant Brain Imaging; Role of Ultrasound and Computed Tomography.* Chicago: Year Book Medical Publishers, 1984
4. Rumack CM, Wilson S, Charboneau JW. Neonatal and infant brain imaging. In Carol M, ed. *Diagnostic Ultrasound*, 2nd edn. St Louis: Mosby-Year Book, 1998
5. Babcock DS. Sonography of the brain in infants: role in evaluating neurologic abnormalities. *Am J Roentgenol* 1995;165:417–23
6. Cohen HL, Haller JO. Advances in perinatal neurosonography. *Am J Roentgenol* 1994;163:801–10
7. Rumack CM, Johnson ML. Neonatal brain ultrasonography. In Sarti DA, ed. *Diagnostic Ultrasound: Text and Cases*, 2nd edn. Chicago: Year Book Medical Publishers, 1987
8. DeMeyer W. Classification of cerebral malformations. *Birth Defects* 1971;7:78–93
9. Volpe JJ. Normal and abnormal human brain development. *Clin Perinatol* 1977;4:3–30
10. Babcock DS. The normal, absent and abnormal corpus callosum: sonographic findings. *Radiology* 1984;151:450–3
11. Kier EL, Truwit CL. The normal and abnormal genu of

corpus callosum. *Am J Neuroradiol* 1996;17:1631–41
12. Atlas SW, Shkolnik A, Naidich TP. Sonographic recognition of agenesis of the corpus callosum. *Am J Roentgenol* 1985;145:167–73
13. Taylor GA. New concepts in the pathogenesis of germinal matrix intraparenchymal hemorrhage in premature infants. *Am J Neuroradiol* 1997;18:231–2
14. Kirks DR, Bowie JD. Cranial ultrasonography of neonatal periventricular/intraventricular hemorrhage: Who, why and when? *Pediatr Radiol* 1986;16:114
15. Rumack CM, Manco-Johnson ML, Manco-Johnson MJ, *et al*. Timing and course of neonatal intracranial hemorrhage using real-time ultrasound. *Radiology* 1985;154:101
16. Boal DK, Watterberg KL, Miles S, *et al*. Optimal cost effective timing of cranial ultrasound in low-birthweight infants. *Pediatr Radiol* 1995;25:425–8
17. Carson SC, Hertzberg BS, Bowie JD, Burger PC. Value of sonography in diagnosis of intracranial hemorrhage and periventricular leukomalacia: a postmortem study of 35 cases. *Am J Roentgenol* 1990;155:595–601
18. Barr LL, McCullough PJ, Ball WS, *et al*. Quantitative sonographic feature analysis of clinical infant hypoxia: a pilot study. *Am J Neuroradiol* 1996;17:1025–31
19. Grant EG, Schellinger D, Smith Y, *et al*. Periventricular leukomalacia in combination with intraventricular hemorrhage: sonographic features and sequelae. *Am J Neuroradiol* 1986;7:443
20. Barkovich AJ, Sargent SK. Profound hypoxia in the premature infant: imaging findings. *Am J Neuroradiol* 1995;16:1837–46
21. Manco-Johnson ML, Thieme G. 3D US of the neonatal brain. Paper presented at the *2nd World Congress on 3D Ultrasound*, Las Vegas, October, 1999

Non-gynecological three-dimensional ultrasound

A. Kratochwil

Introduction

Nearly 10 years after three-dimensional (3D) sonography became available, this technique is now accepted as an additional and powerful tool in obstetrics[1-4]. However, only a few attempts have been made to use this examination technique in other medical disciplines, such as internal medicine, surgery, urology, pediatrics, orthopedics or ophthalmology, although in these specialities as well additional information can be anticipated. In these medical specialities, however, sonography competes against computerized tomography (CT) and magnetic resonance imaging (MRI). The question to be answered is simply: what are the expected advantages and benefits?

Advantages and benefits of three-dimensional sonography

Besides its easy and inexpensive availability, the power of 3D sonography is to produce organ-optimized scans. This is achieved by optimal utilization of volume translation and rotation. Another important capability of 3D sonography is that an unambiguous sonographic diagnosis is based on showing the pathology in two planes perpendicular to each other. In two-dimensional (2D) examination, this is sometimes unobtainable, for different reasons. In 3D examination, however, where the volume is represented in the form of three orthogonal planes, the cursor is placed at the lesion in question. In any of the related scanning planes, the information is immediately updated.

A further advantage of 3D scanning is the capability of simultaneously storing gray-scale and Doppler information on the disk. Thus the tortuous path of vessels can be followed inside the organs. The use of the angiographic mode in combination with an echo enhancer and second harmonic imaging forms the basis for studying tumor vascularization.

The possibility of storing the entire volume on a hard disk has several advantages. Primarily the examination time for the patient is shortened, as volume acquisition needs an average of not more than 10–15 s. The stored volume is analyzed in the absence of the patient and therefore resembles the reading of an X-ray film. This virtual scanning has another benefit. In difficult cases, to obtain a second opinion, it used to be necessary to perform a second examination, or to pass one's judgement on prints or a tape taken during the examination. Now, for the first time, the second opinion is based on the same information as available to the original examiner. As the volume can be compressed, the volume may be sent via the Internet to a distant expert[5].

Live three-dimensional sonography

An upcoming benefit will be live 3D sonography, where the examination is refreshed every second by new pictures. At the moment, only three pictures are shown per second. For real live 3D sonography, at least 16 frames/s will be necessary. This aim will be reached in the near future. The possibility of live scanning will not only improve diagnosis, but also accomplish 3D ultrasound-guided interventions.

Disadvantages of three-dimensional sonography

The disadvantages of 3D sonography are principally the same as in 2D sonography, governed by physical properties. Additional problems are encountered in rendering due either to an unfavorable position, or to a large amount of gas in front of the examined region. Also, there is a problem in surface rendering without liquid in front of the organ.

A prerequisite for 3D sonography, as in all imaging methods, is an excellent knowledge of topographic anatomy. As detailed information on the use of 3D sonography in specialities other than obstetrics is beyond the scope of this chapter, only a brief description, based on clinical examples, will follow.

Gynecology

In gynecology, 3D sonography is already successfully used to examine the uterus – to measure the endometrial volume, to diagnose uterine anomalies and to locate uterine fibroids[6,7]. Because of the accurate volume calculation by 3D sonography the technique has been applied to estimate ovarian volume and the number of ovarian follicles[8,9]. Three-dimensional angiography has been used to study tumor vascularity[10]. It seems that, with the advent of live 3D sonography, hysterosalpingography (HSG) will be replaced by 3D sonography, because of the more detailed anatomical and functional information and the reduction in radiation exposure.

Pelvic floor examination

The anatomical condition of the pelvic floor is of the utmost interest in diagnosing elementary defects or anomalies responsible for urinary stress incontinence. The first attempts to use 3D sonography for this application were reported by Athanasiou and colleagues[11] and Wisser and colleagues[12].

The aim of the 3D examination of the pelvic floor is to demonstrate, in detail, the female urethra, the rectum and the muscles.

The female urethra

The approach to this region is transperineal, transvaginal or transrectal. The last approach is favored, to minimize compression of the urethra induced by the vaginal probe and to demonstrate vaginal suspension. To attain a satisfactory result the probe frequency should be either 5 or 8 MHz[13].

From both available endocavitary probes the rectal probe is preferred, even if it is vaginally applied. The preference for the rectal probe is because the sonic waves are emitted perpendicularly to the longitudinal axis of the shaft. This guarantees that all anatomical structures of interest are oriented perpendicular to the insinuated wave, assuring optimal reflection. This is clearly demonstrated in comparison of the frontal anatomical drawing of the region with the frontal scan of the urethra achieved by 3D examination. Further support for this application is achieved by the comparison between the transverse ultrasonic scan of the urethra and the gross histological drawing (Figures 1 and 2). The vaginal probe, on the other hand, is an end-firing probe; the insinuated wave front therefore runs parallel to the anatomical structures of interest, producing no reflection. The difference in the scans performed with the rectal or vaginal probe, provoked by the difference in propagating ultrasonic waves along or perpendicular to the muscle fibers, is clearly demonstrated by both scans shown side by side (Figures 3 and 4). In 2D examination, one scanning plane demonstrates 360° of the pelvic floor. At the moment, unfortunately, in 3D examination only an opening angle of 180° is possible. Urethral and rectal

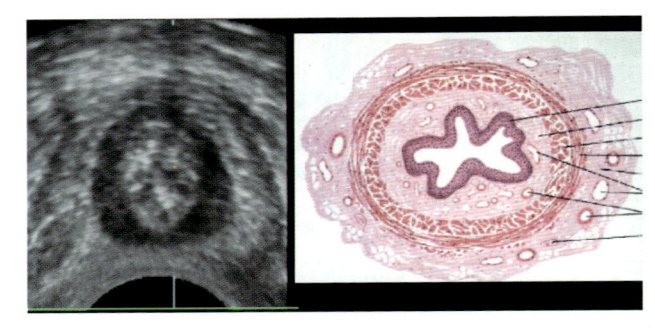

Figure 2 Comparison between the transverse ultrasonic display of the urethra and a gross histological specimen of the same region

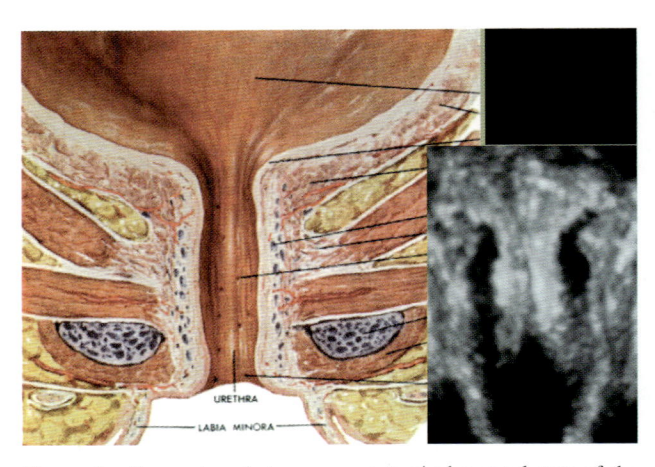

Figure 1 Comparison between an anatomical coronal scan of the bladder and urethra and a three-dimensional ultrasonic coronal scan

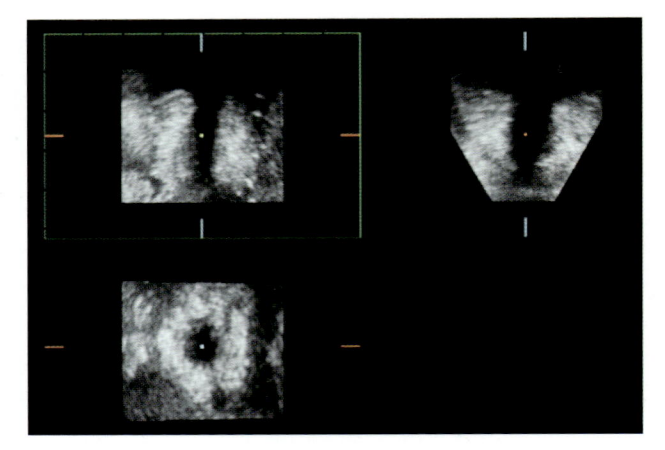

Figure 3 Transvaginal three-dimensional examination with an end-firing vaginal probe. Note that the aspect of the urethra is completely different from scans performed with the rectal transducer

anatomy therefore have to be examined by two different volumes.

In analyzing and comparing anatomy and 3D sonography, a nearly perfect congruity is achieved (Figures 1 and 2). In a transverse scan the anechoic rhabdosphincter surrounds the urethral lumen. That the thickness of the rhabdosphincter is not uniform in all parts is easily perceivable (Figure 5).

In none of the published papers, however, was the coronal scan, only achievable by 3D scanning and niche mode, utilized. One of the main advantages of 3D examination is the fact that the three presented planes on the monitor are always perpendicular to each other. This makes identification of anatomical structures much easier. For instance, in the transverse scan, if the cursor is placed centrally in the lumen of the urethra, the entire extent, not only of the urethra, but also of the rhabdosphincter, is displayed in the coronal scan (Figure 6). The aspect of the rhabdosphincter is curved and anechoic, resembling a Greek lyre surrounding the urethra. The entire length of the urethra is seen from the detrusor muscle to the slightly widening outlet at the introit.

Additional information is extracted from the niche mode. This mode displays a pseudo-3D reproduction of the examination, demonstrating anatomical structures in relation to the longitudinal and transverse aspects. It is thus possible to look at the anatomy from above and below, from the front or the back (Figure 7).

Utilizing all possibilities of 3D scanning, distance and volume measurements of the displayed anatomical structures is performed[14,15]. To measure the rhabdosphincter volume in the transverse scan, two steps are necessary. First, the entire volume of the urethra is calculated. In different transverse scans, the area of the structure is measured. The interval between the measured areas is notified by the equipment. The volume is given by multiplying the area by the distance. Second, the volume of the inner content, surrounded by the sphincter, is calculated. Subtraction of the inner

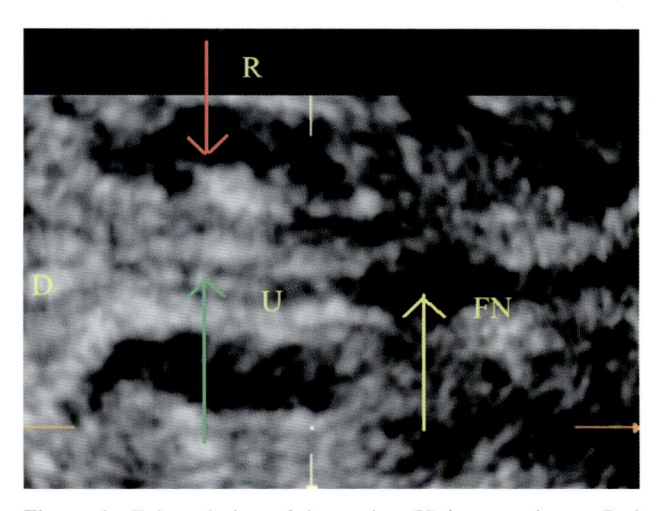

Figure 6 Enlarged view of the urethra (U) in coronal scan. Red arrow, rhabdosphincter (R); green arrow, lumen of the urethra; yellow arrow, navicular fossa (FN); D, detrusor muscle

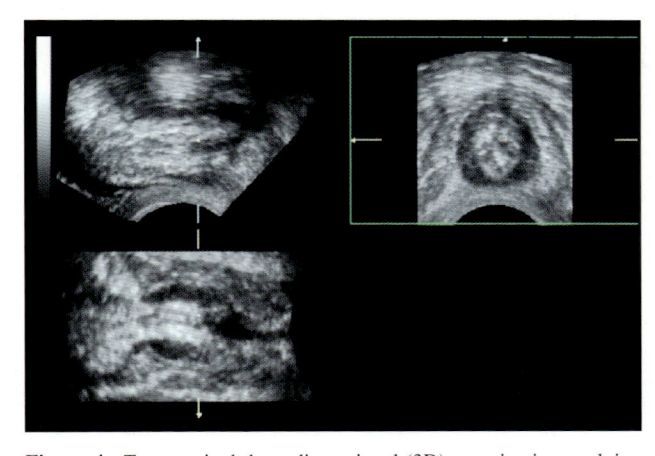

Figure 4 Transvaginal three-dimensional (3D) examination applying the rectal probe vaginally. Upper left, longitudinal scan; upper right, transverse scan; lower left, coronal scan. 'Bird's eye view' not available in two-dimensional examinations. The 3D scan planes are always orthogonal

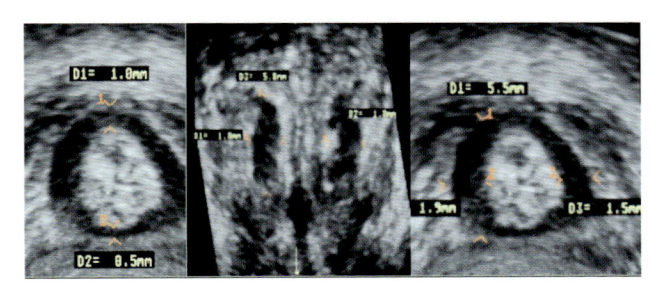

Figure 5 Measurement of the rhabdosphincter in its different portions. Left, anterior and posterior; middle, length of the muscle; right, lateral muscle. The entire volume is accessible

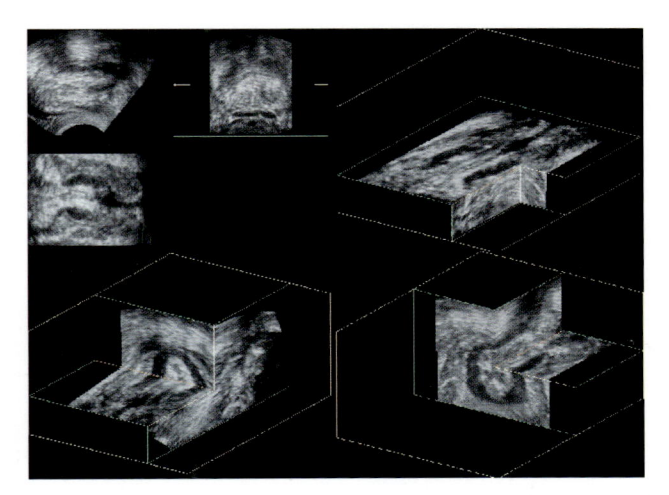

Figure 7 The niche mode provides different displays of the organ of interest. Upper left, original scan; upper right, coronal scan of the urethra; lower left, course of the urethra towards the bladder; lower right, the niche is placed in such a way to display the entire aspect of the rhabdosphincter in longitudinal direction. The front displays the transverse scan of the urethra

content from the calculated total volume gives the volume of the rhabdosphincter. Because of the great number of scans, ultrasonic volume estimation has a statistical error of only ± 4%.

Rectal examination: demonstration of the levator ani

To demonstrate rectal anatomy either the vaginal or the rectal approach can be chosen. The best display in women is achieved if the rectal probe is used vaginally. The probe is rotated through 180°, so that the groove of the transducers faces the perineum. A volume sweep of 90° with an opening angle of 180° is performed. If the patient is sufficiently prepared, with an empty rectum, the entire rectum and levator muscle is ideally displayed (Figure 8). Not only the levator muscle but also the internal sphincter is demonstrable in its longitudinal extent by the niche mode (Figure 9). Three-dimensional examination of the pelvic floor, urethra and levator ani will become a demand in the future, not only for diagnosis but also for evaluation of the result of therapy.

Gynecological tumors

It has already been pointed out that 3D examination may be used for the same indications as for 2D examination, but the incentive for other applications is primarily accurate volume estimations. The question to answer was: who benefits most from such accurate measurements? From the first, it was clear that these measurements are able to reflect the therapeutic success of chemo- or radiation therapy. As ultrasonic examinations are relatively inexpensive and harmless, repeated performance during therapy is possible.

Cervical carcinoma

The first organ of choice in which to evaluate this procedure was the uterus, especially in patients suffering from cervical carcinoma. Soon, however, problems appeared, limiting the primary enthusiasm. Principally, the emerging problems arose from two different sources. One source is the transducer and the second is the tumor itself.

With the use of an electronic vaginal transducer the region of sight is limited, compared to the mechanical transducers used in 2D sonography with an angle of 240°. The electronic probe is end-firing, emitting the waves from the tip of the probe straight forward in a rather limited angle. Therefore, in only rare cases, if the uterus is in a more or less stretched position, can

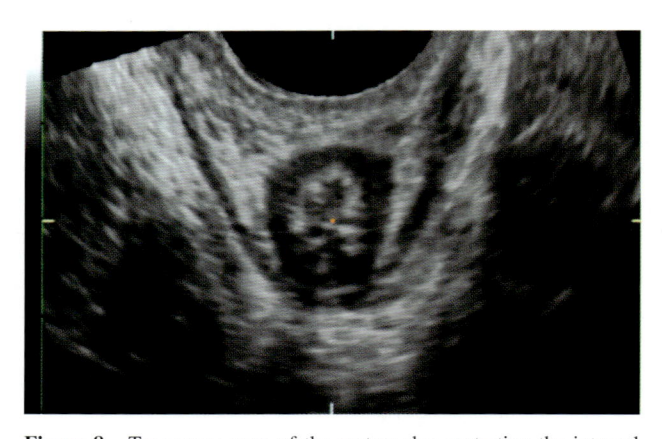

Figure 8 Transverse scan of the rectum demonstrating the internal sphincter and the less echogenic band of the levator muscle. The rectal transducer is placed transvaginally

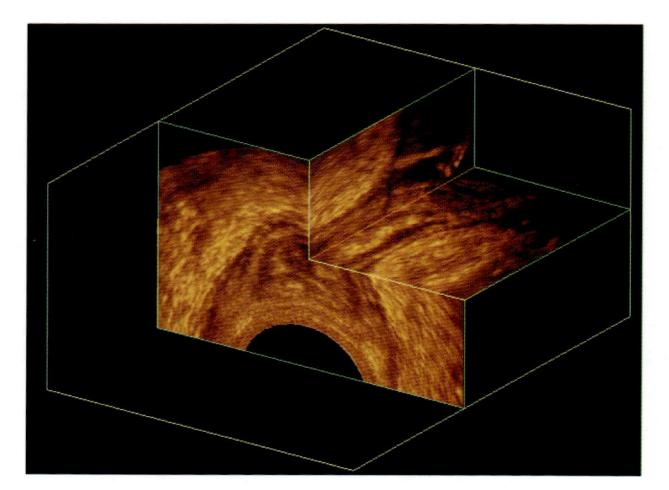

Figure 9 Niche mode demonstration of the rectum, exhibiting the internal sphincter

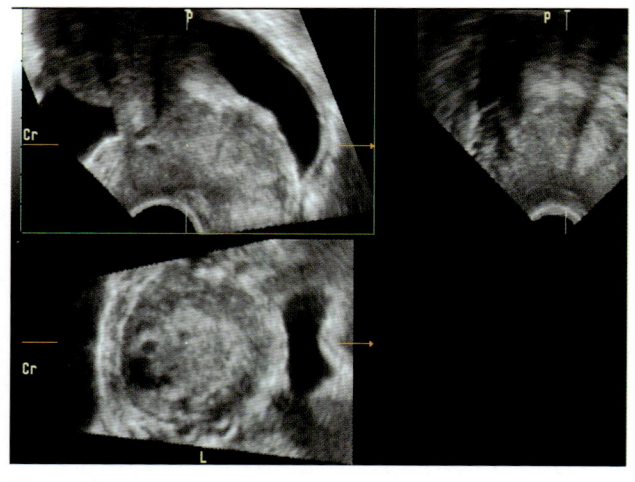

Figure 10 Three-dimensional aspect of a cervical carcinoma. Upper left, longitudinal scan (the cervix is enlarged); upper right, coronal scan; lower left, transverse scan of the portio. There is a minimal amount of fluid in the pouch of Douglas

the entire uterus be displayed (Figure 10). Otherwise, either the cervix or the corpus is shown. If the probe is placed too close to the cervix, even if a volume sweep of 90° is used, parts of the cervix may not be depicted.

Other limitations in demonstrating a cervical cancer by 3D sonography may be due to changes dependent on age, hormonal status, inflammatory changes and tumor necrosis. It is often noted that the uterus in aged patients is less demonstrable than in the generative phase. This might be dependent on altered blood flow in the uterus, governed by hormonal parameters. The uterus is not only smaller, containing no endometrial echo, but also seems less penetrable for sound. Smaller cervical tumors limited to the cervix, as in early development, show as anechoic and defined lesions inside the cervix. Focusing the examination on this region, with the different tissue propagation of sonic waves in tumor, fibrous and muscle tissue, allows visualization of the infiltration process (Figure 11). As soon as the tumor has contact with the surface, infection is possible. The tumor changes its appearance and becomes hyperechoic, almost indistinguishable from the surrounding tissue. Furthermore, in advanced stages, with apparent necrotic changes, air bubbles are trapped in the tumor clefts. These bubbles make ultrasonic examination difficult, as they form shadows, thus extinguishing relevant information in their path (Figure 12).

Additional information in cancers might be obtained by demonstrating neovascularization within the tumor by the angiographic mode (Figure 13). This mode is able to demonstrate vessels smaller than 1 mm in diameter and register flows of less than 1 cm/s.

Three-dimensional examination of cervical cancers also includes transrectal examination for the inspection of the parametrium and the pelvic wall. This possibility is extremely important in localizing tumor relapse at the pelvic wall.

Regarding recurrent tumors, examination of primary cervical carcinomas has not been satisfactory. However, 3D examination has demonstrated its benefits in the diagnostic approach to recurrences, and specially after radical operation, both for cervical and for endometrial cancers.

Tumor volume estimation and therapeutic impact

The tumor volume is easily assessable, as already demonstrated. The second method is an automatic feature, recently implemented in the instrument. Exact measurement of the target volume, calculated by software, taking the spatial orientation of the tumor into account, was recently performed[16], and compared suc-

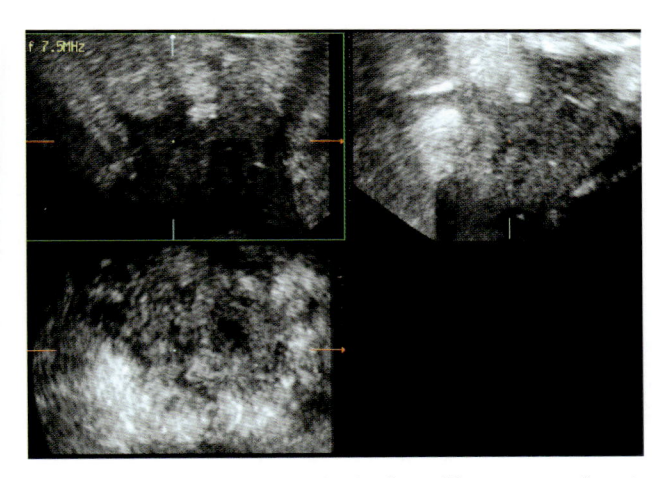

Figure 11 Focusing on the cervix, the finger-like processes of carcinomatous tissue infiltrate the stronger reflective muscle structure

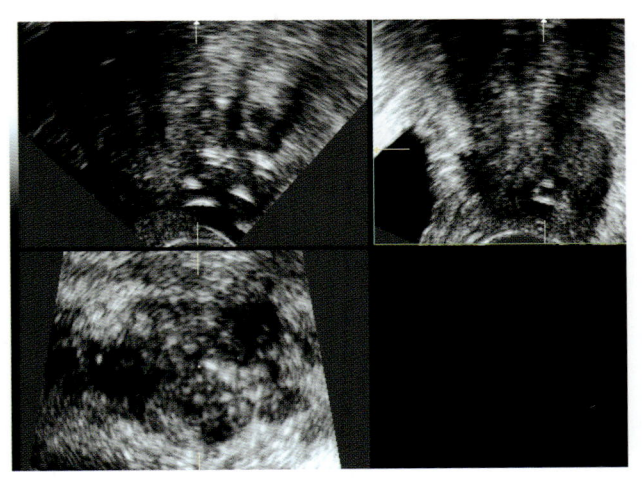

Figure 12 Highly reflective air bubbles in the clefts of a progressed and necrotic cervical cancer block the ultrasonic waves. Shadows are the consequence

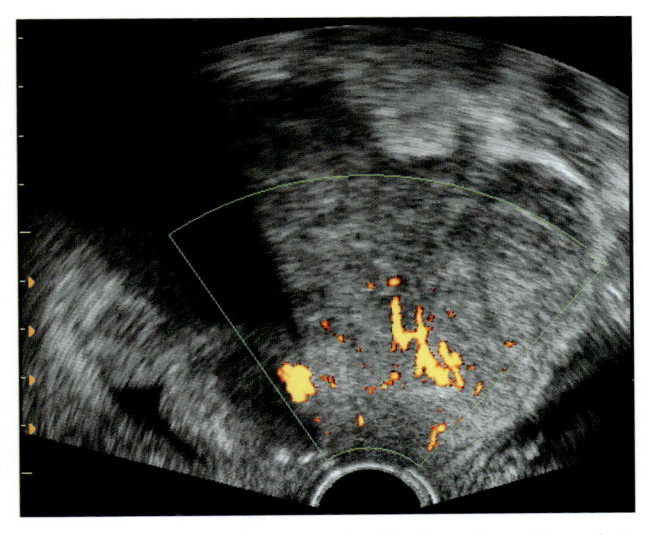

Figure 13 Cervical carcinoma examined by the angiographic mode to demonstrate neovascularization of the tumor

CLINICAL APPLICATION OF 3D SONOGRAPHY

cessfully with other available imaging modalities: CT and MRI.

The therapeutic result of radiotherapy is demonstrated by two clinical cases. The first case shows the transverse scan of a recurrence at the pelvic wall after radical operation for cervical carcinoma (Figure 14). The parallel structure inside the tumor shows the stent in the ureter to relieve hydronephrosis. The second volume (Figure 15) was assessed at the end of therapy. Comparing both scans shows the therapeutic success.

The relationship of the tumor to neighboring structures

In cancer, it is not only the tumor location and measurement that are of priority in radiotherapy, but also the relationship to neighboring structures and organs. The special aim is to minimize the sequelae of planned brachy- or radiotherapy.

Of special interest is the relationship of the tumor to the bladder, ureter, rectum and sigmoid. Even small changes such as slight thickening of the bladder wall

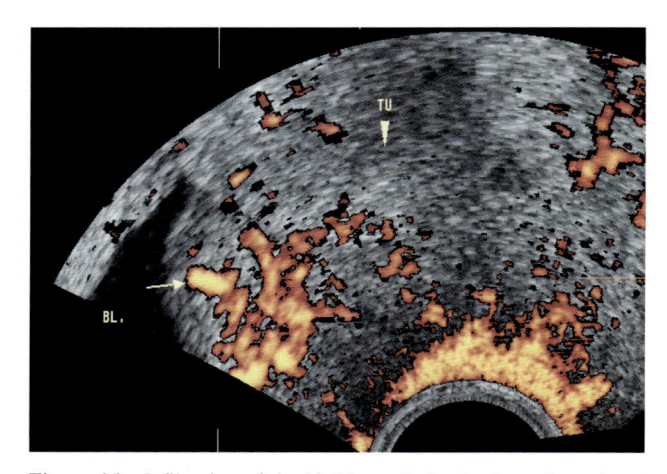

Figure 16 Infiltration of the bladder wall. In the three-dimensional scan, the bladder wall is seen to be slightly thickened. Applying the angiographic mode, however, the tumor supply by small vessels becomes visible

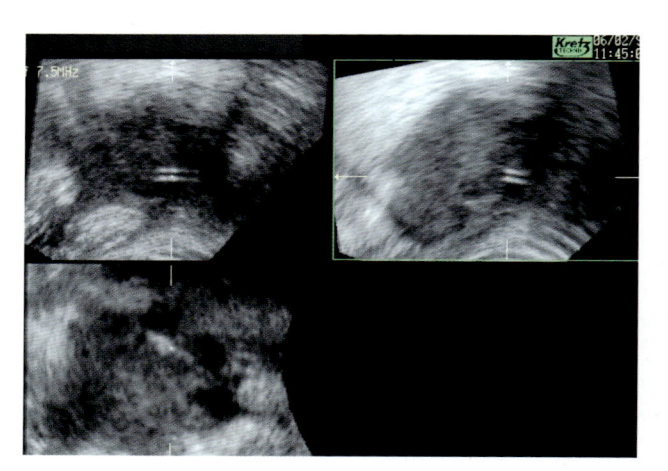

Figure 14 Recurrence after radical operation for a cervical cancer. The tumor blocks the ureter. The parallel structure in the middle of the tumor corresponds to the stent. Before radiation therapy

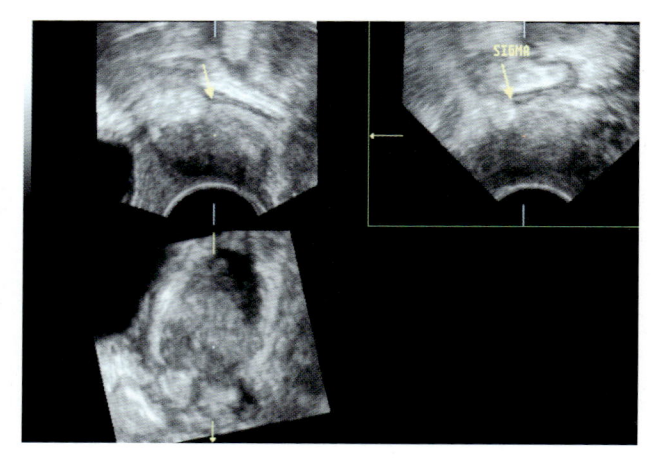

Figure 17 Three-dimensional examination reveals the relationship of the tumor to neighboring organs, such as the sigmoid (arrow). This relationship is important in calculating the target doses for radiotherapy

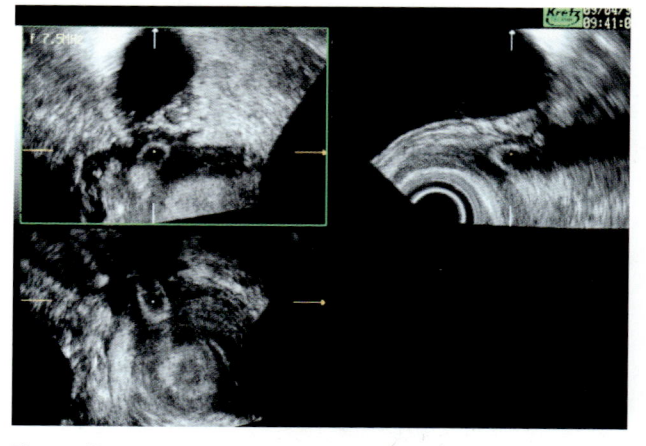

Figure 15 The same recurrence as in Figure 14, after radiotherapy. Only the stent and some strands of tumor tissue are visible

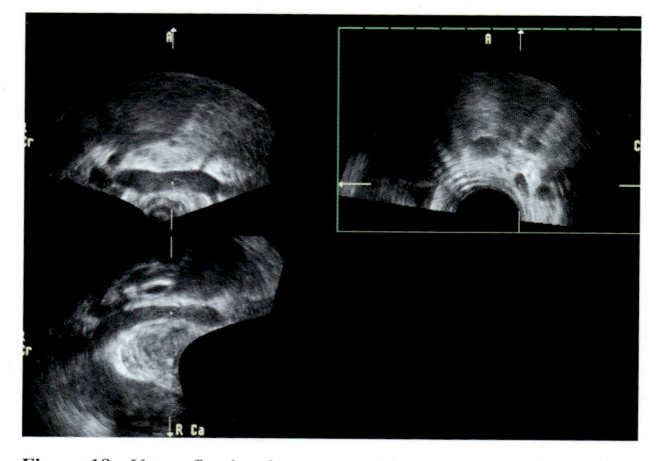

Figure 18 Ureter fixed and compressed by a recurrence of a cervical carcinoma at the pelvic wall. The resulting hydroureter is clearly depicted

are unmasked as a recurrent tumor if the angiographic mode is able to reveal small feeding tumor vessels (Figure 16). A recurrent tumor after an ovarian cancer presents, in 3D examination, a recognizable adhesion and infiltration to the sigmoid (Figure 17). If the examination is supplemented by a transrectal scan, then it is possible to diagnose recurrent tumors at the pelvic wall and to display the hydroureter, caused by tumor compression (Figure 18). In such cases immediate expansion of the examination to the upper abdomen is mandatory, for gynecologists to inspect the kidneys.

Internal medicine

Because of the limited size of the volume box, and the limitation of the volume sweep to 70° (i.e. 35° to the left and 35° to the right of center), it is necessary to take more than one volume. This causes no problems with the large available storage capacity.

The impact of 3D sonography in the upper abdomen is, besides demonstration of a multiplanar scan, the ability to produce organ-optimised scans. Acquiring a volume primarily oriented longitudinally, the longitudinal scan clearly displays the liver and the abdominal aorta. In the coronal scan, however, only a part of the vessel is displayed (Figure 19). This is caused by the fact that, in the longitudinal scan, the vessel crosses the x axis at an increased angle. To display the entire course of the vessel in the coronal scan as well, it is necessary to rotate the longitudinal scan in such a way that the vessel coincides with the x axis. The maneuver results in an optimal visualization in the coronal scan (Figure 20).

In the longitudinal scan a small vessel branching off the aorta is seen (Figure 21). In this scan, at first glance, it is unclear whether this branch is the mesenteric superior artery or the celiac axis. If, however, the

Figure 19 Three-dimensional demonstration of the liver and aortic vessel. Upper right, the long axis of the aorta crosses the x axis; therefore, in the coronal scan the aorta is not fully exposed

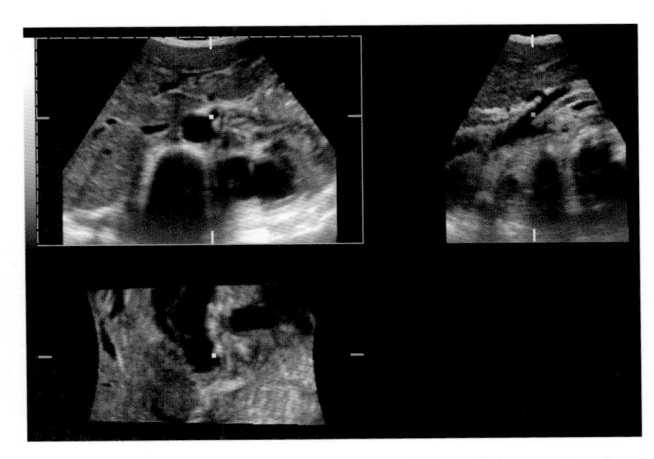

Figure 21 Similarly to Figure 19, an aortic branch is crossing the x axis, upper right. Is it the mesenteric superior artery, or the celiac axis?

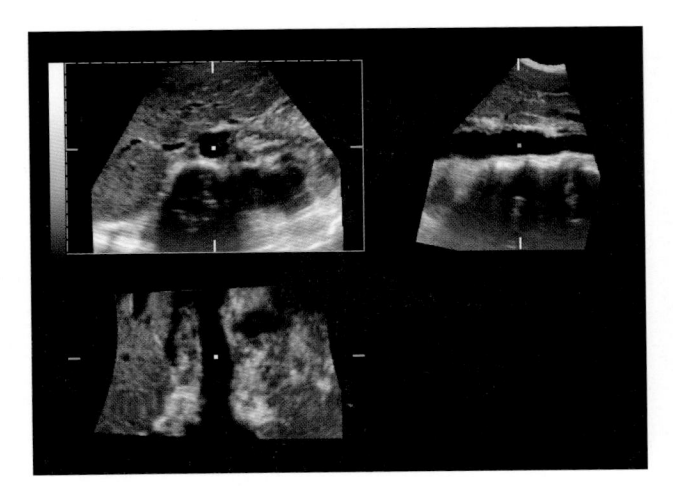

Figure 20 Rotating the scan, so that the long axis of the aorta coincides with the x axis, the vessel is totally exposed in the coronal view

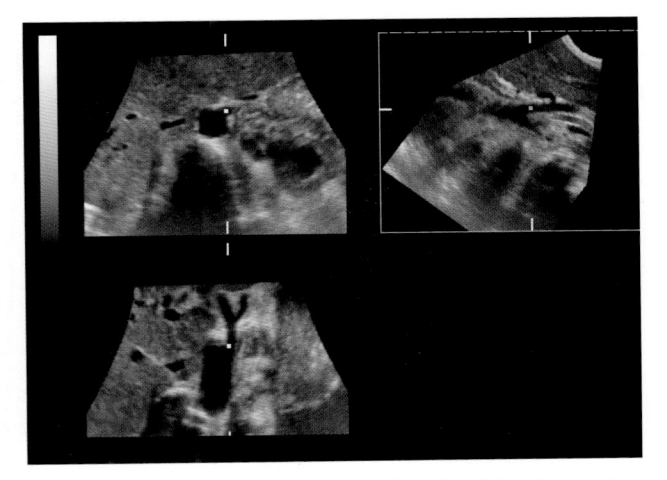

Figure 22 Optimizing the scan by rotation, visualizing the structure in the x axis, the coronal scan reveals the celiac trunk, together with the common hepatic artery and the splenic artery

branch, as shown above, is rotated, so that its run coincides with the *x* axis, the coronal scan immediately shows that the branch is the celiac axis, splitting into the common hepatic and mesenteric artery (Figure 22). Similar maneuvers are feasible at any point of the stored volume to produce an organ-optimized aspect.

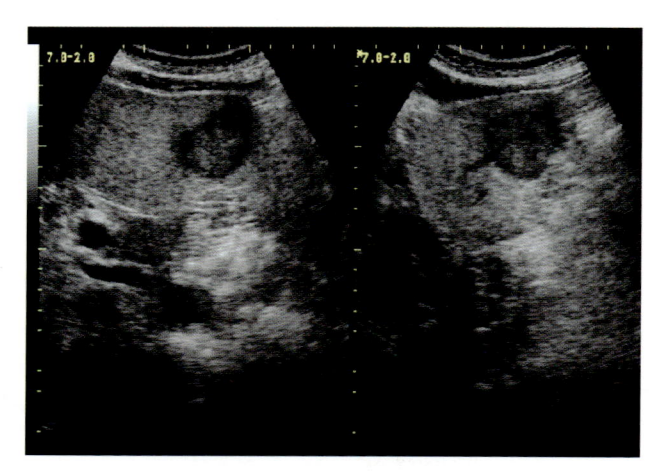

Figure 23 Large liver metastasis in the left lobe of the liver

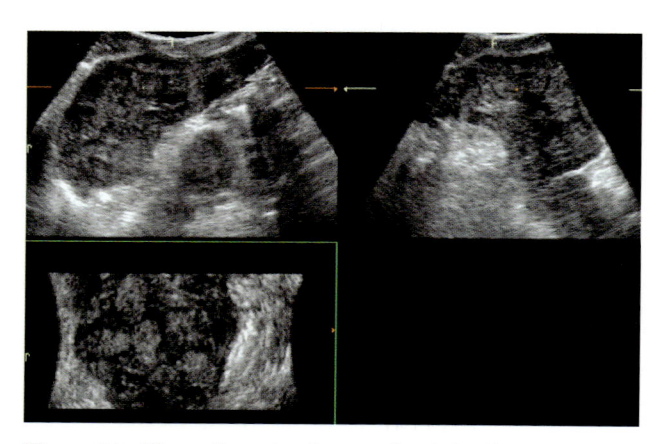

Figure 24 Three-dimensional scan of nodular liver metastases. Impressive picture of the pathology in the coronal scan, bottom left

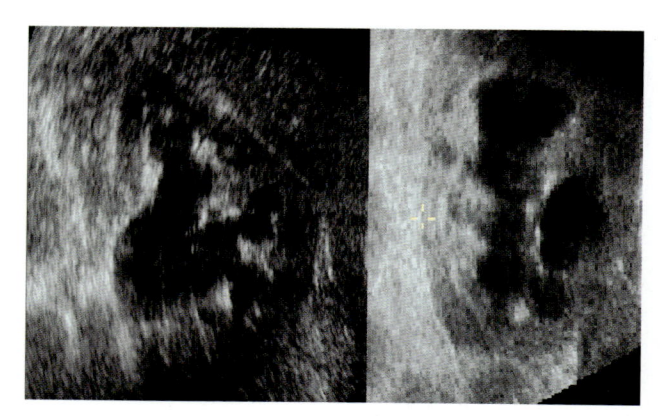

Figure 25 Extrapelvic hydronephrosis, due to the obstruction of the ureter. For three-dimensional reconstruction a combination of X-ray mode and minimum mode was used

Examination of the upper abdomen in patients suffering from a tumor of different origin

For every colleague engaged in ultrasonic diagnosis in oncology, at least a limited knowledge of upper abdomen anatomy and pathology related to cancerous disease is mandatory. In gynecology, prior to any therapy, the liver, kidneys and all lymph nodes accessible to sonography must be inspected.

Liver metastases

These are quite easily demonstrated by sonography, especially by 3D sonography using optimized tissue imaging (OTI), or tissue harmonic imaging. In the first feature, ultrasonic tissue velocity is selected to adapt for solid, cystic, fatty and normal lesions. Liver metastases show as round or irregular areas, either singular or multiple throughout the liver tissue. Segmental localization is guaranteed by relation to the vessels (Figures 23 and 24). Demonstration of such lesions is sometimes improved by angiographic mode, if necessary in combination with echo contrast medium.

Kidney changes due to tumors

As seen in the section dealing with gynecological tumors, pelvic recurrences may compress the ureter, causing hydronephrosis. It needs just a matter of seconds to change the examination area from the pelvis to the upper abdomen. Performing a volume scan including the kidney, and applying rendering of surface mode and minimal mode together, dilatation of the calyces by fluid is easy discernible (Figure 25). In

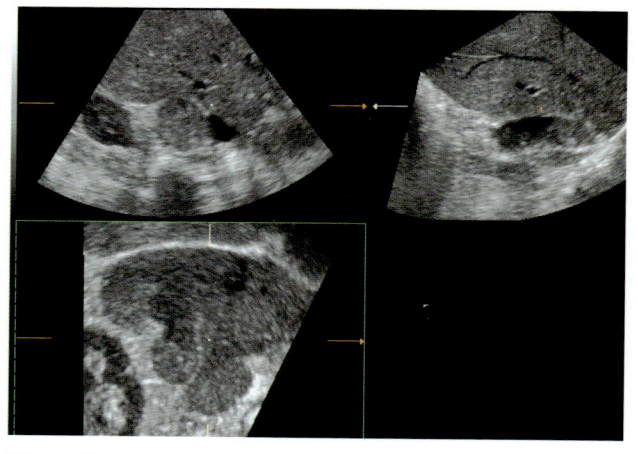

Figure 26 Three-dimensional aspect of a suprarenal metastasis

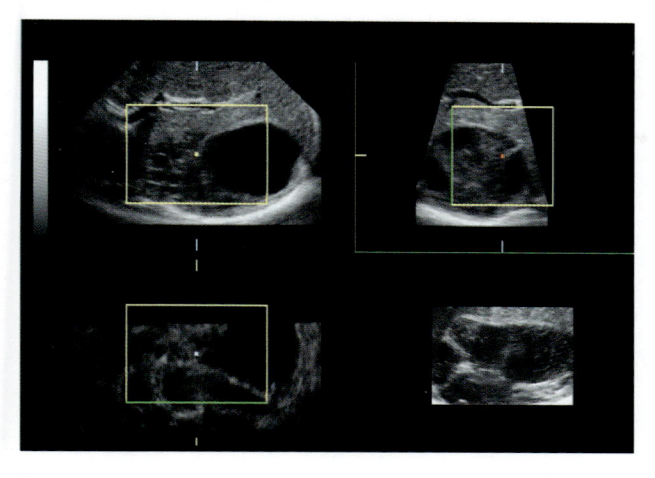

Figure 27 *Echinococcus* cyst of the liver. The rendering box is set

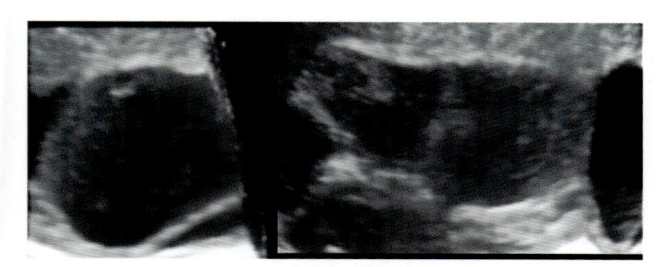

Figure 28 Three-dimensional rendered image of the *Echinococcus* cyst

rare cases even suprarenal metastases are demonstrable (Figure 26).

Gastroenterology

One should be aware that 3D sonography, in spite of competing with MRI and CT, has a place in the examination of the upper abdomen in internal diseases, especially in gastroenterology.

The indication for the search for liver metastases has been pointed out. Other circumscribed lesions in the liver that are clearly recognizable are cysts of different origin, such as amebic abscesses and postoperative infections. One lesion, seldom causing acute problems and therefore often unknown to the patients, is the small liver cyst, or *Echinococcus* cyst[17] (Figures 27 and 28).

Gallbladder

The merit of sonography in diseases of the gallbladder and bile ducts is indisputable. The multiplanar demonstration of the acquired volume helps in differentiating small concretions from polyps located on the gallbladder wall. Rendering allows direct inspection of the

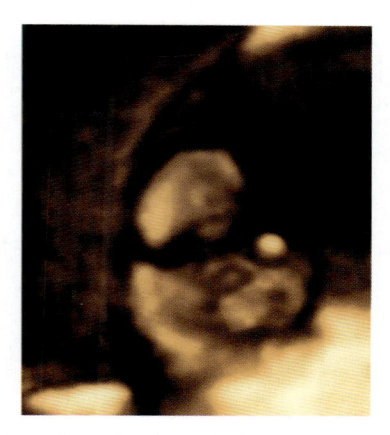

Figure 29 Three-dimensional examination of gallstones. The surface-rendered image displays the stones and wall of the gallbladder

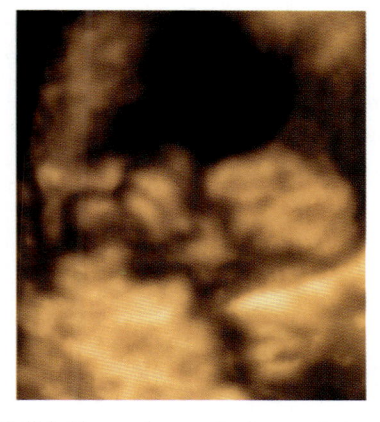

Figure 30 Gallbladder carcinoma. Surface rendering. Irregular and papillomatous structures in the wall

gallbladder wall (Figure 29). Of special interest in this connection is the observation of the coronal scan, or bird's eye view, during translational movement. In 2D examination shadows produced by the calculi block the inspection of the gallbladder walls. Using the coronal scan to scroll through the volume, there is no restriction in the observation of the walls. Even small lesions of the wall, such as atheromatous polyps covering the entire inner surface, are detectable. Of much more importance is the observation of irregular gallbladder wall thickening in cases of suspected malignant tumors (Figure 30). Scanning optimization is useful not only to demonstrate the course of vessels, but also to show the bile ducts, especially for differentiating between the cystic and common bile duct. This maneuver skillfully performed provides evidence of the cause of obliteration, either tumor or stone. If the blockage is due to a stone, 3D sonography contributes to the diagnosis of the MIRIZZI syndrome, by correct stone location.

In dealing with jaundice, the advantage of 3D sonography for correct placement and control of the transjugular intrahepatic portosystemic shunt (TIPS)

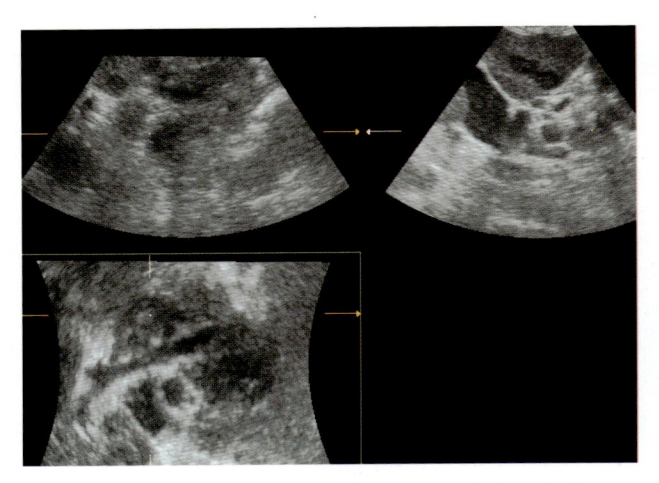

Figure 31 Progressive carcinoma of the pancreatic head infiltrating superior mesenteric vessels. Note that this information is only accessible by the coronal view, bottom left

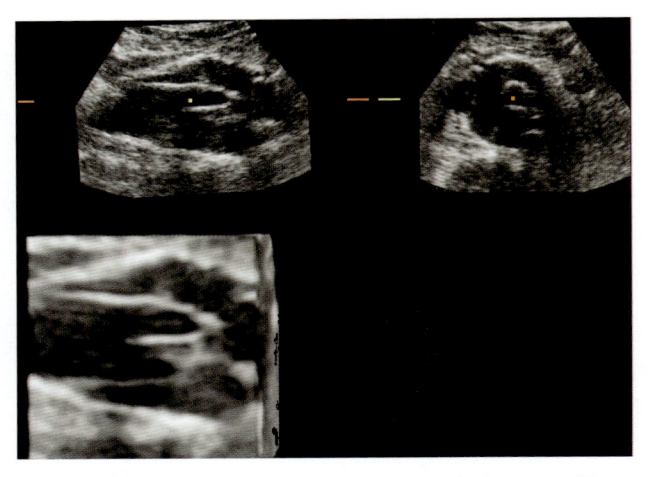

Figure 32 Aortic prosthesis surrounded by thrombotic masses. Upper left, longitudinal scan; upper right, transverse scan; lower right, three-dimensional reconstruction

must be stressed. The placed stent is clearly visible. By injection of an echo contrast medium the correct function of the TIPS can be evaluated.

Pancreas

Provided that the patient is correctly prepared, 3D sonography provides an ideal view of the organ. Organ-optimized scanning should be aimed at.

Tumors usually present as anechoic and irregularly limited regions. In advanced disease vessels may become infiltrated by the tumor; this knowledge is not unimportant. This difficult situation can be solved by 3D scanning (Figure 31). In the coronal scan infiltration of the mesenteric vessel is clearly recognizable.

In some cases, not only the main pancreatic duct, but also the branches of first and second order are observed. This is extremely important in the diagnosis of chronic pancreatic disease such as calcifications, which start in the periphery of the gland. In rare cases even the papillae of Vater can be demonstrated.

Aortic aneurysms

The potential of 2D sonography in demonstrating the situation in aortic aneurysm is exceeded by 3D sonography. The rendering capability demonstrates the entire course of the infrarenal aorta and common iliac vessels. According to the chosen angle for rendering, the vessel is seen from different positions. Positioning of the cursor in any vessel lumen guarantees proper differentiation in the multiplanar scan (Figure 32). A case of aortic aneurysm, supplied with an Endo prosthesis, showed in three dimensions not only the prosthesis, but also a partial thrombosis (Figures 33 and 34).

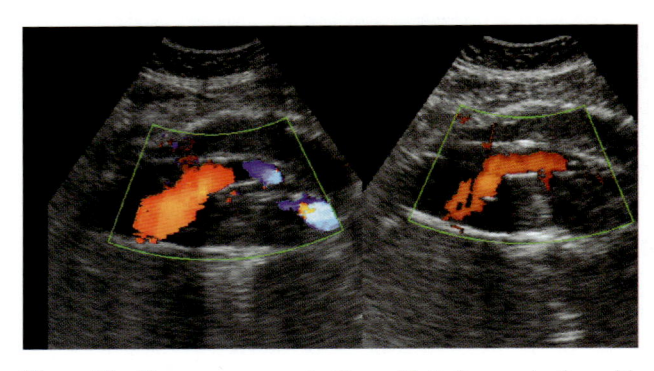

Figure 33 The same case as in Figure 32. Left, examination with CFM; right, with angiographic mode. Only a small and irregular lumen is visible, surrounded by thrombotic masses

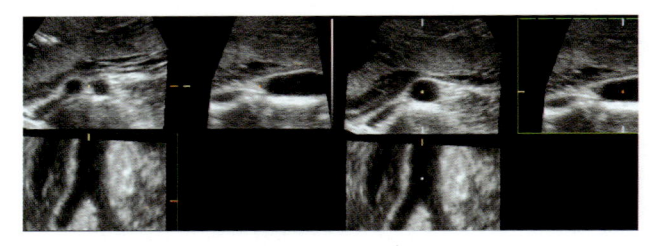

Figure 34 Different aspects of the aorta and common iliac artery in three-dimensional scans. Left, the cursor is positioned exactly at the bifurcation in the iliac arteries; right, the cursor is placed in the lower aorta, above the separation

Lymph nodes

Enlarged lymph nodes

Abdominal lymph nodes are detectable by sonography only over a size of 1 cm, if not covered by intestinal gas. In most cases the detection of enlarged nodes is limited to the para-aortic region, and infradiaphragmal region. Following the course of the vessels, other lymph nodes become detectable. As the aortic bifurca-

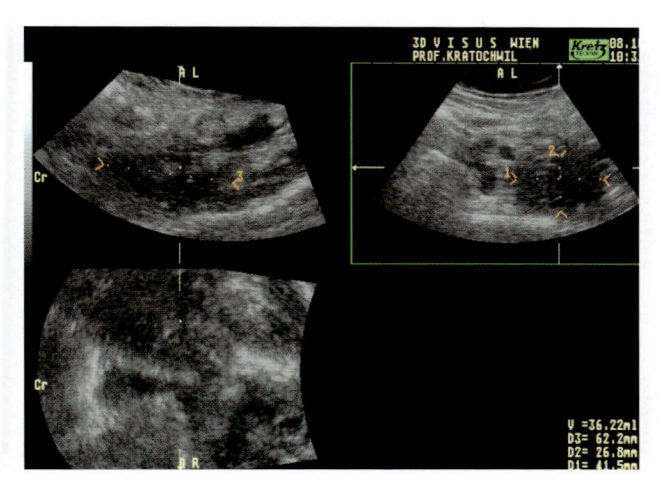

NON-GYNECOLOGICAL THREE-DIMENSIONAL ULTRASOUND

Figure 35 Enlarged lymph nodes in the right iliac region. Volume measurement of the pathology for radiation

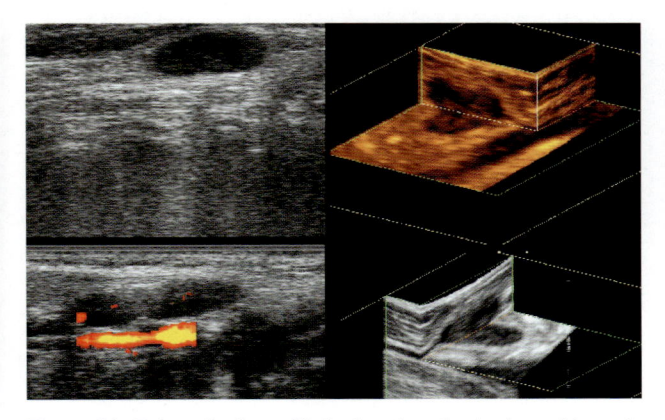

Figure 36 Enlarged submandibular lymph node. Angiographic mode exposes the vessel supply. Similar information is given by the niche mode (upper and lower right). The niche mode demonstrates the feeding tumor vessel

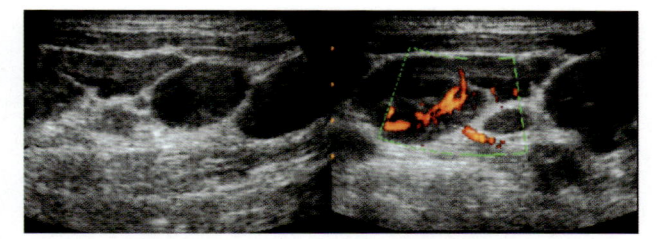

Figure 37 Enlarged lymph nodes in the lower jugular group in a case of Hodgkin's disease. Right, tumor vessels demonstrated by angiographic mode

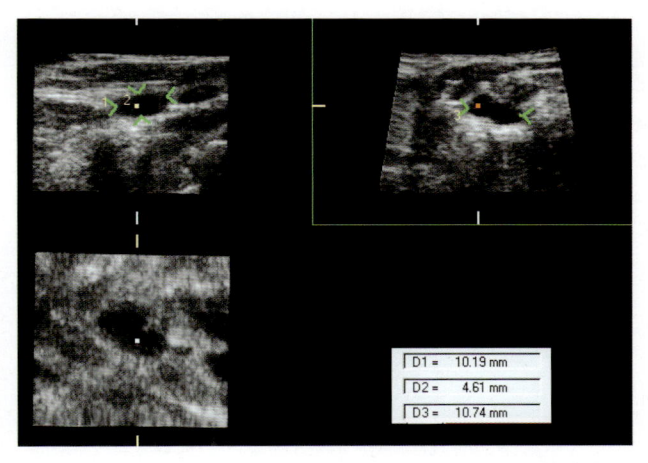

Figure 38 Small retroauricular node in a case of non-Hodgkin's lymphoma

tion is quite easy to inspect, it is possible to follow the course of the iliac vessels and to detect enlarged lymph nodes in this area. It is necessary only to orient the transducer according to the run of the vessels (Figure 35). The simultaneous availability of normal scanning and Doppler examination makes differentiation between small and oval tumor masses from vessels, much easier.

Lymph nodes involved in the superficial region

In cases of cancers originating from the ear, nose and throat region, the necessity arises to include superficial lymph node stations along the neck vessels and the submandibular region in the course of the examination (Figure 36). Inspection of the supra- and infraclavicular region and axilla is mandatory in patients who have undergone operation and are presenting with palpable masses either for restaging or for differentiation between reactive changes or lymph node metastasis. Of course, such examinations are routinely performed by 2D sonography, but the new 3D small-part probes are more efficient, because of the higher frequency available; resolution is superior, and the relationship of the tumor to the surrounding tissues is displayed much easier.

In superficial lymph nodes, 3D sonography is able, by scan optimization and niche mode demonstration, to identify the blood supply of the nodes. Especially in combination with the angiographic mode, identifying neoangiogenesis is very successful. Simultaneous availability of 3D and CFM or angiographic mode makes differentiation between small solid areas, sometimes mimicking the transverse aspect of a vessel, much easier and more reliable. This applies to enlarged lymph nodes in systemic diseases such as Hodgkin's and non-Hodgkin's disease (Figure 37). Even extremely small superficial lymph nodes of only 2–3 mm in size, located in the submandibular or retroauricular area, are detected (Figure 38).

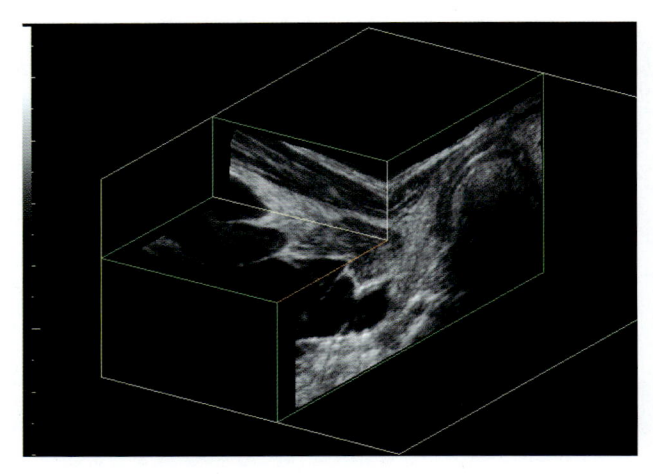

Figure 39 Pseudo-three-dimensional aspect of larynx, trachea, thyroid and vessels

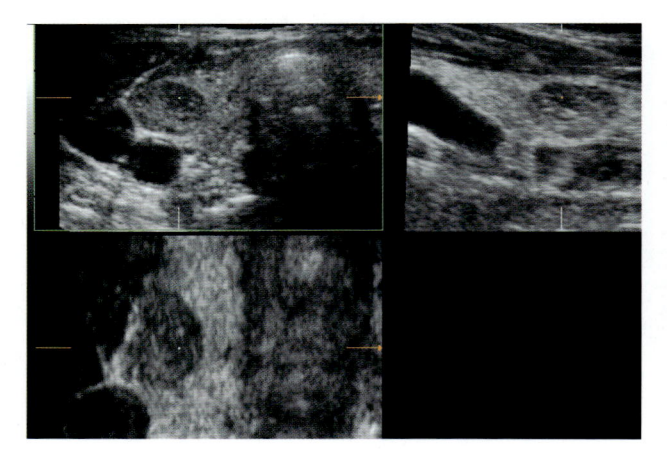

Figure 40 Benign adenoma of the thyroid. Upper left, transverse scan; upper right, longitudinal scan; lower left, coronal scan

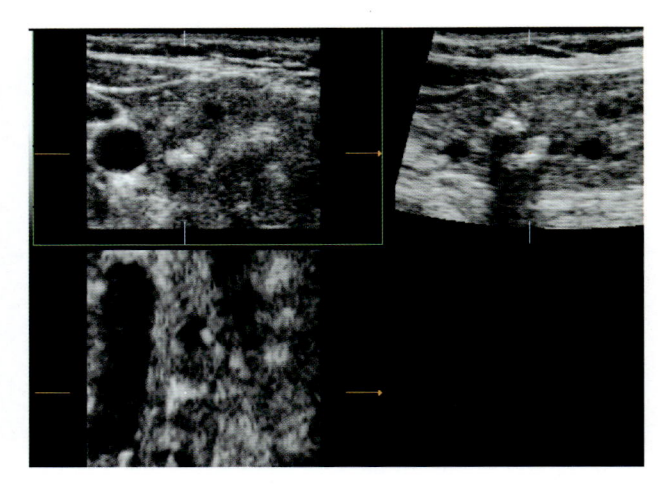

Figure 41 Calcified structures in the thyroid

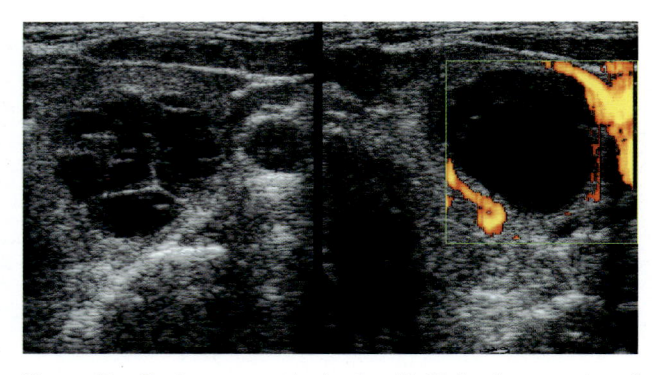

Figure 42 Cystic structures in the thyroid. Right, demonstration of vessels around the cyst, by angiographic mode

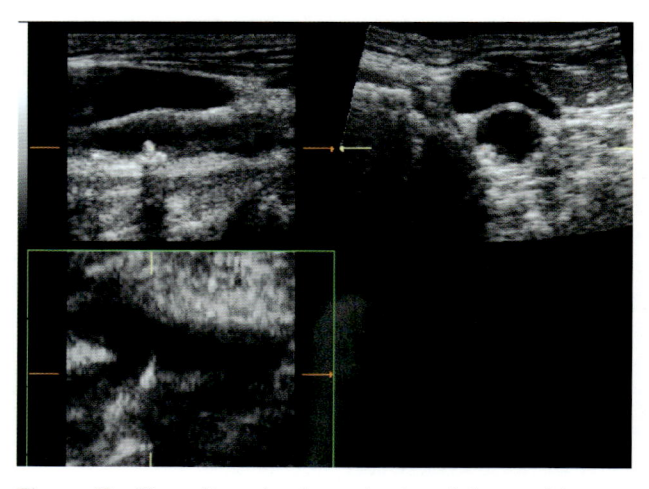

Figure 43 Three-dimensional examination of the carotid artery, demonstrating an atheromatous plaque. Upper left, longitudinal scan, showing a shadow behind the lesion; upper right, transverse scan

The neck

Thyroid gland

In examining the neck for lymph nodes it is obvious that one asks for the possible benefits of 3D sonography in diseases of the thyroid. At first it must be mentioned that, because of the small footprint and the limited sweep angle of 30°, the entire gland is not currently demonstrable in the transverse scan in three dimensions. One lobe of the thyroid, however, is easily demonstrable. The superb resolution is due to the frequency of 12 MHz in combination with the high line density in the slow volume sweep. The examination also benefits from the organ-optimized aspect of the gland. The niche mode demonstrates the transverse scan of the trachea, the thyroid and lateral vessels and, in front, the superficial muscles of the neck (Figure 39). Small, benign adenomas are clearly outlined (Figure 40). In the lower left, the scan demonstrates an ideal frontal scan of the area with the hypoechogenic area of the trachea in the middle flanked by the right lobe of the thyroid containing the small adenoma. Likewise, calcified structures are identified (Figure 41). Again, the angiographic mode facilitates differentiation between cystic structures, solid nodes and degenerated and non-degenerated adenomas (Figure 42).

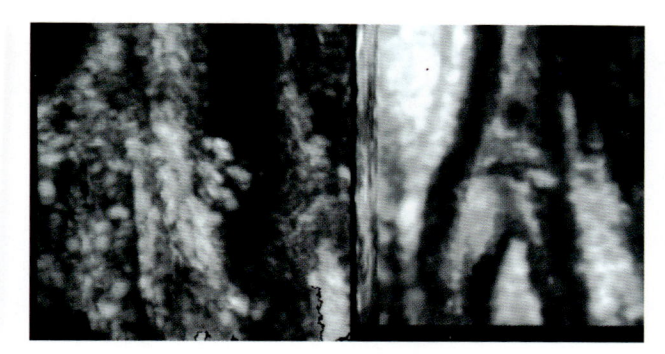

Figure 44 Rendered images of the plaque in the carotid artery. Left, surface and minimum rendering; right, surface and light

Figure 45 Comparison between a transverse scan of the prostate in three-dimensional examination and a schematic drawing of the same region

Carotid plaques

Looking for neck lymph nodes and the thyroid gland, it is unavoidable also to become engaged with the examination of the carotid artery and the question of whether 3D sonography offers a new advantage. The findings are rather promising. Considering just the multiplanar information, calcifications due to atheromatous plaques are discernible at first glance (Figure 43). Optimization of the scan demonstrates a perfectly rendered picture, showing the lesion from different angles (Figure 44). Combining 3D sonography with the angiographic mode shows either the gray-level aspect and color-coded carotid artery in combination, or only the 3D aspect of the artery alone, without surrounding tissue.

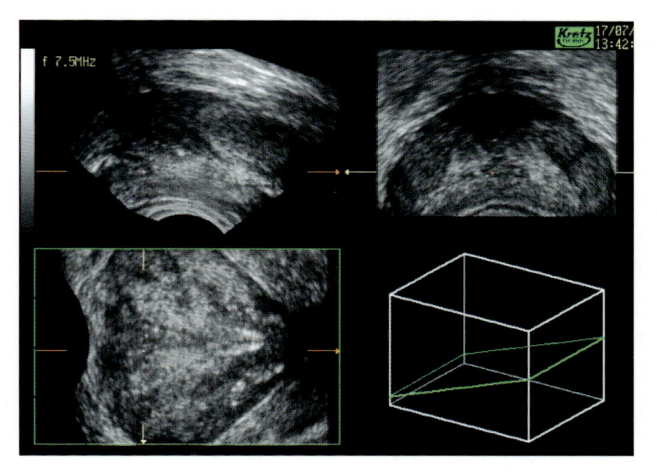

Figure 46 Three-dimensional scan of the prostate with a frequency of 5–8 MHz. Upper left, longitudinal scan; upper right, transverse scan; lower left, coronal scan of the gland, not achievable by two-dimensional scanning

Prostate gland

Difference between two- and three-dimensional examination

The difference from the 2D examination again is the benefit of simultaneous interpretation of the three scanning planes, resulting in better correlation of anatomical details and volumetric measurements. By scrolling the volume by translation, the organ is examined in fractions of millimeters. Just one volume scan gives all the necessary information, including inspection of the junction between the prostate and seminal vesicles. The screen shows the longitudinal scan at the top left, the transverse scan at the top right and the frontal aspect of the gland at the bottom left. The frontal scan is not accessible by 2D examination and adds additional information. The technique for the first time clearly demonstrates the different prostatic zones (Figure 45). The quality of the 3D examination

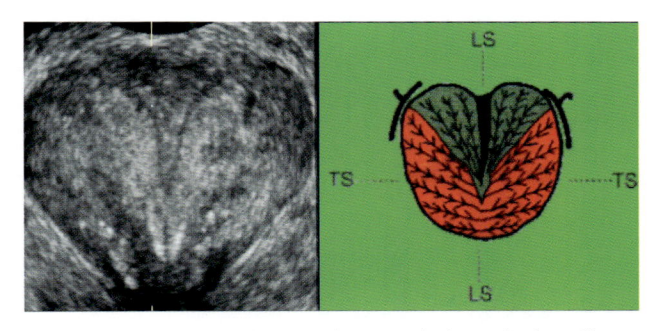

Figure 47 Comparison between the coronal ultrasonic three-dimensional scan and a schematic drawing of the region

is stressed by comparing scans with anatomical drawings and slices[18]. Full accordance between the ultrasonic transverse scan and the drawing is shown in Figure 46, and for the coronal scan and the corresponding anatomical drawing in Figure 47. By volume rotation, aspects of the organ can be displayed in accordance with those of anatomic textbooks. The cumulus as well as the central zone with the urethra, even its bend, is demonstrated. Sometimes even ejacu-

CLINICAL APPLICATION OF 3D SONOGRAPHY

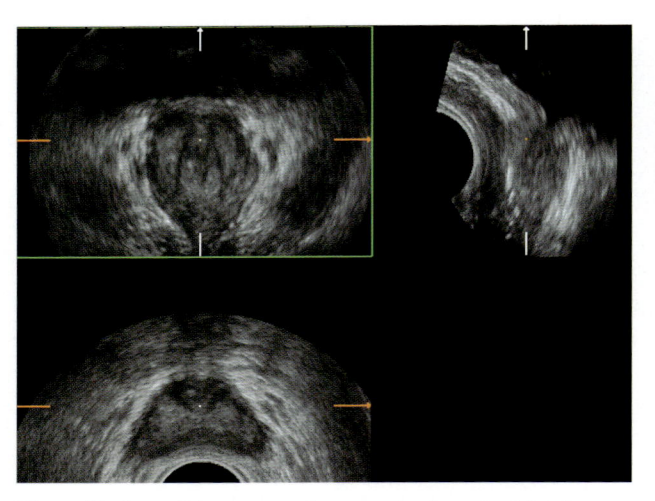

Figure 48 Scan of the prostate, demonstrating intraglandular ducts

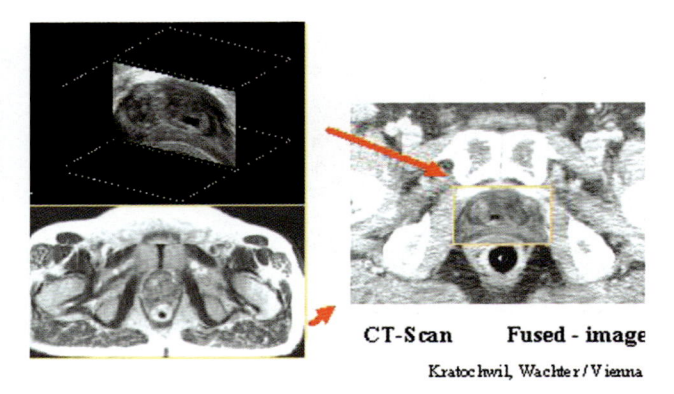

Figure 50 Fusion of ultrasonic three-dimensional examination and computerized tomography dose distribution in radiating prostatic cancers

latory ducts heading for the colliculus seminalis are perceptible (Figure 48). Likewise, seminal vesicles and deferent ducts are demonstrable in their full extent. Only in cases presenting with severe prostatic hypertrophy is it sometimes necessary to take a second volume to demonstrate these appendices.

Volume computation

For volume computation of the organ, different formulae are applicable. From measuring about 200 prostate glands the following conclusion is drawn. The most unreliable measurement is based on a rotational ellipsoid; deviation of more than 25% of the actual volume is frequent. More reliable is the formula based on measuring the largest diameter of the transverse, anteroposterior and longitudinal planes. The standard deviation is roughly about 10%. The best result is achieved by measuring the organ's contour in about 8–10 areas. These measurements are easily and correctly obtained by 3D guidance. The standard deviation is only 3–4%. These advantage is comprehensible as the irregular contours are manually traced in the volume.

Recently, a new calculation for 3D volumes was developed: the automatic volume calculation (VOCAL) mode (Figure 49). With this method the volume is arranged in such a way that the cursor is nearly central in all scans. With activation of the mode, two cursors, in the form of arrows, appear. These cursors are placed on the recognizable organ border. On pressing of the command button, the volume is calculated automatically in 6–120 planes, depending on the preset angle of rotation. The calculated contour can be checked in any plane, and if necessary modified. The estimation is less reliable than with manual contour following – deviations of 6–8% but much quicker. The effort of precise volume estimation is based on the demand of radiotherapy for precise location of the target doses in order to minimize radiation sequelae to radio-sensitive neighboring structures, such as the rectum and bladder (Figure 50).

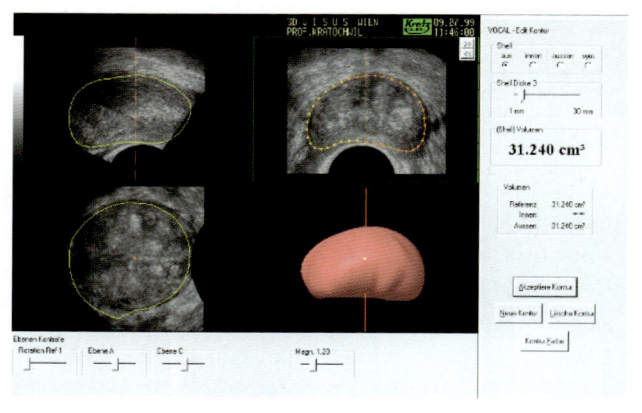

Figure 49 Automatic volume calculation (VOCAL mode) in three-dimensional examination

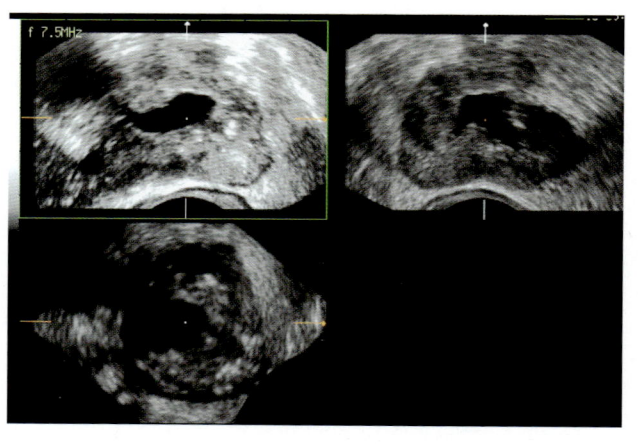

Figure 51 Three-dimensional aspect of tansurethral prostatic resection. Typical central defect

NON-GYNECOLOGICAL THREE-DIMENSIONAL ULTRASOUND

Clinical application: benign hypertrophy

In daily clinical routine, 3D examination is quite helpful in benign hypertrophy, to measure not only the total gland, but also the pathological changes. This should be of interest in conservative treatment of benign hypertrophy, for checking the result. In patients treated by transurethral resection, the defect caused by the operation is demonstrable (Figure 51).

Prostatic carcinoma

The benefit of ultrasonic examination in prostatic cancer is in question, owing to the fact that about one-third of the tumors are isodense and sonographically not accessible. The other tumors are either hyper-reflective or anechoic. The latter group is more easily detectable than the former (Figure 52). In a transverse scan the anechoic lesion is well demarcated. Another useful aspect is the niche mode (Figure 53). If hyperechoic lesions are located close to benign focal disease, considerable diagnostic problems arise. Another reason for misdiagnosis is the multi-focal tumor location, sometimes difficult to interpret. Difficulties in interpreting scans are also induced by anti-androgen blockage, or as a result of radiotherapy.

Tumor staging

In primary tumors, 3D examination is successful in tumor staging. Staging primarily benefits from stepping through the volume and observing the coronal scan. For instance, tumor invasion to the capsule is much more clearly perceptible in the coronal, than in the longitudinal or transverse scans (Figure 54). Bladder infiltration is better recognizable in the frontal scan (Figures 55 and 56). The infiltration to the rectum is presented in Figure 57. The magnification in the lower right corner is convincing. It has already

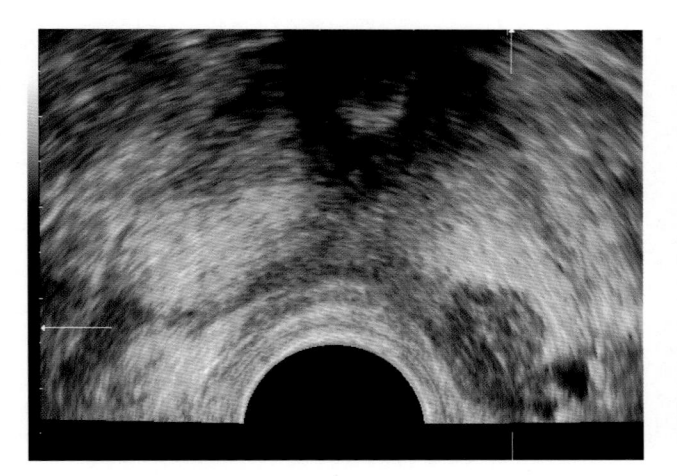

Figure 52 Prostatic cancer in the peripheral zone of the left lobe

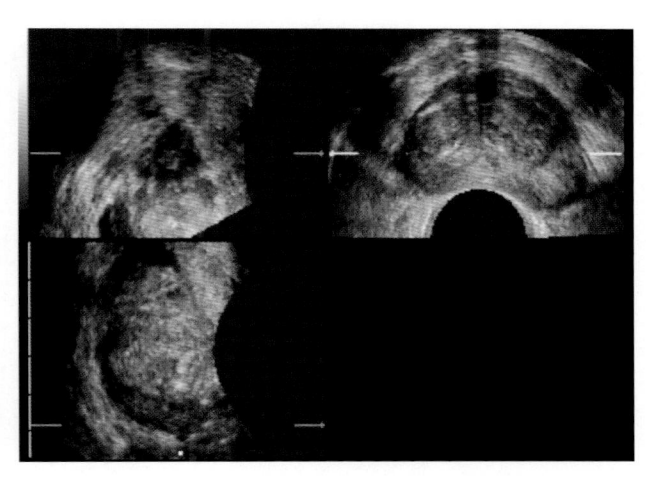

Figure 54 Three-dimensional examination of cancer infiltration of the prostatic capsule

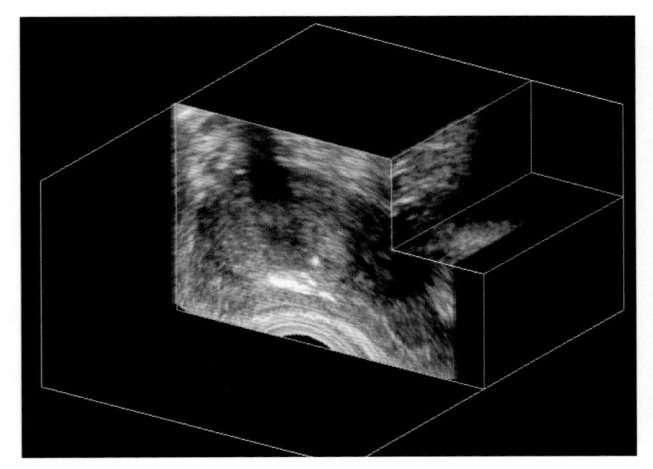

Figure 53 Pseudo-three-dimensional aspect of a prostatic cancer located in the peripheral zone (left). At the same time, niche mode exposes the transverse, longitudinal and coronal aspects

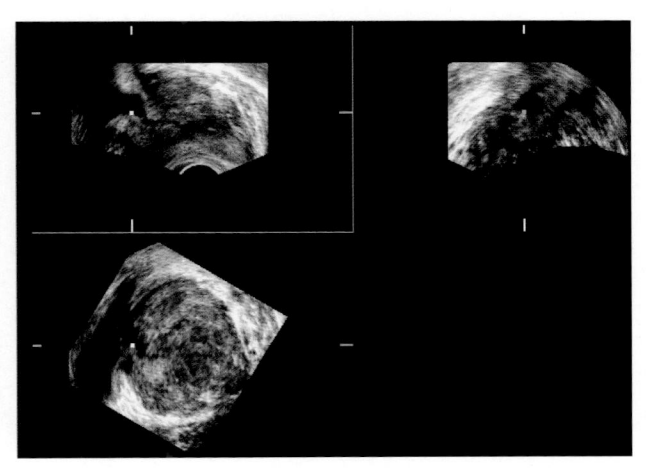

Figure 55 Bladder infiltration by prostatic cancer. Infiltration is best revealed by the coronal plane (lower left), not accessible by two-dimensional examination

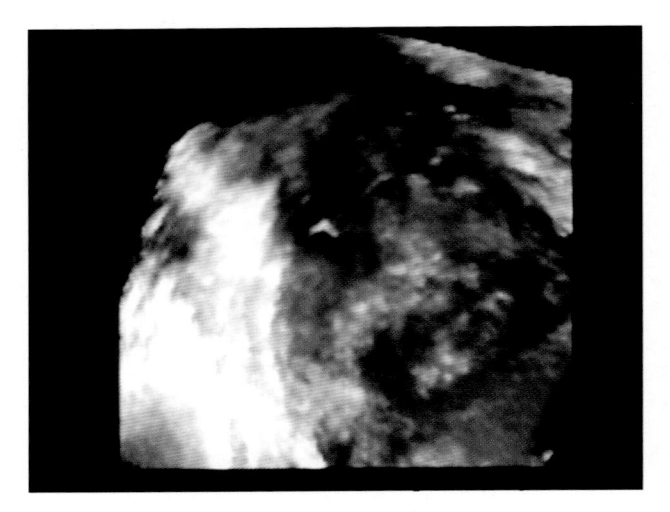

Figure 56 Surface rendering of cancer in Figure 55

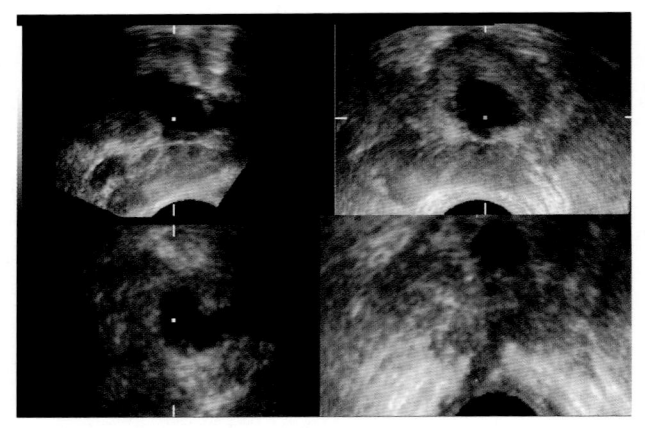

Figure 57 Three-dimensional examination of a prostatic cancer infiltrating the rectum. Best demonstrated in the zoom (lower right)

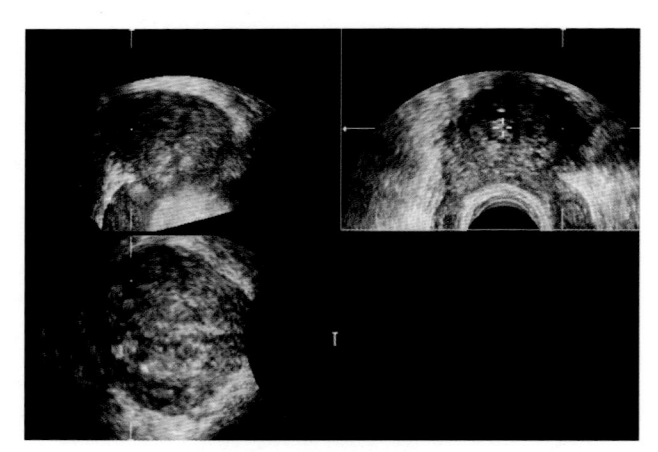

Figure 58 Prostatic cancer infiltrating seminal vesicles. Upper left, longitudinal scan. Left seminal vesicle is fairly enlarged and irregular. This is reflected in the transverse scan, upper right

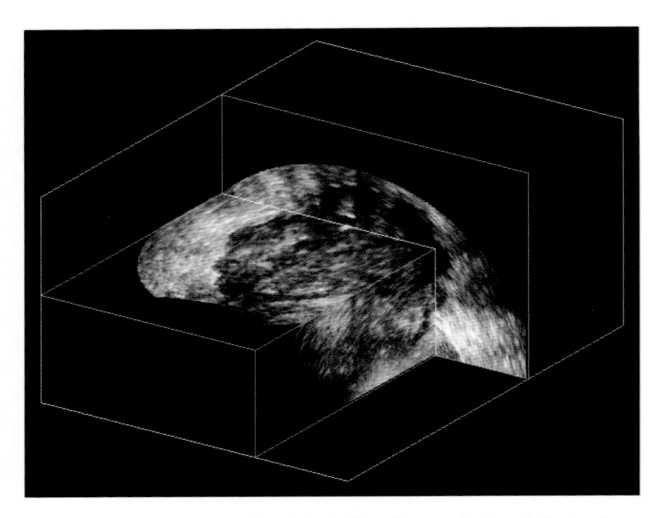

Figure 59 The relationship of the infiltrating seminal vesicles is clearly demonstrated in the niche mode of the same area as in Figure 58

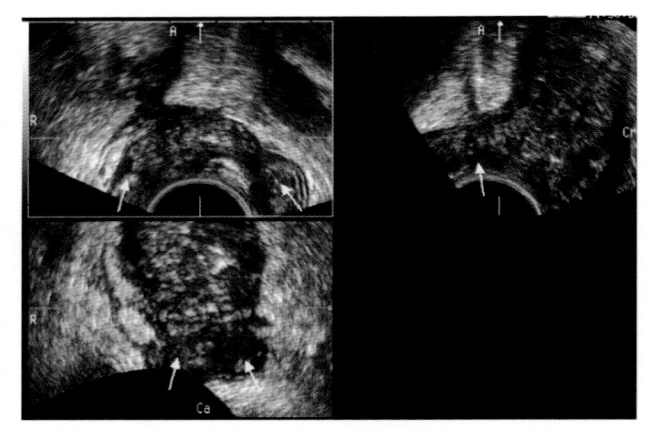

Figure 60 Infiltration of seminal vesicles (arrow) by a rectal cancer

been mentioned that the vesicle–prostatic junction is easy to access and to inspect by translating and rotating the volume. The irregularity and echogenicity of the seminal vesicles in Figure 58 are highly suspicious of tumorous infiltration. Even more convincing is the niche mode in Figure 59. Occasionally the vesicles may be infiltrated from tumors descending from other organs such as the rectum (Figure 60). The reliability of ultrasonic diagnosis has been cross-checked by CT and MRI results. Accordance, mainly with MRI, was the incentive to fuse image information of MRI, CT and ultrasound for improving location of the target doses to prostatic carcinomas (Figure 50).

Diagnosis of recurrences after radical operation

The critical inspection of the region of interest after operation or radiotherapy is primarily based on the again-rising level of prostate-specific antigen (PSA). Despite a recorded change in PSA level it is often a difficult task to locate the suspected recurrent tumor. In this search 3D sonography is successfully integrated, especially in the follow-up of patients who have undergone operation. Transrectal 3D sonography is

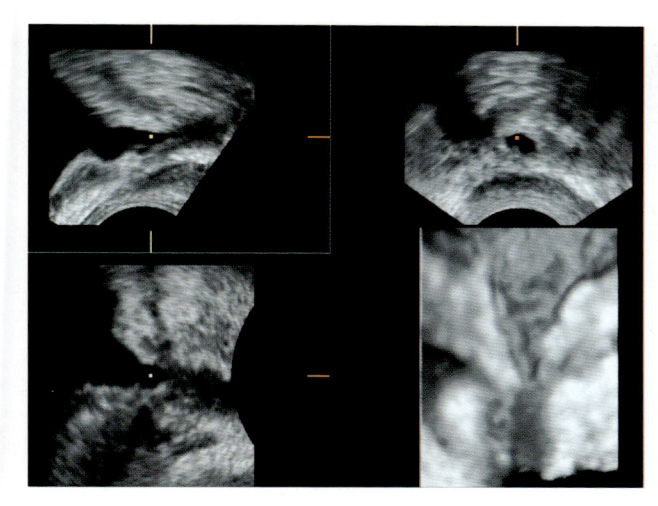

Figure 61 Normal anastomosis after radical prostatectomy. Upper left, bladder neck and the newly formed urethra; upper right, transverse scan of the region; lower left, coronal aspect; lower right, three-dimensional rendered image clearly demonstrates the bladder neck and anastomosis, and the muscles of the pelvic floor

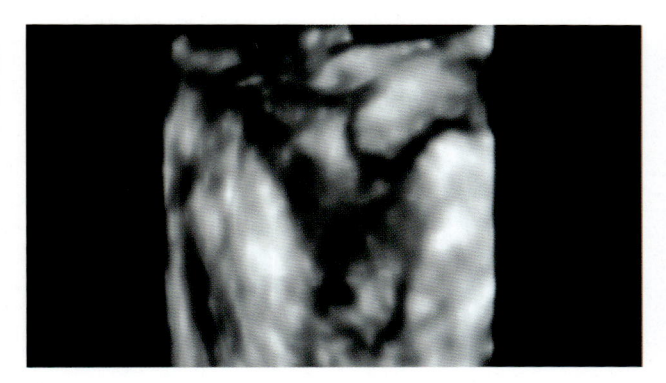

Figure 62 Recurrent tumor after radical operation. The tumor develops at the anastomosis. Papillary parts at the left wall

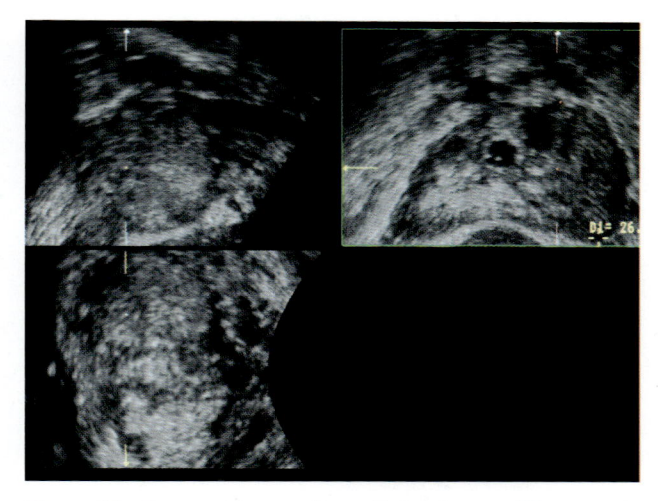

Figure 63 Recurrent tumor after radiation therapy. The tumor is

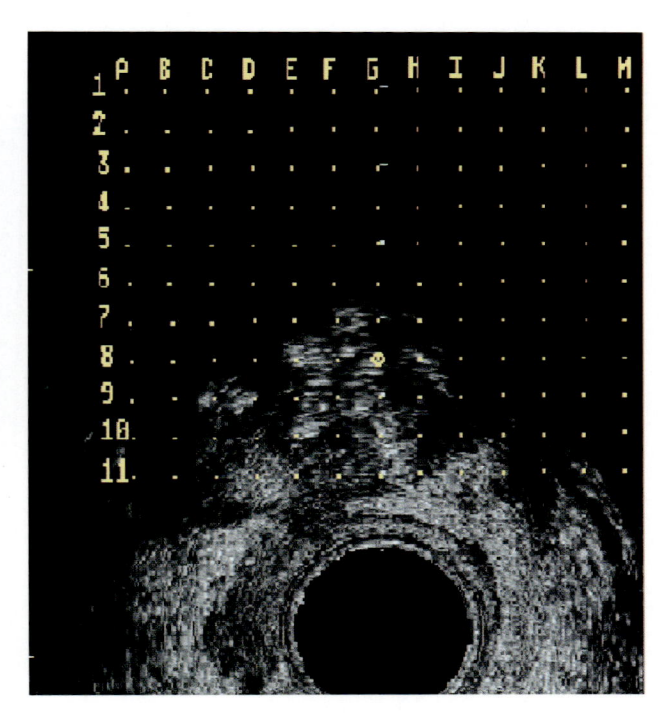

Figure 64 Electronic grid for ultrasonic biopsy and ultrasound-guided interventions

extremely useful in evaluating the postoperative prostatic area and for inspecting the anastomosis of the newly formed urethra. This new structure is followed caudally from the bladder (Figure 61). If the operation was performed relatively recently, sonography is even able to recognize sutures around the urethra neck. The bladder wall is without any noticeable growth. The levator muscle can be followed towards the pelvic wall. More convincing than the scan with multiple, orthogonal planes is a rendered volume of the region demonstrating the entire pelvic floor.

In patients suffering from a recurrence, the findings are quite different. Normally in the prostatic region, structures of nodular, irregular and anechoic appearance are discernible at any site. Sometimes the relapse penetrates to the bladder, levator or rectum. In only a few cases, it seems that recurrence originates in the urethra, near the anastomosis, growing to the bladder lumen and infiltrating the bladder wall (Figure 62).

RITA study

Treatment of recurrences is particularly difficult in cases where radiotherapy has reached its tolerable limits (Figure 63). The hope in these cases rests on destroying the relapse by heat (radiointerstitial tumor ablation; RITA)[19]. By means of a needle, the tissue is heated to 120°C. The heating is controlled by a thermoprobe placed between the rectum and prostate. The therapeutic success depends on the precise location of the tumor and correct placement of the thermic needle.

207

CLINICAL APPLICATION OF 3D SONOGRAPHY

Both targets can be achieved by 3D transrectal sonography. The 3D machine is equipped for ultrasound-guided biopsy. A template with a grid of 64 drill holes is mounted on the transducer shaft (Figure 64). The grid is presented on the monitor, overlying the prostatic scan. For treatment planning, the holes are marked before therapy is started. By activating the biopsy line, the path of the needle and distance to the lesion can be read from the monitor. Acquisition of a single volume needs only a few seconds, as soon as the correct placement is checked. The achieved results are best demonstrated by comparing the photograph of the hook-wired needle with the ultrasonic scan (Figures 65 and 66). The length of the needle is recognizable in the longitudinal plane. In the coronal plane, taken from a bird's eye view, two of the three wires are demonstrated. In the near future, this maneuver, applicable also for placing radioactive seeds in the organ, will be facilitated by live 3D sonography (Figure 67). By this mode, refreshing the volume every second, almost real-time examination is achieved, making targeting of a lesion possible in a few seconds. This will lead to a further reduction of operation time.

Rectal carcinoma

In examination of the prostate gland, the question is: what results can be achieved using 3D sonography? Although my experience of rectal carcinoma is limited to only a few cases, the results seem to be promising. As the transrectal probe has a frequency of 5–10

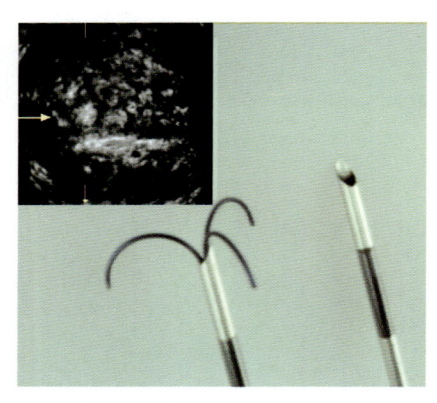

Figure 65 Thermo needle for heat ablation of recurrent tumors. The left upper corner shows a part of the three-dimensional scan, demonstrating the hooks of the needle (arrow)

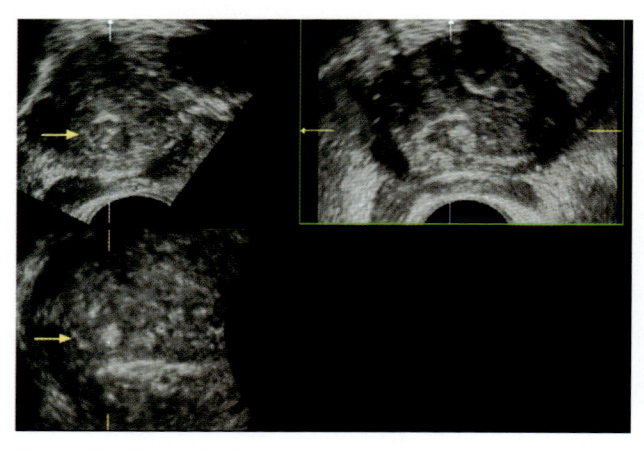

Figure 66 The needle hooks are demonstrated by three-dimensional examination. Best aspect in the coronal scan (lower left)

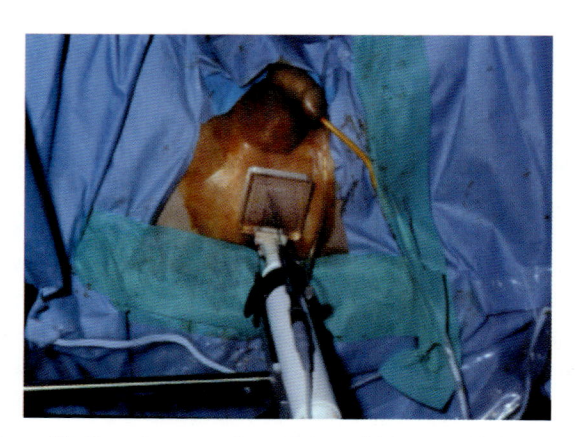

Figure 67 Operation set-up for radiointerstitial tumor ablation

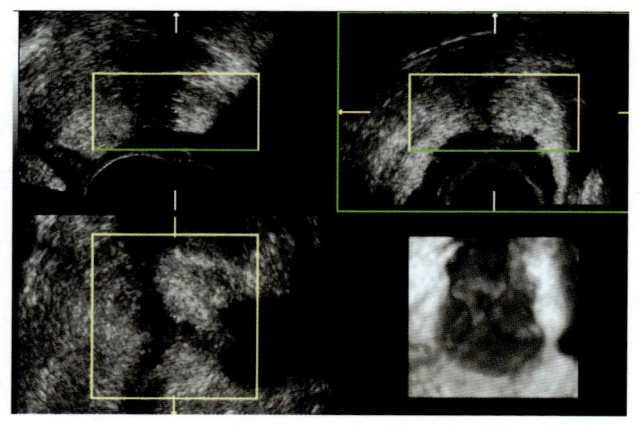

Figure 68 Three-dimensional aspect of a rectal cancer. Rendering box is set. Below right, surface and minimum mode

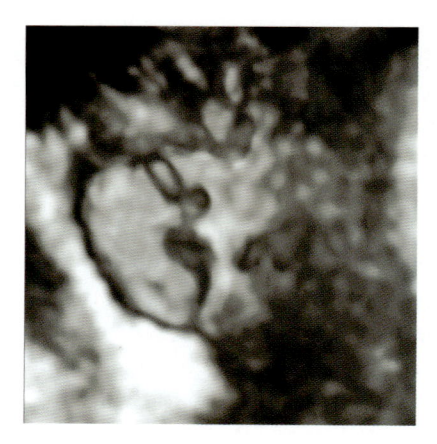

Figure 69 Surface smooth mode and light grading demonstrates the same tumor as in Figure 68

MHz, the layers of the rectal wall and muscles, as demonstrated in the section on the pelvic floor, can be sufficiently differentiated. The only limitation is that only a volume of 180° is demonstrable at once. If the tumor is located more laterally, at least two volumes must be acquired. The same applies to the anal canal. Extension and tumor growth is demonstrated both in the multiplanar view and in the niche mode (Figures 68 and 69). In this far-advanced case, the tumor has already invaded the seminal vesicles. It is interesting that 3D examination is still applicable in stenotic tumors, where other imaging methods are at their limit. In these tumors, nearly completely occluding the lumen, the end-firing vaginal probe helps to surpass the problem[20].

As already pointed out, 3D examination is employed in the diagnosis and follow-up of anal carcinomas. Furthermore, 3D sonography has the potential to clarify an uncertain situation caused, for instance, by a rectal abscess or fistulas.

Other possible, but still not fully realized three-dimensional applications

Pediatrics

Pediatrics is one of the specialties where 3D sonography will probably play an important role in the future. One of the main advantages is that the examination is stored and analyzed in the absence of the patient. The first effect is a reduction in examination time for the children and a calmer environment for volume analysis. The examination is even easy to perform in premature babies in the incubator.

Brain ventricle measurement

Successful examinations of the neonatal brain were performed to study the ventricular development in premature newborns. During these examinations vessel anomalies were detected[21].

Examination of the fetal hip

Three-dimensional examination has been informative in studying the fetal hip. Measurements of the structures relevant for the diagnosis of fetal dysplasia are displayed at ease, even if the fetus is not correctly

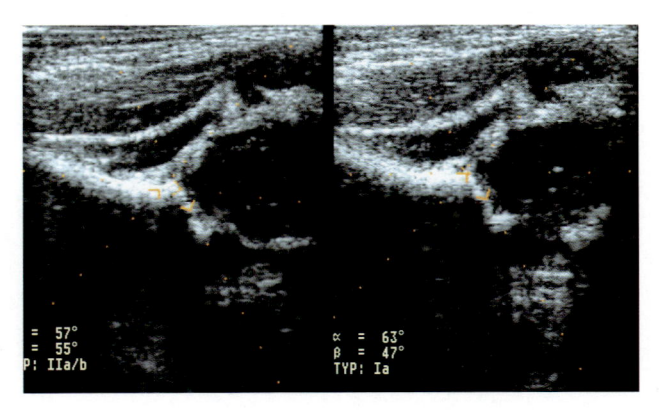

Figure 70 Fetal hip by three-dimensional examination. Demonstration of two-dimensional planes, and the possibility of measurement

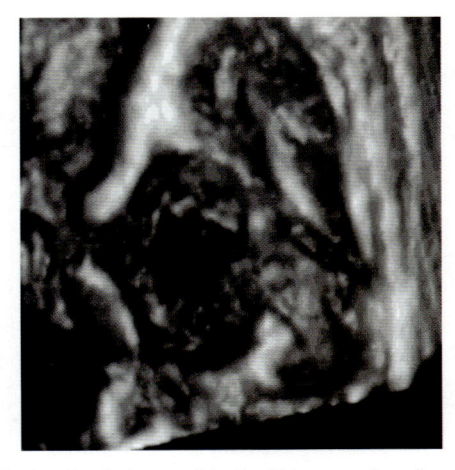

Figure 71 Rendered picture of the fetal hip, smooth surface

placed. Besides measuring the different angles, a rendering is performed to show the situation (Figures 70 and 71).

A further application of 3D sonography in pediatrics is the examination of the upper abdomen in internal diseases and in surgical cases. This applies not only in newborns with malformations, but also in patients undergoing organ transplants. Especially in transplant surgery, 3D sonography in combination with the demonstration of spatial vessel distribution and the use of ultrasonic contrast media will open a wide diagnostic field.

Orthopedics and traumatology

In this specialty the employment of the small-part transducer seems promising in different applications. Although a transducer not primarily developed for this indication was used, some astonishing results were attained. It is worthwhile to consider the application in this field of medicine. Some early experiences are here documented.

CLINICAL APPLICATION OF 3D SONOGRAPHY

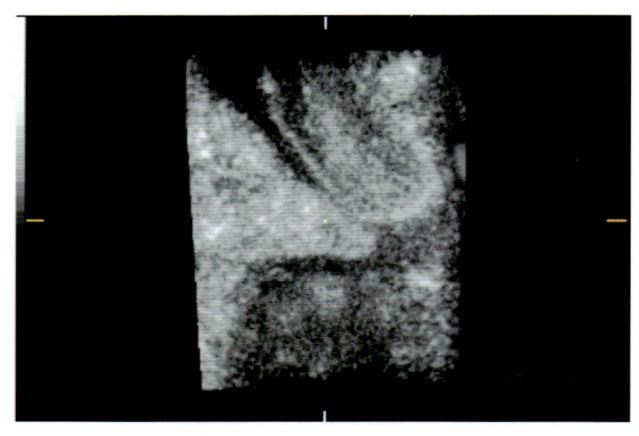

Figure 72 Three-dimensional aspect of the meniscus. Between the femur condylus and the tibial condylus the triangular shape of the meniscus

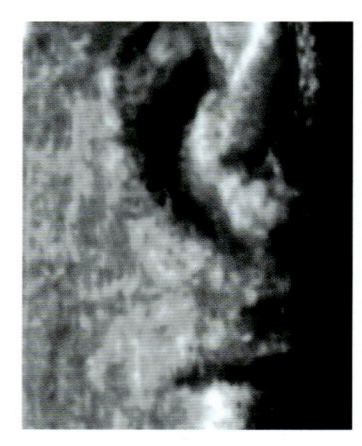

Figure 75 Three-dimensional rendering of the case illustrated in Figure 73 and 74, clearly showing the effusion and its extension

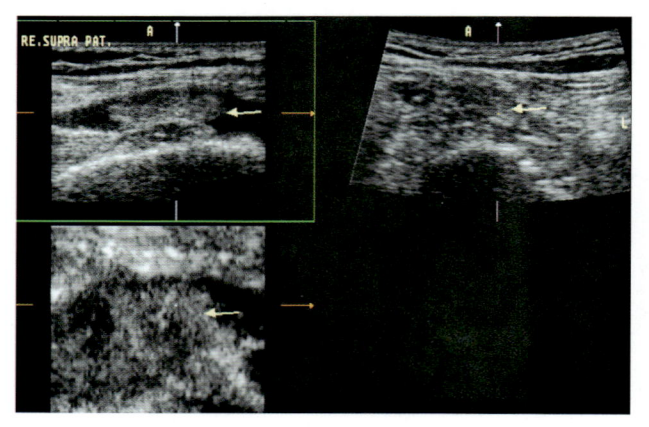

Figure 73 Effusion in the knee. Inside the effusion a solid part is visible. Upper left, longitudinal scan; upper right, transverse scan; lower left, coronal scan

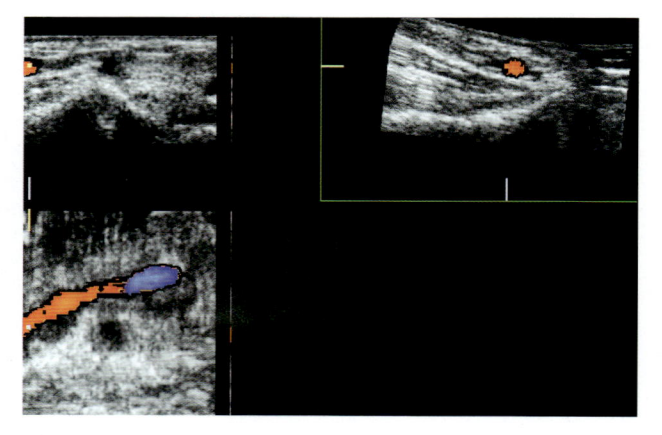

Figure 76 Small-part probe (10–12 MHz) clearly demonstrates the course of the radial artery in CFM. Color and gray-scale information is stored together. This enables the spatial distribution of vessels

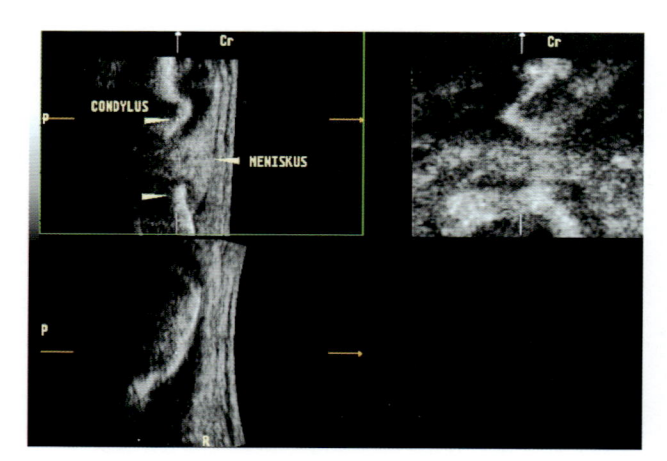

Figure 74 The same case as in Figure 73, from another aspect

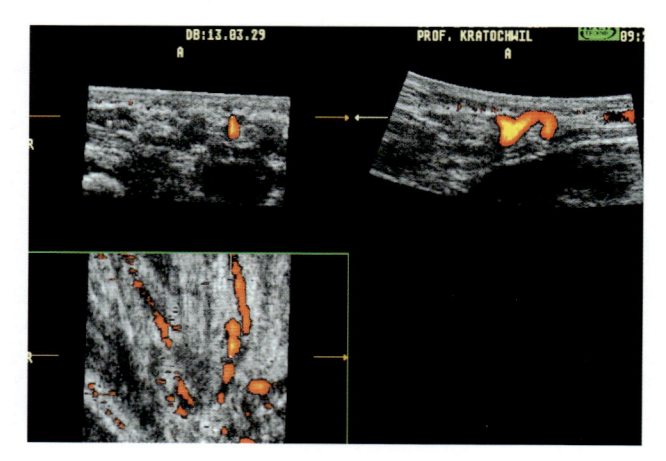

Figure 77 The small-part probe is located in the palm. Angiographic mode demonstrates the arteries of the palm and fingers

A sportsman, suffering from a knee problem, gave the incentive for 3D examination of the region. The examination of the unaffected knee clearly demonstrated the knee joint and the triangular meniscus (Figure 72). In the other knee, a large effusion was detected (Figures 73–75). Unfortunately, it was not possible to demonstrate the posterior horns. By applying a 12-MHz probe, a penetration of only 3–4 cm is possible – not enough to penetrate the muscle volume of a sportsman in the poplitea.

One can imagine applying this technique for location and measurement of muscle hematomas, and

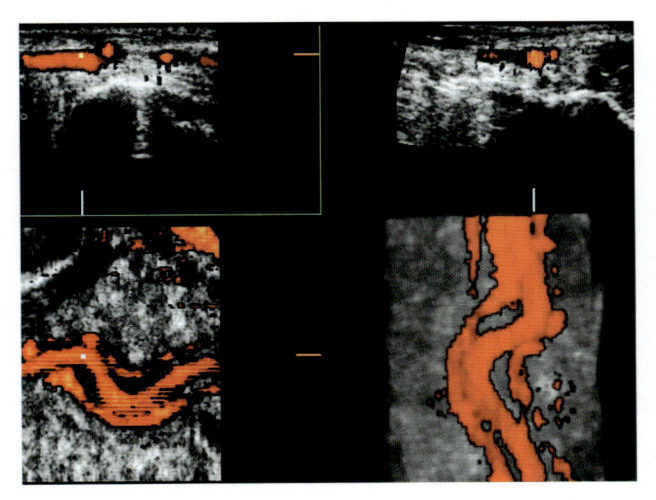

NON-GYNECOLOGICAL THREE-DIMENSIONAL ULTRASOUND

Figure 78 Three-dimensional demonstration of the course of the posterior tibial artery, twining around the ankle

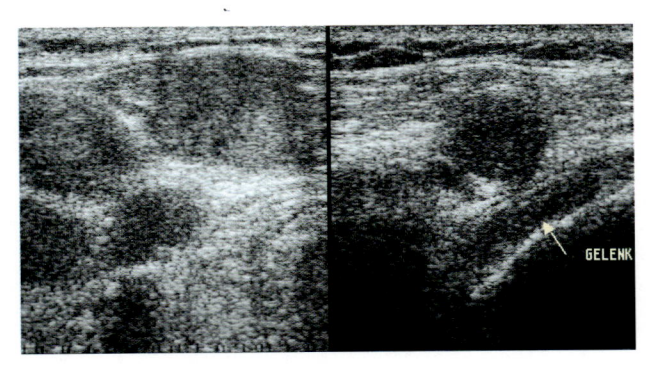

Figure 79 Metastatic deposit of a lung cancer in the muscle tissue around the humeroclavicular joint

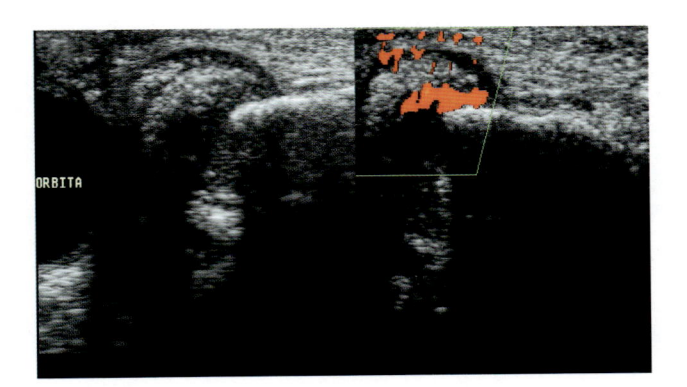

Figure 80 Local recurrence in a case of cancer located in the maxilla. The tumor shows a tendency to grow towards the orbit (left). Inside the tumor, vessels are visible

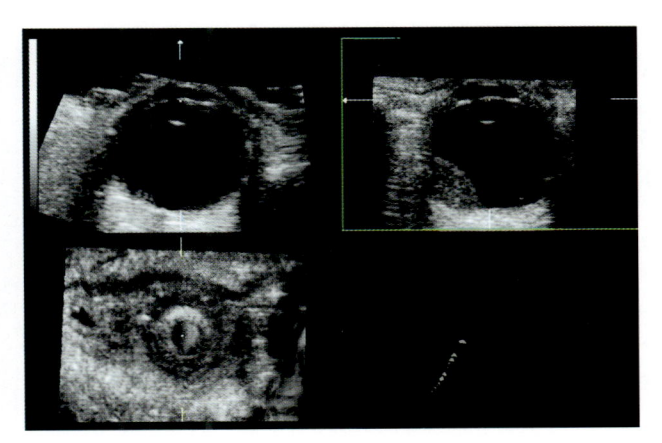

Figure 81 Three-dimensional scan of the eye. The cursor is positioned inside the lens. Note especially the coronal scan (lower left)

the hand, along the fingers and around the ankle (Figures 76–78).

Skeletal and soft tissue metastasis

The small-part transducer is a perfect tool for locating metastases in superficial structures, such as ribs and muscle tissue.

In the first example, a bronchus carcinoma was disseminated to the muscle tissue. For a long period the patient complained of pains in the shoulder. Three-dimensional sonography succeeded in demonstrating a small, anechoic lesion near the humerus head (Figure 79).

In the second example, a metastasis is shown of a maxillary sinus carcinoma located in the orbit (Figure 80).

The examination is also ideal for the examination of limb stumps in the postoperative course, for differentiation between scar tissue and a possible metastatic spread or recurrence.

Ophthalmology

Because of its superficial position, limited size and tissue composition, the eye is an ideal organ for sonography. Indeed, it was the first organ to be examined primarily by a scan and very late by the B-scan technique. The preference for and still enduring use of the A-scan technique in ophthalmology is caused by the necessity of using high frequencies to differentiate the layers of the eye. The other reason is the transducer size.

As the small-part transducer has a frequency of 12 MHz, it should fulfill the demands. The probe was tested in this application; although the footprint is 4

demonstrating the Archilles tendon in three dimensions. Demonstration of muscles and joints is also feasible in the upper extremity. Of special interest is the examination of the hand and the carpal tunnel, tendons and bones.

A further advantage in all the mentioned regions is the spatial distribution of the tortuous course of superficial vessels, such as the radial vessels, the vessels in

CLINICAL APPLICATION OF 3D SONOGRAPHY

cm, the transducer fits into the orbital margins. The first 3D examinations of the eye were performed with a vaginal transducer with a center frequency of 8 MHz. Because of the long shaft, however, the handling of the probe is tiresome.

Using such frequencies, a water delay bath can be ignored. The transducer is coupled by only a thick film of contact jelly to the closed eye. Correct arrangement of the technical parameters for an optimal examination is stored in the probe's program and is always available for further examinations.

Acquisition time for one scan is only some seconds. The entire eye, from the lens to the top of the orbit, is presented, with the optical nerve in its middle (Figure 81). As mentioned in every part of this chapter, additional information is contributed by the coronal scan and the choice of the translation movement. Shifting the coronal scan from the surface to the posterior part successively, the different portions of the eye are demonstrable. The examination can be supplemented either by the niche mode technique, demonstrating the eye in a pseudo-3D demonstration, or by a rendered examination, showing the structure of interest from different angles in the form of a cine loop (Figure 82).

The first clinical experiences with this new technique were collected in cases of chorion melanoma of the eye undergoing radiotherapy. The location of the tumors is rather easy, even if they are small. It is important, however, that concomitant retinal abruption, measuring only 1–3 mm in extent, is undoubtedly demonstrable (Figures 83 and 84), as is the relationship of the tumor to the optic nerve. All cases were followed after therapy for evaluating the therapeutic effect in 2-monthly intervals. To demonstrate the potential of 3D sonography, some images of a lymphoma, located in the eyelid, are shown (Figure 85).

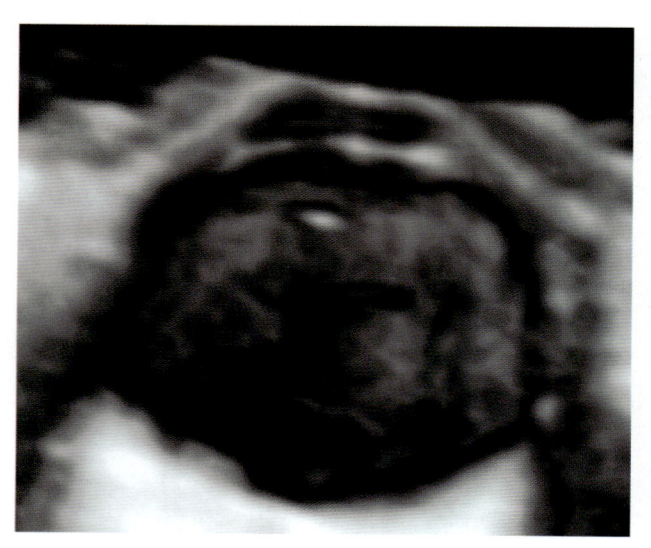

Figure 82 Surface rendering of the eye, smooth and light mode in combination

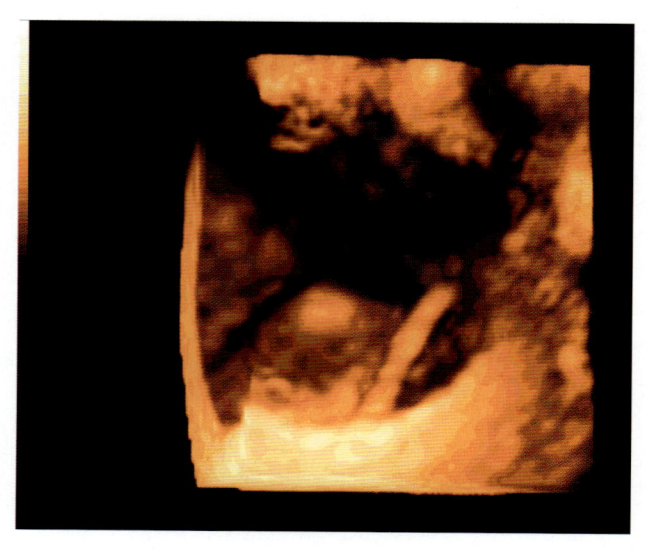

Figure 84 Surface rendering of the choroid melanoma and retinal detachment

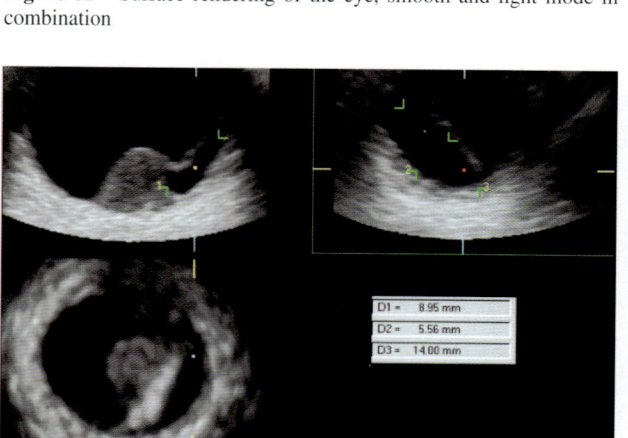

Figure 83 Melanoma of the choroid membrane, three-dimensional aspect. Besides the tumor, detachment of the retina is visible

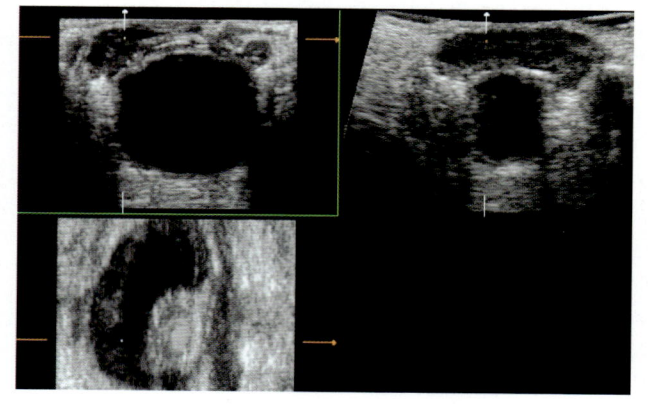

Figure 85 Three-dimensional examination of lymphoma located in the eyelid

References

1. Kratochwil A. Versuch der dreidimensionalen Darstellung in der Geburtshilfe. *Ultraschall Med* 1992;4:149–202
2. Merz E, Machiella D, Bahlmann F, Weber G. Three-dimensional ultrasound in the evaluation of fetal malformation. *Ultrasound Obstet Gynecol* 1992;2(suppl 1):137
3. Pretorius DH, Nelson TR. Three-dimensional ultrasound imaging in patient diagnosis and management: the future. *J Ultrasound Obstet Gynecol* 1991;1:381–3
4. Benoit B. Three dimensional surface mode for demonstration of normal fetal anatomy in the second and third trimester. In Merz E, ed. *3D Ultrasound in Obstetrics and Gynecology*. Philadelphia: Lippincott Williams and Wilkins, 1998:95–100
5. Scherzer O, Schoisswohl A, Kratochwil A. Wavelet compression of 3D ultrasound data. *3rd International Austrian–Israeli Technion Symposion*, Hagenberg, April 1999
6. Weinraub Z, Herman A. Three dimension hysterosonography. In Merz E, ed. *3D Ultrasound in Obstetrics and Gynecology*. Philadelphia: Lippincott Williams and Wilkins, 1998:57
7. Jurkovich D, Gruboeck K. Three-dimensional ultrasound of the uterus. In Baba K, Jurkovic D, eds. *Three-dimensional Ultrasound in Obstetrics and Gynecology*. Carnforth, UK: Parthenon Publishing, 1997:75–83
8. Zaidi J, Kyei-Mensah A, Campbell ST. Three-dimensional transvaginal ultrasonography: applications in infertility. In Baba K, Jurkovic D, eds. *Three-dimensional Ultrasound in Obstetrics and Gynecology*. Carnforth, UK: Parthenon Publishing, 1997:85–94
9. Feichtinger W. Follicle aspiration with interactive three dimensional digital imaging (Voluson): a step toward real time puncturing under three-dimensional ultrasound control. *Fertil Steril* 1998;70:374–7
10. Kratochwil A. Three-dimensional power Doppler: present and future. In Kurjark A, ed. *Three-dimensional Power Doppler in Obstetrics and Gynecology*. Carnforth, UK: Parthenon Publishing, 1999:13–17
11. Athanasiou S, Khullar V, Cardozo L. Three-dimensional ultrasound in urogynecology. In Baba K, Jurkovic D, eds. *3D Ultrasound in Obstetrics and Gynecology*. Carnforth, UK: Parthenon Publishing, 1997:95–105
12. Wisser J, Schär G, Kurmanavicus J, Huch R, Huch A. Use of 3D ultrasound as a new approach to assess obstetrical trauma to the pelvic floor. *Ultraschall Med* 1999;20:15–18
13. Umek W, Kratochwil A, Obermair A, Stutterecker D, Hanzal E. 3-dimensional ultrasound of the female urethra – comparing transvaginal and transrectal scanning. Presented at the *24th Annual Meeting Urogynecology Association*. Denver: Springer Verlag, 1992:(suppl 1);42
14. Lee A, Sator M, Kratochwil A, Deutinger J, Bernaschek G. Endometrial volume change during spontaneous menstrual cycle: volumetry by transvaginal three-dimensional ultrasound. *Fertil Steril* 1997;68:831–5
15. Lee A, Kratochwil A, Stümpflen I, Deutinger J, Bernaschek G. Fetal lung volume determination by three dimensional ultrasonography. *Am J Obstet Gynecol* 1996;715:588–92
16. Wachter S, Lorang T, Gengler M, *et al.* A PC based compatible PACS environment suitable for CT, MRI, and 3D US in radiotherapy. In Piqueras J, Carreno JC, Lucaya J, eds. *Proceedings of the 16th Eoro PACS Annual Meeting*, Barcelona,1998:215–19
17. Ockenga J, Gebel M, Caselitz M, *et al.* 3D-Ultrasound in imaging, diagnosis and follow-up of an atypical hydatid cyst. *Z Gastroenterol* 1998;36:599–603
18. Hammerer P, Huland H. Anatomie und Sonographie der Prostata. *Urologe A* 1989;28:311–16
19. Djavan B, Susani M, Zlotta AR, Silverman DE, Schulman CC, Marberger M. Transperineal radiofrequency interstitial tumor ablation (RITA) of the prostate. *Tech Urol* 1998;160:411–18
20. Hühnerbein M, Schlag PM. Three-dimensional endosonography 63 for staging of rectal cancer. *Ann Surg* 1997;225:432–8
21. Csutak R, Rohrmeister K, Weninger K, Wandl-Vergesslich K. Erstellung standardisierter normwerte des ventrikelsystems bei früh und neugeborenen mittels dreidimensionaler (3D) meßtechnik. *Ultraschall in Medizin* 1998;(suppl 2);49

Three-dimensional sonography of the breast

C. F. Weismann

Introduction

Two-dimensional (2D) mammasonography, mammography and magnetic resonance-mammography are widespread, well-established breast imaging modalities. Three-dimensional (3D) mammasonography is the most recent development in breast imaging, providing additional aspects to conventional 2D sonography: completely new superior diagnostic information such as the ability to study a breast mass and the surrounding tissue in three orthogonal planes, or to obtain new information about the mean blood flow intensity or vascularization of breast lesions by evaluation of the 3D color histogram.

The demonstrated cases were investigated with a linear array 2D and 3D ultrasound volume transducer, 5–13 MHz, with a 30° volume sector (Figure 1) combined with the Voluson 530D machine (Medison-Kretztechnik, Zipf, Austria). The 3DVIEW™, a workstation-like integrated computer system designed by Medison-Kretztechnik, was the basis for volume calculation and Shell™ imaging. All 2D and 3D ultrasound investigations were performed with the patients in the supine position with elevated arms. The typical 2D ultrasound analysis of breast lesion shape, width/depth ratio, margin characterization, lesion compressibility, lesion echogenicity and echo texture followed. Additional 3D ultrasound information first displayed in the multiplanar mode offers the new aspect of the coronal plane, and allows marking of the different breast masses by retracting and compressing the lesion patterns, as described by Rotten and co-workers[1,2].

The following section mainly concentrates on solid benign and malignant breast lesions, comparing the characteristics of 2D and 3D ultrasound aspects.

Basic segmental anatomy of the breast

Superficial and deep layers of the fascia superficialis envelope the breast tissue. Cooper ligaments (Figure 2) embodied in the subcutaneous tissue connect superficial and deep fascial layers, and structure a variable amount of 15–20 glandular lobes, stromal and fatty breast tissue. The terminal ducts are the smallest branches of ducts ending bluntly in the lobules. An intralobular and extralobular portion of the terminal duct are differentiated. Both portions together are called the terminal duct lobular unit (TDLU) (Figure 3). The TDLU is the breast structure where the cells are especially influenced by hormones. It is postulated that most benign and malignant breast neoplasms arise in the terminal duct[3,4]. The terminal ducts join subsegmental ducts and all subsegmental ducts of a lobe form the major collecting duct, which reaches the nipple in a radial fashion. Inside the nipple the collecting ducts widen to form the lactiferous sinus surrounded

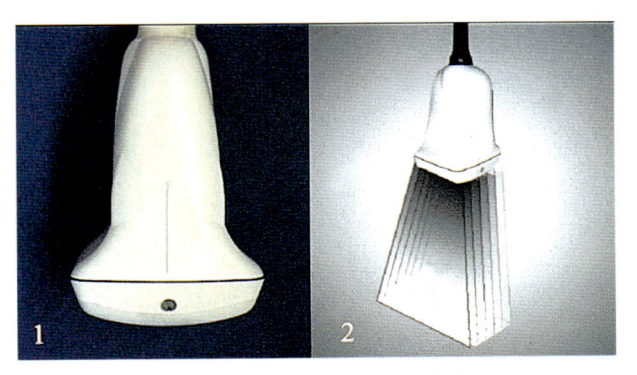

Figure 1 Small parts linear volume probe 5–13 MHz (1), small parts linear volume probe and drawing of volume acquisition (2)

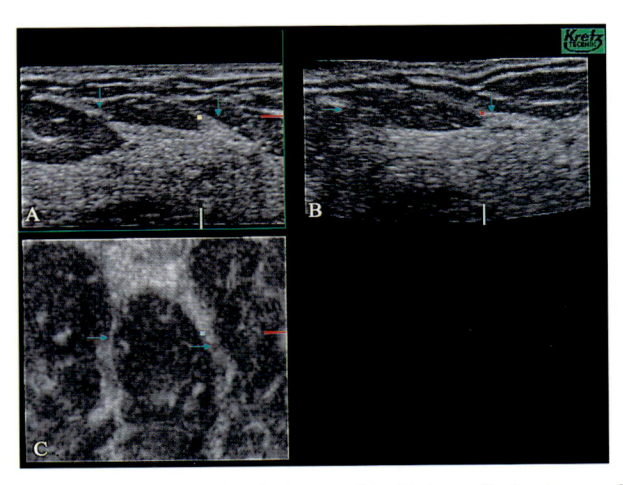

Figure 2 Three-dimensional ultrasound multiplanar display image of Cooper ligaments (arrow). A, sagittal plane; B, transverse plane; C, coronal plane

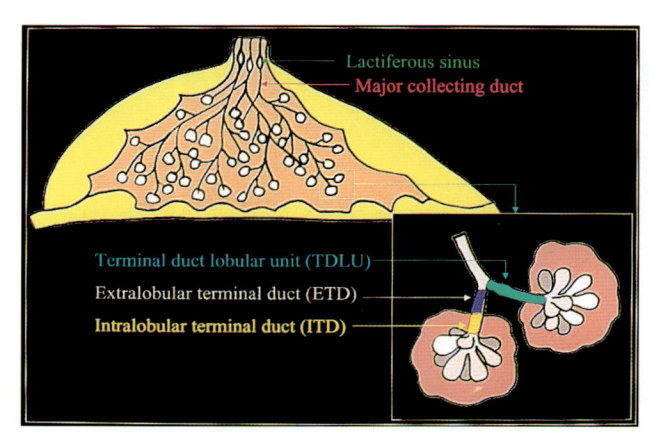

Figure 3 Basic segmental anatomy of the ductal system

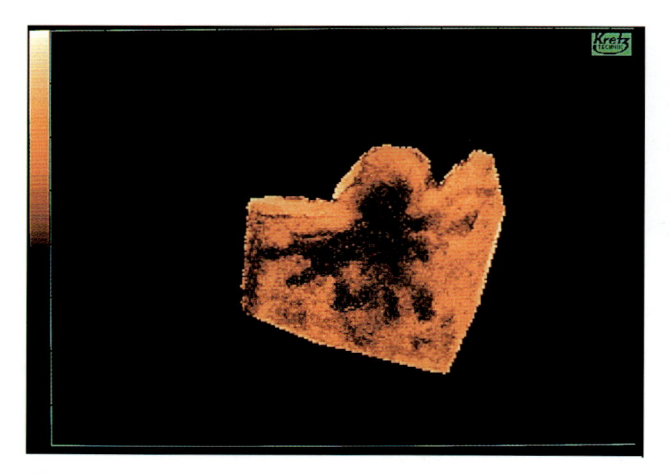

Figure 4 Three-dimensional ultrasound surface reconstruction of the nipple and the retroareolar region with partly ectatic major collecting ducts

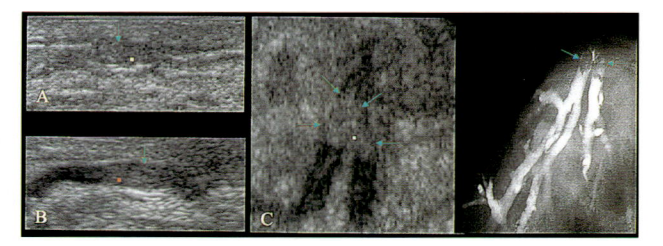

Figure 5 Three-dimensional ultrasound multiplanar display image of a 0.9-cm papilloma (arrow) compared with ductography

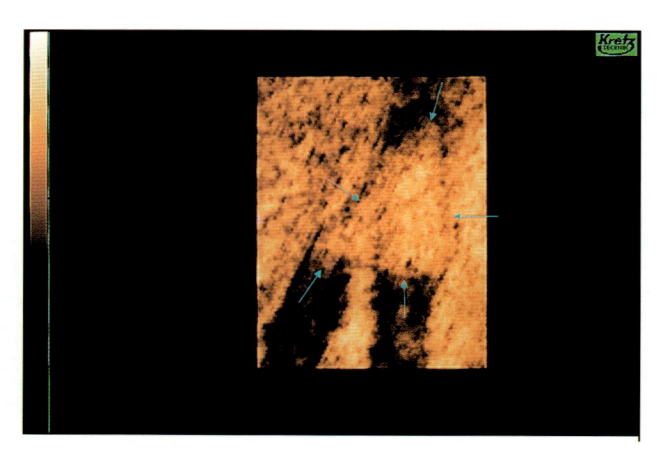

Figure 6 Three-dimensional ultrasound surface-minimum mode reconstruction of the papilloma (arrow) in Figure 5; volume of the papilloma: 0.084 cm³

by collagen and smooth muscle. About 15–20 ducts terminate on the nipple surface. Sometimes ductography reveals branching between different collecting ducts. This information is important, because in case of malignancy an intraductal tumorous spread from one glandular lobe to another in different quadrants may occur.

The retromamillary and subareolar region: intraductal papilloma

Three-dimensional ultrasound offers the data acquisition of the entire nipple area and the retromamillary region in one volume. An optimal time-gain adjustment is necessary to reduce shadowing behind the nipple, and to get full diagnostic information on the collecting ducts (Figure 4). The coronal plane shows the spatial relationship of the ducts branching out in a radial fashion. A 3D rendering using the transparency mode and fading between a maximum and minimum mode adjustment gives reliable information on ductal anatomy. Additionally, an animated study distinctly illustrates ductal branching or intraductal pathological structures. In the case of the latter, for example a centrally located papilloma (Figure 5), a second 3D ultrasound volume will be taken from the papilloma in a mamilloradial plane. A surface-minimum mode reconstruction of the papilloma gives additional spatial information (Figure 6). Spontaneous single duct serous or bloody nipple discharge requires an accurate investigation of the subareolar region, because solitary papillomas are usually found in that area and ductography is positive in 91%[5]. Cardenosa and Eklund[5] described cases of multiple central papillomas in 19%, and multiple peripheral papillomas in 18%. Three-dimensional ultrasound not only shows the pathological findings of an intraductal papilloma outlined by secretions, it also offers an exact volume calculation of the lesion.

The fibroadenoma

The fibroadenoma is the most common benign solid lesion of the breast, especially in younger women (20–30 years). The enlarging volume of the intralobular connective tissue causes stretching and compres-

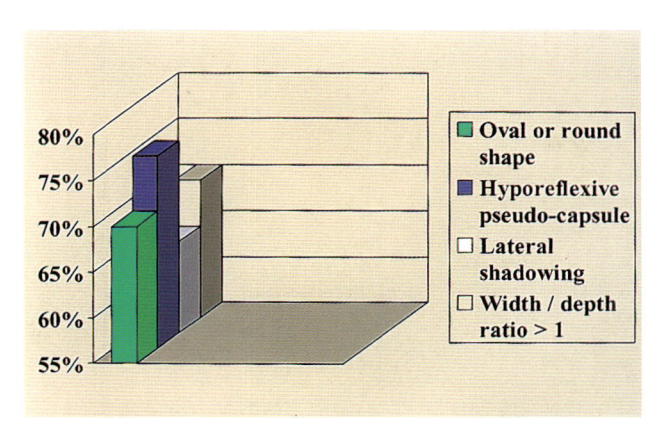

Figure 7 Ultrasound characterization of the fibroadenoma

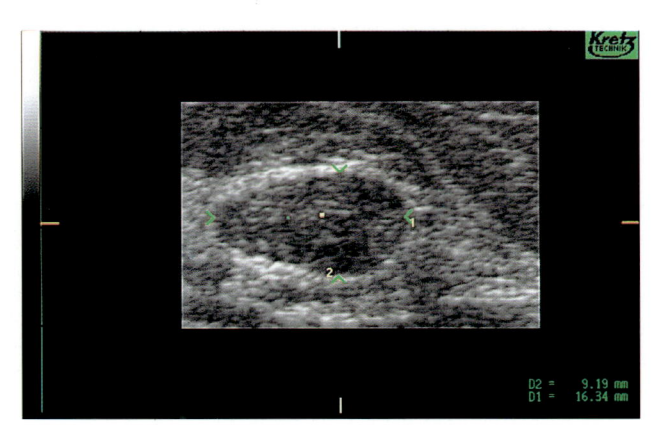

Figure 8 Two-dimensional ultrasound image of a fibroadenoma: transverse width/depth ratio 1.77

sion of the acini and the terminal duct. A sometimes palpable mass with well-defined margins of ovoid and/or lobulated shape may develop. The surrounding breast tissue will be compressed by the smooth surface of the growing fibroadenoma. This growth pattern produces a movable lesion.

The typical 2D sonographic appearance of a fibroadenoma is a well-defined ovoid or round (70%) (Figure 7), partly lobulated, homogeneous hyporeflexive mass (76%), with sometimes a thin hyperechogenic boundary to the surrounding tissue, forming a pseudocapsule. Lateral shadowing (65%) and hyperreflexivity behind the fibroadenoma (in 25–38%)[6-8] may be visible. In 10%, dorsal hyporeflexivity is seen[6]. The typical 2D cross-sectional ovoid shape with the long axis diameter parallel to the skin and a transverse width/sagittal depth ratio of > 1 can be found in about 70% (Figure 8). In 30% a lobulated polycyclic fibroadenoma with slightly heterogeneous internal echogenicity may occur. The short axis depth diameter can be compressed in about 20% (Figure 9). As described by Rahbar and co-workers[9], the most reliable 2D ultrasound features characterizing a benign lesion are a round or oval shape (94% benign), circumscribed margins (91% benign) and a width/depth (anteroposterior dimension) ratio greater than 1.4 (89% benign).

Three-dimensional ultrasound gives reliable information on the shape of the lesion. Fibroadenomas often show a round base, like a coin positioned parallel to the skin, embedded in breast tissue (Figure 10). Owing to their transverse width/sagittal depth ratio of > 1 on 2D cross-sectional images, they have a more cylindrical morphology than is assumed by conventional 2D ultrasound. Also, real-time 2D ultrasound is usually not enough to give a clear understanding of the 3D aspect of the lesion in cases of the more complex fibroadenomas with lobulation of their surfaces and dumbbell-like or irregular aspects (Figure 11). In

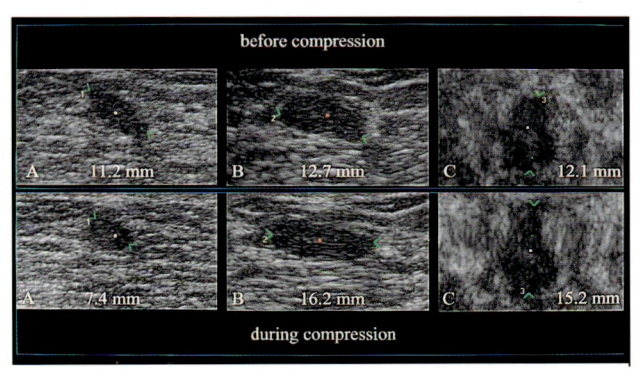

Figure 9 Three-dimensional ultrasound multiplanar display information of morphological changes before and during compression of a fibroadenoma

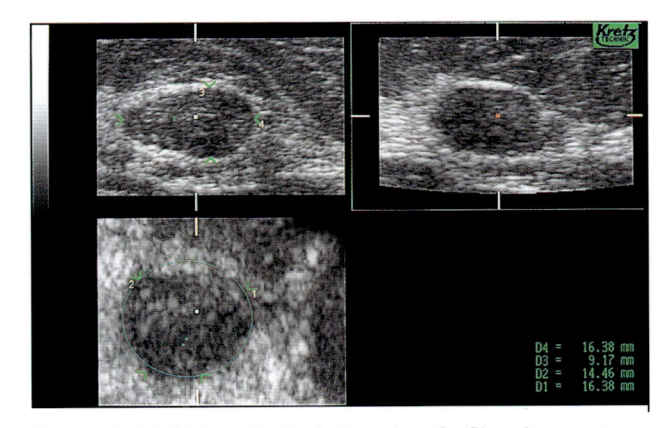

Figure 10 Multiplanar display information of a fibroadenoma: transverse width/sagittal depth ratio 1.78

about 3–4 s the Voluson 530D machine (Medison-Kretztechnik) offers a 3D multiplanar image of the fibroadenoma without any dependence on the diameter of the long or short axis of the lesion or angulation. Different measurements of width and depth can be accurately obtained, guided by all three planes.

According to Friedrich[10], the 2D ultrasound-guided study of lesion compressibility combined with echo palpation in the case of a compressible and elastic

CLINICAL APPLICATION OF 3D SONOGRAPHY

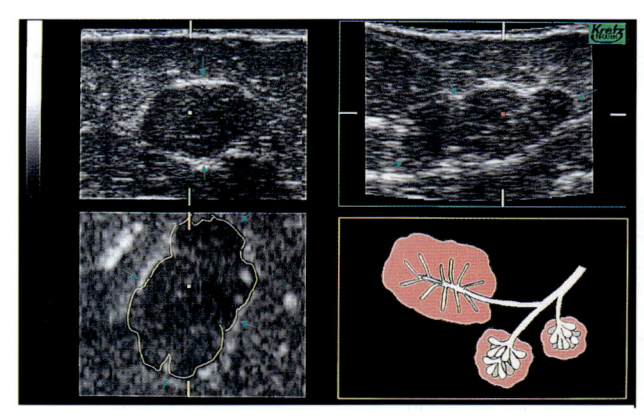

Figure 11 Multiplanar display image of a lobulated fibroadenoma (arrow); yellow frame: drawing of enlarged volume of the intralobular connective tissue stretching and compressing the acini and the terminal duct

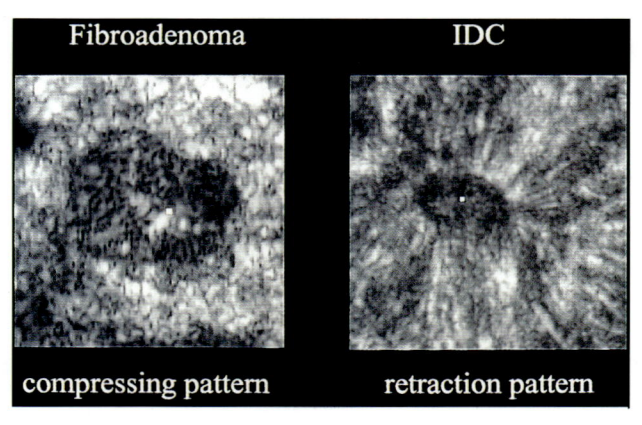

Figure 12 Coronal view of a fibroadenoma with compression pattern and an invasive ductal carcinoma (IDC) with retraction pattern

workable lesion (depth–axis diameter more than 30% compressible) makes a benign lesion 25 times more probable than a malignant lesion.

Three-dimensional ultrasound volume data sets show more objective lesion compressibility than 2D ultrasound, because during echo palpation a well-defined embedded lesion is movable and the probability increases that 2D ultrasound causes depth–axis diameter measurement in different positions, with the consequence of measuring incorrect distances. Comparing the 3D morphology of the lesion before and after compression with 3D ultrasound data sets provides correct measurements of comparable slices.

Rotten and colleagues[1,2] described two predominant tissue patterns surrounding the breast lesion and visible in the coronal plane: the compressive pattern associated with benign lesions such as fibroadenomas and the retraction pattern (Figure 12), which was highly suggestive of malignancy. The 3D statistical performance of differentiating malignant from benign by the criteria of compressive and retraction patterns showed high specificity (0.938), high sensitivity (0.914) and high predictive values (positive 0.869, negative 0.960)[2].

The compressive pattern of a fibroadenoma shows a thin or different wide hyperechogenic boundary to the surrounding tissue caused by a space-occupying lesion. Sometimes forming a pseudocapsule, developed by distortion and compression of the surrounding structures, a fibroadenoma does not infiltrate the neighboring tissue.

Three-dimensional ultrasound reconstructions and display modes such as the niche mode and other rendering options give clear information about the spatial distribution of echo texture related to echo-different areas within a fibroadenoma, e.g. calcifications in an involuting fibroadenoma (Figure 13).

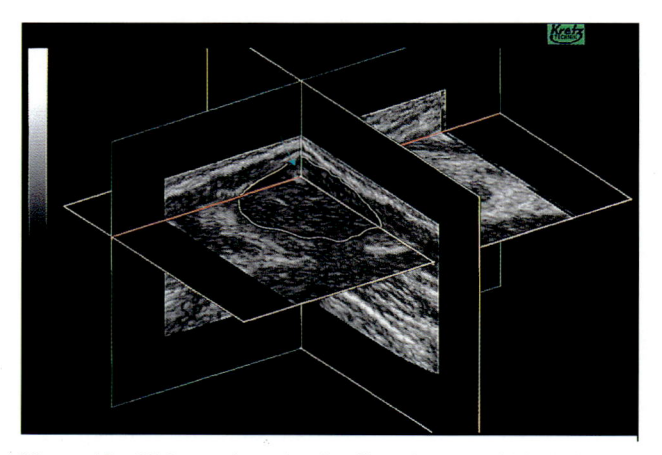

Figure 13 Niche mode study of a fibroadenoma with calcification (arrow)

Volume calculation of well-defined lesions

The 3DVIEW™ is a workstation-like integrated computer system designed by Medison-Kretztechnik that offers volume calculations (VOCAL™). The basic principle of VOCAL is to combine geometric surface information with the volume data set of a lesion (Figure 14). On the condition that the lesion is circumscribed with clear contours, the VOCAL software enables automated or manual volume calculation. The surface geometry is defined by rotation of an image plane around a fixed axis. The surface geometry can be visualized as a colored surface, a wire mesh model or a rendered gray-scale surface (Figure 15). Well-defined lesions including fibroadenomas, papillomas or rare, well-defined breast cancers such as medullary or mucous carcinomas can be evaluated by VOCAL.

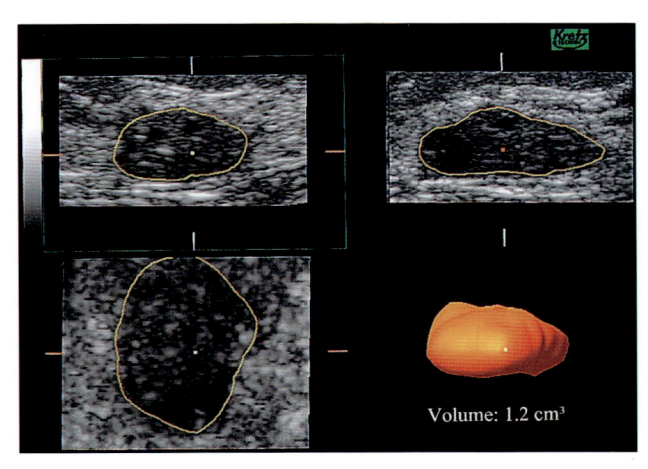

Figure 14 Volume calculation (VOCAL™) of a fibroadenoma with surface reconstruction

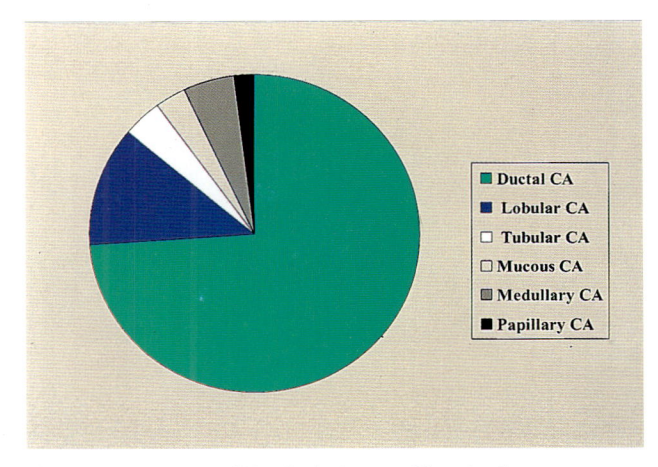

Figure 16 Incidence of histological types of invasive breast cancer

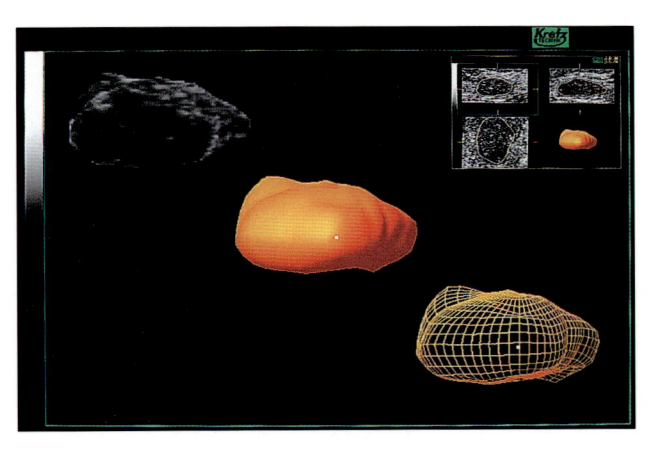

Figure 15 Volume calculation (VOCAL™) of the fibroadenoma of Figure 14 with gray-scale, color and wire mesh surface reconstruction

Invasive breast carcinoma

The macromorphological growth pattern of breast cancer is heterogeneous. Invasive breast cancer can show a stellate and/or nodulary aspect, a circumscribed mass or a diffuse infiltrating growth pattern; it can also develop as a papillary carcinoma or a rare intracystic carcinoma.

Of invasive breast cancers, 75% are invasive ductal carcinomas (Figure 16), frequently arising in the extralobular portion of the terminal duct. Macropathologically, they usually appear as a solid nodulary mass with stellate margins due to the tumorous infiltration into the surrounding tissue followed by a fibroplastic reaction, with architectural distortion. Additional intraductal tumorous spread combined with intraductal microcalcifications can often be found. In 10–15%, invasive lobular carcinomas arise from the epithelial layer of the lobule. They tend to grow diffusely along ducts, vessels and Cooper ligaments like wallpaper combined with architectural distortion, and frequently form diffuse palpable lesions, skin thickening (15%) and skin retraction (21%)[11]. The invasive tubular carcinoma can be found in 2–6% and is a slowly growing, so-called special type of invasive breast carcinoma like the mucous carcinoma (3%). The growth pattern of the tubular carcinoma is usually characterized by a stellate morphology. In contrast, the invasive mucous carcinoma and the invasive medullary carcinoma (5–7% of all invasive breast cancers) show smooth marginated borders with a pseudocapsule and imitate benign lesions such as a fibroadenoma. In 2% of invasive breast cancers a papillary carcinoma is diagnosed. It is a slowly growing tumor that has frequently developed in the subareolar region and the central parts of the breast, tending to form a multinodulary lesion. As a rarity, an intracystic papillary carcinoma can be found. Of all invasive breast cancers (most of them invasive ductal carcinomas), 1–4% produce a so-called inflammatory carcinoma with lymphangitic tumor cell spread into the skin.

Multifocal breast cancer results from different invasive cancer origins of the ductal system of one glandular lobe and is a common finding (Figure 17). Some authors[12,13] showed the ductal tumorous connection between multiple neighboring cancer foci proved contiguous ductal tumorous spread. Multicentricity is unusual and indicates carcinomatous growth in more than one glandular lobe system.

The stellate and/or nodulary macromorphological aspect is typical of the invasive ductal carcinoma (Figure 18). In particular, a stellate pattern can be found in tubular carcinomas more rarely than in invasive lobular carcinomas. The more stellate type is characterized mainly by strands of fibrous tissue and interspersed tumor cells; the more nodulary type is marked by an increasing amount of tumor cells. Subgroups have been defined: carcinoma solidum medullare with a predominance of tumor cells; carcinoma solidum simplex with a balanced situation of

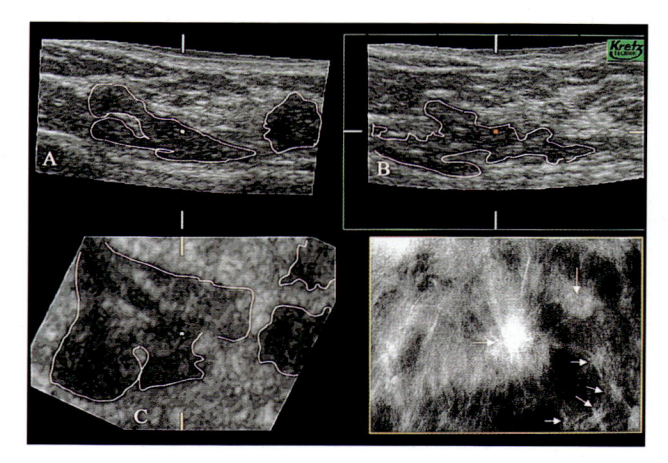

Figure 17 Three-dimensional ultrasound multiplanar display image of a multifocal and diffusely growing invasive ductal carcinoma particularly visible in the coronal plane; yellow frame: corresponding mammography (arrow points to multifocal breast cancer)

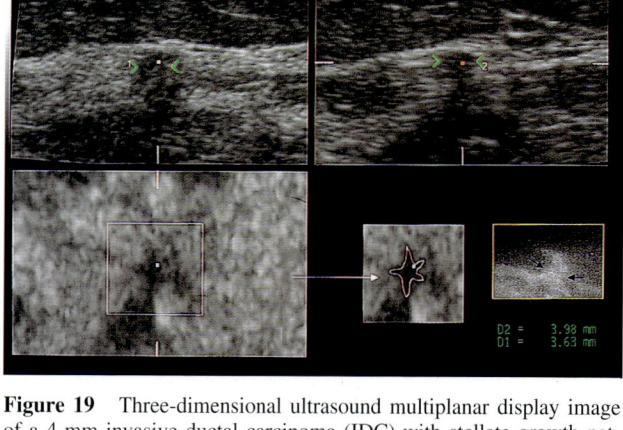

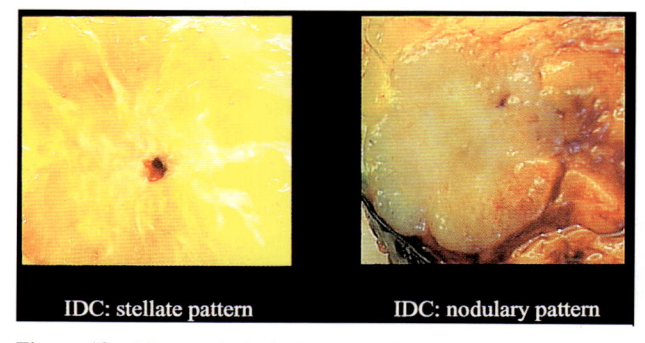

Figure 18 Macropathological aspect of a stellate and a nodulary growth pattern of invasive ductal carcinoma

Figure 19 Three-dimensional ultrasound multiplanar display image of a 4-mm invasive ductal carcinoma (IDC) with stellate growth pattern; yellow frame: mammographical tumor appearance (arrow)

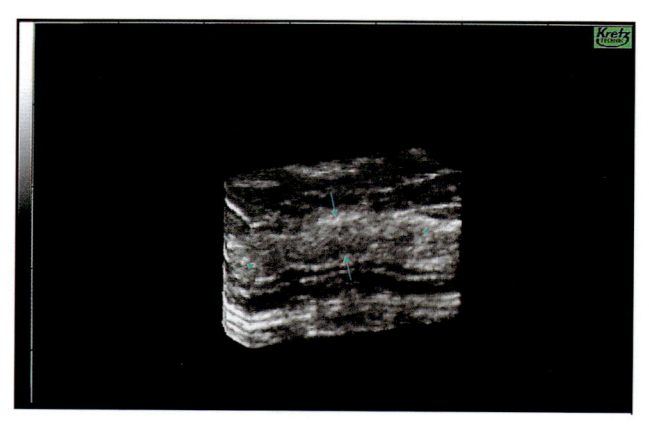

Figure 20 Three-dimensional ultrasound surface reconstruction of an invasive lobular carcinoma (ILC) (arrow) without dominating mass, partly hypoechogenic, partly isoechogenic (long axis tumor diameter 1.5 cm)

tumor cells and fibrous tissue reaction; and carcinoma solidum scirrhosum with mainly fibrous tissue.

The 2D and 3D ultrasound aspect is influenced by the histological composition, as described by Teubner and colleagues for 2D sonography[14]. According to the study of Rahbar and colleagues[9] 2D ultrasound features that characterize lesions as malignant are irregular shape (61% malignant), microlobulation (67% malignant), spiculation (67% malignant) and a width/depth (anteroposterior dimension) ratio of 1.4 or less (40% malignant). Most of the time the tumor center is characterized by a homogeneous echo-poor fibrohyalinosis followed by a dorsal shadowing due to ultrasound energy absorption. The echo-rich margins are the expression of many different tissue components of tumor cells, fibrous strands, fatty tissue and surrounding glandular parenchyma, indicating the tumorous growth and infiltration zone. Mammography clearly shows this stellate infiltration pattern with the architectural distortion of the neighboring structures.

Three-dimensional ultrasound is the first ultrasound imaging modality that simultaneously offers the coronal, transverse and sagittal planes for eliminating architectural distortion, as in mammography. Although 2D ultrasound shows signs of disrupted connective tissue layers and changes of the shape and disruption of the superficial fascia in the transverse and sagittal planes[15], these signs are less impressive compared with the tissue distortion presented in the coronal plane. Even in stellate carcinomas smaller than 1 cm in diameter (Figure 19), the retraction pattern is visible in the coronal plane.

In particular, invasive lobular carcinomas sometimes develop without a visible dominating mass (Figure 20). In this case mammasonography occasionally reveals an echo-rich or isoechogenic area without the typical echo-poor center combined with architectural distortion. This kind of sonographic aspect can be found in 5–10% of all carcinomas (Figure 21).

In such a situation the coronal plane helps to visualize the architectural distortion and enables understanding of the underlying pathology. Therefore dense, palpable, especially asymmetrical breast tissue should be investigated by 3D ultrasound. Mammography depicts architectural distortion in lobular invasive carcinomas in 16% and only parenchymal asymmetry in 11%; 16% are radiographically negative[16].

When invasive lobular carcinoma forms a more circumscribed mass or tends to produce multifocal lesions, these tumorous lesions have a similar ultrasound aspect to that of an invasive ductal carcinoma. Although Rotten and associates[1,2] described the retraction pattern that is highly characteristic of malignant masses, we have to consider benign differential diagnoses such as the radial scar or postoperative scarring. Neither with mammography nor with 2D and 3D mammasonography in most cases of radial scarring is it impossible to rule out carcinoma (Figure 22). If it is not caused by surgery, an architectural tissue distortion always needs further evaluation. Either a large-core needle biopsy combined with 3D targeting, as described below, or an open surgical biopsy should be performed.

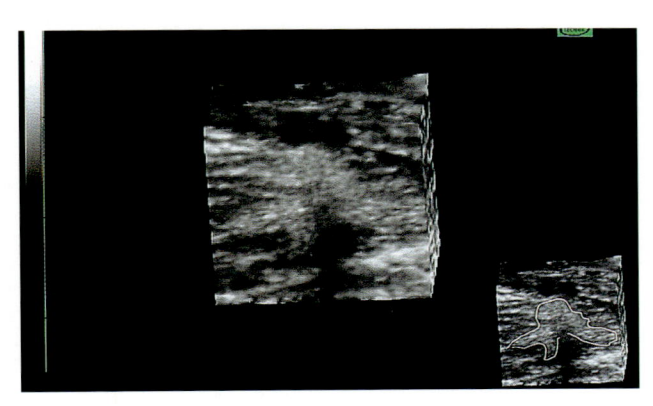

Figure 21 Three-dimensional ultrasound surface reconstruction with a surface-maximum mode of a 1.4–cm hyperechogenic invasive ductal carcinoma

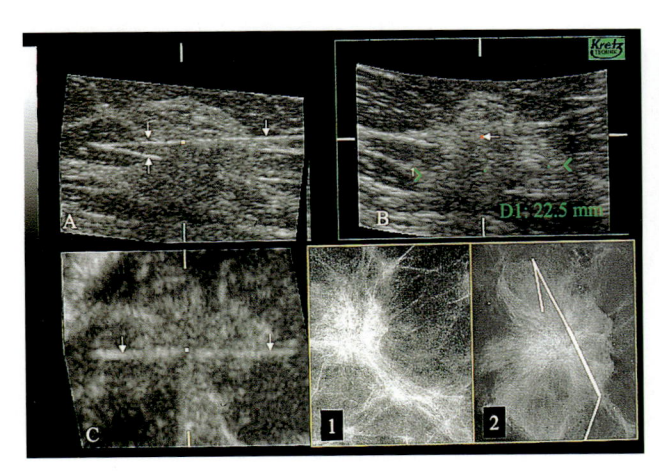

Figure 22 Three-dimensional (3D) ultrasound multiplanar display image and 3D targeting: the hookwire (arrow) penetrates a hyperechogenic retracting mass of sclerosing adenosis in all three planes; yellow frame: mammography before hookwire placement (1) and specimen radiography with hookwire (2)

Three-dimensional targeting technique

The sonographic visibility of a suspicious lesion is the basis for an ultrasound-guided biopsy. Three-dimensional breast ultrasound examination offers a correlation of typical freehand ultrasound-guided core or fine-needle biopsy as described by Parker and co-workers[17] in order to optimize tissue sampling. First a 3D ultrasound volume data set is acquired, to study the morphology of the lesion. The multiplanar scan analysis offers comprehensive information on the lesion and the surrounding structures.

For large-core needle biopsy (14-gauge) with local anesthesia, a 3-mm skin incision is performed. A 13-gauge coaxial cannula is placed near the longer width of the linear transducer. The footprint of the linear volume transducer measures 4.5×5.5 cm with a slight curve on the surface. It may be an added advantage of this broader model to make a more effective breast tissue compression during core needle stroke.

In typical freehand 2D ultrasound guidance the needle path should be as close to horizontal as possible, to optimize visualization of the needle length and needle tip (Figure 23). Via the 13-gauge coaxial cannula, a 14-gauge core needle is positioned in front of the lesion. After a 22-mm core-needle stroke using a BIP (high-speed multi) biopsy gun (Biomed Instrumente und Produkte GesmbH, Türkenfeld, Germany) the Voluson 530D machine (Medison-Kretztechnik) offers the option of acquiring a 3D ultrasound volume data set with the same transducer without freehand movement of the probe. In about 4 s the system acquires the entire 3D data volume set (about 10 MB) and displays the information of needle position accurately in a mul-

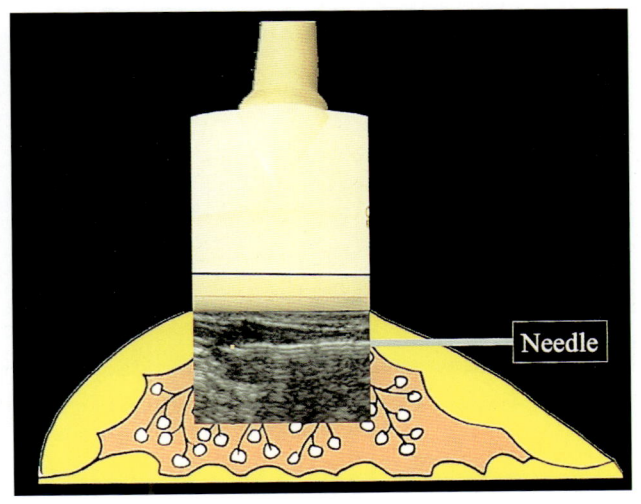

Figure 23 Freehand two-dimensional ultrasound guidance with needle path as close to horizontal as possible, to optimize needle visualization

tiplanar imaging display mode (Figure 24). This needle position check in all three planes is called 3D targeting.

Three-dimensional ultrasound is a reliable and objective tool, demonstrating correct or incorrect fine- or core-needle position during the biopsy procedure. Three-dimensional targeting checks the quality of tissue sampling during biopsy[18-21]. The results of 3D targeting suggest a reduction of core biopsies is possible in cases of 3D ultrasound-proven lesions without a loss of quality.

Live three-dimensional ultrasound breast biopsy

Newly developed software by Medison-Kretztechnik allows live 3D ultrasound needle guidance during breast biopsy. The permanently acquired live 3D ultrasound volume data are displayed in a multiplanar scan plane analysis mode. Compared to conventional freehand 2D ultrasound needle guidance, live 3D offers permanent information of all three planes in the multiplanar display mode, a rendered image of the breast lesion and needle position (Figure 25). The 3D permanent analysis of lesion position as well as needle position in all three planes allows one to navigate the core needle in an optimal prefiring position. After the core needle stroke, 3D targeting follows, unveiling the correct or incorrect needle position. Live 3D breast biopsy is even feasible, but at this time it is reflected in work in progress.

Three-dimensional power Doppler breast mass investigations

The vascularization of a breast lesion can be investigated using the 3D technique with power Doppler (amplitude-based color Doppler sonography) and frequency-based color Doppler sonography. The neovascularization[22-24] of a carcinoma with an irregular vascular pattern, arteriovenous shunts and missing vessel autoregulation, in contrast to normal breast tissue vessels, is the background for many studies with 2D ultrasound[25-35] and computer-assisted quantitative color Doppler analysis[36] aiming at a differentiation between malignant and benign breast lesions. Continuous wave and duplex ultrasound studies have shown a higher blood flow velocity in carcinomas than in benign lesions. The resistance index does not show a significant difference between malignant and benign lesions. In the literature there is inconsistent information about resistance index and pulsatility index[37,38] in breast cancer. On the one hand, this may be explained by a chaotic irregular vascular pattern and pathological vessels in malignant tumors, with a decrease in intratumoral blood flow resistance; on the other hand, a loss of intratumoral tissue elasticity may lead to an increase of blood flow resistance. The computer-assisted quantitative assessment with color Doppler as described by Huber and co-workers[36] is a step towards the understanding of the color pixel density and mean color value of benign and malignant breast lesions, for better differentiation.

Two-dimensional power Doppler is sensitive for

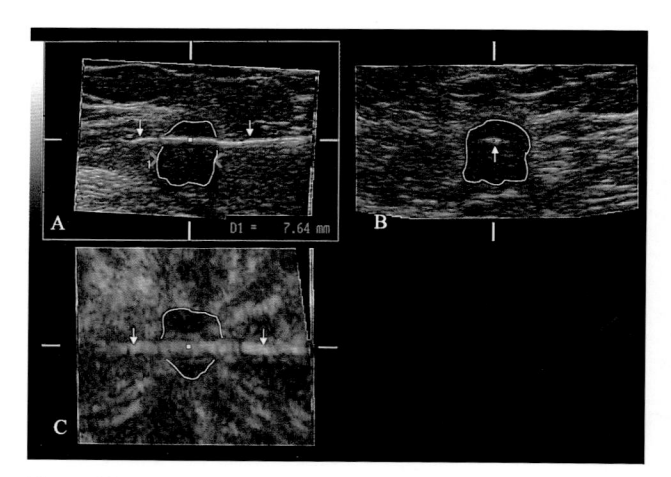

Figure 24 Multiplanar display mode and three-dimensional targeting: 14-gauge core needle penetrates in all three planes the 8-mm echo-poor center of the invasive ductal carcinoma (arrow)

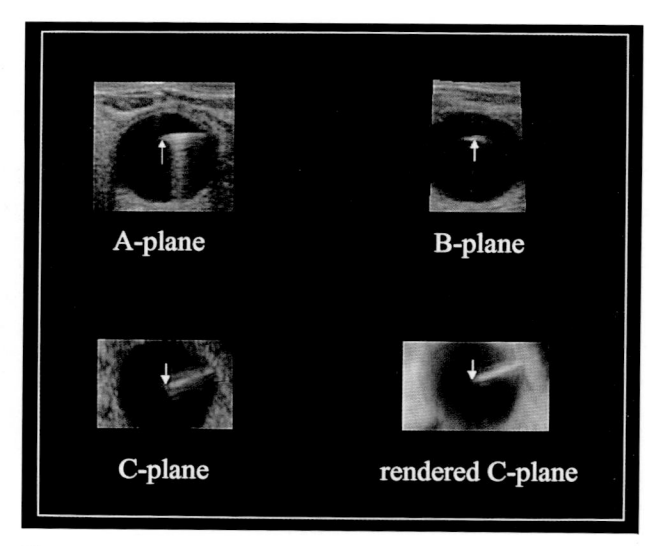

Figure 25 Multiplanar display mode information and rendered C-plane image during live three-dimensional ultrasound breast biopsy of a fine needle within a cyst

THREE-DIMENSIONAL SONOGRAPHY OF THE BREAST

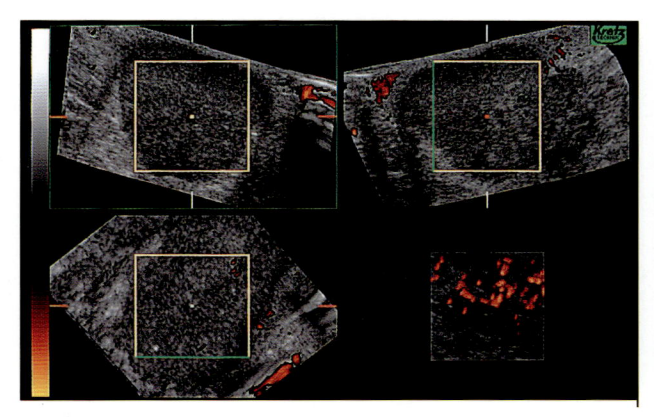

Figure 26 Multiplanar display mode information and rendered image of a three-dimensional power Doppler volume of an invasive ductal carcinoma

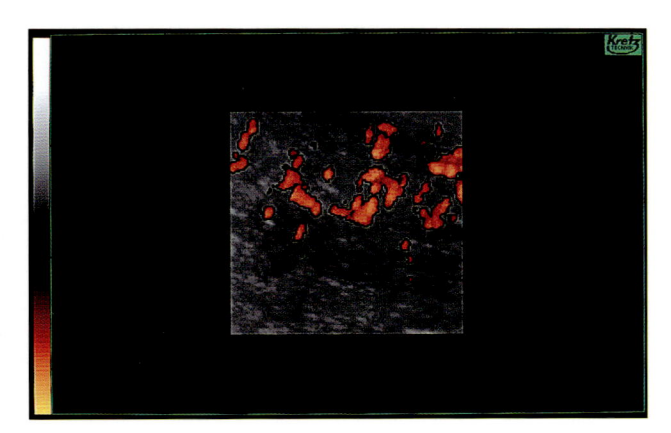

Figure 27 Rendered image of the three-dimensional power Doppler volume of the invasive ductal carcinoma of Figure 26, demonstrating the irregular vascular pattern

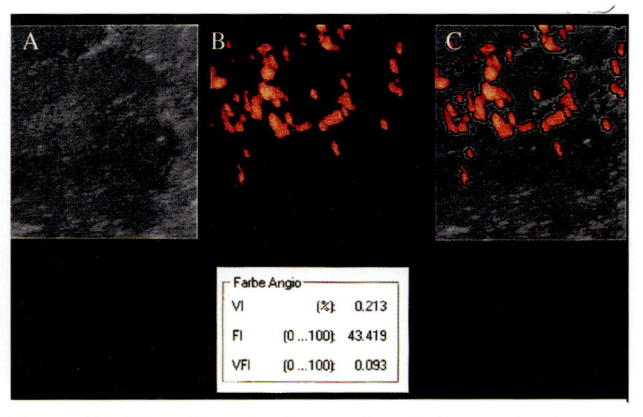

Figure 28 Three-dimensional power Doppler image of an invasive ductal carcinoma (IDC) and color histogram parameters: VI, vascularization index; FI, flow index; VFI, vascularization–flow index. (A, gray-scale volume information; B, color volume information; C, context of gray-scale and color volume information)

detecting low blood flow volume and low flow velocities, and is less angle-dependent than frequency-based color Doppler. The morphological pattern of tumor vessels and tumor feeding vessels is an approach for 3D power Doppler studies (Figure 26). During volume data acquisition, 3D power Doppler is less sensitive than 2D power Doppler, because scanner movement produces color artifacts and therefore the color settings and thresholds are slightly less sensitive. The advantage of 3D power Doppler is in imaging and analyzing blood flow and vascularization patterns of the entire tumorous lesion without the limitation of scanning only 2D planes, including the potential problem that the most representative slice might not be scanned (Figure 27).

Three-dimensional power Doppler volume information, combined with the 3DVIEW software (Medison-Kretztechnik), offers an effective tool to evaluate the color histogram and the spatial distribution of the vessels inside and outside the malignant or benign tumor (Figure 28). Three-dimensional reconstructions of the color volume data are an effective tool for studying the 3D vessel distribution and the potential irregularities in vessel shape. An important aspect of stored 3D power Doppler volumes is the possibility of comparing at different times, the color histogram information of a lesion acquired with completely similar settings, for example before and after neoadjuvant chemotherapy, with an additional feature of ruling out responder from non-responder. The color histogram gives information about the vascularization index (VI), the flow index (FI) and the vascularization–flow index (VFI) inside a user-defined volume of interest. The VI gives information about the percentage of color values (vessels) in that volume of interest. The VI is calculated by dividing the color values by the total voxels and subtracting the background voxels of the selected volume of interest. The dimensionless FI measures the mean blood flow intensity, which ranges from 0 to 100. The FI is calculated as the ratio of weighted color values (weighted by their amplitudes) to the number of the color values. The VFI gives combined information on vascularization and the mean blood flow intensity. This index is also dimensionless and ranges from 0 to 100. It is calculated by dividing the weighted color values (weighted by their amplitudes) by the total voxels and subtracting the background voxels.

Echo-enhancing agents increase the sensitivity of 2D frequency-based color Doppler sonography[39–41] and 2D power Doppler[42] as well as 3D frequency-based color Doppler sonography and 3D power Doppler. In addition, microbubble contrast agent application allows the investigation of the degree of tumor vessel enhancement, the evaluation of the time of maximum enhancement[43] as well as the wash-out effect of the decreasing signal enhancement.

CLINICAL APPLICATION OF 3D SONOGRAPHY

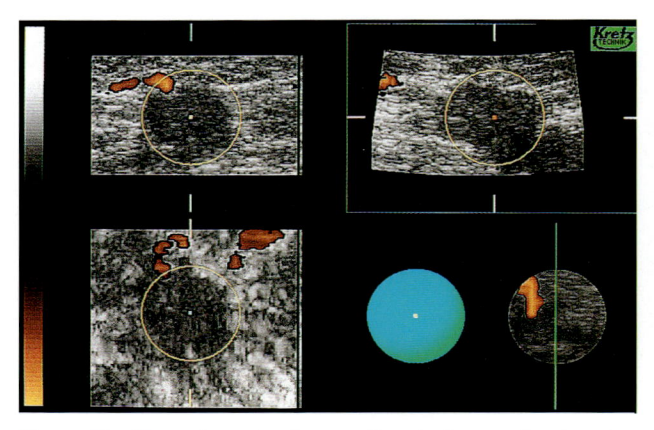

Figure 29 Three-dimensional power Doppler image of an invasive ductal carcinoma (IDC) combined with spherical volume calculation (VOCAL™) with surface contour reconstruction (blue surface) and contour-defined original gray-scale and color presentation

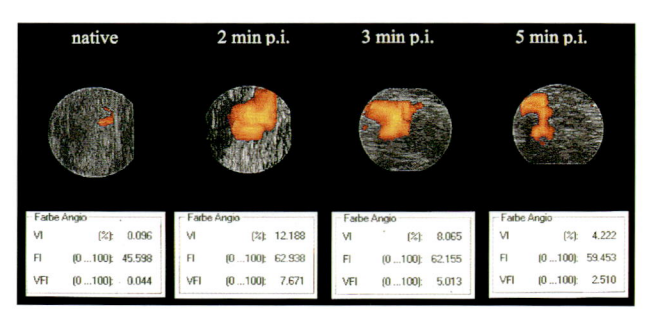

Figure 30 Comparison of four VOCAL™ three-dimensional power Doppler studies of an invasive ductal carcinoma before and after 8 ml Levovist® 300 mg/ml intravenously combined with color histogram

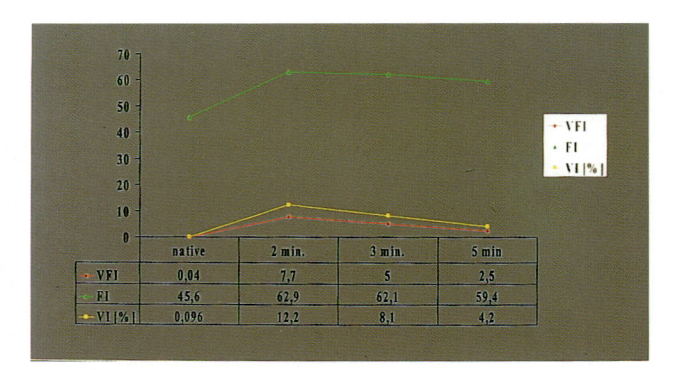

Figure 31 Color histogram evaluation of the case described in Figure 30

Comparison of different three-dimensional power Doppler volumes

In the case of a well-circumscribed lesion the 3D contours are defined in the same way as described above for volume calculation (VOCAL). This VOCAL-defined surface geometry includes the stored 3D power Doppler and gray-scale information. The color histogram parameters (VI, FI, VFI) of this volume of interest are immediately available. The volume of interest of a second stored 3D power Doppler data set from the same lesion may be acquired, for example, 1 week later, with the completely identical ultrasound system adjustments, and can be defined with VOCAL in the same way. Therefore, the histogram figures may be directly compared.

If different 3D power Doppler volumes of an irregular-shaped, ill-defined lesion should be compared, a ball-like volume of interest, presented as a circle, can be customized so that all interesting tumor vessel structures are embedded in that spherical contour. The center of the circle and the center of the tumor are matched (Figure 29). The color histogram parameters inside that spherical volume of interest can be correlated with color histogram parameters obtained from a second 3D power Doppler data set of that lesion, if the other 3D power Doppler data set is acquired in the same way, with the same settings and an identical diameter and position, centered again in the tumorous lesion (Figures 30 and 31).

Three-dimensional power Doppler and Shell™ imaging

After defining a volume of interest either with manual contour tracing of a well-circumscribed lesion or with a spherical contour of an ill-defined mass, as mentioned above, we can create different shells with varying shell thicknesses. The shell is defined by 'parallel' contours and shell geometry consists of an outside and inside surface with a calculated volume between them (Figure 32). The 3D ultrasound information inside the defined shell, such as the color histogram parameters or gray-scale parameters, are immediately available. Additionally, the 3DVIEW software allows varying of the shell position in relation to the defined volume of interest: inside, outside or symmetrical. This software feature enables the comparison of a significant amount of color histogram information from different areas of a lesion, for example the marginal lesion zone with the entire lesion or a combination of the surrounding tissue zone and the neighboring tumorous zone. These correlations can be obtained and compared with each acquired 3D power Doppler data set, and from data sets at different times in the same lesion, for example, before and after the application of echo-enhancing contrast agents. In 1997, Madjar and Jellins[39] described the contrast enhancement flow from the periphery to the center of malignant as well as benign tumors by 2D ultrasound studies. In that study the carcinomas showed this pattern more prominently, with

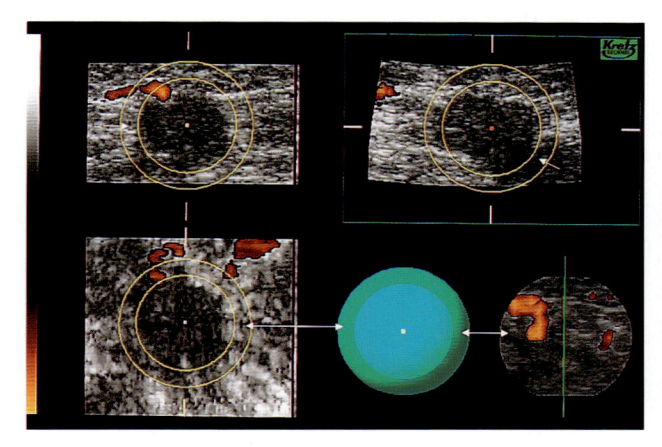

Figure 32 Spherical volume calculation (VOCAL™) combined with a 2-mm shell (↔), with shell geometry reconstructions (blue surface contour and original gray-scale and color reconstruction)

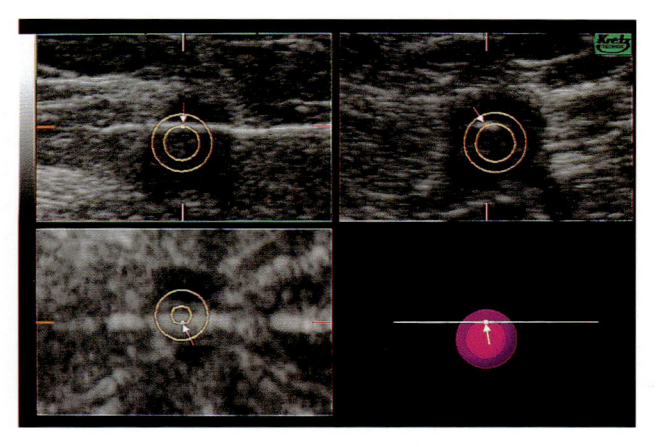

Figure 33 Three-dimensional Shell™-targeting with the three-dimensional 'hunting target' positioned in the center (arrow) of an invasive breast cancer

the malignant neovascularization revealed as having a distinct radiating pattern and a vascular corona, equivalent to the growth zone of the tumor, visible in the echo-dense rim seen on B-mode ultrasound. Three-dimensional power Doppler combined with the presentation of 3D vessel architecture, VOCAL, Shell imaging, color histogram and the additional option of intravenous application of microbubble contrast agents such as Levovist® (Schering AG, Germany), are important tools for further studies of tumor neoangiogenesis, to determine the diagnostic efficacy for differentiation of benign and malignant lesions.

Three-dimensional Shell™ targeting versus three-dimensional targeting

Three-dimensional targeting, as described above, is a typical bedside procedure, fast and accurate, demonstrating correct or incorrect needle position in relation to the lesion during biopsy. Three-dimensional Shell-targeting is the most objective method for demonstrating the relationship between needle and lesion position. Three-dimensional Shell-targeting is a little more time-consuming, and therefore best suited for investigating cases of discordant results of core-needle specimen histology or fine-needle cytology, and for imaging the characteristics of a lesion. In such a situation the question arises of whether the core needle or the fine needle has missed the lesion or not. Three-dimensional Shell-targeting works with the same 3D ultrasound volume data set that is acquired for 3D targeting. Three-dimensional Shell-targeting is a combination of Shell imaging and 3D targeting. The system allows navigation through the entire volume acquired, conducting parallel interactive movement through the image slices. In all three planes of the multiplanar display mode, colored dots (A plane, yellow; B plane,

orange; C-plane, blue) indicating an identical voxel, are directed in every activated plane into the center of the lesion. Afterwards, a 3D spherical volume of interest is created (Figure 33). The center of the volume is identical with the center of the lesion, and the definition of a shell inside, with the shell thickness being a quarter of the diameter of the volume of interest, produces a 3D 'hunting' target. It is crucial to define the diameter of the volume of interest minimally shorter than the shortest axis diameter of the lesion, so that the outside surface of the shell contour is always localized inside the lesion in all three planes. The inside shell contour defines the inner circle of the 3D 'hunting' target. In all three planes, the colored points are positioned in the needle reflexes, and are navigated along the needle reflexes in synchronous real-time parallel image movement in the corresponding orthogonal planes. In the case of a central lesion hit, the colored voxel will enter the outer shell surface, crossing the center of the lesion and leaving the 3D Shell target and the lesion at the direct opposite side (Figure 34). This relationship of central needle position related to the 3D Shell target offers the highest probability of correct tissue sampling and proves at a later date the correct needle position. If the needle passes the volume defined by the outer and inner surface of the shell without penetrating the center of the lesion, there still exists a high probability of correct tissue sampling (Figure 35). If the colored voxel following the needle reflexes does not cross the outer shell surface, the probability of correctly sampled tissue decreases dramatically.

Although Shell-targeting shows correct tissue sampling, discordant results of core-needle specimen histology or fine-needle cytology and imaging characteristics of a lesion may still exist. In 1999 Jackman and co-workers[44] published a paper about stereotactic, automated, large-core needle biopsy of non-palpable

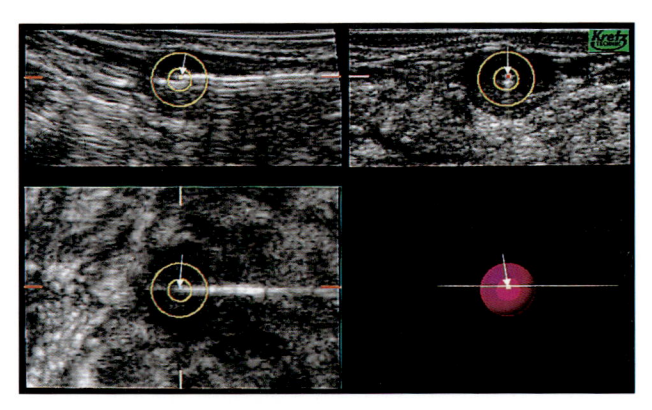

Figure 34 Three-dimensional Shell™-targeting shows the 14-gauge core needle (arrow) penetrating the inner circle and confirms the central lesion hit of a 1.2-cm fibroadenoma (needle in colored surface reconstruction)

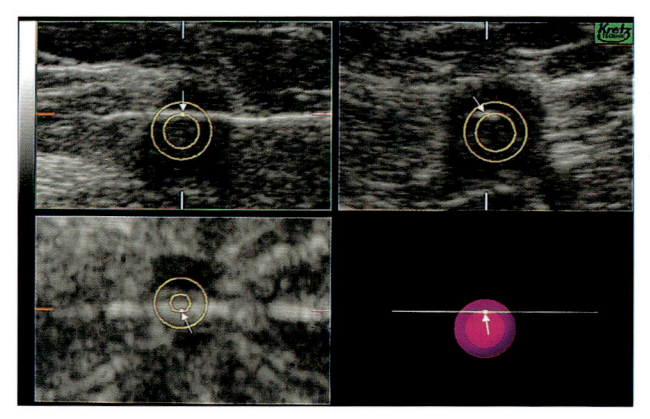

Figure 35 Three dimensional Shell™-targeting shows the 14-gauge core needle (arrow) close to the inner circle and confirms the lesion hit of the invasive breast cancer of Figure 33 (needle in colored surface reconstruction)

breast lesions and the false-negative and histological underestimation rates after long-term follow-up. They found that, on the basis of the histological diagnosis of carcinoma, at surgical biopsy the diagnosis with the large-core needle was not correct in 14 (58%) of 24 ADH lesions and two of five radial scars. They concluded that the presence of carcinoma in ADH and radial scar lesions was often underestimated. In this study the false-negative rate with large-core needle biopsy was 1.2%[13]. In the literature the false-negative rate with large-core needle biopsy ranges from 0.3 to 8.2%[45-52].

Conclusion

These 3D ultrasound techniques are new, reliable and objective tools, demonstrating more comprehensive information than 2D ultrasound: anatomical details, pathological structures, 3D vascular architecture of benign and malignant tumors, more accurate lesion measurements and correct or incorrect fine- or core-needle position during biopsy. They influence biopsy procedure in every case. Three-dimensional mammasonography is a helpful diagnostic and interventional imaging tool, fit for daily diagnostic practice and an important addition to 2D breast ultrasound examination, offering new diagnostic aspects for differentiating benign from malignant breast lesions.

Acknowledgements

I thank Ms Lynda Weese for her assistance with the English version of this manuscript, Mr Helmut Brandl for his assistance with the figure preparation and Mr Josef Steininger for technical support. The research project 'Live 3D Core-Needle Biopsy of Breast Lesions in Comparison to 2D Ultrasound Guided Biopsies' was supported by a grant from the Medison-Kretz Foundation.

References

1. Rotten D, Levaillant J-M, Zerat L. Use of three-dimensional ultrasound mammography to analyze normal breast tissue and solid breast masses. In Merz E, ed. *3-D Ultrasonography in Obstetrics and Gynecology*. Philadelphia: Lippincott Williams & Wilkins, 1998:73–8
2. Rotten D, Levaillant J-M, Zerat L. Analysis of normal breast tissue and of solid breast masses using three-dimensional ultrasound mammography. *Ultrasound Obstet Gynecol* 1999;14:114–24
3. Wellings SR, Jensen HM. On the origin and progression of ductal carcinoma in the human breast. *J Natl Cancer Inst* 1973;50:1111
4. Kopans DB. *Breast Imaging*. Philadelphia, PA: Lippincott Williams and Wilkins, 1998:3–27
5. Cardenosa G, Eklund GW. Benign papillary neoplasms of the breast: mammographic findings. *Radiology* 1991;181:751–5
6. Friedrich M. Gutartige Mammatumore. In Schneider J, Weitzel H, eds. *Lehratlas der Mammasonographie*.

Stuttgart: Wiss. Verl.-Ges., 1999:157–98
7. Teubner J, van Kaick G, Junkermann H, et al. *5 MHz Realtime-Sonographie der Brustdr se Teil2: Untersuchungstechnik und diagnostische Wertigkeit. Radiologe.* Heidelberg: Springer, 1985:457–67
8. Weismann CF. Histopathologische Korrelation von Mammographie und Mammasonographie. Linz: *IBUS-Seminarbook*, 1996:7–12
9. Rahbar G, Sie AC, Hansen GC, et al. Benign versus malignant solid breast masses: US differentiation. *Radiology* 1999;213:889–94
10. Friedrich M. Differential diagnostische kriterien in der mammasonographie. In Schneider J, Weitzel H, eds. *Lehratlas der Mammasonographie.* Stuttgart: Wiss. Verl.-Ges., 1999:75–89
11. Dronkers DJ, Hendriks JHCL, Holland R, et al. *Radiologische Mammadiagnostik.* Stuttgart: G Thieme Verlag, 1999:15–38
12. Holland R, Hendriks JHCL, Verbeck ALM, et al. Extent, distribution and mammographic/histological correlations of breast ductal carcinoma *in situ. Lancet* 1990;335:519–22
13. Ohtake T, Abe R, Izoh K, et al. Intraductal extension of primary invasive breast carcinoma treated by breast conservative surgery. *Cancer* 1995;76:32–45
14. Teubner J, Bohrer M, van Kaick G, et al. Correlation between histopathology and echomorphology in breast cancer. In Madjar H, Teubner J, Hackelöer B-J, eds. *Breast Ultrasound Update.* Basel: Karger, 1994:63–74
15. Nishimura S, Matsusue S, Koizumi S, et al. Optimal combination of diagnostic items in breast ultrasonography. In Madjar H, Teubner J, Hackelöer B-J, eds. *Breast Ultrasound Update.* Basel: Karger, 1994:75–82
16. Andersson I. *Introduction to Mammography.* Lund: Studentlitteratur's Printing Office, 1992:19–21
17. Parker SH, Jobe WE, Dennis MA, et al. US-guided automated large-core biopsy. *Radiology* 1993;187:507–11
18. Weismann CF. 3D-Breast ultrasound (US) correlation of 2D-US guided core needle biopsy and hookwire localization. Seoul: *11th ICUEB Abstract Book*, 1999:390
19. Weismann CF. 3D-Breast ultrasound: a new quality approach to breast imaging and breast biopsy. Freiburg: *IBIU Book of Manuscripts*, 1999:113–15
20. Weismann CF, Forstner R, Kainberger P. 3D-Mammasonographie: Eine neue Dimension zur Objektivierung der Biopsienadellage und Drahth kchenmarkierung in der Brust (abstr). *Ultraschall Med* 1999;(suppl 1):32
21. Weismann CF, Forstner R, Kainberger P. 3D-Sonographie: Eine neue Dimension in der bildgebenden Diagnostik und Nadelbiopsie der Mamma. *Fortschr Röntgenstr* 1999;171:S9
22. Folkman J. Tumor angiogenesis. *Adv Cancer Res* 1985;43:185–203
23. Folkman J, Merler E, Abernathy C. Isolation of a tumor factor responsible for neovascularisation. *J Exp Med* 1970;133:275
24. Horak ER, Leek R, Klenk N, et al. Angiogenesis assessed by platelet/endothelial cell adhesion molecule antibodies, as indicator of node metastases and survival in breast cancer. *Lancet* 1992;340:1120–4
25. Jellins J. Combining imaging and vascularity assessment of breast lesions. *Ultrasound Med Biol* 1988;14 (suppl 1):121–30
26. Madjar H, Sauerbrei W, Münch S, et al. Continuous-wave and pulsed Doppler studies of the breast: clinical results and effect of transducer frequency. *Ultrasound Med Biol* 1991;17:31–9
27. Madjar H, Vetter M, Prömpeler HJ, et al. Studies on the normal vascularisation of the female breast via Doppler ultrasound. *Ultraschall Med* 1992;13:171–7
28. Madjar H. Breast examinations with continuous wave and color Doppler. *Ultrasound Obstet Gynecol* 1992;2:215–20
29. Madjar H, Prömpeler HJ, Sauerbrei W, et al. Color Doppler flow criteria of breast lesions. *Ultrasound Med Biol* 1994;20:849–58
30. Madjar H, Mundinger A, Prömpeler HJ. Doppler-sonographie der Mamma (abstr). *Ultraschall Med* 1999;(suppl 1):30
31. Huber S. Dopplersonographie in der Mammadiagnostik. *IBUS Seminar Book.* Linz: International Breast Ultrasound School, 1996:13–19
32. Hollerweger A, Rettenbacher T, Macheiner P, et al. New signs of breast cancer: high resistance flow and variations in resistive indices evaluation by color Doppler sonography. *Ultrasound Med Biol* 1997;23:851
33. Delorme S, Anton HW, Knopp MV, et al. Breast cancer: assessment of vascularity by color Doppler. *Eur Radiol* 1993;3:253–7
34. Cosgrove D, Bamber JC, Davey JB, et al. Color Doppler signals from breast tumors. *Radiology* 1990;176:175–80
35. Fournier D, Dreyer JL, Hessler C, et al. Color Doppler sonography in breast diseases: is the so-called tumoral flow specific? (abstr). *Imaging* 1993;60(suppl 2):52
36. Huber S, Delorme S, Knopp MV, et al. Breast tumors: computer-assisted quantitative assessment with color Doppler US. *Radiology* 1994;192:797–801
37. Konishi Y, Hamada M, Shimada K, et al. Doppler spectral analysis of the intratumoral wave-form in breast diseases (abstr). *Imaging* 1993;60(suppl 2):18
38. Sohn C, Stolz W, Grischke EM, et al. Die dopplersonographische Untersuchung von Mammatumoren mit Hilfe der Farbdopplersonographie, der Duplexsonographie und des CW-Dopplers. *Zentralbl Gynäkol* 1992;14:249–53
39. Madjar H, Jellins J. Role of echo-enhanced ultrasound in breast mass investigations. *Eur J Ultrasound* 1997;5:65–75
40. Kedar RP, Cosgrove D, McCready VR, et al. Microbubble contrast agent for color Doppler US: effect on breast masses. *Radiology* 1996;198:679–86
41. Schröder RJ, Hadijuana J, Hidajat N, et al. Farbkodierte signalverstärkte Duplexsonographie raumfordernder intramamm rer Prozesse. *Fortschr Röntgenstr* 1998;168:444–50
42. Blohmer JU, Reinhardt M, Kissner L. Kontrastmittel und Mammasonographie (abstr). *Ultraschall Med* 1999;(suppl 1):30–1
43. Stuhrmann M, Aronius R, Roefke C, et al. Vaskularisation von Mammatumoren: Einsatz des Ultraschall-kon-

trastmittels in der Dignitätsbeurteilung. Vorl ufige Ergebnisse. *Fortschr Röntgenstr* 1998;169:360–4

44. Jackman RJ, Nowels KW, Rodriguez-Soto J, *et al.* Stereotactic, automated, large core needle biopsy of nonpalpable breast lesions: false-negative and histologic underestimation rates after long-term follow-up. *Radiology* 1999;210:799–805

45. Nguyen M, McCombs MM, Ghandehari S, *et al.* An update on core needle biopsy for radiologically detected breast lesions. *Cancer* 1996;78:2340–5

46. Fajardo LL. Cost-effectiveness of stereotaxic breast core needle biopsy. *Acad Radiol* 1996;3:21–3

47. Dahlstrom JE, Jain S, Sutton S, *et al.* Diagnostic accuracy of stereotactic core biopsy in a mammographic breast cancer screening programme. *Histopathology* 1996;28: 421–7

48. Lee CH, Egglin TK, Philpotts L, *et al.* Cost-effectiveness of stereotactic core needle biopsy: analysis by means of mammographic findings. *Radiology* 1997;202:849–54

49. Libermann L, Dershaw DD, Glassman JR, *et al.* Analysis of cancers not diagnosed at stereotactic core breast biopsy. *Radiology* 1997;203:151–7

50. Acheson MB, Patton RG, Howisey RL, *et al.* Histologic correlation of image-guided core biopsy with excisional biopsy of nonpalpable breast lesions. *Arch Surg* 1997;132:815–21

51. Meyer JE, Smith DN, Lester SC, *et al.* Large-needle core biopsy: nonmalignant breast abnormalities evaluated with surgical excision or repeat core biopsy. *Radiology* 1998;206:717–20

52. Fuhrman GM, Cederbom GJ, Bolton JS, *et al.* Image-guided core-needle breast biopsy is an accurate technique to evaluate patients with nonpalpable imaging abnormalities. *Ann Surg* 1998;6:932–9

The role of three-dimensional and power Doppler ultrasound in evaluation of breast lesions

I. Bekavac, E. Cosmi and S. Kupesic

Public awareness of the potential benefits of early detection of breast cancer has increased in recent years. More women seek the advice of a physician after detecting a breast mass. For the diagnosis of breast lesions, mammography and sonography have made undisputed diagnostic contributions.

In the recent literature (1995–99), the cancer detection rate by ultrasound is reported to be the same as or even better than that of X-ray mammography; ultrasound-guided punctures are reported to be better and less costly than stereotactic procedures and ultrasound detection of microcalcifications is becoming better and better[1–5].

Three-dimensional (3D) ultrasound analysis provides more precise information on the structure of breast lesions. 3D ultrasound with power Doppler facilities allows the physician to evaluate arbitrary planes not available with two-dimensional (2D) ultrasound, to measure the dimensions and volume of structures, and to obtain anatomic and blood flow information, to improve the assessment of complex structural abnormalities of the breast.

Here we discuss the use of 3D ultrasound in the detection of breast masses and the differentiation between benign and malignant lesions.

Gray-scale criteria

The characteristic sonographic findings of benign tumors include a round or oval, slightly hypoechoic lesion with smooth borders or a pseudocapsule, homogeneous internal echoes, no central posterior acoustic shadowing and a normal appearance of the surrounding tissue[6–9].

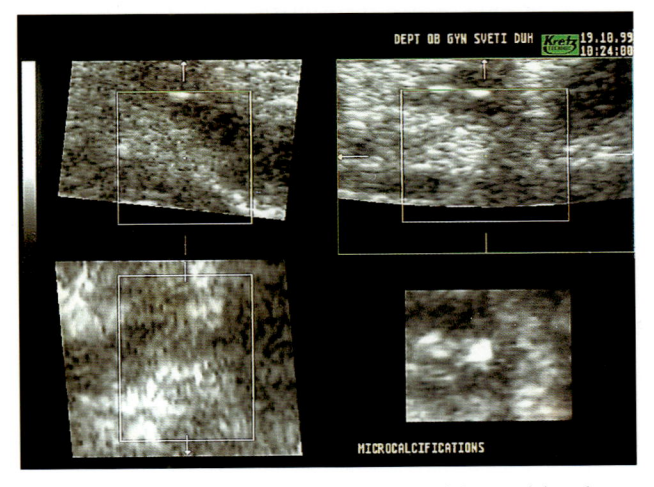

Figure 1 Three-dimensional ultrasound scan of the suspicious breast lesion. Note the posterior acoustic shadowing caused by microcalcification, best visualized by surface rendering mode

The typical features of malignancy include irregular shape, irregular margins, hypoechogenicity, a surrounding echogenic halo and posterior acoustic shadowing[6–9] (Table 1; Figure 1).

However, the sonographic characteristics used to differentiate benign from malignant lesions overlap somewhat. An oval or round shape was found in 82.5–86% of benign tumors and in 24–42% of malignant tumors[9–11]. Contour is one of the most important tumor features, but irregular contour has been reported in 25–27% of fibroadenomas[10–12]. Posterior shadowing has been reported to be an important sonographic feature suggesting a malignant tumor, and present in 72–97% of breast carcinomas[12–14]. An internal echo pattern and echogenicity have low discriminating value.

Table 1 Ultrasound characteristics of benign and malignant breast lesions

Ultrasound characteristics	Benign	Malignant
Shape	oval, round	irregular
Margins	smooth, sharp	spiculated
Echogenicity	hyperechoic	hypoechoic
Internal echo pattern	homogeneous	heterogeneous
Retrotumor acoustic shadowing	none	posterior shadowing
Compressibility	compressible	non-compressible

Three-dimensional ultrasound

With 3D analysis the images are stored as a volume set and the equipment allows any section through this set to be selected and displayed. Importantly, it allows the display of planes at any angle, and sections that cannot be acquired in a conventional sonographic examination. With this technique, images are displayed automatically in orthogonal planes, allowing accurate measurements to be made of the volume of complex structures.

The images from a number of adjacent sections can be combined in a volume-rendered display, using translucency to give depth perception. This perception is enhanced by rotation of the image, which gives better appreciation of the 3D geometrical relationship[15].

Using 3D ultrasound one can evaluate the periphery of breast lesions precisely and estimate the local infiltration in patients with breast malignancy. Furthermore, it provides more information on the internal structure of the tumor, the existence and form of intracystic structures and the existence of multifocal disease. This helps to separate benign from malignant lesions.

In their recent work, Blohmer and co-workers[16] examined 50 patients presurgically (19 with breast cancer and 31 with benign lesions). The suspected diagnoses and their correspondence with postsurgical findings were compared to the results obtained by 2D sonography. 3D ultrasound produced four cases with a false-positive diagnosis of breast cancer, while 2D sonography gave two false-negative findings. Those four false-positive results obtained by 3D ultrasound were due to the irregular contour of fibroadenomas, and a heterogeneous internal echo pattern. The authors stressed the importance of 3D ultrasound in providing more information on the internal structures of a tumor, especially the presence and form of intracystic structures. Three-dimensional sonography provided excellent visualization and delineation in the case of intracystic papilloma, intracystic papillar carcinoma *in situ* and non-puerperalis mastitis.

In three of five cases, multifocal disease was successfully recognized with 3D sonography, while 2D ultrasound detected only one case. This was because 3D sonography allows a cross-sectional display of planes at any angle, which cannot be provided by conventional sonography (Figure 2). Also, the 3D geometrical relationship provides new perspectives and possibilities on the sonographic appearance of breast tissue and tissue peripheral to the breast lesions.

Similar results were obtained by Sohn and co-workers[17]. They provided a correct diagnosis in 95% of the cases of malignant breast tumors and 80% of the benign tumors by 3D ultrasound imaging. This was demonstrated by the examples of 35 malignant and benign tumors of the breast. The main criteria used were the margins of the lesion. In their opinion, owing to the possibility of defining the organ limits, 3D imaging enables the physician to predict the nature of the tumor.

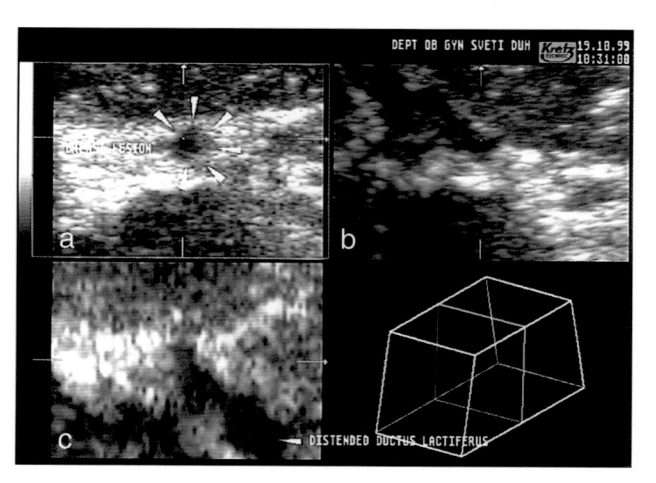

Figure 2 Three orthogonal planes of the breast lesion. Note the cystic appearance of the structure in plane (a), while the remaining two orthogonal planes (b) and (c) demonstrate an elongated regular structure indicative of a distended ductus lactiferous

Ultrasonographic 3D analysis includes planar images with selected orientations, and surface and/or rendering modes that optimize the presentation of anatomy[18]. In the study of Rotten and colleagues[18], two types of planar section were used: orthogonal planar reformatted sections and parallel planar reformatted sections. A total of 186 solid hyperechoic breast masses were analyzed by 2D and 3D ultrasonography. Orthogonal planar reformatted sections closely resembled the original 2D images. Parallel planar reformatted sections provided two types of information in addition to the usual sonographic findings.

Wall continuity in benign tumors and margin jagging in malignant tumors were clearly apparent, enabling mass margins to be analyzed with greater accuracy. The authors stressed the importance of the tissue surrounding the central lesion. Two main patterns were described. In the compressive pattern, the hyperechoic bands of surrounding fibrous tissue appeared to be smoothly pushed aside from the central image. When present, this pattern could be seen surrounding the breast mass, from the polar planes to the equatorial plane of the mass. This pattern was predominantly associated with benign lesions. In the converging pattern, thick hyperechoic bands converged according to a stellar pattern, towards a hyperechoic, irregular rim, surrounding the hypoechoic central core of the mass (Figure 3). This pattern was associated with carcinomas. The converging/compressive pattern

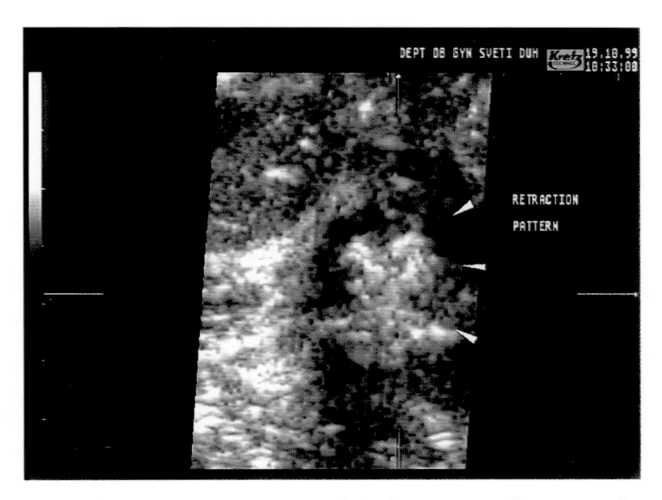

Figure 3 The converging pattern of the tissue surrounding a centrally located lesion; this finding is highly suspicious of a malignant structure

of the peripheral tissue had a higher specificity than the usual 2D characteristics. The authors concluded that 3D reconstruction, in particular parallel planar reformatted sections, represented a valuable adjunct to the characterization of breast masses.

Retrospective analysis[19] was performed for 56 mixed cystic–solid breast masses. The lesions were classified into two major patterns: tumor with cysts and intracystic tumors. Fifty-eight percent of malignant lesions were shown to have a tumor with a cystic pattern and 42% demonstrated an intracystic pattern. Owing to the overlap in sonographic findings between benign and malignant lesions, the lack of a defined 3D contour was the most important criterion for breast malignancy.

Owing to the multimodal imaging, 3D computerized reconstructions of breast cancer are capable of advancing our understanding of the structure of ductal carcinoma *in situ*, lesions simulating microinvasive breast carcinoma, surgical clearance of high-grade calcifying ductal carcinoma *in situ*, and the 3D growth patterns of invasive forms of breast carcinoma[20].

Postoperative changes in the breast may cause shadowing and mimic a recurrent tumor. Hematomas do not always appear as fluid collections and may mimic a solid mass.

The presence of gas in an abscess can give rise to a combination of shadowing and ring-down artifact. The 3D reconstruction and simultaneous observation of three orthogonal planes allow easier recognition of the latter artifact generated by the presence of air-filled spaces inside the lesion.

The role of three-dimensional ultrasound in surgery and biopsy

Three-dimensional ultrasonic images acquired in the operating room just before surgical resection augment visualization for the guidance of breast-conservative cancer surgery. By combining an optical 3D position sensor, the position and orientation of each ultrasonic section are precisely measured to reconstruct geometrically accurate 3D tumor models from the acquired ultrasonic images. Similarly, 3D position and orientation of a video camera are obtained to integrate video and ultrasonic images in a geometrically accurate manner. Superimposing 3D tumor models into live video images of the patient's breast enables the surgeon to perceive the exact 3D position of the tumor, including irregular cancer invasions which cannot be perceived by touch. Using the resultant visualization, the surgeon can determine the region for surgical resection in a more objective manner, minimizing the risk of relapse and maximizing breast conservation[21].

Three-dimensional ultrasound may also be important during fine-needle biopsy for documenting the exact location of the tip of the needle.

In the future, computerized image fusion techniques may be able to take advantage of multimodal imaging of breast cancer, thus correcting primary imaging artifacts, improving robustness and combining complementary information.

Three-dimensional power Doppler

A constantly growing malignant tumor needs nutrient supplies from blood vessels that are usually presented as tumor neovascularization. The vascular network of a malignant tumor is different from that of normal tissues. Previous angiographic studies of breast cancer have revealed abnormalities in the vascular structures as tumor stains, irregular and large-caliber vessels as well as delayed and rapid emptying of vessels due to arteriovenous shunts[22]. These findings are absent in benign lesions and in normal breasts (Figure 4). It has been shown that a cancer as small as 10 mm in diameter was positive for blood flow detection[23].

Color and pulsed Doppler flow profiles analyzed by the resistance index (RI) and systolic/diastolic frequency ratio were higher in carcinomas than in benign breast lesions, but the overlap of the values was wider than the flow velocity measurements[24,25]. Madjar and associates[26] showed that, using the vessel number and the total tumor vascularity, 90% of all lesions could be differentiated.

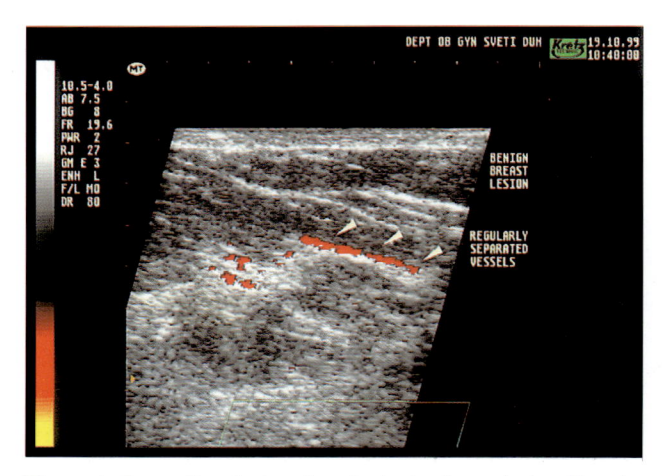

Figure 4 Power Doppler imaging of a benign breast lesion. Note the regularly separated vessels at the periphery

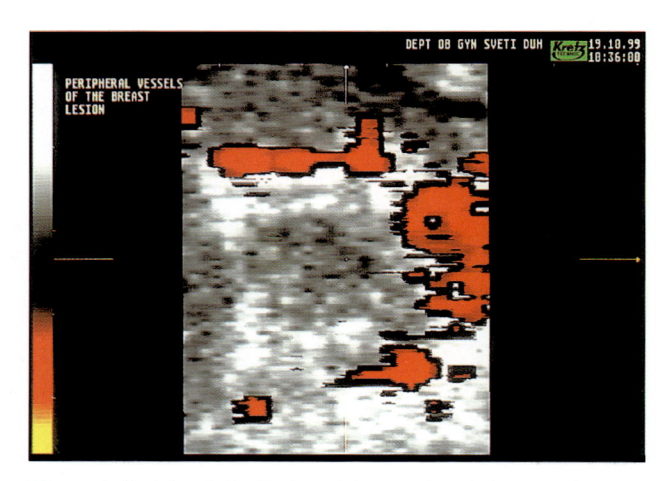

Figure 6 Peripheral distribution of the vessels and absence of a penetrating pattern are typical findings in benign breast lesions and may assist in their differentiation from malignant tumors

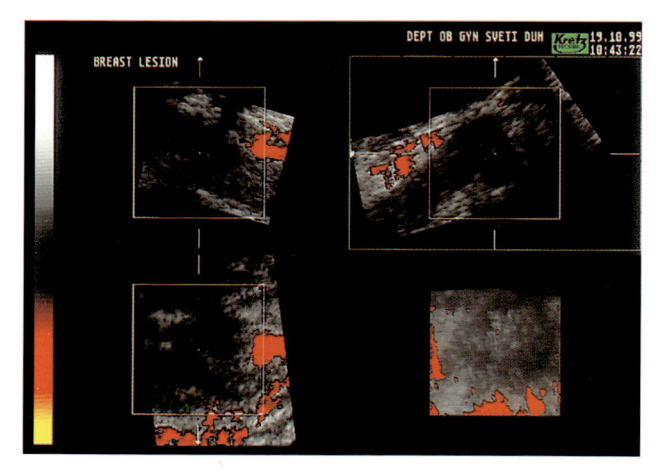

Figure 5 Three-dimensional power Doppler scan of a benign breast lesion. Note the peripheral distribution of the vessels in all three orthogonal planes as well as in surface rendering mode

Power Doppler sonography is regarded as a very sensitive method for detecting low-velocity and low-volume blood flows. The main question is whether increased vascularity in breast carcinomas can be visualized by power Doppler sonography, and whether criteria for differentiating benign and malignant lesions can be found. Power Doppler imaging[27] seems to be better at differentiating benign from malignant breast lesions than conventional (color) Doppler imaging. A total of 100 women with solid breast lumps were investigated. Color Doppler showed a sensitivity of 62 and 42%, and specificity of 62 and 62%, respectively, while power Doppler showed a sensitivity of 76 and 51%, and specificity of 56 and 48%, respectively (Figure 5).

Milz and colleagues[28] examined 315 patients by ultrasound. If a suspicious lesion was found, it was evaluated further by power Doppler sonography. Compared to normal breast parenchyma, a focal increase in blood flow signals was observed. In 97 cases the sonographic findings were correlated with histology or cytology. There were 50 benign lesions, 42 cases of invasive and five cases of *in situ* carcinoma. Of the benign lesions, 73.5% showed no or just minimal increase in flow signal; 81% of invasive cancer presented middle or high flow increases compared to normal breast parenchyma. The extent of flow increase was linked to tumor size in invasive cancer. The results showed power Doppler sonography to be a promising diagnostic tool in the differential diagnosis of breast tumors (Figure 6).

This technique allows detection of blood flow, analysis of vessel arrangement and vascularization extent, and definition of the number of vascular poles. The difficulty encountered is that few cancers have very low flow values and some of the proliferative benign lesions may present increased flow[26].

The 3D display of the color and/or power flow data can be rotated to facilitate the study of the architecture of tumor vessels in various projections. Views of the volume in different projections of malignant lesions clearly show the feeding vessel and the entire neovascular network within the mass. Highly suspicious of malignancy are irregular vessel calibers, serpiginous courses, penetration of the tumor margin and irregular reticular vascularization.

Carson and co-workers[29] showed that good 3D displays were achieved on larger pulsatile vessels, from images obtained during systole and selected for minimal noise. Two methods of potentially improving the detection and assessment of breast cancer vasculature by color flow Doppler ultrasonography were studied: continuous wave Doppler and 3D display.

Contrast agents improve analysis of the vascularization pattern[30]. Ninety-two patients with 110 tumor-like

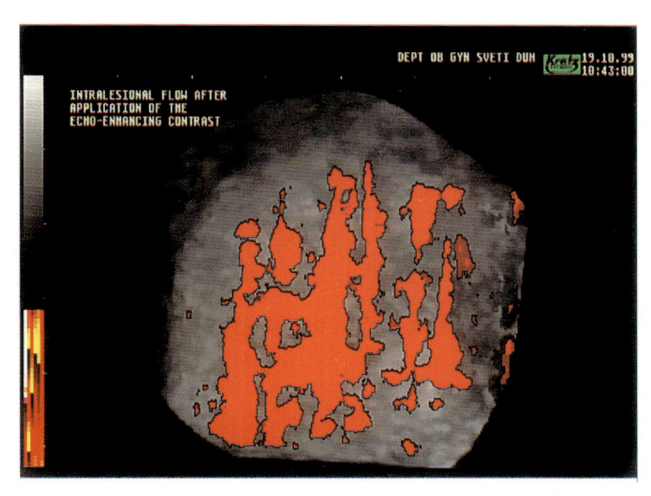

Figure 7 Echo-enhanced three-dimensional power Doppler scan of a malignant breast tumor. Note the massive intralesional vascularization characterized by randomly dispersed vessels with irregular branching and arteriovenous shunts

lesions of the breast were investigated by unenhanced and enhanced color and power Doppler ultrasound. The sonographic aspects of vascularization were analyzed. D-galactose-enhanced color Doppler sonography was found to provide more reliable differential diagnostic information than unenhanced power and/or color Doppler ultrasound in tumor and tumor-like lesions. Signal enhancement resulted in improved sensitivity and specificity ($p < 0.01$). Enhanced vascular network 3D display allows better visualization and detection of abnormal vascular morphology (Figure 7).

Axillary lymph node status is the most important pathological determinant of prognosis in early breast cancer. Determination of axillary status is crucial in clinical decision-making. Because of the 30–40% prevalence of lymph node metastasis in breast cancer, routine axillary operations result in dissection of non-metastatic lymph nodes in 60–70% of patients[31]. Axillary lymph node dissection is major surgery and is associated with increased operative morbidity and cost. New surgical approaches, such as sentinel node dissection or selective node dissection, have been proposed to reduce the number of unnecessary axillary dissections, and are under investigation.

Ultrasonographic studies of axillary lymph nodes in breast cancer have demonstrated that the sensitivity and specificity of B-mode ultrasonography were lower than 90% even using the best criterion under optimal conditions[32,33].

Finally, using 2D and 3D power Doppler analysis, we can assess the lymph node vascularity[34]. The vascular pattern of lymph node metastases is usually different from that of lymph nodes that are altered because of lymphadenitis. Lymph nodes that are altered because of lymphadenitis have hilar vessels which, in larger lymph nodes, branch off on the periphery. In contrast, there are no typical hilar vessels in lymph node metastases. Instead, there are vessels on the periphery that break through the lymph node capsule.

Conclusions

Interest in screening sonography arises because approximately 15% of breast tumors presented as palpable masses are not identified by mammography but are often evident on sonography[35]. In addition, sonography occasionally identifies tumors that are occult to both palpation and mammography.

Ultrasound is superior for the detection of tumors in the breasts of pregnant or lactating women, in surgically altered breasts, near prostheses or at the periphery of the breast. Ultrasound is recommended for screening non-palpable breast cancers in women under 35 years of age (sensitivity to radiation exposure), especially those with a familial history of breast malignancy[4].

3D ultrasound with power Doppler facilities improves visualization of the tumor vessels and helps to differentiate between benign and malignant breast lesions – one of the major controversies in breast imaging.

References

1. Laine H, Rainio H, Arko T, Tukeva T. Comparison of breast structure and findings by X-ray mammography, ultrasound, cytology and histology. *Eur J Ultrasound* 1995;2:107–15
2. Cleverley JR, Jackson AR, Bateman AC. Preoperative localization of breast microcalcification using high-frequency ultrasound. *Clin Radiol* 1997;70:924–6
3. Yang WT, Suen M, Ahuja A, Metreweli C. *In vivo* demonstration of microcalcification in breast cancer using high resolution ultrasound. *Br J Radiol* 1997;70:685–9
4. Huang CS, Wu CY, Chu JS, Lin JH, Hsu SM, Chang

KJ. Microcalcifications of non-palpable breast lesions detected by ultrasonography: correlation with mammography and histopathology. *Ultrasound Obstet Gynecol* 1999;13:431–6
5. Richter K, Heywang-Kobrunner SH, Winzer KJ, *et al.* Detection of malignant and benign breast lesions with an automated US system: result in 120 cases. *Radiology* 1997;205:823–30
6. Bamber JC, Gonzales LD, Grosgrove DO, Simons P. Quantitative evaluation of real-time ultrasound features of the breast. *Ultrasound Med Biol* 1988;14(suppl): 81–7
7. Leucht WJ, Rabe DR, Humbert KD. Diagnostic value of different interpretative criteria in real time sonography of the breast. *Ultrasound Med Biol* 1988;14(suppl):59–73
8. Fornage BD, Lorigan JG, Andry E. Fibroadenoma of the breast: sonographic apperance. *Radiology* 1989;172: 671–5
9. Vlaisavljevic V. Differentiation of solid breast tumors on the basis of their primary echographic characteristics as revealed by real-time scanning of the uncompressed breast. *Ultrasound Med Biol* 1988;14(suppl):75–80
10. Cole-Beuglet C, Soriano RZ, Kurtz AB, Goldberg BB. Fibroadenoma of the breast. Sonomammography of the breast correlated with pathology in 122 patients. *Am J Roentgenol* 1983;140:369–75
11. Chao TC, Lo YF, Chen SC, Chen MF. Prospective sonographic study of 3093 breast tumors. *J Ultrasound Med* 1999;18:363–70
12. Skane P, Engedal K. Analysis of sonographic features in the differentiation of fibroadenoma and invasive ductal carcinoma. *Am J Roentgenol* 1998;170:109–14
13. Kossoff G. Causes of shadowing in breast sonography. *Ultrasound Med Biol* 1988;14(suppl):211
14. Dastous FT, Foster FS. Frequency dependence of ultrasound attenuation and back-scatter in breast tissue. *Ultrasound Med Biol* 1986;13:795
15. Kossoff G. Three-dimensional ultrasound – technology push or market pull? *Ultrasound Obstet Gynecol* 1995; 5:217–18
16. Blohmer JU, Bollman R, Henrich G, Paepke ST, Lichtenegger W. Die dreidimensionale ultraschalluntersuchung (3D-sonographie) der weiblichen Brustdruse. *Geburzsh Frauenheilk* 1996;56:161–5
17. Sohn CH, Stolz W, Kaufmann M, Bastert G. Three-dimensional ultrasound imaging of benign and malignant breast tumors – initial clinical experiences. *Geburzsh Frauenheilk* 1992;52:520–5
18. Rotten D, Levaillant JM, Zerat L. Analysis of normal breast tissue and of solid breast masses using three-dimensional ultrasound mammography. *Ultrasound Obstet Gynecol* 1999;14:114–24
19. Omori LM, Hisa N, Okhuma K, *et al.* Breast masses with mixed cystic–solid sonographic appearance. *Clin Ultrasound* 1993;21:489–95
20. Davies JD, Chinyama CN, Jones MG, Astley SM, Bates SP, Kulka J. New avenues in 3D computerized imaging of breast cancer. *Anticancer Res* 1996;16:3971–81
21. Sato Y, Nakamoto M, Tamaki Y, *et al.* Image guidance of breast cancer surgery using 3-D ultrasound images and augumented reality visualization. *Trans Med Imaging* 1998;17:681–93
22. Feldman F. Angiography of cancer of the breast. *Cancer* 1969;23:803–8
23. Cosgrove DO, Bamber JC, Davey JB, McKina JA, Sinnett HD. Color Doppler signals from breast tumors. *Radiology* 1990;176:175–80
24. Schelling M, Gnirs J, Braun M, *et al.* Optimized differential diagnosis of breast lesions by combined B-mode and color Doppler sonography. *Ultrasound Obstet Gynecol* 1997;10:48–53
25. Madjar H, Sauerbrei M, Prompeler HJ, Wolfarth R, Gufler H. Color Doppler and duplex flow analysis for classification of breast lesions. *Gynecol Oncol* 1997;64:392–403
26. Madjar H, Prompeler HJ, Sauerbrei W, Mundiger A, Pfeider A. Differential diagnosis of breast lesions by color Doppler. *Ultrasound Obstet Gynecol* 1995;6:199–204
27. Wright IA, Pugh ND, Lyons K, Webster DJ, Mansel RE. Power Doppler in breast tumors: a comparison with conventional color Doppler imaging. *Eur J Ultrasound* 1998;7:175–81
28. Miz P, Kesser M, Linemann A, Opitz N, Reiser M. The demonstration of blood flow in focal breast lesions by power Doppler sonography. A new approach to assessment? *Radiology* 1998;169:236–44
29. Carson PL, Adler DD, Fowlkes JB, Harnist K, Rubin J. Enhanced color flow imaging of breast cancer vasculature. Continuous wave Doppler and three-dimensional display. *J Ultrasound Med* 1992;11:377–85
30. Schroeder RJ, Maeurer J, Vogl TJ, *et al.* D-galactose-based-single-enhanced color Doppler sonography of breast tumors and tumor-like lesions. *Invest Radiol* 1999;34:109–15
31. Morrow M. Axillary dissection: when and how radical? *Semin Surg Oncol* 1996;12:321
32. Tateishi T, Machi J, Feleppa EJ, *et al. In vitro* B-mode ultrasonographic criteria for diagnosing axillary lymph node metastasis of breast cancer. *J Ultrasound Med* 1999;18:349–56
33. Yang WT, Ahuja A, Tang A, *et al.* High resolution sonographic detection of axillary lymph node metastases in breast cancer. *J Ultrasound Med* 1996;15:241
34. Dixon JM, Walsh J, Paterson D, Chetty U. Colour Doppler ultrasonography studies of benign and malignant breast lesions. *Br J Surg* 1992;79:259–60
35. Gordon PB, Goldberg SI. Malignant breast masses detected only by ultrasound. *Cancer* 1995;76:626–30

Three-dimensional ultrasonography in hepatogastroenterology

G. Esmat

Three-dimensional (3D) ultrasonography represents a development of non-invasive, diagnostic, real-time two-dimensional (2D) ultrasonography. The use of transparent rotating scans, comparable to a block of glass, generates a 3D effect[1]. The clinical use of 3D ultrasound in the hepatogastroenterology system has revealed some of its possible applications[2-4].

Although the risks associated with X-ray carcinogenesis are relatively low at diagnostic dose levels, concerns remain for individuals in high-risk categories. In addition, the cost and portability of computed tomography (CT) and magnetic resonance imaging (MRI) machines can be prohibitive. In comparison, ultrasound can provide portable, low-cost, non-ionizing imaging[5].

The major advantage of 3D ultrasonography is the ability to obtain ultrasound sections which are impossible to see on a routine scan and the ability to perform accurate volume measurements. In addition, it allows interactive manipulation of volume data using rendering, rotation and zooming on localized features, displaying images of anatomy and organs in a straightforward manner[6].

However, the problem with 3D sonography is not its efficiency but rather its efficacy: what role can this technique play in diagnosis and what information can it add to that from 2D imaging?[7].

The liver

Ultrasound plays an extremely important role in evaluating liver diseases worldwide. In developed countries CT, MRI and ultrasound all have both complementary and competing roles in assessing the liver[8,9]. The limitations of 2D ultrasound include a lesser ability to give an overall panoramic view of large structures, such as the liver, and a sensitivity to artifacts, because of degradation by gas, bone and, to a lesser extent, fat[10].

It is necessary to image the patient in different positions at different phases of respiration. Typically, one must scan from at least three different scanning positions to obtain an adequate examination, because the liver is too large to be seen from any single perspective. The examiner must visualize exactly which portions of the liver have been imaged from each transducer location to be sure the entire organ has been evaluated. This can be challenging. A good 3D ultrasound system should document exactly which portions of the liver were evaluated, and therefore facilitate a more thorough examination[11].

Liver volume

In a clinical context, measurements of organ volume are often performed in the diagnosis and follow-up of patients with a variety of diseases. Ultrasonography is a cheap, widely available and non-hazardous imaging modality to use for estimation of volumes. Using 2D ultrasound, the simplest method of calculating the volume of an organ is based on the multiplication of three diameters perpendicular to each other. These 2D methods are often based on geometrical assumptions, which may introduce significant errors in volume estimation. Therefore, volume estimation based on 3D ultrasound has been developed to increase the accuracy and precision[12].

Knowing the true volume of the entire liver is sometimes clinically important. Both native and transplanted liver tissue have the ability to regenerate, and imaging is often used to monitor this regeneration process following surgery[13].

To date, MRI and volumetric CT are the modalities most frequently employed for these assessments[13,14]. Three-dimensional ultrasound has the potential to replace CT and MRI in this role, if the technical problems in acquiring high-quality data sets can be overcome. This would be desirable, as assessment could be carried out more frequently, since ultrasound is more readily available, uses non-ionizing radiation and is less expensive[15].

Diffuse liver disease

Wagner and colleagues[11] studied 93 patients with chronic liver disease and compared 3D ultrasound with the conventional 2D ultrasound. They found that

CLINICAL APPLICATION OF 3D SONOGRAPHY

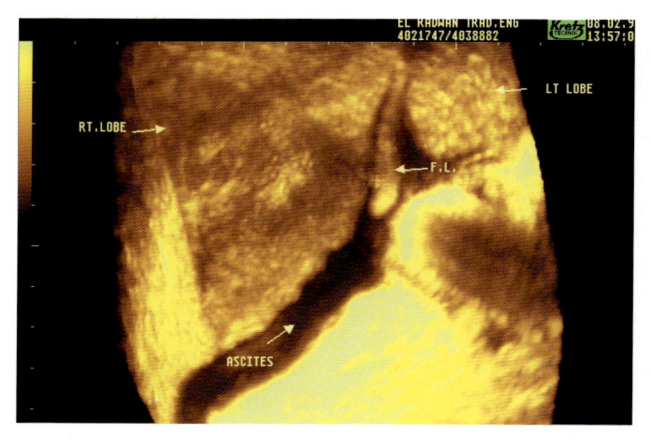

Figure 1 Falciform ligament (F.L.) seen between both lobes of a cirrhotic liver with irregular hepatic edge and ascites

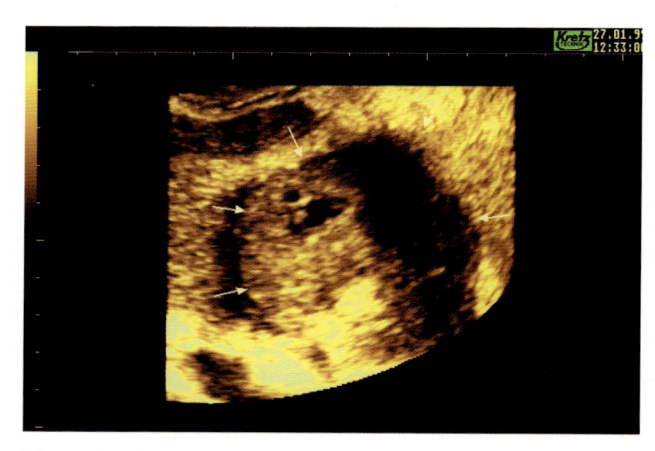

Figure 3 Solid hepatic focal lesion (hepatocellular carcinoma; arrows) with central breakdown

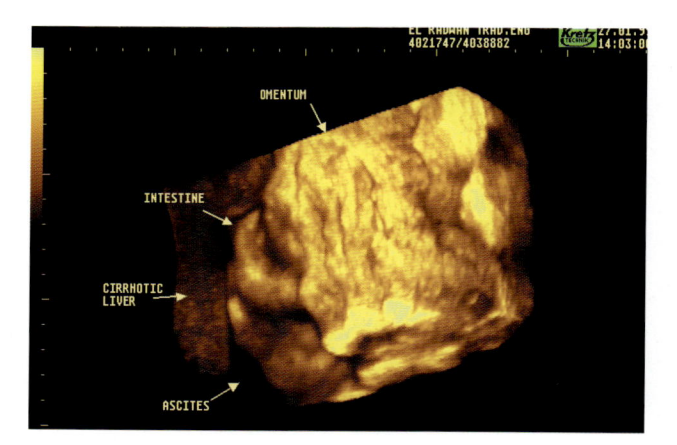

Figure 2 Omental surface seen in a case of liver cirrhosis with ascites

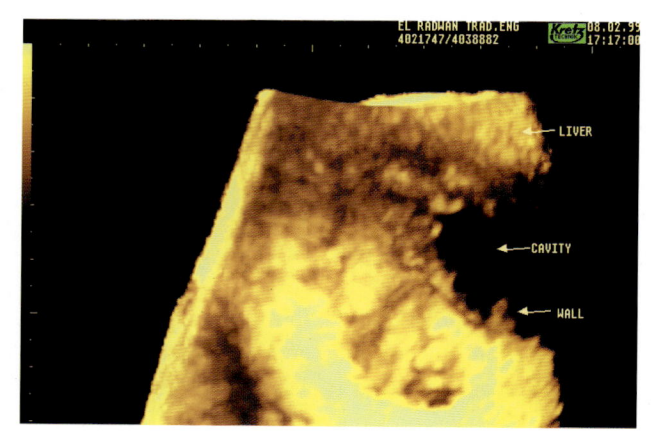

Figure 4 Irregular wall of hydatid cyst of the liver

3D imaging was superior to routine sonography in the anatomical assessment of complex vascular and biliary duct alterations. Three-dimensional ultrasonography was found to be better in the diagnosis of Budd–Chiari syndrome and primary sclerosing cholangitis. However, 3D imaging did not add important information in diffuse liver disease.

In our personal experience, 3D ultrasound has been valuable in demonstrating the irregular surface of liver cirrhosis and rounded edges in a view very similar to the laparoscopic view. Visualization of the falciform ligament (Figure 1) and the omentum (Figure 2) could also be demonstrated.

Hepatic focal lesions

Liess and colleagues[16] showed that 3D ultrasound provided more accurate and repeatable measurements of focal liver lesions than either 2D ultrasound or CT in sequential studies.

This is an extremely important finding, as it is crucial to have an accurate measurement of the volume of liver lesions that are to be treated with minimally invasive therapies. The amount of therapy given to the patient is usually directly proportional to the volume of the lesion. For example, with alcohol ablation of hepatocellular carcinoma in cirrhotic patients, the dose of alcohol injected into the lesion is directly proportional to the volume of the tumor[17].

As regards the accuracy of volume measurement, 3D ultrasound is comparable to CT but more precise than 2D ultrasound. This indicates that 3D ultrasound may be applied in the follow-up of tumor patients as an alternative diagnostic procedure to CT (Figure 3). Lang and colleagues[18] showed that the volume measurement using 3D ultrasound provided comparable results to those of CT. Clinically, 3D ultrasound could be helpful in the follow-up of patients with non-resectable tumors or in planning for liver resection, by assessing the volume of the liver tissue remaining after resection or by better visualization of the topography of the liver tumor or the major hepatic structures[19].

Three-dimensional ultrasonography was found to be a helpful imaging technique in the detection of

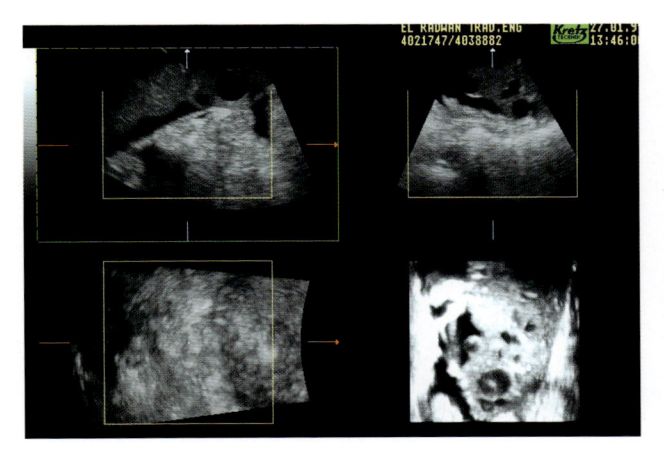

Figure 5 Multiplanar view and interactive three-dimensional ultrasound for countless splenic cysts in a case of vascular malformations

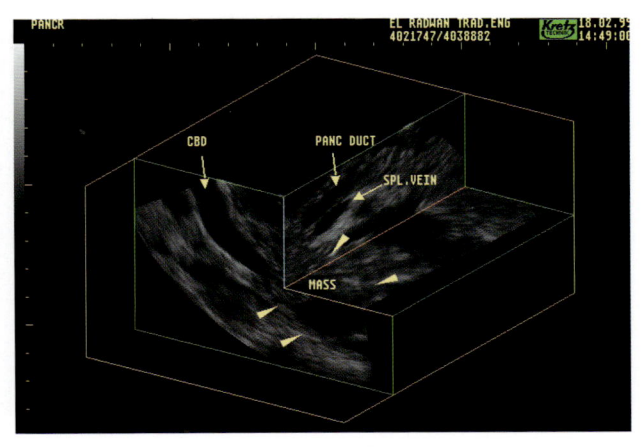

Figure 6 Dilated pancreatic duct (PANC DUCT) and common bile duct (CBD) owing to pancreatic head mass

hepatic hydatid cyst (Figure 4) and in the measurements of its volume. The effect of alcohol injection by the percutaneous–aspiration–injection and reaspiration (PAIR) technique could be demonstrated in the form of detachment of the membrane.

Four-dimensional (upgraded 3D) ultrasonography is useful in providing guidance for interventional procedures in the liver, including the taking of biopsies, aspirations or injections of therapeutic materials.

Hepatic vasculature

Three-dimensional power Doppler ultrasonography of the portal vein produces relatively clear images of the portal venous system when viewed in volume-rendered mode. In addition, assessing the patency of the portal systemic shunts and transjugular–intrahepatic–portosystemic shunt (TIPS) procedures may be more elegantly displayed in three dimensions, essentially with 3D power rendering. The role of contrast enhancement of liver tumors using three dimensions holds great promise, although this is still untested[20].

Three-dimensional Doppler ultrasound was a useful addition in diagnosing the cause of chronic liver disease in patients with ascites due to venoocclusive disease, where the hepatic veins were occluded, with minimal irregular blood flow[21].

The spleen

Diffuse splenomegaly is the most commonly diagnosed abnormality within the spleen. Focal splenic abnormalities including cysts (Figure 5), and benign and malignant tumors are easily demonstrated[22]. Splenic volumes can be calculated automatically after serial slices have been obtained. Each has a manually drawn region of interest assigned around the spleen.

Three-dimensional ultrasonography is potentially superior to 2D ultrasonography for evaluation of irregularly shaped objects such as the spleen, and can provide improved accuracy over that of the traditional technique[23]. High-quality 3D power Doppler images of the spleen are relatively easily obtained and this type of evaluation may assist in evaluating splenic infarctions and trauma[20].

The pancreas

Sackmann and co-workers[24] used 3D ultrasound to visualize pancreatic lesions and stones, and they concluded that this imaging procedure could be helpful in identification of the extension of tumors and the invasion of the surrounding tissues (Figure 6). Stones and stone fragments in the pancreas were also visualized.

Three-dimensional ultrasound may also be helpful in deciding the extent of peripancreatic cystic diseases due to either pseudocyst formation or tumors and may help in measuring intrapancreatic lesions more accurately, which may be clinically useful in following the pseudocyst.

Selner and Machacek[25] commented on the importance of tumor volume in the prognosis of radically periampullary cancer. They found that the larger the cancer, the worse the prognosis. Whether 3D ultrasound will provide more accurate measurements than CT or endoluminal ultrasound is currently unknown.

The gallbladder and biliary tract

Knowing the exact location of the gallbladder is important prior to surgery or radiological intervention

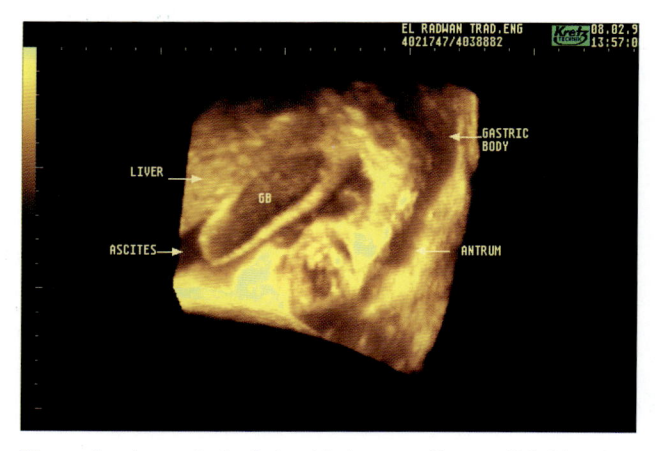

Figure 7 Anatomical relationship between liver, gallbladder (GB) and stomach in a case of ascites

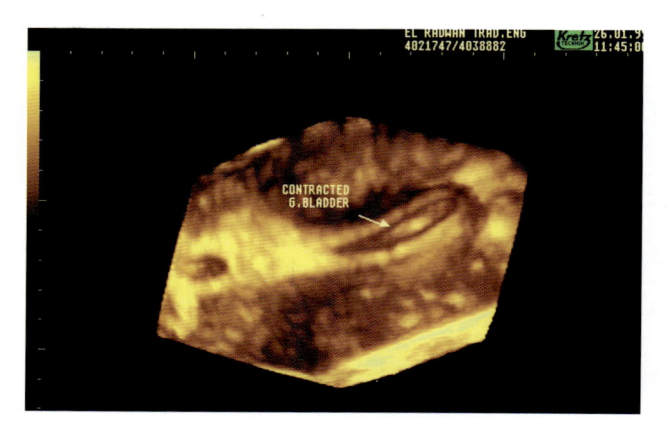

Figure 8 Contracted gallbladder with a thick wall

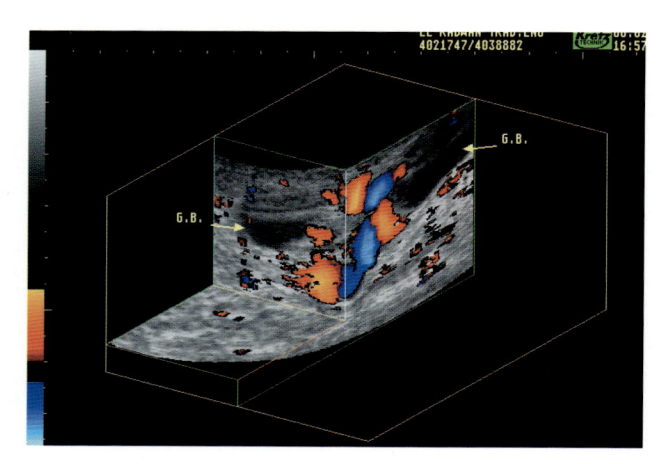

Figure 9 Niche mode showing gallbladder (G.B.) wall collaterals in a case of portal hypertension

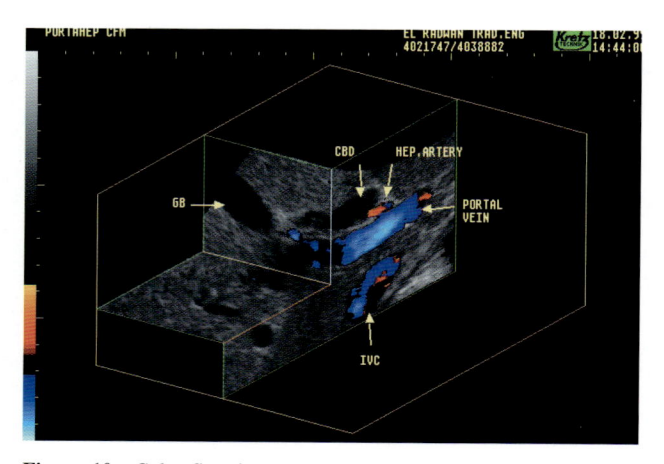

Figure 10 Color flow image. Dilated common bile duct (CBD) and its relationship to the gallbladder (GB), portal vein, hepatic artery and inferior vena cava (IVC)

(Figure 7). Although extremely rare, anomalies in gallbladder location such as a left-sided gallbladder or intrahepatic gallbladder may make laparoscopic cholecystectomy and other procedures extremely challenging. These anomalies might be better appreciated in 3D ultrasound examination, when a more panoramic view of the gallbladder and the surrounding structures is present. Obtaining a clear perspective of the pericholecystic region may also be desirable in assessing the appropriate surgical approach for gallbladder masses, either carcinoma or metastatic disease[22].

Three-dimensional ultrasonography accurately measures gallbladder volume and emptying (Figure 8), and has produced a significantly smaller systematic bias and closer limits of agreement with the true volume[26].

Sackmann and associates[24] demonstrated the use of 3D ultrasound in evaluating the gallbladder wall and gallbladder stones. In our experience, in a case of portal hypertension, portosystemic collaterals could be visualized surrounding the wall of the gallbladder (Figure 9).

Wagner and colleagues[11] evaluated the role of 3D ultrasound in detecting the extent of biliary tract alterations in primary sclerosing cholangitis. A dilated common bile duct and its relation to the gallbladder, portal vein, hepatic artery and inferior vena cava are shown in Figure 10.

The gastrointestinal tract

Recent studies have illustrated that endoluminal ultrasound produces detailed imaging of the gastrointestinal wall and adjacent structures. Three-dimensional imaging may improve visualization of topographic relationships and the nature of pathological lesions.

Transcutaneous sonography has been reported to be clinically useful in assessing focal mass lesions, diffuse lesions of the bowel wall and intraluminal pathologies[22].

Hydrosonography using 3D ultrasound can be performed in the diagnosis of hollow organ pathology.

THREE-DIMENSIONAL ULTRASONOGRAPHY IN HEPATOGASTROENTEROLOGY

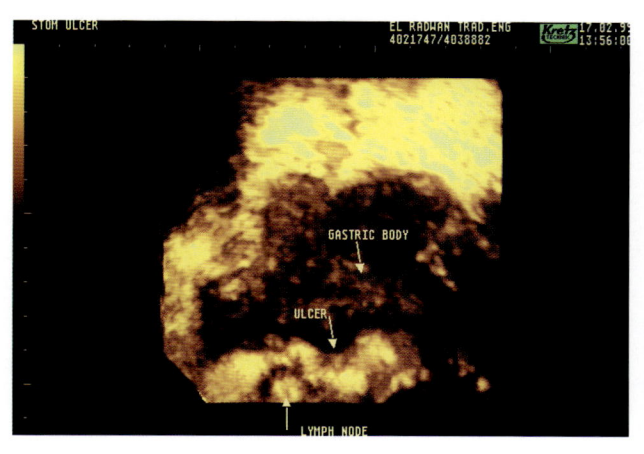

Figure 11 Three-dimensional hydrosonography showing a gastric ulcer on the greater curvature with nodal involvement

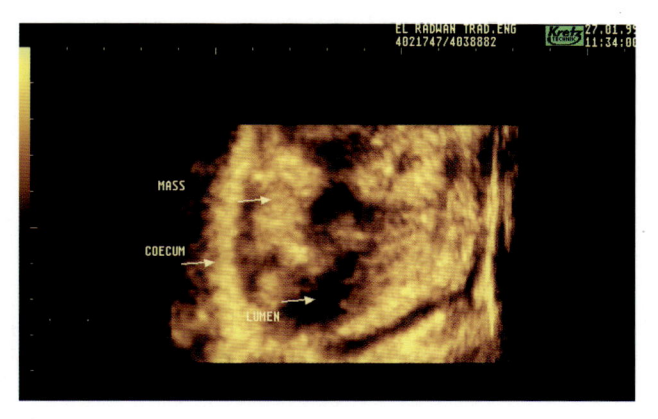

Figure 12 Tuberculous mass in the cecum (confirmed by colonoscopy)

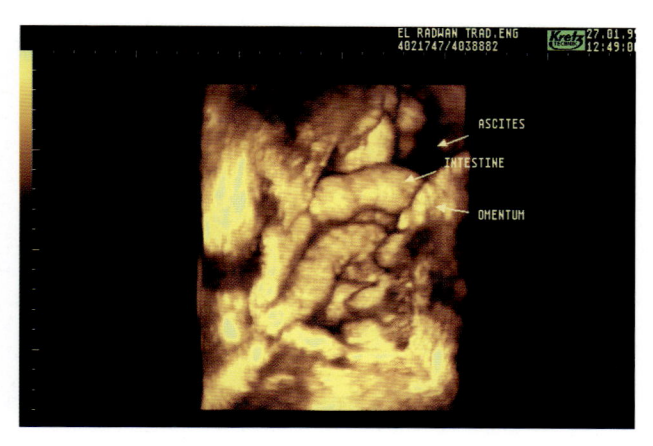

Figure 13 Smooth surface of the intestinal loop as seen in an ascitic patient with liver cirrhosis

vature of the stomach with nodal involvement (Figure 11). By this technique a mass in the cecum and the ascending colon was demonstrated (Figure 12), and it was confirmed by colonoscopy and histopathology to be of tuberculous etiology[21]. The loops of the small bowel, visceral peritoneum, and greater as well as lesser omentum can be visualized in ascitic patients (Figure 13).

Hunerbein and co-workers[30] assessed the role of 3D endosonography in examining 100 patients with rectal cancer. They concluded that the technique allowed visualization of the lesions in different planes, which would be impossible with conventional 2D ultrasound imaging.

This was found to be more accurate than 2D ultrasound because of the multiple cuts that can be made and also because of more accurate orientation[21]. Three-dimensional ultrasound can be extremely helpful in assessing overall tumor volume and for measuring some distances (e.g. the distance from a rectal tumor to the external sphincter, which may dictate how and when surgery is planned)[22]. The use of three-dimensional ultrasound in the esophagus was shown to be technically possible, and it added potential for improving cancer staging[27].

Molin evaluated the usefulness of 3D reconstruction for interpretation and quantitative analysis during stent deployment in cancer of the esophagus[28]. In assessment of intragastric distribution and gastric emptying, 3D ultrasound magnetic scanhead tracking showed excellent *in vitro* accuracy, calculating emptying rates more precisely than by 2D ultrasound and enabling estimation of the intragastric distribution of soap meal[29].

Three-dimensional hydrosonography of the stomach demonstrated a malignant ulcer on the greater cur-

Ascites

The best 3D ultrasound images have been obtained from anatomical and pathological conditions with a liquid content and structures surrounded by liquid (e.g. hydrocele and ascites)[31].

Esmat and El Raziky[21] studied 39 ascitic patients. Ascites was found to be beneficial for 3D ultrasound examination because it facilitated the visualization of the intestinal surface as well as the parietal peritoneum. They evaluated the role of 3D ultrasound in the etiological diagnosis of ascites. Peritoneal nodules were seen in most of the ascitic cases, owing to local causes. They found that 3D ultrasound was helpful in the differentiation between tuberculous nodules (Figures 14 and 15) and malignant nodules (Figure 16) in 80% of the cases. A typical pattern was described for tuberculous ascites (Figure 17).

CLINICAL APPLICATION OF 3D SONOGRAPHY

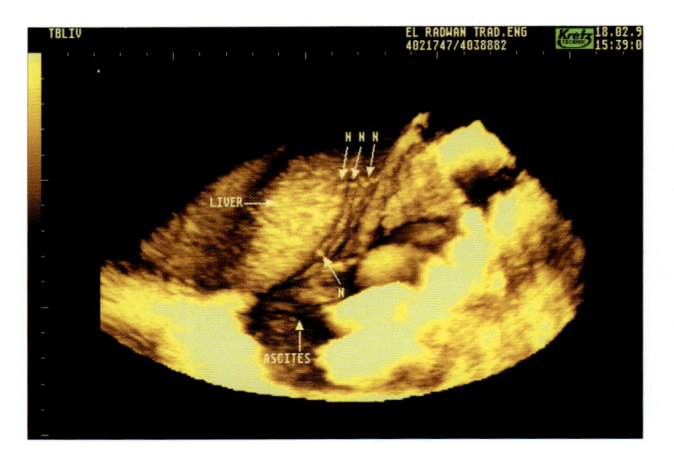

Figure 14 Non-cirrhotic liver covered by tuberculous nodules (N) in a case of tuberculous ascites

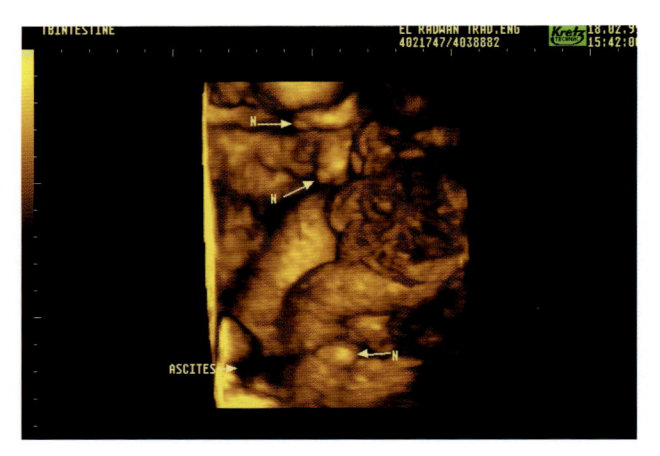

Figure 16 Multiple variable-sized nodules on the visceral peritoneum in a case of malignant ascites

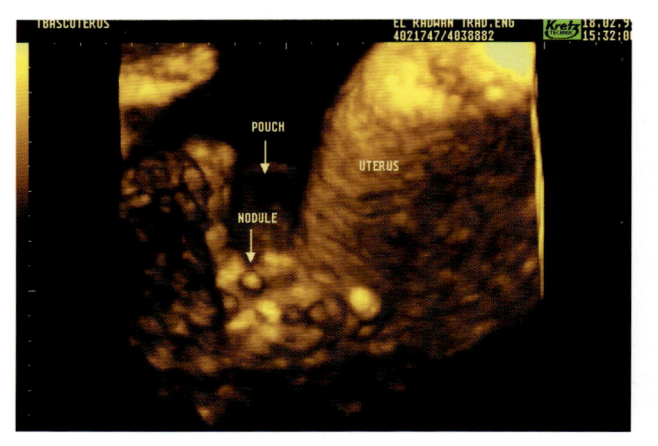

Figure 15 Tuberculous nodules on the pouch of Douglas. The nodules are characteristically surrounded by a hypoechoic margin

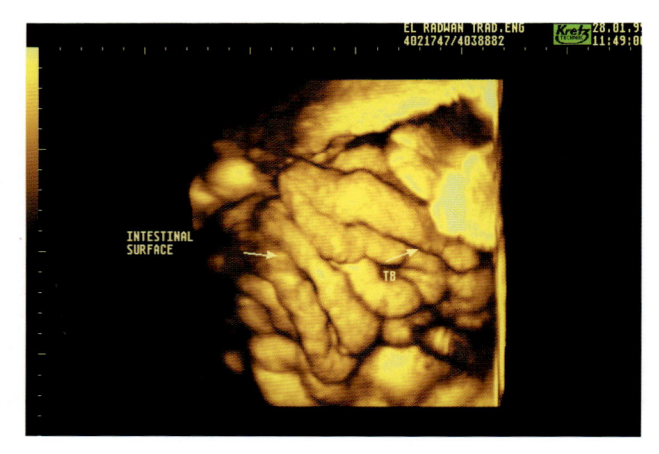

Figure 17 Fine nodularity of the intestinal surface in tuberculous ascites.

References

1. Zoller W, Liess H, Roth C, Umgelter A. Clinical application of three-dimensional sonography in internal medicine. *Clin Invest* 1993;71:220–32
2. Liess H, Roth C, Umgelter A, et al. Improvements in volumetric quantification of circumscribed hepatic lesions by three-dimensional sonography. *Z Gastroenterol* 1994;39:488–92
3. Pauletzki J, Sackmann M, Holl J, et al. Evaluation of gall bladder volume and emptying with a novel three-dimensional ultrasound system: comparison with the sum of cylinders and the ellipsoid methods. *J Clin Ultrasound* 1996;24:277–85
4. Wolf G, Lang H, Prokop M, Schreiber M, Zoller W. Volume measurements of localized hepatic lesions using three-dimensional sonography in comparison with three-dimensional computed tomography. *Eur J Med Res* 1998;3:157–64
5. Morimoto A, Krumm J, Kozlowski D, et. al. High definition 3D ultrasound imaging. *Stud Health Technol Inform* 1997;39:90–8
6. Thomas R, Dolores H. Interactive acquisition, analysis and visualization of sonographic volume data. *Int J Imaging Technol* 1997;35:40–7
7. Riccabona M, Nelson T, Pretorius D, Davidson T. Distance and volume measurement using three-dimensional ultrasonography. *J Ultrasound Med* 1995;14:881–6
8. Ferrucci J. Liver tumor imaging: current concepts. *Am J Roentgenol* 1990;155:473–84
9. Ohahsi I, Ina H, Okada Y, et al. Segmental anatomy of the liver under the right diaphragmatic dome: evaluation with axial CT. *Radiology* 1996;200:779–83
10. Cosgrove D. Why do we need contrast agents for ultrasound? *Clin Radiol* 1996;51(suppl 1):1–4
11. Wagner S, Gebel M, Bleck J, Manns M. Clinical application of three-dimensional sonography in hepatobiliary diseases. *Bildgebung* 1994;61:104–9
12. Gilja O, Hausken T, Perstand A, Odegaard S. Measurements of organ volumes by ultrasonography. *Proc Inst Mech Eng* 1999;213:247–59
13. Chari R, Baker M, Sue S, Meyers W. Regeneration of a

transplanted liver after right hepatic lobectomy. *Liver Transpl Surg* 1996;2:233–4
14. Caldwell S, de Lange E, Gaffey M, *et al*. Accuracy and significance of pretransplant liver volume measured by magnetic resonance energy. *Liver Transpl Surg* 1996; 2:438–42
15. Henderson J, Macky G, Kutner M, Noe B. Volumetric and functional liver blood flow are both increased in the human transplanted liver. *J Hepatol* 1993;17:204–8
16. Liess H, Roth C, Umgelter A, Zoller W. Improvements in volumetric quantification of circumscribed hepatic lesions by 3D-US. *Z Gastroenterol* 1994;32:488–92
17. Alexander D, Unger E, Seeger S, *et al*. Estimation of volumes of distribution and intra-tumoral ethanol concentrations by CT scanning after percutaneous ethanol injection. *Acad Radiol* 1996;3:49–56
18. Lang H, Wolf G, Prokop M, Nuber B, Weimann A. 3-D sonography for volume determination of liver tumor – report of initial experiences. *Chirurgie* 1999;70:246–50
19. Lang H, Wolf G, Prokop M, Nuber B, Weimann A. Volumetry of circumscribed liver changes with 3D US in comparison with 3D CT. *Langenbecks Arch Chir Suppl Kongressbd* 1998;115:1478–80
20. Downey D, Fenster A. Vascular imaging with a 3D power Doppler system. *Am J Roentgenol* 1995; 156:665–8
21. Eamat G, El Raziky M. Etiological diagnosis of ascites by 3D utlrasonography. *Medical Imaging International*, 2000;10:18–19
22. Nelson T, Downey D, Pretorius D, Fenester A. Abdomen. *Three-dimensional Ultrasonography*. Philadelphia, PA: Lippincott Williams and Wilkins, 1999:151–67
23. De Odoricio I, Spaulding K, Pretorius D, *et al*. Normal splenic volumes estimated using 3D ultrasonography. *J Ultrasound Med* 1999;18:231–6
24. Sackmann M, Pauletzki J, Zwiebel F, Holl J. Three-dimensional ultrasonography in hepatobiliary and pancreatic diseases. *Bildgebung* 1994;61:100–3
25. Sellner F, Machacek E. The importance of tumor volume in the prognosis of radically treated periampullary carcinomas. *Eur J Surg* 1993;159:95–100
26. Pauletzki J, Sackmann M, Holl J, Paumgartner G. Evaluation of gall bladder volume and emptying with a novel three-dimensional ultrasound system: comparison with the sum-of-cylinders and the ellipsoid methods. *J Clin Ultrasound* 1996;24:277–85
27. Kallimanis G, Garra B, Tio T, *et al*. The feasibility of three-dimensional endoscopic ultrasonography: a preliminary report. *Gastrointest Endosc* 1995;41:235–9
28. Molin S. Usefullness of three-dimensional reconstruction for interpretation and quantitative analysis during stent depolyment in esophageal cancer. Presented at the *8th International Congress of Interventional Ultrasound,* Copenhagen, September 1, 1999:56
29. Gilja O, Detmer P, Jong J, *et al*. Intragastric distribution and gastric emptying assessed by three-dimensional ultrasonography. *Gastroenterology* 1997;113:38–49
30. Hunerbein N, Dohmoto M, Haensch W, Schlag P. Evaluation and biopsy of recurrent rectal cancer using 3D endosonography. *Dis Colon Rectum* 1996;39: 1373–8
31. Cesarani F, Isolato G, Capello S, Pianchi S. Tridimensional ultrasonography. First clinical experience with dedicated devices and review of the literature. *Radiol Med (Torino)* 1999;97:256–64

Advantages, limitations and future developments of three-dimensional ultrasound in gynecology and obstetrics

A. Kurjak and S. Kupesic

Three-dimensional (3D) ultrasound has recently been introduced into clinical practice[1,2], overcoming some of the limitations of two-dimensional (2D) sonography. Although 2D transvaginal ultrasound has been established as a reliable, cost-effective and non-invasive technique for the evaluation of organs of the lower pelvis[3], a disadvantage of this technique is that the examination of the organ is usually limited to transverse and longitudinal sections, which give an incomplete view of the structure.

The major advantages of 3D ultrasound are the ability to obtain ultrasound sections which are impossible to see on a routine scan, and the ability to perform accurate volume measurements. In addition, 3D anatomical reconstruction of the organs of interest is possible[4]. Once the complete volume has been stored, the data can be accessed and re-examined at any time, even after the patient has been discharged. Equivocal findings can be scrutinized without time pressure and without causing the patient any discomfort, and even a second or third examiner can read and interpret the stored volume independently of the first examiner. Table 1 lists the benefits of the use of 3D ultrasound in gynecology and obstetrics.

Three-dimensional ultrasound offers four different display options:

(1) Two-dimensional multiplanar display of orthogonal image planes;

(2) Niche view;

(3) Three-dimensional surface-rendering view;

(4) Transparent view in the maximum or X-ray mode[3].

With the orthogonal display, all three perpendicular planes are displayed simultaneously on the monitor, enabling an accurate assessment to be made of the acquired volumes. Rotation controls can be used to rotate stored organs into the position most favorable for the examiner, and the tomographic exploration of the pelvic organs can be initiated from the same starting position. The coronal section has not only become the plane of choice in the diagnosis of uterine anomalies[5,6], but it can also be used to determine the position of an intrauterine device (IUD)[7,8]. It is suited for the detection of uterine masses and irregularities within the endometrium[9,10], and is particularly useful in women receiving long-term tamoxifen therapy.

Saline solution may be infused for evaluation of the uterine cavity and serves as an aid in the investigation of endometrial polyps[4,10,11]. Three-dimensional ultrasound is superior to the conventional ultrasound for the identification of spreading of endometrial carcinoma into the myometrium and for the detection of tumor extension towards the cervix. As tumor size is a major prognostic factor in cervical carcinoma, the simultaneous display of all three orthogonal planes on the monitor provides the optimum conditions for an accurate determination of tumor volume[12]. Three-dimensional ultrasound offers advantages in the evaluation of complications in early pregnancy, such as an ectopic gestational sac, even in intramural pregnancies, and the intrauterine remnants of an incomplete abortion. In 3D ultrasound imaging of the ovaries, the simultaneous display of all three sectional planes affords a view of ovarian morphology and provides high accuracy in calculating the ovarian volume[13].

The niche view provides a cutaway or 'cut-open' view of an organ, removing one-quarter of the structure electronically, in order to view the interior of the organ. This view can be used in obstetrics and for determination of tumor spread (eg. in cases of uterine malignancy to predict parametrial invasion).

The surface mode is used in the assessment of superficial structures. If a cystic ovarian mass is found, 3D transvaginal ultrasound offers new possibilities for surface evaluation and the differentiation between benign and malignant disease[14,15].

The fluid-distended urinary bladder allows accurate evaluation of both the surface of the structure and the size of a tumor (endometriosis, carcinoma) projecting into the bladder lumen[3]. At present, the outer surfaces of the organs can be delineated by 3D ultrasound only if they are surrounded by fluid. A new technique allowing the precise electronic separation of adjacent organs ('electronic scalpel') has recently been introduced.

Table 1 Possible benefits of three-dimensional ultrasound

Imaging of previously inaccessible planes
Improved demonstration of complex anatomy
More standardized investigations, offering an improved tool for a second opinion
Low inter- and intraobserver variability
More accurate measurement, especially in irregularly shaped organs
More accurate guidance of interventional procedures using multiplanar and rendered images
More accurate placement of the needle and/or catheter during an invasive procedure

Table 2 Advantages of three-dimensional compared to two-dimensional ultrasound in obstetrics

Improved comprehension of fetal anatomy by families
Improved maternal–fetal bonding
Improved identification of fetal anomalies using planes unobtainable with two-dimensional ultrasound
Improved recognition of anomalies by less experienced physicians
More accurate identification of the extent and size of anomalies in spite of anatomic constraints or fetal position
Possibility of a retrospective review or consultation with specialists if an anomaly is subtle or difficult to assess, or after the patient has finished the examination

The transparent mode can effectively scrutinize indeterminate echogenic areas in structures such as dermoid cysts or breast, to detect calcifications and/or proliferative lesions.

Comparing three- and two-dimensional ultrasound in a preliminary study of 348 patients, Merz found that, in 52% of patients, the four different display modes provided by 3D ultrasound yielded additional or superior information to the 2D technique[3]. Furthermore, 3D transvaginal ultrasound offers the opportunity to store and investigate the pelvic organs with three different volumes such as the uterus, left adnexa and right adnexa. The total examination time for the patient is considerably reduced.

In this chapter we overview the limitations and benefits of 3D ultrasound and 3D power Doppler in routine practice in both gynecology and obstetrics. Further developments are also listed (Tables 1 and 2).

Clinical applications of three-dimensional ultrasound in gynecology and infertility

Detailed assessment of the uterine cavity and myometrium is important in the conditions of uterine malformations, endometrial pathology (synechia, polyps, hyperplasia, carcinoma) and uterine myomas.

The coronal plane of the uterus assessed by 3D ultrasound allows the physician to view both horns of the endometrium and the cervix at the same time. Three-dimensional ultrasound permits the shape of the uterus to be more clearly demonstrated, thus optimally displaying congenital anomalies of the uterus. Two-dimensional ultrasound is helpful in identifying the two horns of the uterus, but the distinction between a septate and bicornuate uterus cannot be made, because the contour of the myometrium cannot be imaged in the transverse plane. Hysterosonography (HSG) displays the uterine cavity very well, but cannot differentiate between a septate and bicornuate uterus because the myometrium and external contour of the uterus cannot be precisely evaluated. Until recently, infertile patients required hysteroscopy, laparoscopy or even magnetic resonance imaging (MRI) to assess the shape of the uterine cavity and myometrium, after a hysterosalpingogram had suggested an endometrial abnormality. In this light, 3D ultrasound provides a cost-effective alternative to MRI and/or invasive methods of investigation.

Conventional 2D ultrasound has been used as a screening test to evaluate patients for the possibility of endometrial cancer. The thickness of the endometrium has been traditionally measured on a sagittal plane through the uterus. Limitations of this technique were due to varying thickness and coexistent pathology, such as endometrial polyps, which may be displayed as focal areas of thickening. Patients with endometrial hyperplasia and cancer show a significant overlap in endometrial thickness. That is why volume measurements of the endometrium may be much more helpful in distinguishing endometrial cancer from benign pathology[16]. Invasion of endometrial carcinoma into the myometrium may also be examined with 3D ultrasound[17]. Simultaneous display of the transverse plane with 3D ultrasound allows possible visualization of cervical or endometrial carcinoma infiltrating the bladder or rectum. Three-dimensional ultrasound may be able to replace computerized tomography (CT) scans currently performed for the staging of tumors.

Three-dimensional ultrasound is helpful in the delineation of endometrial polyps and synechiae, as well as in determining their location. This technique assists in distinguishing between small polyps and synechiae, and, in cases of bridging synechiae, the degree of cavity obliteration is readily assessed.

By use of the simultaneous display of three perpendicular planes, the exact location of myomas can be demonstrated within the uterus. Accurate measurement of leiomyoma size may be obtained using volumetric data. The precise relationship between each myoma and the uterine cavity and its size can be assessed more accurately with 3D ultrasound than with 2D ultrasound. Three-dimensional ultrasound gives information that is critical in planning the type of myomectomy, and in post-myomectomy assessment of the cavity. One limitation of scanning the uterus with myomas, true for both 3D and 2D ultrasound, occurs when there is significant shadowing from calcification. Patients who are on medical therapy to reduce the size of leiomyomas may be followed to estimate the volume of the leiomyomas and therefore evaluate the effectiveness of the therapy.

Two-dimensional ultrasound has been used to identify the location of IUDs within the uterus for many years, but occasionally it may be difficult to locate an IUD accurately with this technique. Three-dimensional ultrasound allows for accurate location using multiplanar display, whereas the coronal plane often visualizes a large portion of the IUD. Multiplanar imaging and volume rendering are helpful in determining the exact location of a malpositioned IUD[6]. Rotation of rendered images of the IUD permits recognition of the small arms of the IUD, and can demonstrate incomplete opening of the two arms of the device after insertion.

HSG is typically performed with conventional 2D ultrasound, but 3D ultrasound has several advantages. Three-dimensional ultrasound provides more accurate information about the location of abnormalities, very important for preoperative assessment and the distinguishing of pathologies. During HSG performed with the 2D technique, uterine distension may be uncomfortable, but the 3D ultrasound volume can be acquired in only a few seconds and reviewed later, allowing the uterus to be distended for a shorter period of time than on 2D ultrasound examinations. The use of saline contrast 3D HSG is a useful non-invasive method for assessment of uterine anomalies, submucous myomas and polyps, but in cases of intrauterine synechiae, the use of echogenic contrast media (Echovist) is probably more accurate than saline-contrast 3D HSG.

Three-dimensional ultrasound offers potential information in evaluating adnexal masses. It is superior to 2D ultrasound in evaluating papillary projections, showing the characteristics of cystic walls, identifying the extent of capsular infiltration of tumors and calculating ovarian volume. The transparent minimum–maximum mode of surface rendering may be useful in evaluating dermoid tumors, because it makes it easier to identify teeth, bones and calcification.

Three-dimensional ultrasound is also available for evaluating ovarian enlargement from multiple follicles and lutein cysts, in differentiating ovarian cysts from hydrosalpinges and for accurate volume measurement of irregularly shaped follicles, which are often distorted by adjacent follicles. In geometrically shaped objects, 2D volume calculations are accurate (ellipsoid calculation), whereas irregularly shaped objects pose a great challenge to 2D ultrasound.

Three-dimensional ultrasound may improve the diagnostic accuracy of polycystic ovaries. Increased ovarian stroma is an essential criterion for the morphological diagnosis of polycystic ovaries[18]. Using 3D ultrasound we can assess accurate ovarian stromal volume by subtracting the volume of all the follicles from the total ovarian volume. The follicular size and follicular fluid volume are related to oocyte maturity, oocyte retrieval rate, fertilization rate and pregnancy rate. Therefore, the estimation of follicular volume is more accurate using 3D measurement, which is not influenced by the shape or size of the follicles[19]. Follicular aspiration using 3D ultrasound has been reported, but until now this has not become routinely used[20]. Measuring endometrial volume by 3D ultrasound is highly reproducible[13], but it remains to be seen whether it is useful in predicting the chances for implantation. Three-dimensional power Doppler technology during hysterosalpingocontrast sonography (HyCoSy) helps to visualize the complete length of the Fallopian tube together with the uterine cavity and free spillage of contrast medium. Two-dimensional ultrasound requires freezing of the image, therefore the dynamic process of bubbles passing out of a tube may be overlooked.

Three-dimensional sonography obtains additional information about the urethra and periurethral tissues, owing to the availability of transverse planes as well as to the possibility of demonstrating irregular surface structures three-dimensionally. It allows accurate volume measurements to be made of the bladder and urethral sphincter, which are irregular structures.

Three-dimensional power Doppler sonography is a promising tool in the evaluation of the angiogenesis of pelvic tumors, especially when a malignant neoplasm is suspected, and contrast agents are another possibility for enhancing the 3D power Doppler examination by increasing the detection rate of small vessels. Power Doppler sonography has been found to be superior to frequency-based color Doppler sonography, especially in the situations of low blood flow (low velocities)[21], with the potential to detect alternations in blood flow[22]. Three-dimensional power Doppler ultrasound detects characteristic structural abnormalities of malignant tumor vessels such as microaneurysms, arteriovenous shunts, tumoral lakes, disproportional calibration, elongation, coiling and dichotomous branching. In these cases, the tumor vessels are usually randomly dispersed within the stroma and periphery, and the course of the main tumor vessel is 'thorn-like' and irregular, with more complicated branching[23]. In addition, the resolution of current power Doppler is sufficient to detect vessels of about 1 mm in diameter[24]. The appeal of the 3D display is that it is more comprehensive and allows physicians to understand the 3D architecture of the microcirculation interactively. The indices provide quantitative values for the measurement of blood flow and vascularization, characterizing the physiological and pathological conditions of neoangiogenesis.

This technique is especially useful in the evaluation of complex ovarian lesions (such as ovarian dermoids, endometriomas and fibromas), which may give an incorrect impression of malignancy under conventional transvaginal sonography and color Doppler ultrasound[15,25]. The use of a contrast agent in 3D power Doppler sonography appears to improve the sensitivity for differentiating benign from malignant ovarian lesions, by allowing better detection of the intralesional flow than is obtained by imaging without contrast. To determine the practical value of contrast-enhanced 3D power Doppler, comparative studies need to be performed.

Three-dimensional power Doppler examination of the adenomyotic uterus is able to demonstrate the perfusion in adenomyotic foci and to trace the course of these vessels. The good results achieved by 3D power Doppler ultrasound examination of uterine lesions can be explained by the improved recognition of the anatomy, characterization of the surface features, detection of the tumor infiltration and precise depiction of the size and volume. Three-dimensional power Doppler imaging can detect structural abnormalities of the malignant tumor vessels, and therefore, it enhances and facilitates the morphological and functional evaluation of both benign and malignant pelvic tumors[26].

Obstetric applications of three-dimensional ultrasound

Three-dimensional sonography has gained significant popularity among specialists interested in prenatal diagnostics[27]. This technique not only offers the third plane that is not available with 2D ultrasound, but also provides the examiner with a tomographic approach and with the possibility of viewing the fetus in a true 3D surface image. The main advantages of 3D ultrasound over 2D ultrasound in obstetrics are listed in Table 2. The orthogonal display presents all three orthogonal planes simultaneously, allowing a detailed tomographic examination to be performed of the embryo or fetus in a non-moving position. The surface mode provides realistic images of the fetal surface. Unfavorable structures adjacent to the region of interest (placenta, umbilical cord, limbs or uterine wall) can be easily removed with an 'electronic scalpel', thus allowing free access to the region to be rendered. This technique enables the examiner to 'cut' the fetus into slices in order to demonstrate inner surfaces. The transparent mode enables a selective view of the fetal skeleton. All presented modes provide a detailed demonstration of the normal and abnormal anatomy of the fetus. Three-dimensional ultrasound offers advantages in assessing the embryo in the first trimester, owing to the ability to obtain multiplanar images through endovaginal volume acquisition. Using this method, one can calculate gestational sac and yolk sac volumes, which significantly correlate with gestational age and pregnancy outcome[28]. Three-dimensional ultrasound imaging can also be used to evaluate the developmental anatomy of the cerebral cavities and is complementary to pathological and histological findings. Rotation of the embryo enables a systematic review to be carried out of anatomic structures such as cord insertion and limb buds. Furthermore, it has the potential for improved anomaly detection during the first trimester. Three-dimensional ultrasound offers several advantages over 2D ultrasound, especially in the detection of specific small defects of the brain, face, spine and hands, and also for detection of the gender.

Three-dimensional ultrasonography has the potential to provide improved visualization of the fetal face anatomy, including lips, nose, chin and eyes, over current 2D ultrasound, owing to its demonstration on a single image as a coherent structure rather than as many cross-sectional images produced by 2D ultrasonography[29]. Some of the facial abnormalities seen on 3D ultrasound and not on 2D ultrasound include cleft lip/palate, facial dysmorphia, dysplastic ears and micrognathia. Three-dimensional ultrasound is superior to 2D ultrasound in evaluating the fetal face, owing to better presentation of curvature, continuity and the profile. Data can be reviewed later, for network consultation; features can be enhanced and views can be optimized.

Three-dimensional ultrasonography is superior to conventional ultrasonography in the visualization and evaluation of fetal tooth germs, and therefore has the potential for antenatal detection of syndromes associated with oligodontia or anodontia[30].

The fetal spine and thorax contain many different structures that are curvilinear in nature, and, therefore, 3D sonography provides additional information about the fetal thoracic skeleton to that gained by 2D sonography, by presenting the thorax as a coherent structure rather than as a series of cross-sectional slices[31,32]. Three-dimensional power Doppler sonography has potential use in the study of the process of placentation and evaluation of the development of the embryonic and fetal cardiovascular systems. Three-dimensional sonographic imaging of the fetal heart provides both anatomic and functional information regarding the valves, myocardium, great vessels and chamber dynamics[33,34]. The technique may become useful for the screening and diagnosis of congenital cardiac defects in the future.

Nuchal translucency (NT) thickness, which is considered to be the most accurate marker of fetal chromosomal abnormalities between 10 and 14 weeks' gestation, can be measured by 3D transvaginal ultrasound, because it allows an almost ideal mid-sagittal view of the fetus, owing to its ability to reorient the fetal position using multiplanar imaging. The new generation of 3D ultrasound units allows volumetric measurement of nuchal edema[35].

Growth analysis forms the basis for the diagnosis of intrauterine growth restriction (IUGR). Three-dimensional ultrasound is superior to 2D ultrasound for accurate volume measurements of irregular objects, whereas they compare closely for volume measurements of regular objects. Therefore, 3D ultrasound can be used to evaluate birth weight, since arm and thigh volumes assessed by 3D ultrasound correlate well with birth weight.

Three-dimensional ultrasound imaging of the fetal and neonatal brain offers great promise in obtaining axial and oblique images through the brain. Conventional 2D ultrasound is limited to image planes that are perpendicular to the anterior fontanelle, whereas the coronal and sagittal views are the primary planes used to evaluate intraventricular and parenchymal anatomy. Undoubtedly, owing to patients' acceptance and the sensitivity of diagnosis, 3D ultrasound already has its place in everyday obstetric practice (Table 2).

Limitations and possible problems of three-dimensional ultrasound

Users of the 3D ultrasound technique will agree that there are many difficulties to be overcome. Table 3 reviews the limitations of 3D ultrasound. Several of these difficulties have been improved, largely because of technological developments, but also because of increased experience in the application of the technique, such as the orientation in the scanning process and the storage of volume. The first commercially available 3D endovaginal transducer was a forward-scanning sector probe equipped with a motor to enable 180° rotation of the 2D scan plane about the long axis of the probe. This produced a forward scan volume in the shape of a truncated cone[9,36–38]. All of the sectional planes intersected at the center created an overlap effect that led to the degradation of image quality[9]. In the current transvaginal 3D probe the rotary principle has been abandoned and replaced by a mechanism that deflects the forward scan plane in a fan-shaped pattern, comparable to the mechanism of a transabdominal 3D transducer. This eliminates the overlap effect, and quadruples the speed at which volume data are acquired.

However, there are still problems with 3D ultrasound. The first issue concerns the overall performance of 3D systems. In image quality, the image resolution was a major point of low acceptance of three-dimensions. The possible advantage of three-dimensions in superior imaging was hampered by suboptimal surface delineation and tissue differentiation compared to available 2D high-end technology. It is possible to produce the appearance of tissue or bone defects merely by moving the threshold up to the point at which echos should be displayed. The operator must be aware of possible pitfalls that can mimic false-positive scans.

Table 3 The limitations of three-dimensional ultrasound

Distortion of a measured object during acquisition (by pressure or motion)
Distortion of the transducer
Motion during acquisition (breathing, pulsation, movement)
Reconstruction mistakes
Size and borders of the measured object
Increased time necessary for processing
Reduced portability of some systems

Motion artifacts are of special importance in prenatal ultrasound, but also in gynecological applications if 3D power Doppler sonography is used to look at low-flow compartments. Motion artifacts have been reduced as a consequence of shorter acquisition time which, along with overall time consumption, was reduced by new developments in computer technology. Transducer artifacts are not as important and can be overcome by repeated scans in the absence of even minimal motion.

More important is the time consumption. Mean values for a 3D scan of one region of interest in obstetric and gynecological applications are 5.3 min for the scan and 4.5 min for processing and evaluation, giving 9.8 min total time[3]. On average, 1.9 attempts were needed to obtain an image of sufficient quality. In 85% data acquisition was successful at the first attempt.

True 3D real-time scanning should be of great interest, and it should illustrate the reality of a fetus, with its proportions and movements, and provide the option of freezing the image as for the conventional 2D scanning.

The size of the volume visualized is limited in the system using systematic scans and so is the volume of interest, although it would be desirable to image the entire fetus. Especially important would be measurements such as placental volume, amniotic fluid volume and the fetal volume, which might revolutionize the assessment of fetal weight and growth, or the assessment of fetal well-being or fetal compromise.

The experience of the operator is crucial for successful application of 3D ultrasound, and this is one of the major reasons for its limited application to date.

The following issues are quite new and represent an overview of developments such as automatic volume measurements and the ability to transfer data between different systems and via the Internet. Solutions for the problems discussed above are worked out primarily by the industry. Technical developments, such as improvements in focusing and digital beam formation, will provide better image quality. Reduction of motion artifacts will be achieved by much more rapid data acquisition. Finally, education and training are most important for the spread of any technique, and training courses are already in place for 3D ultrasound.

Further developments

The clinical applications of 3D ultrasound continue to expand, while its clinical acceptance and use will be determined by the availability and the ease of use of the equipment. Future areas of investigation in 3D ultrasound include 3D color/power Doppler analysis of neovascularization patterns in gynecological tumors, automated computer programs for tumor volume acquisition and the visualization of tumor surfaces in three dimensions, which has been feasible by the introduction of the 'electronic scalpel'.

Three-dimensional color/power Doppler enables us to image blood flow, thus allowing 3D ultrasound angiography. Three-dimensional power Doppler sonography may be useful not only for imaging vascular structures but even for providing non-directional information about the amount of moving blood cells in a given volume. Conventional 2D pulsed Doppler, in addition to vessel diameter measurement, allows quantification of blood flow, but there is a significant error in the estimation of about 20% and even more in large vessels in obstetric applications, and it is not suitable for low-flow compartments, such as tumors. Computer analysis of 2D ultrasound data is also hampered by the impossibility of accurate volumetric measurement. The presence of low-velocity blood flow can be detected quantitatively by 3D power Doppler. This method allows investigation of the morphological patterns and vessel distribution as well as application of some mathematical models[23]. The 3D approach improves the following of the course of vessels and enables overlapping vessels to be differentiated. However, criteria for analyzing blood flow are too subjective. Recently, a more objective method based on measurements and mathematics has been introduced: the 3D color histogram[39,40].

After 3D visualization of the vessels, the cube (volume) enclosing the vessels of interest should be defined. This cube is analyzed using a computer program giving color and size information for the indices. These indices describe the vascularization in terms of color percentage in the cube and the blood flow in terms of mean (amplitude) color value. Three-dimensional power Doppler sonography displays blood flow in a varying color scale according to its amplitude. To enclose the volume of interest, which contains the color information to be measured, a cube can be placed within the tissue block excluding blood vessels that do not demonstrate low velocity, such as vessels with high velocity flow (iliac vein), excluding artifacts due to tissue, patient or probe movements, and including tumor vessels. Artifacts are common, because of the high sensitivity of the amplitude-based color Doppler. Three-dimensional color histogram indices are:

(1) The vascularization index (VI), which indicates the color percentage within the volume of interest and therefore reflects the number of vessels that can be detected within the tissue block;

(2) The flow index (FI), which is a mean amplitude value, reflecting the number of blood cells that are displaced during the 3D sweep;

(3) The vascularization–flow index (VFI);

(4) The flow/vessel quotient (FVQ), which is a combination of the VI and FI, combining the information of vessel presence and amount of flow[39].

Measuring blood flow and vascularization can be useful in all fields of neoangiogenesis, for example in physiological conditions such as angiogenesis in follicle growth, corpus luteum formation, endometrial growth, embryo implantation, placentation, fetal growth, or even in tumors where the 3D approach enables the whole pathological process to be analyzed in contrast to the 2D measurements, which depict only a slice of the tumor. Initial results[40] have shown a significant difference in some of the histogram indices between benign and malignant ovarian masses. Color histogram calculations might indicate the change of blood flow after chemotherapy for a tumor[41].

The presence of subendometrial and intraendometrial blood flow could be a good predictor for the outcome of *in vitro* fertilization, and since color histogram indices measure flow or flow changes, they might be useful in the field of medically assisted reproduction.

Amplitude-based color Doppler is very sensitive, and is able to detect low-velocity blood flow. Owing to its sensitivity, power Doppler produces motion artifacts. The comparison of index values with those from ultrasound machines of different manufacturers is problematic, and that is why standardization still has to be defined.

Imaging of blood flow vessel anatomy using contrast material is one of the most important areas of ultrasound imaging. Current power Doppler images suffer from reduced spatial and temporal resolution compared with B-mode images, because of the additional processing and signal averaging required to produce high-quality images. In these cases it is possible that small vessels or rapidly moving structures can be blurred, appearing much larger than their actual size.

The future advances in contrast 3D power Doppler include improved image resolution, real-time 3D imaging, quantification (vessel density), improved contrast agents and equipment technology for their better utilization, and determination of perfusion.

The results of cyclic endostatin therapy[41] suggest that drugs targeting angiogenesis and tumor vasculature will become a major new weapon for effectively treating and preventing human cancer. The tumor should neither grow nor regress but should continue to be fed by its established vessels, remaining in a metastable state of proliferation balanced by apoptosis[42]. There is another important question. Could 3D power Doppler help in answering the question about tissue-specific differences in the vasculature and consequently in tumor vessel anatomy that affect a tumor's susceptibility to inhibition or disruption? This is a challenge for ultrasonographers, because the control and perhaps the cure of human cancers are surely on the horizon. Currently, the application of 3D power Doppler in the evaluation of neoplasms is mainly qualitative or semi-quantitative, but in the not too distant future we may use the integrated software for calculating the total extent of the vascularity of an entire mass in the 3D perspective[43–45]. The results reported in the recent literature on 3D color power Doppler are indeed provocative, and raise many new questions about the regulation of tumor angiogenesis, the density of tumor vessels and the differences between vessel architecture in benign and malignant growths.

Three-dimensional ultrasound plays an important role in obstetrics, especially for assessing fetal anatomy. Future progress in computer technology will provide true 3D real-time ultrasound in the near future, offering new diagnostic approaches to fetal behavior, and to the assessment of complex malformations of the fetal heart[27].

Finally, 3D ultrasonography has the potential to be used not only in tertiary centers, but also in primary care settings as networking capabilities become a reality, transferring a volume data set to specialists in tertiary care centers where it can be interpreted on-line, as the necessary images are available in the volume.

Three-dimensional ultrasound is an area undergoing rapid development that represents a natural extension of conventional sonography methods requiring integration of 2D ultrasound slices to develop a 3D impression of anatomy and pathology. Future 3D ultrasound techniques will allow visualization of the anatomy of organs and the fetus as they actually are, so that we feel as if we are holding a model of the organ in our hands.

Interactive visualization technology allows clear recognition of the anatomy by both care givers and consumers. It is expected that development of the new technology will soon enable improved and expanded patient care.

References

1. Jurkovic D, Jauniaux E, Campbell S. Three-dimensional ultrasound in obstetrics and gynecology. In Kurjak A, Chervenak FA, eds. *The Fetus as a Patient*. Carnforth, UK: Parthenon Publishing, 1994:135–40
2. Steiner H, Staudach A, Spitzer D, Schaffer H. Three-dimensional ultrasound in obstetrics and gynecology: technique, possibilities and limitations. *Hum Reprod* 1994;9:1773–8
3. Merz E. Three-dimensional transvaginal ultrasound in gynecological diagnosis. *Ultrasound Obstet Gynecol* 1999;4:81–6
4. Balen FG, Allen CM, Gardener JE, Siddle NC, Lees WR. 3-Dimensional reconstruction of ultrasound images of the uterine cavity. *Br J Radiol* 1993;66:588–91
5. Kupesic S, Kurjak A. Septate uterus: detection and prediction of obstetrical complications by different forms of ultrasonography. *J Ultrasound Med* 1998;17:631–6
6. Bonilla-Musoles F, Raga F, Osborne N, Blanes J. Control of inserted devices (IUDs) by using three-dimensional ultrasound (3D). Is it the future? *J Clin Ultrasound* 1996;24:263–7
7. Lee A, Eppel W, Sam C, Kratochwil A, Deutinger J, Bernaschek G. Intrauterine device localization by three-dimensional transvaginal sonography. *Ultrasound Obstet Gynecol* 1997;10:289–92
8. Raga F, Bonilla-Musoles F, Blanes J, Osborne N. Accuracy of three-dimensional ultrasound diagnosis in congenital mullerian anomalies. *Fertil Steril* 1996;65:523–8
9. Merz E, Weber G, Bahlmann F, Macchiella, D. Transvaginale 3D-Sonographie in der Gynäkologie. *Gynäkologe* 1995;28:276–85
10. Ayida G, Kennedy S, Barlow D, Chamberlain P. Contrast sonography for uterine cavity assessment: a comparison of conventional two-dimensional with three-dimensional transvaginal ultrasound. *Fertil Steril* 1996;66:848–50
11. Weinraub Z, Maymon R, Shulman A, *et al*. Three-dimensional saline contrast hysterosonography and surface rendering of uterine cavity pathology. *Ultrasound Obstet Gynecol* 1996;8:277–82
12. Chou CY, Hsu KF, Wang ST, Huang SC, Tzeng CC, Huang KE. Accuracy of three-dimensional ultrasonography in volume estimation of cervical carcinoma. *Gynecol Oncol* 1997;66:89–93
13. Kyei-Mensah A, Machonochie N, Zaidi J, Pittrof R, Campbell S, Tan SL. Transvaginal three-dimensional ultrasound: reproducibility of ovarian and endometrial volume measurements. *Fertil Steril* 1996;66:718–22
14. Weber G, Merz E, Bahlmann F, Macchiella D. Sonographische Beurteilung von Ovarealtumoren – Vergleich zwischen transvaginaler 3D-Technik und konventioneller 2-dimensionaler Vaginosonographie. *Ultraschall Med* 1997;18:26–30
15. Bonilla-Musoles F, Raga F, Osborne N. Three-dimensional ultrasound evaluation of ovarian masses. *Gynecol Oncol* 1995;59:129–35
16. Jurkovic D, Gruboeck K. Three-dimensional ultrasound of the uterus. In Baba K, Jurkovic D, eds. *Three-dimensional Ultrasound in Obstetrics & Gynecology*. Carnforth, UK: Parthenon Publishing, 1997:75–83
17. Kupesic S, Kurjak A, Zodan T. Staging of endometrial carcinoma by 3-D power Doppler. *Gynaecol Perinatol* 1999;8:1–5
18. Adams J, Franks S, Polson DW, *et al*. Multifollicular ovaries: clinical and endocrine features and response to pulsatile gonadotrophin releasing hormone. *Lancet* 1995;2:1375–9
19. Kyei-Mensah A, Zaidi J, Pittrof R, Shaker A, Campbell S, Tan SL. Transvaginal three-dimensional ultrasound: accuracy of follicular measurements. *Fertil Steril* 1996;65:371–6
20. Fleichtinger W. Follicular aspiration with interactive three-dimensional digital imaging (Voluson): a step toward real-time puncturing under three-dimensional control. *Fertil Steril* 1998;70:374–7
21. Rubin JM, Bude RO, Carson PL, Bree RL, Adler RS. Power Doppler US: a potentially useful alternative to mean frequency-based color Doppler US. *Radiology* 1994;190:853–6
22. Rubin JM, Adler RS, Fowlkes JB, *et al*. Fractional moving blood volume: estimation with power Doppler US. *Radiology* 1995;197:183–90
23. Kurjak A, Kupesic S, Breyer B, Sparac V, Jukic S. The assessment of ovarian tumor angiogenesis: what does three-dimensional power Doppler add? *Ultrasound Obstet Gynecol* 1998;12:136–46
24. Kurjak A, Kupesic S, Anic T, Kosuta D. Three-dimensional ultrasound and power Doppler improve the diagnosis of ovarian lesions. *Gynecol Oncol* 2000;76:28–32
25. Chan L, Lin WM, Verparjoikit B, Hartman D, Reece EA. Evaluation of adnexal masses using three-dimensional ultrasonographic technology: preliminary report. *J Ultrasound Med* 1997;16:349–54
26. Kurjak A, Kupesic S. Three-dimensional ultrasound and power Doppler in assessment of uterine and ovarian angiogenesis: a prospective study. *Croat Med J* 1999;40:51–8
27. Kurjak A, Kupesic S, Banovic I, Hafner T, Kos M. The study of morphology and circulation of early embryo by three-dimensional ultrasound and power Doppler. *J Perinat Med* 1999;27:145-57
28. Kupesic S, Kurjak A. Volume and vascularity of the yolk sac studied by three-dimensional ultrasound and color Doppler. *J Perinat Med* 1999;27:91–6
29. Pretorius D, Nelson TR. Fetal face visualization using three-dimensional ultrasonography. *J Ultrasound Med* 1995;14:349–56
30. Ulm MR, Kratochwil A, Ulm B, Solar P, Aro G, Bernaschek G. Three-dimensional ultrasound evaluation of fetal tooth germs. *Ultrasound Obstet Gynecol* 1998;12:240–3
31. Nelson TR, Pretorius DH. Visualization of the fetal thoracic skeleton with three-dimensional sonography: a preliminary report. *Am J Roentgenol* 1995;164:1485–8
32. Mueller GM, Weiner CP, Yankowitz J. Three-dimensional ultrasound in the evaluation of fetal head and

spine anomalies. *Obstet Gynecol* 1996;88:372–8
33. Nelson TR, Pretorius DH, Sklansky M, Hagen-Ansert S. Three-dimensional echocardiographic evaluation of fetal heart anatomy and function: acquisition, analysis and display. *J Ultrasound Med* 1996;15:1–9
34. Zosmer N, Jurkovic D, Jauniaux E, Gruboeck K, Lees C, Campbell S. Selection and identification of standard cardiac views from three-dimensional volume scans of the fetal thorax. *J Ultrasound Med* 1996;15:25–32
35. Kurjak A, Kupesic S. Three-dimensional ultrasound improves measurement of nuchal translucency. *J Perinat Med* 1999;27:97–102
36. Kirbach D, Wittingham TA. 3D-ultrasound – Kretztechnik Voluson® approach. *Eur J Ultrasound* 1994;13:85–9
37. Fleichtinger W. Transvaginal three-dimensional imaging. *Ultrasound Obstet Gynecol* 1993;3:375–8
38. Merz E, Weber G, Macchiella D, Bahlmann F. 3D-Volumensonographie in der transvaginalen Diagnostik. *Ultraschall Klin Praxis* 1993;8:154
39. Pairleitner H. Three-dimensional color histogram using three-dimensional power Doppler. In Kurjak A, ed. *Three-dimensional Power Doppler in Obstetrics & Gynecology*. Carnforth, UK: Parthenon Publishing, 1999:35–9
40. Pairleitner H, Steiner H, Staudach A. Preliminary findings using three-dimensional power Doppler and three-dimensional color histogram in adnexal masses. *J Ultrasound Med* 2000;in press
41. Boehm T, Folkman J, Browder T. Antiangiogenic therapy of experimental cancer does not induce acquired drug resistance. *Nature (London)* 1997;390:404–7
42. Holmgren L, O'Reilly MS, Folkman J. Dormancy of micrometastases: balanced proliferation and apoptosis in the presence of angiogenesis suppression. *Nature Med* 1995;1:149–53
43. Lencioni R, Pinto F, Armillotta N, Bartolozzi C. Assessment of tumor vascularity in hepatocellular carcinoma: comparison of power Doppler US and color Doppler US. *Radiology* 1996;207:353–8
44. Birdwell RL, Ikeda DM, Jeffrey SS, Jeffrey RB. Preliminary experince with power Doppler imaging of solid breast masses. *Am J Roentgenol* 1997;169:703–7
45. Meyerowitz CB, Fleischer AC, Picken DR, *et al*. Quantification of tumor vascularity and flow with amplitude color Doppler sonography in an experimental model: preliminary results. *J Ultrasound Med* 1996;15:827–33

Telemedicine performed by three-dimensional ultrasound

K. Kettl

Introduction

The definition of telemedicine is the exchange of medical information from one side to another via electronic communications for the health and education of the patient or health-care provider, and for the purpose of improving patient care[1]. It can be defined as the investigation, monitoring and management of patient information, using systems that allow access to expert advice and patient information no matter where the patient or relevant information is located. The Internet will provide the common data channel, replacing the point-to-point and dial-up connectivity. Even in remote rural areas, where the patient and the closest health-care professional can be distant from each other, telemedicine can mean access to health care where little had been available before, and it can significantly reduce the time and costs (Figure 1). To bring telemedicine into the realm of practical reality will require a close collaboration between physicians, medical centers, government and business.

The objectives of telemedicine

(1) The main objective is to exchange all the data from the examination of a patient in a very short time.
(2) The transferred examination data should give the opportunity of performing a post-examination interactively.
(3) Telemedicine should connect different locations to collect information, for example rare cases for multi-case studies in scientific projects.
(4) Telemedicine should provide a discussion forum and an education platform worldwide, connected via the Internet.

Facilities of performance

Videoconference

This can be a live or real-time conference between several locations globally, as long as connection and

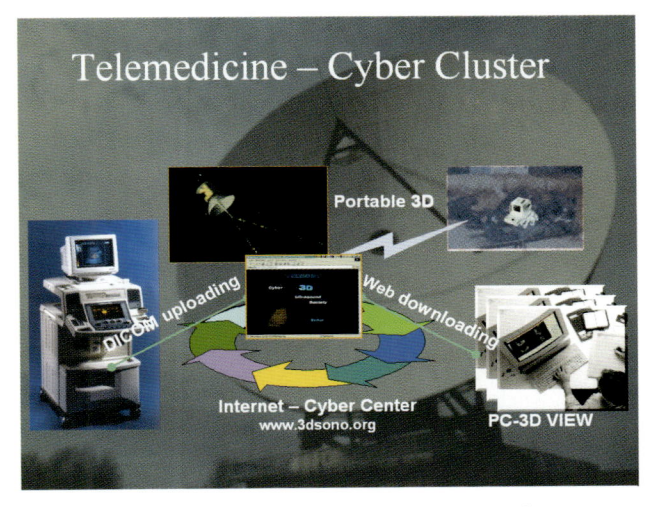

Figure 1 An Internet cyber cluster can connect even rural areas

hardware facilities are available and participants are present, regardless of the local time. When the videoconference is held, all participants can give their comments and interact during the transmission time. The videoconference can be recorded and then used for education purposes. Interactivity is only possible during transmission time and is generally only verbal. Hardware is not available everywhere, and its use is sometimes difficult because of the matching of different systems.

Image transfer

Image transfer has a relatively low cost, and fast transmission depends on compression and small size of the data set. An explanation must be attached to define the examination procedure. There is a major disadvantage in not having the possibility of interactivity.

Volume data set transfer

The major advantage of this system is the possibility of exchanging an entire ultrasound examination of a certain region. These data sets can be used by the receiver to perform a post-examination of the patient interactively. The re-examination is in this case independent of time and location. The limitation will be the size of the volume data set of the examined region of interest. The transfer time depends on the size of the volume and can be shortened by volume compression.

Why three-dimensional volume ultrasound is meant as the initiation to real telemedicine

The above-mentioned objectives are fulfilled by three-dimensional (3D) ultrasound volume data sets, but the following conditions must be considered:

(1) Data accuracy must be ensured by 100% digital ultrasound data, independent of how often the data are transferred, uploaded or downloaded.

(2) Data accuracy must be ensured for geometrical correctness, to enable measurements and the rendering process to be produced.

(3) Short acquisition time must be realized to avoid movement artifacts.

(4) Homogeneous data density must be realized for homogeneous resolution in all three dimensions.

(5) Controlled size of the data set must be effected, to control transmission time and the downloading process.

There are different systems for 3D ultrasound data acquisition: freehand data acquisition and automatic volume data acquisition.

Freehand data acquisition

This is mostly accomplished by integrated 3D acquisition software or by an additional workstation. For the present, these systems do not guarantee geometrical correctness and are useful mainly for viewing images or for viewing rendered 3D images. Most of these systems also need a certain environment and a skilled sonographer to acquire good results (Figure 2). Data transfer of the volume data is highly complicated and time consuming.

Automatic volume acquisition

This is performed by specially designed volume trans-

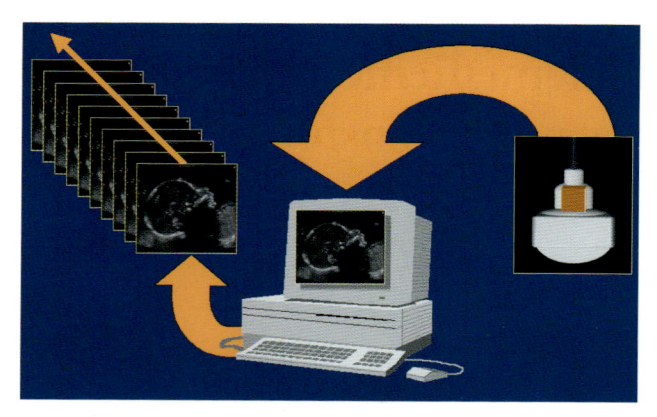

Figure 2 Freehand data acquisition

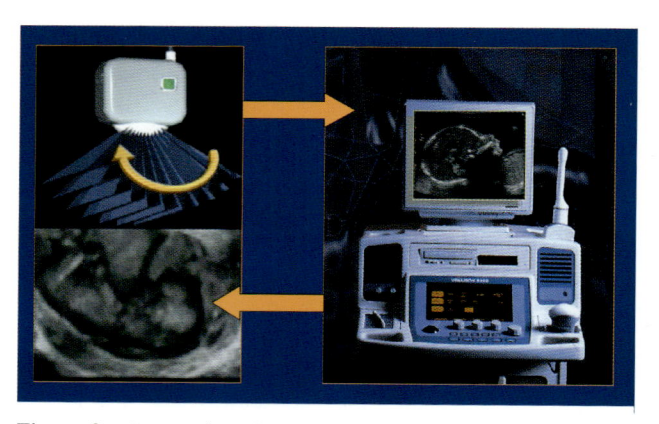

Figure 3 Automatic volume acquisition performed by specially designed volume transducers. Only dedicated volume transducers have a real-time rendering mode, which uses the fourth dimension for movement visualization

ducers, in an integrated system. The acquisition time ranges from 0.5 s to a maximum of 5 s. Immediately after the data acquisition, the volume data are displayed as three orthogonal planes and as a rendered 3D image (Figure 3). The simultaneous image analysis includes all advantages of the conventional two-dimensional (2D) image technique and, additionally, allows the display of any plane within the entire volume block. The images can be shifted or rotated around the three axes in any plane. The multi-parallel planes permit a multi-format display of all three orthogonal planes simultaneously. The planes displayed are always kept in a perpendicular position to each other, no matter which rotation is performed. This allows a unique identification of the displayed anatomic planes. The additional third plane, the coronal plane, gives expanded information for assessment of position, size and spatial relationship between organs or structures. All of these data can be stored or saved in digital mass memories and can be reloaded to the system for further processing, measurements or diagnosis at any time[2,3].

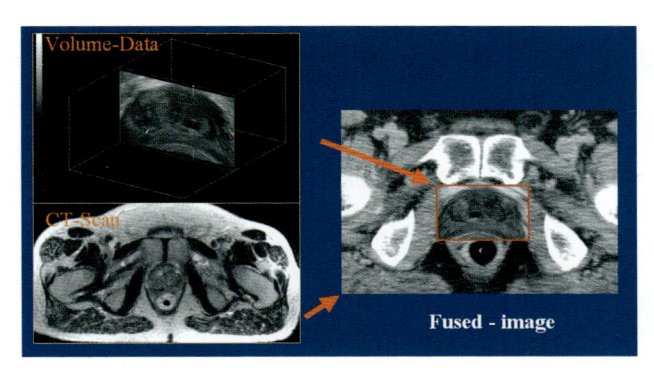

Figure 4 DICOM connected fused-image from computed tomography, magnetic resonance imaging and ultrasound

Data transfer for a global three-dimensional cluster via the Internet

For a global communication, a common language is necessary. The common language in the medical field is DICOM (Digital Imaging and Communications in Medicine). DICOM defines data structures (e.g. ultrasound image objects), service classes (e.g. verification, storage), protocols for data exchange over networks, media storage formats (e.g. for CD storage) and so on. The so-called 'DICOM Conformance Statement' tells what standards are implemented and have to be consulted in order to determine interoperability between DICOM applications (e.g. ultrasound scanner, PACS storage system)[4] (Figure 4).

A mean volume data set contains approximately 2–10 MB. The transfer time of a data set of 6 MB on an ISDN line at 6 KB/s takes approximately 16 min. On a conventional telephone line it takes three to four times longer and amounts to a transfer time of nearly 1 h. This is not acceptable for performing a 3D cluster for exchanging or archiving an entire patient examination, therefore compression is needed.

Why is wavelet compression used?

(1) To save memory space;

(2) To allow volume storage on small media (floppy disk);

(3) To allow faster Internet transactions of volume data.

The fundamental idea behind wavelets is analysis of image or volume data according to scale.

In the early 1800s Joseph Fourier discovered that he could superimpose sines and cosines to represent the original function. Based on his concept, compression methods such as JPEG or MPEG were used to compress images or image sequences. The advantage is the free choice of adapting the analyzing wavelet function to the image behavior (in our application ultrasound images).

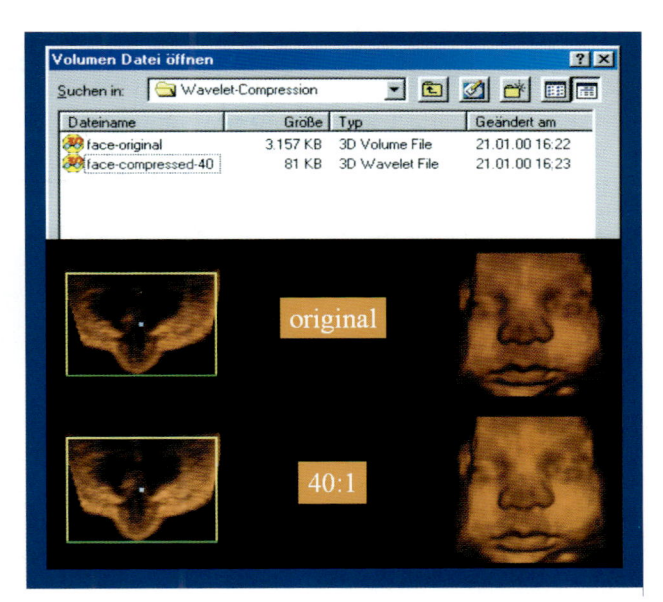

Figure 5 Comparison of a 40 : 1 wavelet compressed volume data set

With wavelet transformation the original data can be represented in a compact form (wavelet coefficient) without loss of information. If lossless wavelet compression is used, standard compression methods are used to compress the wavelet coefficient, with the advantage that this method is more efficient at compressing the original data. A factor of 3 is normally achieved with no loss of information. If semi-lossless wavelet compression is used, the wavelet coefficient is truncated within a certain threshold (depending on the compression rate) and then standard compression methods are used to compress the wavelet coefficient. The truncation of the wavelet coefficient causes a loss of information. With a compression factor between 10 and 50 good results can be achieved[5] (Figure 5).

The usage of semi-lossless wavelet compression is under the user's sole responsibility. Data sets of 6 MB are compressed to 100–300 KB and can be transferred via the Internet even on conventional telephone lines in less than 1 min.

Results

Interactive telemedicine can be performed with 3D ultrasound data sets when the following requirements are fulfilled:

(1) There is 100% digital data acquisition of volume datasets.

(2) Accuracy is ensured by automatic volume acquisition.

(3) DICOM standard for global communication is available.

(4) Wavelet compression for fast Internet transaction and storage is performed.

Re-examination can be achieved anywhere in the world by recalling a data set from, for example, PACS, HIS, the Internet or any type of digital memory (Figure 6). An entire ultrasound examination can be exchanged in the form of a volume data set. Interactively, a post-examination can be performed for a second opinion. With a cyber connection, a meeting point for multi-case studies is possible. An education platform can be established for an ultrasound course with global participation.

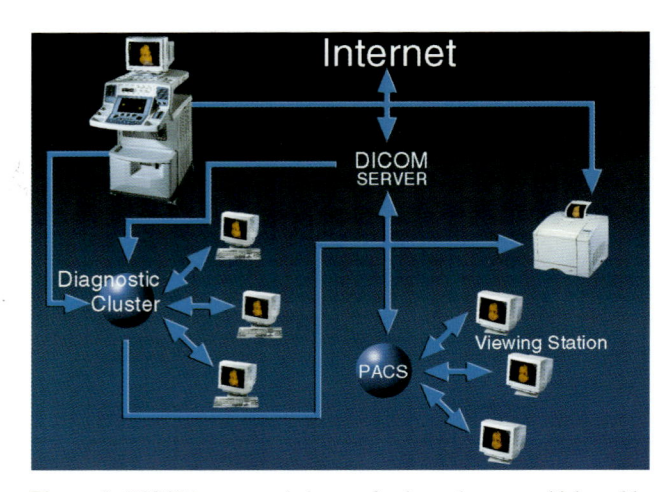

Figure 6 DICOM connected cluster of volume data sets which enable interactive re-examinations

Conclusion

With special software that can download the volume data set from the Internet to a PC, telemedicine is available for everyone. Global transfer of examination data sets that can be interactively re-examined allows for more specific diagnoses to be made in specialist centers.

References

1. American Telemedicine Association, Washington DC 20005. *Telemedicine Report to Congress*, 31 January 1997
2. Kettl K, Gritzky A. *Introduction to Three-dimensional Ultrasound Technology and Future Aspects*. Carnforth, UK: Parthenon Publishing, 1999
3. Kettl K. *Prospects for Three-dimensional Sonography in the Next Millennium*. Carnforth, UK: Parthenon Publishing, 1999
4. Wachter S, Kratochwil A, Pötter R, et al. A DICOM-based compatible PACS environment suitable for CT, MRI and 3D ultrasound in radiotherapy. In Piqieras J, Carreno JC, Lucaya J, eds. *Proceedings of the 16th Euro PACS Annual Meeting*. Barcelona, 1998:215–19
5. Scherzer O, Schoisswohl A, Kratochwil A. Compression of 3D ultrasound data using wavelet bases on intervals. *Report*. Linz: Johannes Kepler University 2000:No 9 (SFB F013)
6. Mayo Foundation for Medical Education and Research. www.mayo.edu

Index

achondroplasia 136
    facial dysmorphism in 131
acrania 135
adenocarcinoma of ovary 30
adenomyosis 58
adhesions, uterine 57
adnexal tumors 35–40
    use of contrast agents in investigation of 35
    vascularity of 36, 37
advantages of three-dimensional ultrasound 29, 39, 191, 243–9
agenesis of corpus callosum 173, 176, 188
angiogenesis 7–17
    advances in tumor therapy and 17
    blood flow quantification in 15
    blood vessel geometry in 14
    data interpretation problems 12
    display methods for study 12
    equipment requirements 12
    functional impairments caused by capillary abnormalities 10
    growth factors in 9
    image acquisition for 12
    imaging techniques for 11
    in pelvic tumors 245
    mathematical basis of 13
    molecular basis of 8
    pathological cf. physiological 7
    quantification of 11
    role in tumor growth 7, 8
    tumor diagnosis from ultrasound study of 13
    tumor neovascularization 9
aorta
    aneurysms 200
    imaging of 197
Apert's syndrome, facial profile in 130
applications of three-dimensional ultrasound 244
arthrogryposis 138
ascites 239
assisted reproduction techniques (ART)
    monitoring of ovulation induction in 67–9
    puncture procedures under three-dimensional ultrasound guidance 72
asymmetrical ventriculomegaly 176
automated scanning systems 1

benefits of three-dimensional ultrasound 191, 244
biliary tract 238
bladder
    imaging of 192
    infiltration of by prostate carcinoma 205
blood flow
    assessment in embryo 116–18
    hepatic 237
    in fetal brain 177
    in hand 210
    quantification of and vascularization 15
blood vessel geometry in angiogenesis 14
brain (fetal) 171–8
    abnormal 173
    agenesis of corpus callosum 188
    asymmetrical ventriculomegaly 176
    calvarial structure 171, 172
    circulatory assessment 177
    intracranial hemorrhage 184
        grade I 184
        grade III 185
        grade IV 186
    normal 173, 183
    periventricular leukomalacia 186
    technique of neurosonography 181
    ventricle measurements 209
    ventriculomegaly 188
breast 215–26
    anatomy of 215
    evaluation of lesions 229–33
        benign 232
        benign cf. malignant 229
        gray-scale 229
        malignant 233
        power Doppler imaging 231
        three-dimensional imaging 230
    fibroadenoma 217–18
    intraductal papilloma 216
    retromamillary region 216
    subareolar region 216
    three-dimensional imaging of 222–6
    volume computation of lesions 218
breast carcinoma
    benign lesions 229, 233
    incidence 219
    invasive 219
    needle biopsy of 221, 222
    power Doppler investigation of 222
    three-dimensional imaging of 222–6
    three-dimensional targeting technique 221

cardiac gating 162
carotid artery
    plaques in 202, 203
central nervous system (fetal), assessment 174
cervical carcinoma 194–7
    imaging of 195
    infiltration by 196
    therapeutic impact measurement 195
    tumor volume estimation 195
choroid plexus cysts

as an ultrasound marker for chromosomal anomalies 145
cirrhotic liver 236
cleft lip 130, 137
clubfoot 138
color Doppler hysterosalpingography 89
contrast agents
    use in adnexal tumor investigations 35
    use in ectopic pregnancy imaging 48
    use in septate uterus 81
    use in tubal patency studies 87
corpus callosum
    agenesis of 173, 176, 188
cystadenocarcinoma of ovary 27, 30
cystadenofibroma of ovary 28
cystic hygroma 140

data acquisition and telemedicine 254
data interpretation, problems with in angiogenesis 12
data presentation 3
data processing for three-dimensional ultrasound 1
data storage 3
dermoid cyst 27
dermoid tumors 245
developments in three-dimensional ultrasound 248
Digital Imaging and Communications in Medicine 255–6
disadvantages of three-dimensional ultrasound 191
Doppler, angiogenesis study 11–17
Down's syndrome, *see under* trisomy 21

Echinococcus cyst in liver 199
echocardiography
    clinical studies 162
    role of networking in 165
    technical considerations for 161
Echovist 81
ectopic pregnancy
    color Doppler findings 47
    three-dimensional ultrasound findings 47
    two-dimensional ultrasound findings 46
embryo, imaging of 109–18
endometrial carcinoma 244, 59–62
endometrial hyperplasia 58
endometrial polyps 56–7
endometrioma, ovarian 26
endometrium, volume measurement 72
equipment for angiogenesis studies 12
eye 211
    choroid melanoma 212
    lymphoma in eyelid 212
    retinal detachment 212

face (fetal) 246
    abnormal anatomy 128–31
    assessment of 127–31
    in achondroplasia 136
    in trisomy 18 136
    normal anatomy 127, 129
Fallopian tube 43–52
    benign tumors of 48

developments in imaging of 86
ectopic pregnancy, imaging of 46–8
hysterosonosalpingography 85–94
malignant tumors of
    color Doppler findings 49
    three-dimensional ultrasound findings 50–2
    two-dimensional ultrasound findings 49
pelvic inflammatory disease, imaging of 43–6
pulsed Doppler in patency studies 89
use of contrast agents in patency studies 87
fetus
    abnormal anatomy in 133–40
        abdomen 137–8
        cardiovascular system 140
        extremities 139
        first trimester 133–4
        head and neck 134
        identification by power Doppler 155–60
        second trimester 134–40
        skeleton 139
        third trimester 134–40
        thorax 137–8
        tumors 140
    advantages of three-dimensional ultrasound in imaging of 246
    brain assessment 171–8
        abnormal 173
        blood flow 177
        normal 173
        three-dimensional ultrasound 171
        two-dimensional ultrasound 172
    cardiac malformations 161–6
    central nervous system assessment 174
    facial anatomy 127–31
        abnormal 128–31
        normal 127, 129
    heart visualization in 162
    intracranial hemorrhage
        grade I 184
        grade III 185
        grade IV 186
    neurosonography 181–9
    normal anatomy of 121–5
    normal brain anatomy 183
    periventricular leukomalacia 186
    placental abnormalities in 167–9
    power Doppler imaging in 155–60
    ultrasound markers for chromosomal anomalies 143–9
        choroid plexus cysts 145
        echogenic foci in heart 144
        hyperechogenic bowel 143
        long bone biometry 144
        nuchal translucency 146–9, 151–4
        renal pyelectasis 145
    umbilical abnormalities in 167–9
fibroadenoma in breast 217–18
follicle aspiration, puncture procedures under three-dimensional ultrasound guidance 72

gallbladder 238
    carcinoma of 199
    stones in 199

gastrointestinal tract 238
gestational sac, imaging of 109–14
growth factors, role in angiogenesis 9

heart (fetal)
    aortic arch 163
    cardiac gating 162
    clinical studies 162
    ductal arch 163
    echocardiography of 161–6
    four-chamber view 162–3
    role of networking in echocardiography of 165
    two-dimensional cf. three-dimensional views 164
    visualization of 162
hepatogastroenterology 235–40
hernia, umbilical 133
hip (fetal) 209
Hodgkin's disease 201
hydranencephaly 135
hydronephrosis 198
hyperechogenic bowel, as an ultrasound marker for chromosomal anomalies 143
hysterosalpingography
    color Doppler in 89
    three-dimensional ultrasound for 91–4
hysterosonosalpingography 85–94
    gray-scale 89
    procedure for 88
    requirements for 87

incontinence (urinary) 103–6
infertility (female)
    application of three-dimensional ultrasound in 244
    assessment of 67–74
    endometrium volume measurement 72
    follicle aspiration 72
    hysterosonosalpingography 85–94
    ovulation induction in 67
    polycystic ovary syndrome 69
    uterine causes of 74
Internet 255
intracranial hemorrhage in fetus 184
    grade I 184
    grade III 185
    grade IV 186
intrauterine devices 97–100
    complications of use 98
    contraindications to use 97
    malposition of 98–100
    three-dimensional ultrasound of 99
    ultrasound and placement of 97
    ultrasound assessment prior to insertion 97
intrauterine synechiae 57

kidney
    fetal cyst 138
    hydronephrosis 198
    metastases in 198

renal pyelectasis 145
knee 210

leiomyoma 62–4, 245
    infertility and 74
leiomyosarcoma 64
leukomalacia (periventricular) 186
levator ani 194
limitations of three-dimensional ultrasound 39, 243–9
liver
    blood flow in 237
    carcinoma 236
    cirrhotic 236
    diffuse disease 235
    Echinococcus cyst in 199
    focal lesions of 236
    hydatid cyst 236
    imaging of 197, 235–40
    metastases in 198
    volume computation 235
long bone biometry 144
lumbar myelomeningocele 137
lung cancer, metastases 211
luteal cyst, angiogenesis to 16
lymph nodes
    enlarged 200
    superficial 201
lymphangioma 140
lymphoma in eyelid 212

melanoma 212
metastases
    lung cancer 211
    to kidney 198
    to liver 198
methodology 1–6
micrognathia, facial profile in 130
myelomeningocele, lumbar 137

neck, imaging of 202
neovascularization
    advances in tumor therapy and 17
    blood flow quantification in 15
    characteristics of 9
    features of 16
    functional impairments caused by 10
    in cervical carcinoma 195
    in endometrial carcinoma 60
    in Fallopian tube malignancy 52
    in ovarian cancer 31–2
    in pelvic tumors 245
    of adnexal lesions 35–9
    power Doppler studies of 7–17
    tumor diagnosis from ultrasound study of 13
networking, use in interpretation of fetal echocardiography 165
neurosonography 181–9
    technique of 181

non-Hodgkin's lymphoma 201
nuchal translucency
    as an ultrasound marker for chromosomal anomalies 146–9
    imaging of 134
    measurement of 151–4
    three-dimensional ultrasound measurement of 114

ophthalmology 211
orthopedics 209
ovarian cancer
    adenocarcinoma 30
    angiogenesis in 31
    cystadenocarcinoma 30
    diagnosis by two-dimensional cf. three-dimensional ultrasound 28
    diagnostic criteria for 24–5
    histopathological characterization 26
    neovascularization in 17, 23
ovary
    adnexal lesions 35–40
        use of contrast agents in investigation of 35
        vascularity of 36, 37
    advantages of three-dimensional ultrasound 29
    assessment of 23–33
    characterization of lesions
        by three-dimensional ultrasound 25
        by two-dimensional ultrasound 24
        histopathological 26
    complex adnexal tumor 29
    cyst 26
    cystadenocarcinoma 27
    cystadenofibroma 28
    cystadenoma 29
    dermoid cyst 27
    endometrioma 26
    fetal cyst 138
    monitoring of ovulation induction 67–9
    polycystic ovary syndrome 69–72, 245
ovulation induction, cycle monitoring in ART 67–9

pancreas 237
    carcinoma of 200
papilloma, intraductal in breast 216
pediatrics 209
pelvic floor examination 192
pelvic inflammatory disease
    color Doppler findings 44
    three-dimensional ultrasound findings 45
    two-dimensional ultrasound findings 43
periventricular leukomalacia 186
placenta percreta 167–8
placenta previa, color Doppler imaging in 156–7
placenta succenturiata 157
placental invasion 167
polycystic ovary syndrome 245
    ovary measurement in 69–72
polydactyly in trisomy 18 139
pregnancy
    ectopic 46–8
    first trimester 109–18
        abnormal anatomy during 133–4

        at 5 weeks 109, 116
        at 6 weeks 110, 116
        at 7 weeks 110, 117
        at 8 weeks 111, 117
        at 9 to 10 weeks 111, 117
        at 11 to 12 weeks 112–14, 117
        embryonic vascularity assessment 116–18
        normal anatomy in 121, 122
        nuchal translucency measurement 114, 151–4
        yolk sac assessment 114
    neurosonography 181–9
    normal fetal anatomy 121–5
    placenta previa in 156, 157
    placental abnormalities 167–9
    power Doppler imaging in 155–60
    second trimester, abnormal anatomy during 134–40
    third trimester
        abnormal anatomy during 134–40
        facial imaging 127–31
        normal anatomy in 122–3
    twin–twin transfusion syndrome 157
    ultrasound markers for chromosomal anomalies 143–9
    umbilical abnormalities 167–9
prostate gland
    benign hypertrophy 205
    carcinoma
        radiointerstitial tumor ablation 207
        recurrence of 206
        staging 205
    two-dimensional cf. three-dimensional imaging 203
    volume computation 204
pterygium syndrome, facial dysmorphism in 131
pyelectasis 145

rachischysis 137
radiointerstitial tumor ablation (RITA) 207
rectal carcinoma 208
renal pyelectasis 145
rhabdosphincter, measurement of 193

sacrococcygeal teratoma 140, 159
sarcoma, uterine 64
scanning procedure 1
    automated 1
    manually moved 3
    mixed 2
scoliosis, fetal 139
septate uterus 74, 77–82
    imaging of 77–80
    management of 80
    obstetric complications and 81
skeleton 211
sonoembryology 109–18
    at 5 weeks 109
    at 6 weeks 110
    at 7 weeks 110
    at 8 weeks 111
    at 9 to 10 weeks 111
    at 11 to 12 weeks 112–14
spleen 237
synechiae, intrauterine 57

telemedicine 253–6
    objectives of 253
    role of three-dimensional ultrasound in 254
teratoma,
    sacrococcygeal 140, 159
three-dimensional ultrasound
    automated scanning systems 1
    basics of 1
    methodology 1–6
    principles of volume rendering for 4
thyroid gland
    benign adenoma of 202
    calcifications in 202
    cystic structures in 202
trauma 209
trisomy 13, nuchal translucency in 146
trisomy 18
    facial dysmorphism in 136
    nuchal translucency in 146
    overlapping fingers in 139
    polydactyly in 139
trisomy 21
    facial profile in 130
    nuchal translucency in 146
    renal pyelectasis in 145
tuberculous ascites 239–40
tuberculous nodules 240
tumors, fetal 140
twin–twin transfusion syndrome 157

umbilical cord
    abnormalities of 168–9
    herniation of 133
    normal insertion 124
    placental insertion
        normal 168
        velamentous 168
urethra (female)
    imaging of 192
    transvaginal cf. transrectal sonography 192
urinary incontinence
    power and color Doppler in 105
    three-dimensional ultrasound in 104
    two-dimensional ultrasound in 103
urogynecology 103–6
    bladder imaging 192
    rhabdosphincter measurement 193
    urethral imaging 192
uterus
    adenomyosis 58
    adhesions 57
    assessment of lesions of 55–64
    endometrial carcinoma 59–62
    endometrial hyperplasia 58
    endometrial polyps
        three-dimensional ultrasound findings 55–7
    endometrial volume measurement 72
    infertility and 74
    intrauterine devices 97–100
    leiomyoma 62–4, 74, 245
    leiomyosarcoma 64
    normal 55
    polyps 244

    septate 56, 74, 77–82
    synechiae 244
    unicornuate 56
    visualization by hysterosonosalpingography 85–94

vasa previa 169
ventriculomegaly 188
asymmetrical 176
videoconferences 253

yolk sac, three-dimensional ultrasound assessment of 114